Natural Products for Cancer Chemoprevention

John M. Pezzuto • Ole Vang
Editors

Natural Products for Cancer Chemoprevention

Single Compounds and Combinations

Springer

Editors
John M. Pezzuto
Arnold & Marie Schwartz College of Pharmacy and Health Sciences
Long Island University
Brooklyn, New York, USA

Ole Vang
Department of Science, Systems & Models
Roskilde University
Roskilde, Denmark

ISBN 978-3-030-39854-5 ISBN 978-3-030-39855-2 (eBook)
https://doi.org/10.1007/978-3-030-39855-2

This Springer imprint is published by the registered company Springer Nature Switzerland AG.
The registered company address is: Gewerbestrasse 11, 6330 Cham, Switzerland

This book is dedicated to the millions of human beings who have suffered the pain and anguish of cancer; had they only been given greater therapeutic options, we would be in a better place.

Foreword

The intense, unrelenting, worldwide burden of suffering and death from cancer demands new approaches to its control. It is almost 50 years since President Nixon declared "War on Cancer," and the war has yet to be won with conventional modalities of treating invasive and metastatic disease. Indeed, alarming and unexplained recent increases in both incidence and death from both adenocarcinoma of the lung in nonsmokers and pancreatic ductal adenocarcinoma now represent particularly new challenges. Because incidence drives mortality, it is common sense that we must find new ways to prevent incidence. That is the subject of this book.

Although immunotherapy of cancer is currently very much in vogue in the oncology community (and very much the darling of the investment world), it has major limitations for control of the worldwide cancer problem. Most tellingly, many immunotherapies cost hundreds of thousands of dollars per patient, and even then they may not always be curative. Immunotherapies are often complicated with serious side effects. Extension of life is not the ultimate goal; it is quality of life that counts for the individual. Moreover, it is not ethically satisfactory that immunotherapy should be available only to those who can afford it, while millions of indigent cancer patients throughout the world go without treatment. Although ultimately we may achieve an effective form of immunoprevention, at present such an approach is a long way from actual implementation.

Therefore, for the present, it should be intuitively obvious that an immediate goal for control of cancer is to find some relatively inexpensive and safe modality to prevent the disease, before a person must undergo all the mental anguish and physical suffering that result from a diagnosis of invasive malignant disease.

Although several approaches to prevention of cancer could be considered, this book will deal with the simplest and perhaps most logical, namely the use of natural products as drugs for chemoprevention. People have been modifying their diet or intake of plant products for thousands of years with the goal of achieving the healthier life that the intake of specific natural products (or combinations of such products) might provide. Indeed, we have been doing spontaneous, unnamed chemoprevention studies on ourselves for many generations. We have been modifying the epigenetic microenvironment of potential cancer cells by what we eat and otherwise ingest for thousands of years and thus have modified patterns of gene expression. Indeed, one might consider that cancer is essentially an epigenetic disease, as Andrew Feinberg has suggested, and that alterations in epigenetics (in its broadest sense) offer a compelling strategy to prevent cancer.

With the advent of the isolation of specific chemicals from plant sources and elucidation of their chemical structures, it is now possible to do chemoprevention in studies in a much more systematic manner, with control of dosage and measurement of both desired endpoints, as well as undesirable side effects, dependent on dosage. Chemicals that are natural products have an intrinsic advantage (as compared to totally new synthetic chemicals) for chemoprevention, in that the basic safety of ingesting these naturally occurring molecules has already been established by hundreds of years of human use, especially if they occur in the diet. However, natural products may also have limitations, especially in terms of their limited potency. In this case, it may be possible to increase potency by using a fundamental naturally occurring molecule as a platform or scaffold for chemical modification, as has been done with new analogs of vitamin D. Another practical example of this has been chemical synthesis of new analogs of oleanolic acid, a natural triterpenoid, found in high amounts in olives. Such new analogs have been shown to have chemopreventive activity for many diseases, including cancer; chemical modification of oleanolic acid has increased anticarcinogenic activity more than 1000-fold.

This book will not only consider the empirical identification and use of natural products for chemoprevention. There will be chapters that will emphasize mechanistic approaches to chemoprevention, by focusing on control of pathways that are uniquely dysfunctional during carcinogenesis. Such pathways can be rather general, such as those involved in inflammation, or more specific, such as EGF receptor signaling. This approach then allows screening of large libraries of potential chemopreventive agents, whether they are natural products or their synthetic derivatives.

A few examples currently exist in which cancer chemoprevention makes an important difference in the general population (e.g., tamoxifen for breast cancer, finasteride for prostate cancer). It is intuitively clear, however, that the impact of chemoprevention could be much more far-reaching. This is especially true for individuals at high risk, such as those who have had a primary tumor surgically resected and then enter a period of wait and watch. Even more broadly, given the overall incidence of cancer, essentially every human being is at risk. It is hoped the information provided in this book will be of some value in promoting the true goal of the "War on Cancer" espoused by the Nixon administration and subsequently by many others, which is to eradicate cancer as a major cause of death.

Dartmouth Medical School
Hanover, NH, USA

Michael B. Sporn

Preface

A good place to start with this book seems to be by remembering the driving force behind the effort. Many papers appearing in the scientific literature lead off with a statement such as "Cancer is the second leading cause of death globally, and was responsible for an estimated 9.6 million deaths in 2018." As dying is inevitable, perhaps around one in six human deaths being due to cancer could be viewed as simply part of the "big picture." Especially when it comes to the elderly. But recently, the issue has reached yet a new crescendo, with the report of Dagenais et al. (2019) indicating that deaths from cancer are now more common than those from cardiovascular disease in some high-income and middle-income countries (including Sweden, Canada, Chile, Argentina, Poland, and Turkey). Thus, the intensity of the scourge intensifies.

It is justifiable to refer to this disease as a scourge? Actually, the word "scourge" is a euphemism. When it comes to the treatment of cancer, of course there are some success stories. This is undeniable. But also undeniable are the nine million plus deaths each year. And let us not forget the circumstances of these deaths. For a start, recall the common side effects of routine treatment regimens. As listed by the National Cancer Institute, common side effects include anemia, appetite loss, bleeding and bruising (thrombocytopenia), constipation, delirium, diarrhea, edema (swelling), fatigue, fertility issues in boys and men, fertility issues in girls and women, flu-like symptoms, hair loss (alopecia), infection and neutropenia, lymphedema, memory or concentration problems, mouth and throat problems, nausea and vomiting, nerve problems (peripheral neuropathy), organ-related inflammation and immunotherapy, pain, sexual health issues in men, sexual health issues in women, skin and nail changes, sleep problems, and urinary and bladder problems (Side Effects of Cancer Treatment 2019). On top of this, individual chemotherapeutic agents, even those approved for use over the past couple of years, have unique toxicities, e.g., pneumonitis, colitis, hepatitis, nephritis, kidney failure, encephalitis, and sometimes, perhaps mercifully but not intentionally, death.

The chances of success or failure with chemotherapy are often not known from the outset, and sometimes the definition of success is nebulous. For example, should prolongation of a moribund condition for a few days be deemed a success? Of course, it is expected that caregivers will use their best judgment in treating cancer patients, while "... remember[ing] that there is art to medicine as well as science, and that warmth, sympathy, and understanding may outweigh the surgeon's knife or the chemist's drug" (Hippocratic Oath) (The Hippocratic Oath Today 2019). Dealing with cancer is a demanding vocation and those who commit themselves to such a life are heroes. Beyond the angst of death with terminally ill cancer patients, ethical and moral dilemmas of witnessing pain and suffering must be faced.

Consider the torment of a friend, relative, loved one, or any patient, who is terminally ill with cancer. Do the circumstances vary so much, irrespective of wealth, beauty, or intellect? Do the circumstances vary so much irrespective of one's lifetime contributions to family or humanity as a whole? The truth of the matter is the pathetic morbidity of the end stage does not vary. The loss of bodily control, the loss of hair, or the loss of coherence does not vary. We try to remain optimistic and try to convince ourselves things are better than in the past. We attempt to control pain, nausea, constipation, or diarrhea. But are control measures really effective? Can we in fact control and maintain the essence of life? Or even self-dignity? Is placing a person into a full or semi-comatose state and waiting for the transition (i.e., from alive to dead) really a humane act?

Looking directly in the face of this dismal reality, the concept of death with dignity (i.e., assisted suicide) becomes an act of kindness. In the classical version of the Hippocratic Oath, it was stated: "I will neither give a deadly drug to anybody who asked for it, nor will I make a suggestion to this effect" (The Hippocratic Oath Today 2019). This pledge no longer appears in the modern version. It is simply absent. After a great deal of debate and consternation, which is still ongoing, assisted suicide is now legalized in some countries (Belgium, Canada, Colombia, Luxembourg, the Netherlands, Switzerland) and in six US states (California, Colorado, Montana, Oregon, Vermont, and Washington State). Specific conditions and regulations apply in each case. However, in the end, relative to simply giving up treatment options with a terminally ill patient and allowing them to undergo terminal decline due to conditions such as cachexia, the availability of such an option seems rational. As an alternative, many terminally ill cancer patients commit suicide (Zaorsky et al. 2019).

So, in reality, is this best we can do? To a limited extent, we can look back over time and say we actually do know what has led to such a state of pathos. For example, after years of lies and self-deceit, we finally agree cigarette smoking leads to cancer. Undoubtedly, primary cancer prevention though cessation of cigarette smoking has been the single most important change leading to cancer reduction. But what else? What else leads to the genesis of cancer with certainty? What else leads to the genesis of cancer that can be readily avoided with the clarity of simply not smoking cigarettes?

It is generally agreed that body fatness is one major promoting factor for cancer development (Lauby-Secretan et al. 2016), so physical activity and weight reduction should reduce the risk of different types of cancer incidence. However, weight reduction is not a simple matter. Perhaps in many cases weight reduction is as difficult as cessation of habitual cigarette smoking.

Some will say abstaining from alcoholic beverage consumption, avoiding certain foods, and so on will reduce the cancer risk. But really? The fact of the matter is that the etiology of many or even most cancers is a mystery. Even people with a "perfect" lifestyle, a "perfect" diet, a "perfect" body mass, etc., die a morbid and miserable death due to the manifestations of cancer. And in many cases we just watch and wait and suffer in the end.

Will society ever wake up and do something about this tragic situation? It is starting to seem like the answer is probably not. But does it need to be this way? Do we have to sit by and simply watch over nine million people waste away and suffer a miserable death every year? Obviously, people will die, and they will die of what we call "natural causes." Is cancer a natural cause of death? Or, the scourge of mankind, like the plagues of the past?

Around 50 years ago, a "War on Cancer" was declared (National Cancer Act of 1971, 2019). Notably, in recent years, some treatment options have been devised that are considered curative, namely, chimeric antigen receptor (CAR) T-cell immunotherapy (Feins et al. 2019). However, the total cost of CAR T-cell therapy, for a single patient, has been estimated at $1.5 million (CAR T-cell Therapy Total Cost Can Exceed $1.5 Million Per Treatment 2019). More typically, the cost of treating one cancer patient for one year may fall in the range of $400,000 (Chap. 1). Obviously, an economic burden of this magnitude is a serious impediment. Even moreover, how many people have died of cancer since the time of declaring a "War on Cancer"? Perhaps 300 million? Equally shocking, it is projected that the global burden is expected to grow to 27.5 million new cancer cases and 16.3 million deaths by 2040 (Global Cancer Facts & Figures 2019). Overall, it is difficult to objectively rationalize major progress in this "War on Cancer."

Around the same time the "War on Cancer" was declared, the concept of cancer chemoprevention was awaken. On an intuitive basis, it is irrational to disagree with the principle of chemoprevention: the arrest or reversal of carcinogenesis during its initiation and in its premalignant stages, before signs and symptoms of malignancy occur (see Foreword and Chap. 1). A great deal of experimental work has been done in the laboratory and with animal models, with many promising results, but is chemoprevention effective with human beings? The short answer is yes. We know it is effective in humans, based on prototype chemopreventive agents such as tamoxifen and finasteride.

Physicians and other healthcare professionals have a limited armamentarium of chemopreventive agents at this time, but would be well advised to use what is available to maximum effect. The purpose of this book is to rekindle interest in the development of classical chemoprevention and help us move toward a world in which all of those at risk of developing primary or secondary cancers have a therapeutic option that offers hope for prevention, delay, or reversal.

In assembling this book, some unique patterns and themes emerged. First, some natural product chemopreventive agents that have been investigated as single drug entities are described. In other cases, combinations of structurally related chemopreventive agents have been studied, or, alternatively, combinations of chemopreventive agents representing different structural classes are included in the book. In most of these cases, pleotropic mechanisms come into play. In addition, certain metabolic and signaling pathways, subcellular networks, or morphological processes are causally related to tumorigenesis, and specific targeting by chemopreventive agents is described. Further, improvements in activity by means of producing structural derivatives or using contemporary formulations are covered.

An overarching theme of the book is chemopreventive agent interactions, with no major effort of breaking this down into additive, complementary, or synergistic effects. This would be especially difficult taking into account concepts such as hormesis, j-shaped curves, etc. It is worth noting, however, one imperative of chemoprevention is low or no toxicity, or alternatively, a highly favorable risk–benefit ratio. It is our hope that this cadre of topics, all converging on the nexus of chemoprevention, will be viewed as enlightening.

As an overview of the chapters, it is fitting that we begin the journey with a contribution by Sporn and Liby (Chap. 1). These authors briefly review the history of cancer chemoprevention, the conceptual framework, challenges, and hope. In addition to single agents, the potential of combinations as well as (semi)synthetic drugs is described. Paradigms and methods offering additional promise are illustrated, some mechanistic insight is provided, and the potential value of attacking one of the most devastating types of cancer, pancreatic, is exquisitely explored.

Of course, all effective chemopreventive agents function through some molecular mechanism, but interestingly, the "one drug, one target" dogma of drug design largely does not apply in the field of chemoprevention. One example is resveratrol, wherein a plethora of effects has been described in the scientific literature (Park and Pezzuto 2015; Pezzuto 2019). Interestingly, most of the chemopreventive compounds described in the book are capable of mediating multifaceted responses. But how does this multiplicity (promiscuity) relate to clinical trials and efficacy?

As described by Brown (Chap. 2), a great deal of meaningful preclinical and clinical work has been completed with resveratrol. Although some open questions still remain, there is now a sufficient body of evidence that supports advancing resveratrol to a phase II efficacy trial in which its ability to reduce colorectal polyp recurrence in high-risk patients can be assessed. The complexity of dose selection, metabolism, mechanistic correlations, etc., as related to clinical trials in cancer prevention, are well illustrated in this chapter.

Next, as described by Levenson (Chap. 3), a structural cousin of resveratrol, pterostilbene, also demonstrates a plethora of effects and broad protective responses. The compound may be viewed as advantageous in terms of bioavailability and utilization in combination regimens.

Both resveratrol and pterostilbene are somewhat unique given that so many studies have been reported using them as single agents, but of course that is an oversimplification, given the ramifications of the microbiome, metabolic conversions, and the subsuming activity of respective metabolites. Some of these topics, generally applicable to all chemopreventive agents, are discussed by Gerk (Chap. 4). In addition to general concepts of pharmacokinetics and bioavailability of natural products, the value of co-administration regimens is described.

In many cases, a single chemopreventive agent may fundamentally be viewed as promising, viz., vitamin D, but this logically progresses to the investigation of diverse structures and combination strategies for improving efficacy. As described by Suh (Chap. 5), vitamin D and its relevant analogs have shown inhibitory effects and mechanisms targeting cancer stem cell signaling. Another agent often considered as a single bioactive agent, silibinin, again is capable of mediating a host of responses. As described by Agarwal (Chap. 6), silibinin and derivatives mediate chemopreventive activity against a large number of tumor types and function through a variety of mechanisms. Palliative and adjuvant measures are of further interest when used in combination therapies.

The remarkable case of curcumin, another widely touted chemopreventive agent, is presented by Lau (Chap. 7). Here, we have a situation in which bioavailability is enhanced through administration as turmeric, serving in an adjuvant role, or by applying specialized formulations. Interaction with the gut microbiota is also discussed, as well the potential to ameliorate chemotherapeutic toxicity. Lessons learned in this case may be applicable to other naturally occurring chemopreventive agents.

As with curcumin, a component of turmeric, it is common to explore chemopreventive effects with natural substances containing a family of active compounds or in the natural milieu. A good example is tea. As described by Yang (Chap. 8), tea shows promise for inhibiting many different types of cancer, and green tea polyphenols, mainly catechins, are generally regarded as the active components. Many targets and potential mechanisms are described, as well as formulations suitable for clinical trials, including tablets.

In a similar vein, a class of compounds associated with cruciferous vegetables, isothiocyanates, capable of inducing cytoprotective enzymes (e.g., NQO1), were instrumental in validating the overall concept of chemoprevention from the beginning. As described by Dinkova-Kostova and Gerhäuser (Chap. 9), a great deal has been learned regarding the structures and actions of isothiocyanates. Working through novel signaling pathways, pro-oxidative and electrophilic mechanisms lead to enhanced expression of cytoprotective enzymes and restoration of cellular redox homeostasis. A host of in vitro and in vitro studies are described that are of translational value, either in the immediate realm of cancer chemoprevention or in an adjuvant setting with chemotherapy.

It is logical to assume that a family of structurally related compounds would function in a different and presumably more efficacious manner than one single entity of the same class. This is nicely exemplified in the chapter by Stevens (Chap. 10), describing the action of xanthohumol and related prenylflavonoids, which may be ingested from beer, for example. In addition, metabolites and derivatives are described, capable of functioning through a host of chemopreventive mechanisms as well as possibly reducing the metastatic potential of cancer cells. Similarly, as presented by Kong (Chap. 11), anthocyanins are an important class of compounds found in many fruits and vegetables, and, as a class, these compounds exert a chemoprevention effect through an array of biological activities and signaling pathways by a variety of mechanisms. Promising results have been obtained with a number of in vivo models.

The next two chapters illustrate a somewhat different approach in which whole foods or extracts containing a variety of structurally diverse chemopreventive agents yield promising activity. As described by Ahmed (Chap. 12), grapes contain over 1600 phytochemicals, with resveratrol, catechin, epicatechin, peonidin, cyanidin, malvidin, kaempferol, isorhamnetin, taxifolin, and quercetin in greatest abundance. In studying tumor angiogenesis and metastasis, considered as pivotal points in tumor progression, inhibitory activity mediated by grapes is likely due to pleiotropic mechanistic actions resulting from this combination of active ingredients.

In the following chapter by Vanden Berghe (Chap. 13), the anticancer activity of pomegranate is discussed. Pomegranate contains a structurally diverse group of phytochemicals as well as some unique components (e.g., estrone and punicic acid). The constituents along with (gut microbiota-derived) metabolites modulate transcription factors, pro- and anti-apoptotic proteins, cell cycle regulator molecules, protein kinases, cell adhesion molecules, pro-inflammatory mediators, growth factors, and other targets in various cancers. In some cases, extracts are more beneficial than purified ingredients.

In sum, as exemplified by these chapters, it is reasonable to suggest that the use of a mixture of active principles, or various structural classes, can lead to additive or even synergistic effects and reduce the opportunity for developing resistance or inducing toxicity.

Next, the book moves into the broader arena of modulating tumorigenesis through interaction with more general and well-defined targets. Remarkably, targets affected by chemopreventive agents are often the same targets associated with chemotherapeutic agents. However, unlike typical chemotherapeutic agents, untoward side effects are not acceptable with chemopreventive agents. But, on a conceptual level, it is interesting to note that a chemotherapeutic agent with little to no toxicity can be used in a chemopreventive setting (e.g., tamoxifen). Also, there are many examples in this book wherein there is a blurry line between the preventative and therapeutic activity of select agents or preparations.

For example, agents typically considered as chemotherapeutic, as well as agents typically considered chemopreventive, might induce apoptosis. In fact, there are numerous metabolic and signaling pathways and processes related to the genesis of a tumor to consider in terms of inhibition and modulation, affected by both chemotherapeutic and chemopreventive agents. Some have been highlighted in the aforementioned chapters (e.g., Ahmad; angiogenesis and metastasis) (Chap. 12). Chemopreventive agents function by diverse mechanisms of action, including through several of the ten hallmarks of cancer described by Hanahan and Weinberg (2011). Thus, we are not advocating solely for the mechanistic approaches described in this book, but it is clear the topics covered in the next four chapters are important.

First, epidermal growth factor receptor (EGFR), playing a critical role in tumor progression, is described by Lee (Chap. 14) as a target for natural product antitumor and chemopreventive agents. Overexpression of EGFR in malignancies makes inhibition of this entity a desirable endpoint. However, the development of resistance to the inhibitory action of drugs is problematic, and it is suggested that the unique attributes of natural products have a role to play in overcoming this shortcoming, either singly or in combination.

As described by Sundar and Firestone (Chap. 15), the cyclin-dependent kinase (CDK) gene family, comprising 21 distinct serine/threonine protein kinases, affects several processes involved in tumorigenesis. A myriad of drug targets is conceivable given, for example, the orchestration of specific sets of cyclins and CDK inhibitor proteins that control the selective phosphorylation of cell cycle target proteins. Signaling pathways regulating CDK activity present additional opportunities for intervention. Therapeutic strategies involving CDK inhibitors have been or are being developed, but a number of well-known natural product chemopreventive agents function through this network as well.

More broadly, natural chemopreventive agents are known to induce apoptosis in cancer cells. In the following chapter, Neophytou (Chap. 16) describes the various processes by which cells undergo apoptosis. Since evasion of apoptosis is also established as a hallmark of cancer, it is reasonable to consider compounds capable of inducing apoptosis under appropriate conditions as antitumor agents. Indeed, a variety of natural product chemopreventive agents capable of inducing apoptosis are discussed, either singly or in combination with other chemopreventive agents or chemotherapeutic agents. In addition, given shortcomings with the pharmacodynamics of chemopreventive agents, nanoformulations (nanochemoprevention) highlighted in this chapter represent an important new future direction.

Finally, in this segment of the book, the global topic of anti-inflammatory activity is discussed by Cuendet (Chap. 17). There is little doubt that inflammation plays a critical role in carcinogenesis, as well as multiple other chronic illnesses, and natural products functioning through anti-inflammatory mechanisms have a global role to play in disease prevention. The anti-inflammatory potential of several agents is described, and the interesting notion of using natural product anti-inflammatory agents in an adjuvant setting to help alleviate cancer chemotherapeutic toxicity is suggested.

The penultimate chapter of the book is presented by Gerhäuser (Chap. 18). Epigenetic mechanisms, including DNA hyper- and hypomethylation, remodeling of the chromatin, modification of histones by histone acetylation and methylation, and noncoding RNAs (miRNA), are clearly related to the genesis of a transformed phenotype. As such, the potential of maintaining or restoring homeostasis with the aid of natural product chemopreventive agents is enormous. An exciting example is the potential of resensitizing ER-negative tumors to anti-hormonal therapy. Captivating examples of how "classical" chemopreventive agents interact with the epigenome are presented. Further, this is a particularly dynamic example of achieving greater efficacy by means of combination chemoprevention.

In the final chapter, we have provided a brief perspective, reiterating the enormous potential of cancer chemoprevention, especially with focus on chemoprevention as a combination effect of multiple compounds, promoting additivity and synergism. Over the years, the conceptual framework originally espoused by iconic scholars such as Michael Sporn, Paul Talalay, and Lee Wattenberg has proven true. We continue to learn and discover and acquire greater insight, but a great deal of information is currently available, and we suggest that now is the time to consider chemoprevention from a holistic point of view. We propose creating a cocktail, perhaps comprising 10–25 chemopreventive agents provided to us by nature, and such a cocktail could ultimately be of great value for promoting the health span of humans.

In the end, together with the dedicated authors of these chapters, we hope this book can provide some inspiration to continue this so-called war on cancer through chemoprevention. Interestingly, in a Commentary advocating for a role of chemoprevention in the war on cancer published over 20 years ago (Pezzuto 1997), it was noted that traveling to the earth's moon and back was a relatively easy task compared with defeating cancer. Traveling to the earth's moon mainly involved established technology, money, and grit. Stopping the plague of cancer is much more daunting.

Recently, the war on cancer has actually been rebranded as the Cancer Moonshot^{SM} (Cancer Moonshot^{SM} 2019). This is quite an odd coincidence given the context of the antithetical relationship discussed in the Commentary (Pezzuto 1997). As we know, the war on cancer cannot be considered a success. Will the Cancer Moonshot^{SM} be any more successful? Obviously, we continue to hope, as we have done for a very long time. But once again it is not apparent that cancer chemoprevention is viewed with much enthusiasm as part of the moonshot. It has been said by some in the scientific community: "That ship (i.e., chemoprevention) has sailed." To the contrary, that ship was never built, but it is not too late. That ship would allow us to reach and cross new horizons.

In the modern version of the Hippocratic Oath, it is stated: "I will prevent disease whenever I can, for prevention is preferable to cure" (The Hippocratic Oath Today 2019). In this context, meaningful progress has been realized in the prevention of cardiovascular disease. There is also progress in cancer. Beyond primary prevention, e.g., avoiding cigarettes or overexposure to UV irradiation from the sun, vaccines are administered to prevent cancer causing infections, such as hepatitis and human papilloma virus (HPV), which are responsible for up to 25% of cancer cases in low- and middle-income countries (Plummer et al. 2016). However, in dealing with "typical" patients, especially those at high risk of developing cancer or having a recurrence, shouldn't chemoprevention have a role to play? The concept of "watch and wait" is frankly obtuse if proactive measures were available. It is incumbent on us to make proactive measures available.

Cancer chemoprevention is not a complicated concept to grasp. For example, it does not need to approach the big data complexity generated by defining the phenotype of every tumor from every cancer patient, although it can benefit through such analyses (cf. Chap. 18). Nonetheless, one factor stunting the development of chemoprevention seems to be a lack of "sexiness." In this context, it is worth recalling an oft-cited quotation from Einstein: "Everything should be made as simple as possible, but not simpler." And, on the flip side, again from Einstein: "A little knowledge is a dangerous thing. So is a lot."

By the time an average reader may complete reading this book, around 50,000 people will have died due to the manifestations of cancer. We can do better.

Brooklyn, NY — John M. Pezzuto
Roskilde, Denmark — Ole Vang

References

Cancer Moonshot^SM. https://www.cancer.gov/research/key-initiatives/moonshot-cancer-initiative. Accessed 16 Oct 2019

CAR T-cell Therapy Total Cost Can Exceed $1.5 Million Per Treatment. https://www.healio.com/hematology-oncology/cell-therapy/news/online/%7B124396e7-1b60-4cff-a404-0a2baeaf1413%7D/car-t-cell-therapy-total-cost-can-exceed-15-million-per-treatment. Accessed 8 Nov 2019

Dagenais GR et al (2019) Variations in common diseases, hospital admissions, and deaths in middle-aged adults in 21 countries from five continents (PURE): a prospective cohort study. Lancet. https://doi.org/10.1016/s0140-6736(19)32007-0

Feins S, Kong W, Williams EF, Milone MC, Fraietta JA (2019) An introduction to chimeric antigen receptor (CAR) T-cell immunotherapy for human cancer. Am J Hematol 94:S3–S9

Global Cancer Facts & Figures. https://www.cancer.org/research/cancer-facts-statistics/global.html. Accessed 16 Oct 2019

Hanahan D, Weinberg RA (2011) Hallmarks of cancer: the next generation. Cell 144:646–674

Lauby-Secretan B et al (2016) Body fatness and cancer-Viewpoint of the IARC Working Group. N Engl J Med 375:794–798

National Cancer Act of 1971. https://www.cancer.gov/about-nci/legislative/history/national-cancer-act-1971. Accessed 16 Oct 2019

Park E-J, Pezzuto J.M (2015) The pharmacology of resveratrol in animals and humans. Biochim Biophys Acta 1852:1071–1113

Pezzuto JM (1997) Plant-derived anticancer agents. Biochem Pharmacol 53:121–133

Pezzuto JM (2019) Resveratrol: twenty years of growth, development and controversy. Biomol Ther 27(1):1–14

Plummer M, de Martel C, Vignat J, Ferlay J, Bray F, Franceschi S (2016) Global burden of cancers attributable to infections in 2012: a synthetic analysis. Lancet Glob Health 4(9):e609–e616. https://doi.org/10.1016/S2214-109X(16)30143-7

Side Effects of Cancer Treatment. https://www.cancer.gov/about-cancer/treatment/side-effects. Accessed 16 Oct 2019

The Hippocratic Oath Today. https://www.pbs.org/wgbh/nova/article/hippocratic-oath-today/. Accessed 16 Oct 2019

Zaorsky NG, Zhang Y, Tuanquin L, Bluethmann SM, Park HS, Chinchilli VM (2019) Suicide among cancer patients. Nat Commun 10:207. https://doi.org/10.1038/s41467-018-08170-1

Contents

Chapter 1
Chemoprevention of Cancer: Past, Present, and Future

Michael B. Sporn and Karen T. Liby

Abstract We present a brief review of the history of chemoprevention of cancer, the present status of this field, and its prospects for the future. Topics covered are the scientific basis for chemoprevention of cancer, drugs in current use for chemoprevention of cancer, the need for new synthetic drugs, and the challenges ahead. The special relevance of chemoprevention of pancreatic cancer is emphasized, and the importance of the use of combinations of drugs for effective prevention is also stressed.

Keywords Chemoprevention · Cancer · Selective estrogen receptor modulators (SERMs) · Rexinoids · Triterpenoids · Pancreatic cancer

1.1 Introduction

In 1997 the Nobel Laureate, Michael Bishop, predicted "a new era, in which prevention will take its rightful place as the premier means by which to control cancer" (Bishop 1997). Sadly, this has not yet happened in spite of continuing interest in chemoprevention of this disease. In this brief mini-review, we present a broad, but not detailed, overview of the chemoprevention of cancer, which is the arrest or reversal of carcinogenesis during its initiation and in its premalignant stages, before signs and symptoms of malignancy occur.

This chapter is partially derived from a paper that appeared in *Progress in Chemistry* **25** (9): 1421-1428, 2013, with permission.

M. B. Sporn (✉)
Molecular and Systems Biology/Active Emeritus, Dartmouth Medical School, Lebanon, NH, USA
e-mail: michael.sporn@dartmouth.edu

K. T. Liby
Pharmacology & Toxicology, Michigan State University, East Lansing, MI, USA
e-mail: libykare@msu.edu

J. M. Pezzuto, O. Vang (eds.), *Natural Products for Cancer Chemoprevention*,
https://doi.org/10.1007/978-3-030-39855-2_1

Table 1.1 Deaths for 2018 are estimated

Total cancer deaths in men, USA			Total cancer deaths in women, USA		
Site	1971	2018	Site	1971	2018
Lung	53,000	84,000	Lung	11,000	70,000
Colorectal	22,000	27,000	Colorectal	24,000	23,000
Prostate	17,000	29,000	Breast	31,000	41,000
Pancreas	10,000	23,000	Pancreas	8000	21,000
			Ovary	10,000	14,000

These are total deaths, not rates which are adjusted for population. Data from Siegel R L, et al. *CA Cancer J. Clin.*, 2019, 69: 7–34

The ultimate justification for chemoprevention of cancer is two-fold. The first is the failure of the "War on Cancer" to control the number of cancer deaths (see Table 1.1). This failure makes it necessary to find a practical way to prevent invasive metastatic malignancy by using safe and effective drugs. This would save millions of people from undergoing the pain and suffering that they now endure because we now allow carcinogenesis to proceed to advanced stages of invasion and metastasis with consequent pain, suffering and death.

Secondly, a practical way to prevent cancer by using safe and effective drugs would save billions of dollars now spent to provide the extremely expensive medical and surgical care to millions of cancer patients worldwide. In the present era of personalized, targeted cancer therapy, costs to just a single patient for new anti-angiogenic or signal transduction drugs alone can be in excess of $ several 100,000 per year, although many patients are still not surviving for extended periods despite these costs. The profits that accrue to the pharmaceutical companies that develop and produce such drugs are immense, and these costs are passed on to society as a whole in the form of the high cost of medical insurance and care. Thus, chemoprevention offers dual benefits, both to the individual and to society as a whole.

In spite of this, there has been tremendous reluctance, both on the part of individuals (both patients and doctors) and various institutions (medical schools, hospitals, pharmaceutical companies, and insurance companies) to embrace chemoprevention in a practical, clinically accepted manner. One small example: in spite of the fact that the two selective estrogen receptor modulators (SERMs), tamoxifen and raloxifene, have been clinically proven (and approved by the United States Food and Drug Administration (FDA)) to prevent estrogen-receptor-positive breast cancer in women, neither of these drugs are in widespread clinical use in America, even though they have the potential to save the lives of thousands of women (Davidson and Kensler 2011).

Later in this review we will discuss the practical impediments to clinical chemoprevention of cancer. First we will survey some of the basic research that indicates that chemoprevention rests upon a sound scientific foundation, and then we will briefly discuss some important new approaches that should help to make this vital approach to prevention of disease all the more practical and useful.

1.2 Scientific Basis for Chemoprevention

Beginning in 1976, we have published a series of review articles in which we have summarized the scientific basis for the concept of chemoprevention and then discussed various classes of drugs that could be practically used as chemopreventive agents (Sporn et al. 1976; Sporn 1976, 1996, 2006, 2011; Sporn and Suh 2002; Sporn and Liby 2005; Albini and Sporn 2007; Liby et al. 2007a). A critical conceptual basis for chemoprevention is the long latency period (the time from initiation of carcinogenesis to onset of symptoms) for the development of almost all invasive carcinomas; this has been documented for many years in many studies. During this long latency period it is possible to intervene with drugs to arrest or reverse the process of carcinogenesis. Indeed, we have argued that the disease in reality should be called "carcinogenesis", rather than "cancer"; the actual disease is a continuous, evolving process rather than a static entity fixed in time (Sporn 1991). The overall biology of the evolution of the carcinogenic process in most epithelial target sites is now well understood, and the sequential histological and genetic changes that occur in almost all epithelia throughout the body have been described in many published reviews; pancreatic cancer is an excellent example (Hruban et al. 2000; Hingorani et al. 2003a, b). We now know that by the time that the carcinogenic process has progressed to invasive carcinoma, there may be hundreds of mutations that may have occurred in the tumor. As an example, it has been estimated that in lung cancer cells there is one mutation for approximately every 15 cigarettes smoked (Pleasance et al. 2010). It is simple common sense that measures could and should be adopted to prevent this progression to full-blown malignancy. The long latency period in which drugs could be used and the availability of effective drugs now make this a necessity. The use of drugs for prevention rests on the well-established fact that tissues have endogenous repair mechanisms for reversing the process of carcinogenesis. Thus, it has been known for a long time that cessation of smoking spontaneously can lead to reversal of dysplasia in tracheobronchial epithelium (Sporn 1976), and indeed, smoking does not lead to cancer in all heavy smokers. The use of drugs to arrest and reverse carcinogenic tissue injury, therefore, represents a physiological approach to control cancer by enhancing endogenous mechanisms of repair (Sporn et al. 1976; Sporn 1976).

Other important considerations in the use of drugs for preventing cancer are the use of combinations of chemopreventive agents and the need to consider rest periods (without drugs) during the prolonged, chronic period in which a preventive drug is administered. "Combination chemoprevention" was suggested as early as 1980 as a strategy for increasing potential synergistic efficacy of drugs, while at the same time decreasing the toxicity of the individual agents, which could be given at a lower dose level in a combination regimen (Sporn 1980). The practicality of this approach was clinically proven later, for the first time, in a definitive study which clearly demonstrated that the combination of low doses of difluoromethylornithine (DFMO) and sulindac together was uniquely effective in preventing colon cancer by arresting the progression of adenomas (Meyskens et al. 2008). The abundant evidence that

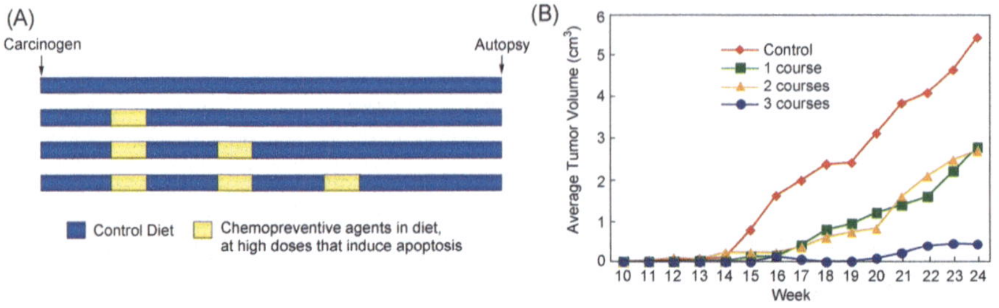

Fig. 1.1 (**a**) Intermittent chemoprevention protocol: the protocol was designed to give high doses of agents for short periods followed by drug-free rests. (**b**) Intermittent chemoprevention is effective in a rat mammary cancer model. Drugs were fed for 2-week intervals, between which rats were fed control diet for 4 weeks. Tumors were measured weekly with calipers. In each course of dosing, drug levels were as follows: arzoxifene, 20 mg/kg diet; and LG100268, 200 mg/kg diet (Rendi et al. 2004). Reprinted from Rendi MH, et al. *Cancer Research*, 2004, 64: 3566–3571

mutations in multiple genes are involved in human carcinogenesis (Pleasance et al. 2010) now argues that further development of new combinations will be essential in order to achieve effective chemoprevention. Studies from our laboratory have repeatedly demonstrated the effectiveness of combinations of SERMs, rexinoids, and synthetic triterpenoids (Liby et al. 2007a; Rendi et al. 2004); later we added a histone deacetylase inhibitor to these combinations (Tran et al. 2013).

Consideration of the use of intermittent, rather than constant dosing of chemopreventive agents is another important new development. This is standard practice for drugs used in chemotherapy, but unfortunately it has not been adopted in clinical chemoprevention trials. It is notable that chronic dosing of the COX2 inhibitors, rofecoxib and celecoxib (for clinical prevention of colon cancer), led to serious cardiovascular side effects, which caused the termination of the respective trials (Solomon et al. 2005; Bresalier et al. 2005). However, these side effects only appeared after many months of constant dosing. One wonders whether intermittent dosing protocols, with mandatory rest periods between dosing, might have avoided these unfortunate events, without sacrificing the beneficial effects of the drugs themselves.

There is ample evidence from studies in experimental animals that such an intermittent approach is effective in preventing cancer (Rendi et al. 2004; Wu and Lippman 2011). If one uses rest periods, then it is possible to give higher doses of drugs than would ordinarily be used during constant administration. Such higher doses can be particularly effective for inducing apoptosis in premalignant cells. In Fig. 1.1, we show results that were obtained in a rat breast cancer model, using the combination of the SERM, arzoxifene, and the rexinoid, LG100268, in an intermittent dosing protocol (Rendi et al. 2004). The overall conclusion of the study was that intermittent dosing of high doses of arzoxifene combined with LG100268 is an effective way to induce apoptosis and prevent breast cancer in rats. Others have subsequently pursued intermittent chemoprevention in experimental animals using drugs that induce synthetic lethality; the results have been promising (Wu and

Lippman 2011). Whether this overall approach of intermittent high dose combination chemoprevention can be clinically applied to high-risk populations remains to be determined.

1.3 Drugs for Chemoprevention of Cancer

By now there is a huge number of drugs that have been used for cancer prevention in experimental animals, and many of these drugs have even been used clinically for prevention. We will not review them all in this article as this topic has been covered in other reviews. Among the most important are the SERMs such as tamoxifen, raloxifene, lasofoxifene and arzoxifene. These compounds have the added benefit of preventing osteoporosis in addition to preventing ER-positive breast cancer in women at risk (Davidson and Kensler 2011; Sporn 2011; LaCroix et al. 2010). Likewise, the androgen analogs, finasteride and dutasteride, have been shown to prevent prostate cancer in men at risk (Andriole et al. 2010). Other significant chemopreventive agents in various stages of clinical trials for chemoprevention include the aromatase inhibitors, anastrozole and exemestane (Davidson and Kensler 2011) (which exert a general, rather than selective, anti-estrogenic action, and therefore can have undesirable effects on bone); aspirin (for a variety of cancers in which inflammation plays a major carcinogenic role) (Chan 2013); and metformin (a drug long used for type 2 diabetes and retrospectively found in a meta-analysis study to cause a 31% reduction in overall risk of cancer (Decensi et al. 2010)). Metformin is now being clinically evaluated prospectively for many different cancers. The above synthetic drugs are all examples of compounds that have been "repurposed"; they were originally developed and used for diseases other than cancer (Umar et al. 2012), and therefore many of the issues of long-term safety and dosage have already been solved before they enter into a clinical chemoprevention trial.

Natural products derived from food, spices, and drink also are in widespread clinical use for chemoprevention (Umar et al. 2012). These include polyphenols (from green tea), flavones and isoflavones (from soy and other foods), lycopene (from tomatoes), omega-3-fatty acids (from fish oil), curcumin (from turmeric), sulforaphane (from broccoli) (Egner et al. 2013), and resveratrol (from grapes and red wine). In contrast to many synthetic drugs, most of these natural products are extremely safe for human administration, and people have been safely ingesting such compounds for thousands of years. However, they all have a major inadequacy in their relative lack of potency; doses well in excess of 10 μM are often needed to show efficacy in cell culture studies. In contrast, many synthetic drugs have pronounced activity in the nM range.

1.4 The Need for New Synthetic Drugs

One of the most pressing needs in the field of chemoprevention is the development of new, more potent, and safer drugs. Quite simply, we do not yet have an adequate number of chemopreventive agents that are totally effective and safe for preventing all the common forms of carcinoma. For any long-term administration to humans, safety is a paramount issue, and therefore, in our laboratory, we have chosen to use a safe natural product scaffold for semi-synthesis of new drugs (Sporn et al. 2007). In this case, the parent triterpenoid scaffold, oleanolic acid, is widely found in many plants (it is a principal constituent of olives), so again, it has been safely consumed by humans for millennia. Using oleanolic acid as a starting material, we have developed a new series of multifunctional drugs for potential clinical use (Sporn et al. 2011; Liby and Sporn 2012). These compounds have anti-oxidative, anti-inflammatory, anti-proliferative, anti-angiogenic, pro-apoptotic, and differentiating activities in a wide variety of cell culture assays (Liby and Sporn 2012). They are also extremely effective in preventing carcinoma in many organs, including lung, breast, and pancreas, in experimental animals, especially if used in combination with other agents such as rexinoids or histone deacetylase inhibitors (Liby and Sporn 2012). Suppression of highly invasive lung carcinomas (in which a clinically relevant KRAS mutation occurs) has been particularly impressive (Liby et al. 2007b) (see Fig. 1.2).

These synthetic oleanane triterpenoids interact with entire physiological networks, rather than solely with single molecular targets (Liby and Sporn 2012; Yore et al. 2011). We have summarized their chemical syntheses and overall biological activities in several reviews (Sporn et al. 2011; Liby and Sporn 2012). Because of their pronounced anti-inflammatory and anti-oxidative activities, they have also been successfully used in experimental animals for prevention of diseases other than cancer, especially for neurodegenerative diseases (Alzheimer's, Parkinson's, Huntington's, amyotrophic lateral sclerosis, and multiple sclerosis) and chronic lung injury (Liby and Sporn 2012). Potency of these agents is seen in nM and even pM levels in cell culture (See Fig. 1.3). Phase 1 clinical studies have shown promise for potential treatment of cancer (Hong et al. 2012), although these drugs have not yet been used clinically for prevention of cancer.

1.5 New Vistas in Chemoprevention

Ultimately, successful clinical chemoprevention of cancer will depend on the synthesis and development of new drugs. The existing chemopreventive agents, although promising, are not yet potent and safe enough to achieve prevention of all carcinomas, which is the true goal. The development of such new drugs will need to rely upon fundamental new advances in cell and molecular biology. Recent advances in these fields are revolutionizing our concepts of how cells and tissues

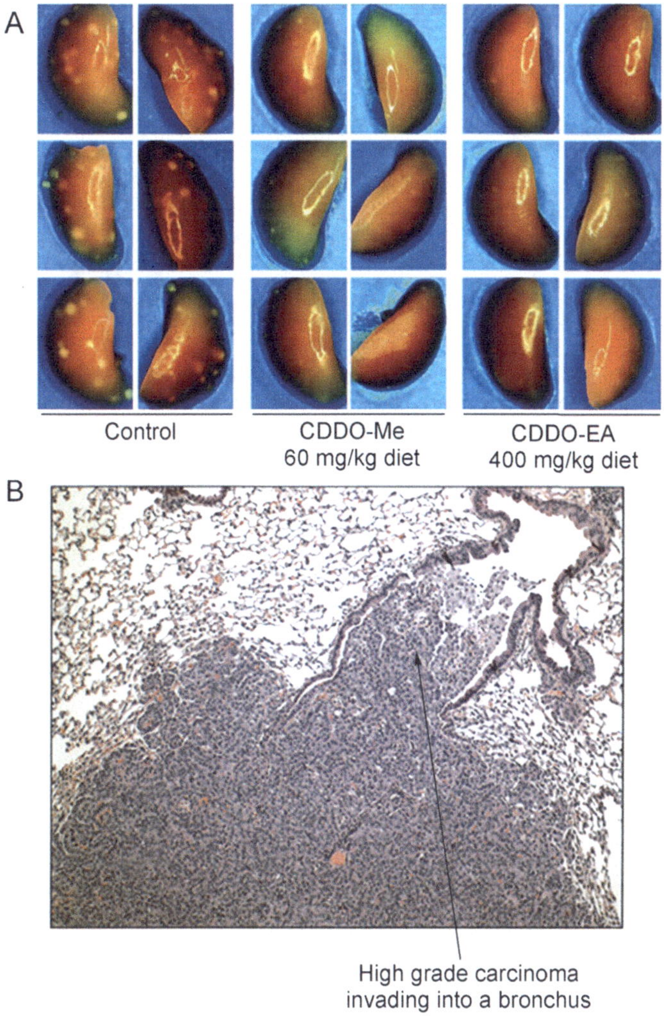

Fig. 1.2 (**a**) Gross appearance at autopsy of representative lungs from six mice in three experimental groups, after treatment of all mice with the carcinogen, vinyl carbamate. Mice were randomized to either control diet, or diet containing either the triterpenoid CDDO-methyl ester (CDDO-Me) or CDDO-ethyl amide (CDDO-EA) and sacrificed 15 weeks later. (**b**) Histopathology of a typical high-grade invasive lung carcinoma induced by vinyl carbamate in a control mouse. Both figures from Liby KT, et al. *Cancer Research*, 2007, 67: 2414–24

actually function. The old linear reductionistic paradigm namely, DNA makes RNA which in turn makes protein, is essentially obsolete, as we are now in a new era of network biology, in which there is an immense array of connectivity between all the molecules of the cell and between cells as well. In many respects, this is hardly new because deep thinkers such as Leslie Foulds wrote about such networks 50 years ago (Foulds 1969). Foulds proposed the concept of "dynamic organization," in which

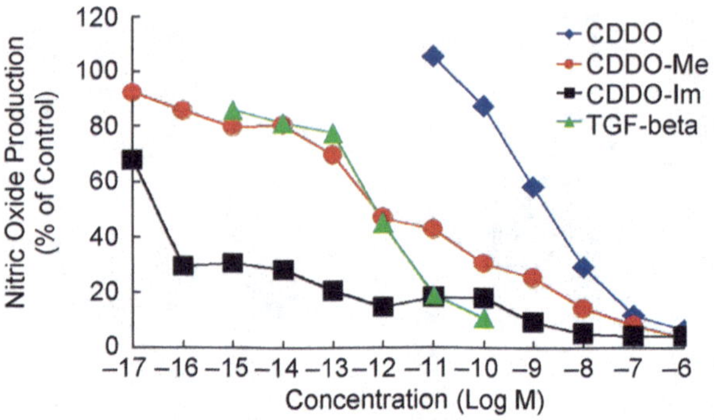

Fig. 1.3 Triterpenoids suppress ability of γ-interferon to induce nitric oxide synthase (iNOS) in primary macrophages. Note exceptional potency of CDDO-Imidazolide (CDDO-Im) in this assay (Sporn et al. 2007). Reprinted from Sporn MB, et al. *Drug Development Research*, 2007, 68: 174–182, which provides experimental details

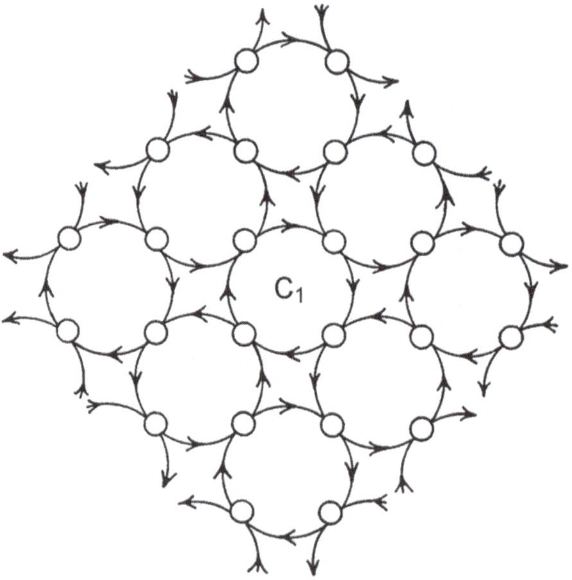

Fig. 1.4 Leslie Foulds' conception of a dynamic biological system with network characteristics (Foulds 1969). Reprinted from *Neoplastic Development*, 1969, page 269

cycles of cellular regulation are linked together in open systems (networks), which interact with the environment (Fig. 1.4). In Foulds' outlook, biological organization is maintained by and because of the flux of metabolites. Thus, cancer may be viewed as a failure of communication between networks, rather than as a failure of specific genes (Clark 1995). A more modern representation of such an outlook is shown in Fig. 1.5, although the intuitive recognition of the importance of networks can be seen in ancient mosaics in which all pathways are interconnected (Fig. 1.6).

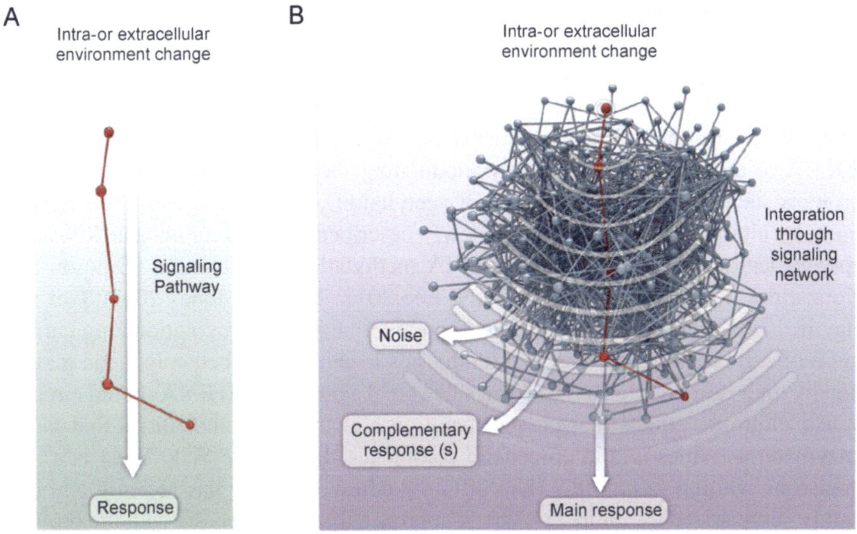

Fig. 1.5 The real contemporary world of network signaling (right panel) contrasted with popular reductionistic views of signal transduction, which are over-simplifications (left panel). Reprinted from Levy ED, et al. *Science*, 2010, 328: 983

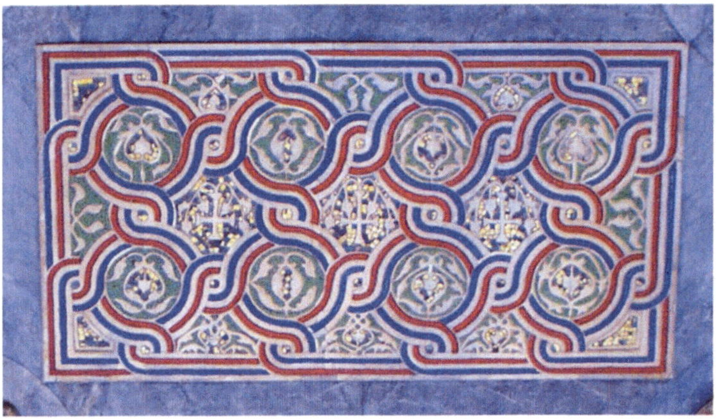

Fig. 1.6 An intuitive view of networks, as seen in this centuries-old mosaic on an exterior wall of Basilica San Marco, Venice, Italy. The creator(s) of this mosaic are unknown. Note that all the pathways surrounding the circles are interconnected. Photo courtesy of Dr. Adriana Albini

Thus, the tumor microenvironment provides a particularly attractive target for new drug development. The ability of networks in the microenvironment either to suppress or enhance carcinogenesis is now recognized to be of great importance (Albini and Sporn 2007; Bissell and Hines 2011). The microenvironment influences promotion of premalignant lesions as well as further progression to invasion and metastasis. Particularly important in this regard are the processes of inflammation and angiogenesis which represent ideal targets for new drug development (Coussens et al. 2013; Albini et al. 2012).

In even more modern terms this will lead to development of new chemopreventive drugs that act by epigenetic mechanisms (Dawson and Kouzarides 2012; Huang et al. 2011; Lee et al. 2013), whether by modulating the post-translational structure of proteins such as histones (alteration of acetylation, methylation, and phosphorylation), by altering the function of the newly described non-coding nuclear RNAs, or epigenetically changing patterns of DNA methylation and function (Dawson and Kouzarides 2012; Guttman et al. 2009; Lee 2012; You and Jones 2012; Tsai and Baylin 2011). This entire area is now in great ferment and is revolutionizing current ideas of cell function. As one investigator has recently described epigenetic regulation by long-non-coding RNAs, "drugs designed against (such) RNAs could circumvent pleiotropic effects that plague many current treatment modalities that target enzymatic activities within epigenetic complexes. Indeed the Wild West is a rich landscape waiting to unfold." (Lee 2012). Andrew Feinberg has recently and elegantly summarized the entire epigenetic approach to carcinogenesis with the provocative and unorthodox statement that "cancer is fundamentally an epigenetic (sic) disease" (Feinberg 2018).

Furthermore, it is not just "driver genes" that are uniquely important for carcinogenesis, in spite of much emphasis on this subject. One must be particularly cognizant of recent and revolutionary genetic analyses, which have proposed that "[chronic] disease risk is largely driven by [many] genes with no direct relevance to disease and is propagated through regulatory networks to a much smaller number of core genes with direct effects.... .referred to as an "Omnigenic model." (Boyle et al. 2017). This approach will clearly require new drugs that will target entire networks of genes and their actions, rather than single targets.

1.6 Chemoprevention of Pancreatic Carcinogenesis as a Special Target

There has been an alarming increase in the number of pancreatic cancer deaths, in both men and women, since the War in Cancer began in 1971. Numbers of deaths have more than doubled (as shown in Table 1.1), which has occurred for no other form of cancer, other than lung cancer in women. Indeed it has been projected that, by the year 2030 in USA, pancreatic cancer will exceed breast, prostate, and colorectal cancer to become the second leading cause of cancer death, surpassed only by lung cancer (Rahib et al. 2014). The reason for this marked increase in pancreatic cancer incidence and death is not fully understood, although obesity and factors related to the microbiome have been implicated (Michaud 2013; Zambirinis et al. 2014; Incio et al. 2016). Underlying all causative factors is an emphasis on inflammation as a critical process for progression of carcinogenesis (Incio et al.

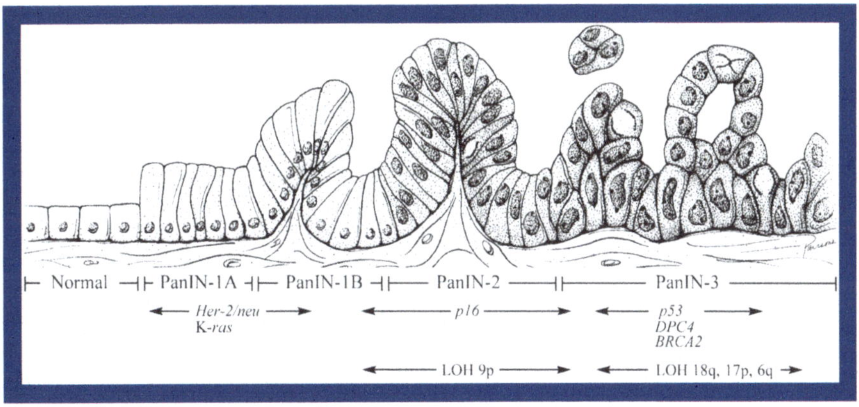

Fig. 1.7 Progression model for pancreatic cancer. The progression from histologically normal epithelium to low-grade PanIN to high-grade PanIN (left to right) is associated with the accumulation of specific genetic alterations (Hruban et al., Am. J. Pathol. 156:1821, 2000)

2016; Guerra et al. 2011), which in both animals and humans proceeds through a well studied series of premalignant lesions, known as "Pancreatic Intraepithelial Neoplasias," also called PanINs [see Fig. 1.7, as well as references Hruban et al. (2000), Hingorani et al. (2003a, b)]. Chronic pancreatitis is a well known risk factor in people. Inflammation can drive progression via either genetic or epigenetic mechanisms, and indeed is essential for progression in some animal models of disease (Guerra et al. 2011). There are abundant macrophages found in PanINs (see Fig. 1.8 and Leal et al. 2016).

Suppressing inflammation in the pancreas thus provides an excellent approach to chemoprevention. It is particularly important that chemoprevention be started at the earliest possible moment during carcinogenesis, because pancreatic cancer cells metastasize very early in the course of disease, particularly by invasion along nerve trunks ("perineural invasion", see Fig. 1.9). Such invasion along nerve trunks may also be partially responsible for the severe pain which is clinically associated with pancreatic cancer. Experimentally, invasiveness has recently been shown to be driven by the hepatocyte growth factor (HGF) /cMet pathway (Nan et al. 2019). HGF has previously been known as "scatter factor", which promotes invasiveness of tumor cells. Thus, targeting HGF, or even other inflammatory cytokines, might represent a useful new approach to chemoprevention.

Actual experimental data showing effective chemoprevention in pancreatic carcinogenesis are scarce. The experimental models in transgenic mice are extremely difficult and costly. Several years ago we showed that the combination of a rexinoid, LG 100268, and a synthetic triterpenoid, CDDO-methyl ester, had some efficacy in delaying death in a very aggressive model in which both Kras and TP53 (highly relevant for human disease) were mutated (Liby et al. 2010). Moreover, an EGF receptor kinase inhibitor, Gefitinib, inhibited carcinogenesis in a less aggressive Kras model (Mohammed et al. 2010). In our own laboratory, we have also shown

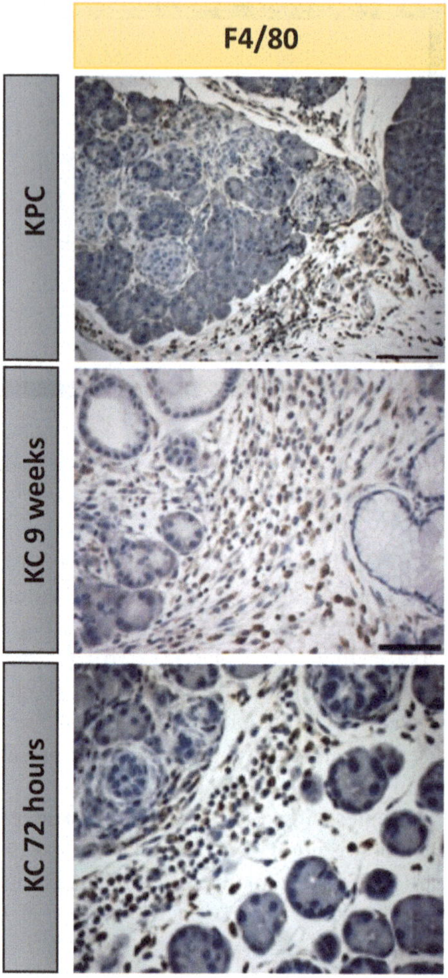

Fig. 1.8 LSL-Kras$^{G12D/+}$; LSL-Trp53$^{R172H/+}$; Pdx-1-Cre (KPC) pancreas immunohistochemistry of 12 weeks old mice. LSL-Kras$^{G12D/+}$; Pdx-1-Cre (KC), caerulein was used to induce pancreatitis. Pancreas was collected 72 h or 9 weeks after cearulein administration. Immunohistochemistry for the spatial localization of macrophages (F4/80) in the pancreas. Scale bar 120 μm. F4/80 antibody used for immunohistochemistry is specific for staining of macrophages. Photomicrographs courtesy of Ana S. Leal

evidence that the triterpenoid, CDDO imidazolide, can strongly suppress inflammation in the pancreas (Leal et al. 2016), but a complete chemoprevention study with this drug has not been performed. Repurposed drugs or natural products, such as metformin or curcumin, have also been studied, but these are unlikely to provide effective prevention of aggressive disease unless used in some future combinations. Considering the genetic and epigenetic complexity of carcinogenesis in the pancreas, effective chemoprevention will probably require combinations of drugs, and unfortunately combinations are even more expensive to study.

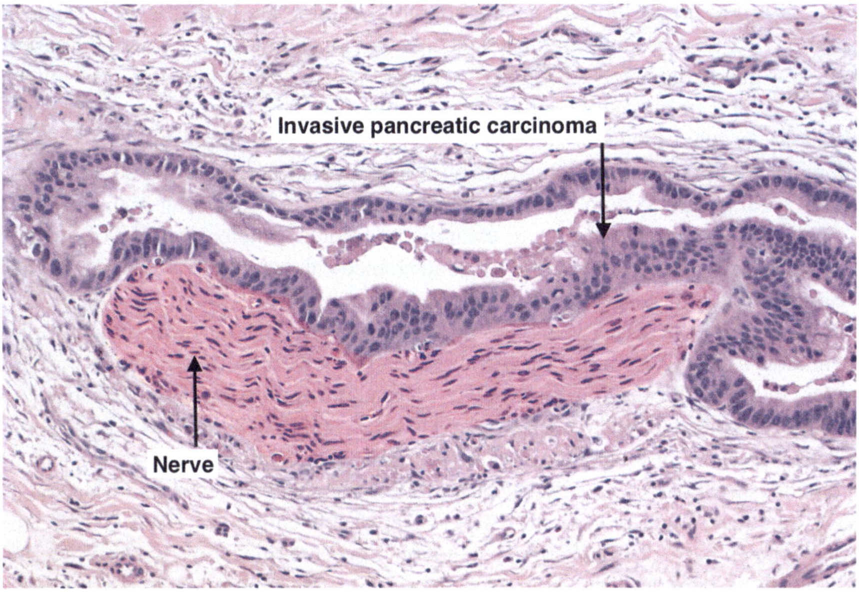

Fig. 1.9 Invasion of pancreatic adenocarcinoma along a nerve trunk ("perineural invasion"). See Nan et al. (2019) for details of importance and mechanism of perineural invasion. Photomicrograph courtesy of Ralph Hruban

1.7 Conclusion and Outlook

It is doubtful whether we will find a general, overall cure for advanced metastatic carcinomas, with their hundreds of genetic lesions, in the foreseeable future. There is simply too much pathology, too much heterogeneity (Gerlinger et al. 2012; Swanton 2012; Longo 2012), to contend with. We must not be fixated on the cancer cell; there are hundreds of different variants within the tumor itself. Advanced malignancy is not just a dragon with a few heads like the Hydra (Sporn 1996), it is a dragon with thousands of heads. There is no reason to assume that any single therapy will solve the cancer problem. Overall, we must be receptive to the concept of polypharmacology (Hopkins 2007; Barabasi 2000).

So we are left with prevention as the only rational, sensible way to deal with the cancer problem. Right now this is not a popular viewpoint. One can only hope that someday reason will prevail and we will eliminate the plague of cancer by finding practical ways to prevent the disease. The use of drugs for chemoprevention should be at the very center of this effort. As summarized above, we now have sufficient basic knowledge that can be expanded for effective clinical prevention of cancer.

A huge question now is, "Do we have the will to use this knowledge?" There is tremendous opposition to chemoprevention of cancer within the community of practicing oncologists, the big pharmaceutical companies, the hospital and insurance industries, and even within women's advocacy groups (Umar et al. 2012; Alberts et al. 1999). Many of those opposing chemoprevention are in a conflict-of-interest situation because of their own financial considerations; they have a vested interest in the status quo. Conversely, the goal of prevention is to keep people out of hospitals.

We can still be guardedly optimistic that someday chemoprevention will become a widely accepted modality for clinical control of cancer simply because such an approach is critically needed. It would appear likely that countries that do not have a private health care system, such as Japan, China, many European countries, and Canada, will be more receptive to eventual widespread implementation of chemoprevention of cancer. The need to control medical care costs, associated with treatment of advanced disease, will also be important.

However, in the past 5 years, the prospects for practical and widespread implementation of clinical studies in chemoprevention have unfortunately not become better. Indeed, with the immense new emphasis on immunotherapy of cancer, the prospects would seem to be even worse. Although immunotherapy has offered some spectacular cures of advanced disease, it is not a practical approach to the cancer problem as a whole, especially because of the huge costs associated with personalizing treatments such as CAR-T. The concept of preventing advanced disease still offers a much more practical approach, not only in economic terms, but also in terms of prevention of morbidity. Moreover, the topic of chemoprevention has not been helped by recent attempts to "rebrand" chemoprevention with a new name and a new marketing gimmick, such as "cancer interception". This unfortunate term misses the entire comprehensive approach of chemoprevention, which is to prevent cancer at all stages of the process of carcinogenesis, all the way from preventing initial, mutagenic DNA damage, to preventing promotion and progression of invasive lesions. Foolish, simplistic diagrams that attempt to portray the process of carcinogenesis as a football, waiting to be intercepted in mid-air, distract from the importance of preventing DNA damage in the first place. It is difficult to intercept a football that has not even been thrown in the first place. It is also frequently mentioned that people are frightened by the "chemo" in chemoprevention, and that chemoprevention is no longer a suitable term. This would seem to be part of the general "chemophobia" which is so prevalent these days, as manifested in widespread skepticism about science in general. Unfortunately, we have come a long way from the old and widely used slogan, "Better things for better living through chemistry."

In spite of the lack of enthusiasm of the pharmaceutical industry (and many practicing oncologists as well) for chemoprevention, the scientific basis for using chemoprevention is on an even stronger footing than it was 5 years ago. Most notably, two major areas have seen huge advances in knowledge, which now make an even stronger case for prevention of early disease. These are the topics of: (1) tumor heterogeneity, and (2) epigenetics. These have been mentioned earlier in this chapter, and there is now a flood of new mechanistic data which lead to the importance of prevention. Tumor heterogeneity and epigenetics now emphasize the difficulty of "personalizing" therapy directed against a single molecular target. Which of the millions of genetic and epigenetic mutations that may exist in a patient's tumors do we wish to target? Prevention of mutation makes much more sense. Epigenetics, of course, places particular emphasis on the ability of natural products to modify DNA structure and function. A recent article, entitled "Intratumor heterogeneity in epigenetic patterns" (Assenov et al. 2018), emphasizes the scientific connection between the two topics; it is discussed in a later Chapter in this book.

The entire situation, regarding the use of chemoprevention to prevent cancer in people, has been elegantly summarized in an editorial by Davidson and Kensler, who wrote in the *New England Journal of Medicine* (Davidson and Kensler 2011), "Women and practitioners now have three options for breast cancer chemoprevention: tamoxifen, raloxifene, and exemestane—agents of proven efficacy that are among the best-studied drugs in the world. Breast cancer is the second most common cause of death from cancer and one of the most feared diagnoses for women in the United States. We have the knowledge and tools to reduce its incidence today. We have run out of excuses. What are we waiting for?"

Acknowledgments We thank all of our colleagues, too numerous to mention individually, for their contributions to this field. Chemoprevention has been a group effort from its very inception. Supported by NIH R01-CA78814, the National Foundation for Cancer Research, the Breast Cancer Research Foundation, and Reata Pharmnaceuticals.

References

Alberts DS, Colvin OM, Conney AH, Ernster VL, Garber JE, Greenwald P, Gudas LJ, Hong WK, Kelloff GJ, Kramer RA, Lerman CE, Mangelsdorf DJ, Matter A, Minna JD, Nelson WG, Pezzuto JM, Prendergast F, Rusch VW, Sporn MB, Wattenberg LW, Weinstein B (1999) Prevention of cancer in the next millennium: report of the chemoprevention working group to the American Association for Cancer Research. Cancer Res 59:4743–4758

Albini A, Sporn M (2007) The tumour microenvironment as a target for chemoprevention. Nat Rev Cancer 7:139–147

Albini A, Tosetti F, Li VW, Noonan DM, Li WW (2012) Cancer prevention by targeting angiogenesis. Nat Rev Clin Oncol 9:498–509

Andriole GL, Bostwick DG, Brawley OW, Gomella LG, Marberger M, Montorsi F, Pettaway CA, Tammela TL, Teloken C, Tindall DJ, Somerville MC, Wilson TH, Fowler IL, Rittmaster RS (2010) Effect of dutasteride on the risk of prostate cancer. N Engl J Med 362:1192–1202

Assenov Y, Brocks D, Gerhauser C (2018) Intratumor heterogeneity in epigenetic patterns. Semin Cancer Biol 57:12–21

Barabasi AL (2000) Linked: how everything is connected to everything else and what it means. Penguin Group, New York

Bishop JM (1997) Cancer: what should be done? Science 278:995

Bissell MJ, Hines WC (2011) Why don't we get more cancer? A proposed role of the microenvironment in restraining cancer progression. Nat Med 17:320–329

Boyle EA, Li YI, Pritchard JK (2017) An expanded view of complex traits: from polygenic to omnigenic. Cell 169:1177–1186

Bresalier RS, Sandler RS, Quan H, Bolognese JA, Oxenius B, Horgan K, Lines C, Riddell R, Morton D, Lanas A, Konstam MA, Baron JA (2005) Cardiovascular events associated with rofecoxib in a colorectal adenoma chemoprevention trial. N Engl J Med 352:1092–1102

Chan AT (2013) Aspirin for the prevention of colorectal cancer. Prog Chem 25:1450–1453

Clark WH Jr (1995) The nature of cancer: morphogenesis and progressive (self)-disorganization in neoplastic development and progression. Acta Oncol 34:3–21

Coussens LM, Zitvogel L, Palucka AK (2013) Neutralizing tumor-promoting chronic inflammation: a magic bullet? Science 339:286–291
Davidson N, Kensler TW (2011) "MAPping" the course of chemoprevention in breast cancer. N Engl J Med 365:2463–2464
Dawson MA, Kouzarides T (2012) Cancer epigenetics: from mechanism to therapy. Cell 150:12–27
Decensi A, Puntoni M, Goodwin P, Cazzaniga M, Gennari A, Bonanni B, Gandini S (2010) Metformin and cancer risk in diabetic patients: a systematic review and meta-analysis. Cancer Prev Res 3:1451–1461
Egner PA, Wang JB, Kensler TW et al (2013) Prevention of liver cancer in Qidong, China: lessons from aflatoxin biomarker studies. Prog Chem 25:1454–1461
Feinberg AP (2018) The key role of epigenetics in human disease progression and mitigation. N Engl J Med 378:1323
Foulds L (1969) Neoplastic development. Academic, London, p 269
Gerlinger M, Rowan AJ, Horswell S, Larkin J, Endesfelder D, Gronroos E, Martinez P, Matthews N, Stewart A, Tarpey P, Varela I, Phillimore B, Begum S, McDonald NQ, Butler A, Jones D, Raine K, Latimer C, Santos CR, Nohadani M, Eklund AC, Spencer-Dene B, Clark G, Pickering L, Stamp G, Gore M, Szallasi Z, Downward J, Futreal PA, Swanton C (2012) Intratumor heterogeneity and branched evolution revealed by multiregion sequencing. N Engl J Med 366:883–892
Guerra C, Collado M, Navas C, Schuhmacher AJ, Hernandez-Porras I, Canamero M et al (2011) Pancreatitis-induced inflammation contributes to pancreatic cancer by inhibiting oncogene-induced senescence. Cancer Cell 19:728–739
Guttman M, Amit I, Garber M, French C, Lin MF, Feldser D, Huarte M, Zuk O, Carey BW, Cassady JP, Cabili MN, Jaenisch R, Mikkelsen TS, Jacks T, Hacohen N, Bernstein BE, Kellis M, Regev A, Rinn JL, Lander ES (2009) Chromatin signature reveals over a thousand highly conserved large non-coding RNAs in mammals. Nature 458:223–227
Hingorani SR, Wang L, Multani AS, Combs C, Deramaudt TB, Hruban RH, Rustgi AK, Chang S, Tuveson DA (2003a) Trp53R172H and KrasG12D cooperate to promote chromosomal instability and widely metastatic pancreatic ductal adenocarcinoma in mice. Cancer Cell 7 (5):469–483
Hingorani SR, Petricoin EF, Maitra A, Rajapakse V, King C, Jacobetz MA, Ross S, Conrads TP, Veenstra TD, Hitt BA, Kawaguchi Y, Johann D, Liotta LA, Crawford HC, Putt ME, Jacks T, Wright CVE, Hruban RH, Tuveson DA (2003b) Preinvasive and invasive ductal pancreatic cancer and its early detection in the mouse. Cancer Cell 4:437–450
Hong DS, Kurzrock R, Supko JG, He X, Naing A, Wheler J, Lawrence D, Eder JP, Meyer CJ, Ferguson DA, Mier J, Konopleva M, Konoplev S, Andreeff M, Kufe D, Lazarus H, Shapiro GI, Dezube BJ (2012) A phase I first-in-human trial of bardoxolone methyl in patients with advanced solid tumors and lymphomas. Cancer Res 18:3396–3406
Hopkins AL (2007) Network pharmacology. Nat Biotechnol 25:1110–1111
Hruban RH, Goggins M, Parsons J, Kern SE (2000) Progression model for pancreatic cancer. Clin Cancer Res 6:2969–2972
Huang YW, Kuo CT, Stoner K, Huang TH, Wang LS (2011) An overview of epigenetics and chemoprevention. FEBS Lett 585:2129–2136
Incio J, Liu H, Suboj P, Chin SM, Chen IX, Pinter MN et al (2016) Obesity-induced inflammation and desmoplasia promote pancreatic cancer progression and resistance to chemotherapy. Cancer Discov 6:852–869
LaCroix AZ, Powles TC, Osborne K, Wolter K, Thompson JR, Thompson DD, Allred DC, Armstrong R, Cummings SR, Eastell R, Ensrud KE, Goss P, Lee A, Neven P, Reid DM, Curto M, Vukicevic S, on behalf of the PEARL Investigators (2010) Breast Cancer incidence in the randomized PEARL trial of Lasofoxifene in postmenopausal osteoporotic women. J Natl Cancer Inst 102:1706–1715
Leal AS, Sporn MB, Pioli PA, Liby KT (2016) The triterpenoid CDDO-imidazolide reduces immune cell infiltration and cytokine secretion in the KrasG12D;Pdx1-Cre(KC) mouse model of pancreatic cancer. Carcinogenesis 37:1170–1179

Lee JT (2012) Epigenetic regulation by long noncoding RNAs. Science 338:1435–1439
Lee JH, Khor TO, Shu L, Su Y, Fuentes F, Kong AN (2013) Dietary phytochemicals and cancer prevention: Nrf2 signaling, epigenetics, and cell death mechanisms in blocking cancer initiation and progression. Pharmacol Ther 137:153–171
Liby KT, Sporn MB (2012) Synthetic oleanane triterpenoids: multifunctional drugs with a broad range of applications for prevention and treatment of chronic disease. Pharmacol Revs 64:972–1003
Liby K, Yore M, Sporn M (2007a) Triterpenoids and rexinoids as multifunctional agents for the prevention and treatment of cancer. Nat Rev Cancer 7:357–369
Liby K, Royce DB, Williams CR, Risingsong R, Yore MM, Honda T, Gribble GW, Dmitrovsky E, Sporn TA, Sporn MB (2007b) The synthetic triterpenoids CDDO-methyl ester and CDDO-ethyl amide prevent lung cancer induced by vinyl carbamate in A/J mice. Cancer Res 67:2414–2419
Liby KT, Royce DB, Risingsong R, Willliams CR, Maitra A, Hruban RH, Sporn MB (2010) Synthetic triterpenoids prolong survival in a transgenic mouse model of pancreatic cancer. Cancer Prev Res 3:1427–1434
Longo DL (2012) Tumor heterogeneity and personalized medicine. N Engl J Med 366:956–957
Meyskens FL Jr, McLaren CE, Pelot D, Fujikawa-Brooks S, Carpenter PM, Hawk E, Kelloff G, Lawson MJ, Kidao J, McCracken J, Albers CG, Ahnen DJ, Turgeon DK, Goldschmid S, Lance P, Hagedorn CH, Gillen DL, Gerner EW (2008) Difluoromethylornithine plus sulindac for the prevention of sporadic colorectal adenomas: a randomized placebo-controlled, double-blind trial. Cancer Prev Res 1:32–38
Michaud DS (2013) Role of bacterial infections in pancreatic cancer. Carcinogenesis 34:2193–2197
Mohammed A, Janakiram NB, Li Q, Madka V, Ely M, Lightfoot S et al (2010) The epidermal growth factor receptor inhibitor gefitinib prevents the progression of pancreatic lesions to carcinoma in a conditional LSL-KrasG12D/+ transgenic mouse model. Cancer Prev Res 3:1417–1426
Nan L, Qin T, Xiao Y, Qian W, Li J, Wang Z et al (2019) Pancreatic stellate cells facilitate perineural invasion of pancreatic cancer via HGF/cMet pathway. Cell Transplant 28:1289–1298
Pleasance E, Stephens P, O'Meara S et al (2010) A small-cell lung cancer genome with complex signatures of tobacco exposure. Nature 463:184–190
Rahib L, Smith BD, Aizenberg R, Rosenzweig AB, Fleshman JM, Matrisian LM (2014) Projecting cancer incidence and deaths to 2030: the unexpected burden of thyroid, liver, and pancreas cancers in the United States. Cancer Res 74:2913–2921
Rendi MH, Suh N, Lamph WW, Krajewski S, Reed JC, Heyman RA, Berchuck A, Liby K, Risingsong R, Royce DB, Williams CR, Sporn MB (2004) The selective estrogen receptor modulator arzoxifene and the rexinoid LG100268 cooperate to promote transforming growth factor β-dependent apoptosis in breast cancer. Cancer Res 64:3566–3571
Solomon SD, McMurray JJ, Pfeffer MA et al (2005) Cardiovascular risk associated with celecoxib in a clinical trial for colorectal adenoma prevention. N Engl J Med 352:1071–1080
Sporn MB (1976) Approaches to prevention of epithelial cancer during the preneoplastic period. Cancer Res 36:2699–2702
Sporn MB (1980) Combination chemoprevention of cancer. Nature 287:107–108
Sporn MB (1991) Carcinogenesis and cancer: different perspectives on the same disease. Cancer Res 51:6215–6218
Sporn MB (1996) The war on cancer. Lancet (London, England) 347(9012):1377–1381
Sporn M (2006) Dichotomies in cancer research: some suggestions for a new synthesis. Nat Rev Clin Oncol 3:364–373
Sporn M (2011) Perspective: the big C—for chemoprevention. Nature 471:S10–S11
Sporn MB, Liby K (2005) Cancer chemoprevention: scientific promise, clinical uncertainty. Nat Rev Clin Oncol 2:518–525
Sporn MB, Suh N (2002) Chemoprevention: an essential approach to controlling cancer. Nat Rev Cancer 2:537–543

Sporn MB, Dunlop NM, Newton DL, Smith JM (1976) Prevention of chemical carcinogenesis by vitamin A and its synthetic analogs (retinoids). Fed Proc 35:1332–1338
Sporn MB, Liby KT, Yore MM, Suh N, Albini A, Honda T, Sundararajan C, Gribble GW (2007) Platforms and networks in triterpenoid pharmacology. Drug Dev Res 68:174–182
Sporn MB, Liby KT, Yore MM, Fu L, Lopchuk JM, Gribble GW (2011) New synthetic triterpenoids: potent agents for prevention and treatment of tissue injury caused by inflammatory and oxidative stress. J Nat Prod 74:537–545
Swanton C (2012) Intratumor heterogeneity: evolution through space and time. Cancer Res 72:4875–4882
Tran K, Risingsong R, Royce DB, Williams CR, Sporn MB, Pioli PA, Gediya LK, Njar VC, Liby KT (2013) The combination of the histone deacetylase inhibitor vorinostat and synthetic triterpenoids reduces tumorigenesis in mouse models of cancer. Carcinogenesis 34:199–210
Tsai HC, Baylin SB (2011) Cancer epigenetics: linking basic biology to clinical medicine. Cell Res 21:502–517
Umar A, Dunn BK, Greenwald P (2012) Future directions in cancer prevention. Nat Rev Cancer 12:835–848
Wu X, Lippman S (2011) An intermittent approach for cancer chemoprevention. Nat Rev Cancer 11:879–885
Yore MM, Kettenbach AN, Sporn MB, Gerber SA, Liby KT (2011) Proteomic analysis shows synthetic oleanane triterpenoid binds to mTOR. PLoS One 6:22862–22863
You JS, Jones PA (2012) Cancer genetics and epigenetics: two sides of the same coin? Cancer Cell 22:9–20
Zambirinis CP, Pushalkar S, Saxena D, Miller G (2014) Pancreatic cancer, inflammation, and microbiome. Cancer J 20:195–202

Chapter 2
Resveratrol for Cancer Prevention: Current Gaps and Opportunities

Karen Brown, Grandezza Aburido, and Robert G. Britton

Abstract The increasing incidence of cancer worldwide, coupled with spiralling treatment costs, presents a situation that is not sustainable for health care systems. Going forward, it is clear there must be a much greater emphasis on prevention strategies. Effective implementation of preventive therapies could have a profound impact on cancer incidence and mortality. Resveratrol (*trans*-3,5,4′-trihydroxystilbene), a constituent of grapes, peanuts, certain berries and red wine, has received considerable attention as a potential agent that can prevent cancer. Hundreds of preclinical studies have attested to its preventive activity in a variety of in vitro and in vivo models across a spectrum of malignancies. The pharmacokinetics, metabolism and safety of resveratrol in humans is now well established through small scale studies, but to date, few clinical trials have attempted to evaluate its effects on endpoints relevant to cancer. This review describes how resveratrol fulfils the requirements of a cancer preventive therapy and highlights the gaps that still need addressing as part of its development. We focus on malignancies where clinical trials have already been conducted or there is a significant weight of evidence supporting the design of trials, namely skin, colorectal, breast and prostate. We also suggest routes to advancing resveratrol towards efficacy studies in high-risk populations; colorectal cancer stands out as having a sufficient body of data that support testing resveratrol in a phase II polyp prevention trial.

Keywords Resveratrol · Cancer · Prevention · Colorectal · Skin · Pharmacokinetic · Prostate · Breast · Trials · Human

---

K. Brown (✉) · G. Aburido · R. G. Britton
Leicester Cancer Research Centre, University of Leicester, Leicester, UK
e-mail: kb20@le.ac.uk

J. M. Pezzuto, O. Vang (eds.), *Natural Products for Cancer Chemoprevention*,
https://doi.org/10.1007/978-3-030-39855-2_2

2.1 The Need for Cancer Prevention

In 2012, there were 14.1 million new cancer cases worldwide (Torre et al. 2015; Ferlay et al. 2013, 2015) and this incidence is increasing. In the European Union for example, by the year 2040 the number of cancers is predicted to increase to 4.75 million cases and 2.55 million deaths, primarily because of population ageing and growth (Wild et al. 2019). This equates to a 32% increase in mortality, or an additional 620,000 people dying every year. Today, the economics of cancer are already astronomical; in 2010 the annual global cost was estimated at US$ 2.5 trillion (Union for International Cancer Control 2014). In the UK the National Health Service costs for cancer services are £5 billion per year, with the cost to society and wider economy estimated at £18.3 billion (https://www.gov.uk/government/publications/2010-to-2015-government-policy-cancer-research-and-treatment). The magnitude of the cancer problem, coupled with spiralling treatment costs presents a situation that is unsustainable for health care systems across the world and it is clear that countries cannot rely on treatment as their only response to cancer. There is an urgent need for alternatives and a greater emphasis on prevention is essential (Forman et al. 2018).

Cancer prevention strategies can take several complementary forms including avoidance of exposure to environmental or occupational carcinogens, implementing lifestyle or behavioural interventions around diet, exercise and smoking, and the use of therapies to actively reduce cancer risk. The latter approach has traditionally been termed chemoprevention, however, experiences in the breast cancer field have shown that this name can evoke inappropriate associations with cancer and chemotherapy, which can deter eligible women from taking what are effective preventive drugs (Cuzick et al. 2011). Consequently, there is a move to use alternative terminology such as therapeutic or medical prevention, which can be defined as the use of natural, synthetic or biological agents to reverse, suppress, delay or prevent either the initial phases of carcinogenesis or the progression of premalignant cells to invasive disease (Serrano et al. 2019).

2.2 Therapeutic Prevention

The long latency for the majority of cancers to progress from premalignant cells to invasive disease offers ample opportunity to intervene with preventive therapies. Moreover, it is becoming increasingly recognised that targeting cells at the premalignant stage when they should theoretically contain fewer genetic alterations, and before the emergence of resistant, heterogeneous clones, presents an exciting window of opportunity that has thus far not been fully exploited (Hait and Levine 2014). Effective implementation of preventive therapies could have a profound impact on cancer incidence and mortality, as illustrated by the way this approach has transformed outcomes associated with cardiovascular disease (CVD) (Hansson

2005). The introduction of drugs that lower blood pressure, suppress cholesterol synthesis or modify platelet aggregation has resulted in a steady fall in death due to heart disease over the past 40 years (Steward and Brown 2013). The major reason for successful uptake of preventive interventions in this setting is the availability of measurable biomarkers of increased risk of disease and death, such as hypercholesterolaemia and hypertension. It is critical that analogous quantifiable risk factors and biomarkers are identified for cancer, to enable preventive therapies to be focused on at-risk individuals, reducing anxieties about potential side effects and providing a surrogate end point of efficacy, which may predict a reduced risk of malignancy.

2.3 Requirements of a Preventive Therapy and Consideration of the Target Population

There are a specific set of requirements when developing therapies for the prevention of cancer, which differ from the main considerations around drugs used to treat cancer (Steward and Brown 2013). Obviously, the agents have to be efficacious and people need to buy into the concept of taking something long term, potentially for years, without knowing whether a particular therapy is going to benefit them personally. Since these target populations are essentially healthy, albeit high-risk, they are not certain to develop cancer, therefore the safety and tolerability of any preventive therapy is paramount. This contrasts with the desired traits of traditional chemotherapeutics and even targeted drugs and immunotherapy for cancer treatment, since these are all associated with significant side effects and long-term risks, which are endured because the potential benefits to the individual greatly outweigh the problems. This means that if preventive agents are to be translated to the clinic, the choice is largely restricted to dietary-derived compounds that are already consumed regularly by human populations, such as resveratrol, and existing drugs that have been in widespread use for other indications and have suitable safety profiles for repurposing (e.g., metformin and aspirin). The therapy also needs to be relatively cheap to make the intervention cost effective and available as an oral formulation or other form that can be easily self-administered, if local or topical application is warranted.

Another integral component to maximize successful cancer prevention is the identification of high-risk populations, as well as individuals that are more likely to benefit from a given intervention. This is a separate, although interrelated area of research, and will not be covered in this article, but it is important to consider the availability of a suitable clinical model to test the therapies in, since this will dictate the feasibility of actually advancing an agent to the clinic. As such, the intended patient group and clinical scenario should be factored in from the outset when selecting preclinical systems for screening and development, to ensure the models represent the patient population and target tissue as much as possible. This could encompass the use of cells harbouring the genetic alterations expected in the patient population, premalignant cells/tissues rather than cancer cell lines to study activity and the inclusion of clinically attainable concentrations in incubations and repeated exposures to mimic human dosing regimens, where possible (Scott et al. 2009).

This review will describe how resveratrol fulfils the requirements of a cancer preventive therapy and highlight the gaps that still need addressing as part of its preclinical and clinical development (Fig. 2.1).

2.4 Resveratrol

Resveratrol (*trans*-3,5,4′-trihydroxystilbene), was first reported to have anticancer activity in the seminal paper from Jang et al., which showed it could impede the three classical stages of carcinogenesis—initiation, promotion, and progression (Jang et al. 1997). Resveratrol was initially identified on the basis of its ability to inhibit the cyclooxygenase activity of COX-1 in a screen of extracts from *Cassia quinquangulata* Rich. (Leguminosae). This enzyme converts arachidonic acid to an array of prostanoids including the pro-inflammatory prostaglandin E2, which has a role in promoting tumour formation, progression and metastasis via a direct action on tumour cells and the surrounding stroma. This potential for anti-inflammatory effects was also borne out in vivo, whereby resveratrol significantly reduced carrageenan-induced pedal edema in rats, both in the acute and chronic phase; such activity may help constrain inflammation-associated tumour promotion. Resveratrol also inhibited events associated with tumour initiation in various cellular systems, namely, free-radical formation and generation of chemical-induced mutations, whilst increasing the activity of quinone reductase, a cytoprotective enzyme that detoxifies carcinogens. Furthermore, the ability of resveratrol to push HL-60 cells towards terminal differentiation and a non-proliferative phenotype was taken as evidence that it can also hinder the progression stage of carcinogenesis (Jang et al. 1997).

Of more direct relevance to cancer prevention, resveratrol inhibited, in a dose-dependent manner, the development of 7,12-dimethylbenz(*a*)anthracene (DMBA)-induced preneoplastic lesions in a mouse mammary gland culture model of carcinogenesis (Jang et al. 1997). More notably, topical application of resveratrol was efficacious in vivo, when employed in the two-stage mouse skin cancer model in which DMBA was used as the initiator and 12-*O*-tetradecanoylphorbol-13-acetate (TPA) as a promoter. Resveratrol reduced the number of tumours occurring per mouse and the percentage of mice that developed tumours; it was particularly potent at the highest dose tested (25 μmol) where it almost completely blocked tumour development (Jang et al. 1997).

Subsequently, a plethora of preclinical studies has attested to the cancer preventive activity of resveratrol in a variety of in vitro and in vivo models across a spectrum of malignancies (Park and Pezzuto 2015; Carter et al. 2014). It is also being pursued for the management of other chronic conditions including diabetes and metabolic syndrome, the pathophysiology of which share overlapping pathways

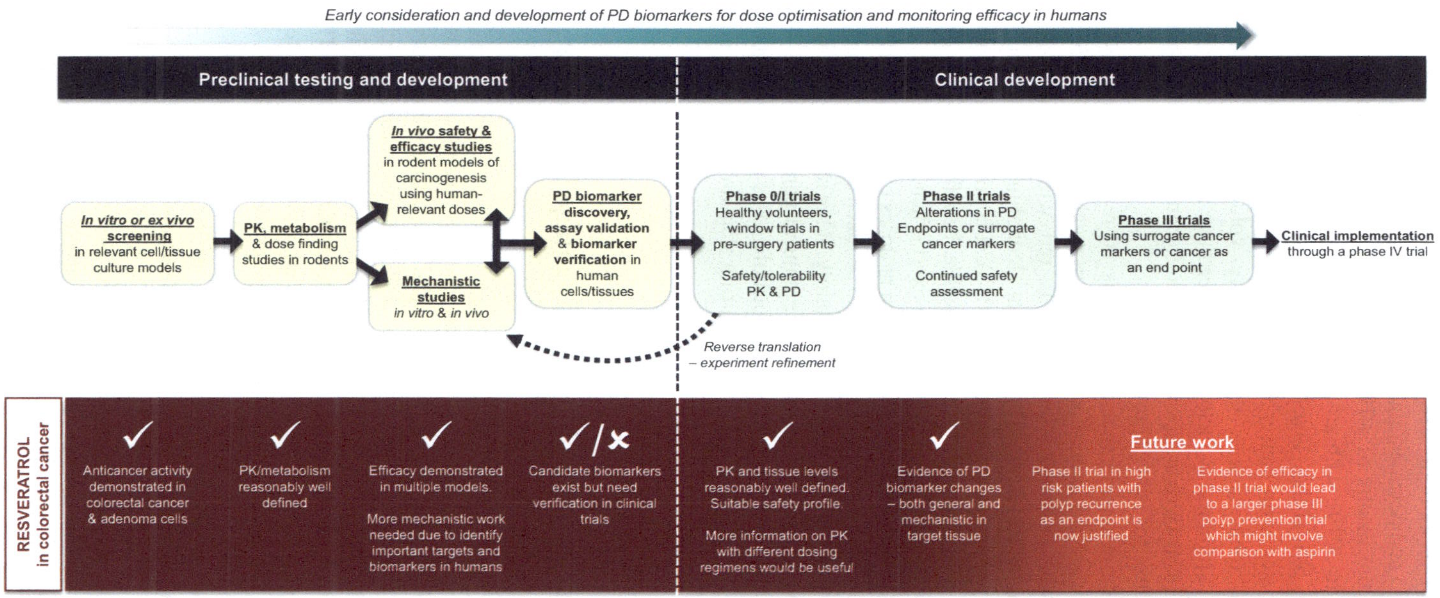

Fig. 2.1 General development pathway for preventive therapies with the supporting evidence for resveratrol in colorectal cancer mapped onto each stage. Also included is an indication of future work needed to assess the preventive efficacy of resveratrol in humans

with cancer, as well as more diverse indications such as neurodegenerative diseases (Turner et al. 2015) and postmenopausal health maintenance (Evans et al. 2016). As of August 2018, the results of ~79 clinical trials had been published involving resveratrol (Pezzuto 2019), with around seven that can be considered to be directly relevant to cancer, in that they involved cancer patients or specifically focussed on biomarkers associated with cancer risk/aetiology (Table 2.1) (Popat et al. 2013). However, several other studies using healthy volunteers or different patient populations with common risk factors for cancer have also provided generic information on safety, pharmacokinetics and biomarker changes that underpin the development of resveratrol for cancer prevention.

It is worth acknowledging that that there is no real evidence that resveratrol consumption through the diet offers protection against cancer. Given that the predominant source of dietary resveratrol is red wine, at least in European populations (Zamora-Ros et al. 2016), and that alcohol increases the risk of several cancers (Griswold et al. 2018; Brown et al. 2018), it is conceivable that the alcohol content of wine would cancel out any possible beneficial effects of low dose resveratrol, if indeed such doses were able to exert efficacy in humans. It is widely envisaged that resveratrol will have to be taken at doses exceeding those commonly consumed via the diet and therefore will have to be taken as a supplement or perhaps rebranded as a drug for some indications. Certainly, if the results of any future cancer trials are to be perceived as credible by the clinical cancer community then the studies must be conducted with resveratrol formulated as an investigational medicinal product with all the associated manufacturing standards and regulatory requirements fulfilled.

2.5 Molecular Promiscuity: An Advantage for Cancer Prevention

Like many other natural products resveratrol is a highly promiscuous molecule, affecting a wide array of biological pathways and interacting with numerous targets (Britton et al. 2015; Pezzuto 2011; Kumar et al. 2018); this makes it mechanistically fascinating but also challenging when it comes to delineating those mechanisms that are important for exerting efficacy in vivo and those that are collateral. The puzzle is further complicated by the fact much of the work described in the literature uses concentrations of resveratrol that are not readily achievable in humans and so may present false leads in the search for key mechanisms of action and pharmacodynamic (PD) biomarkers of activity in humans (Scott et al. 2012).

Confirming and elaborating on the initial effects described by Jang et al., in the context of cancer, it is now well established that resveratrol acts as an antioxidant and anti-inflammatory agent, it can alter immune surveillance, reduce cell proliferation through its ability to induce cell cycle arrest, autophagy, senescence and apoptosis, and regulate cell metabolism and hormone signalling (Jang et al. 1997;

Table 2.1 Biomarkers examined in clinical trials of resveratrol with direct relevance to cancer

Tissue analysed	Biomarkers analysed	Biomarker outcome	Patient or population	Resveratrol dose and duration
Brown et al. (2010)				
Plasma	Fasting IGF-1 and IGFBP-3	Significant reduction in IGF-1 and IGFBP-3, comparing pre and post-dose levels across all patients. Analysis of individual doses revealed significant reductions in IGF-1 at 2.5 g and IGFBP-3 at 1 and 2.5 g.	**Healthy volunteers**	0.5, 1, 2.5 or 5 g daily for 1 month
Cai et al. (2015)				
Colorectal mucosa	NQO1 protein expression and protein carbonyl levels	Both biomarkers were significantly increased by resveratrol at 5 mg daily compared to control untreated patients, but the higher 1 g dose had no effect.	**Colorectal cancer patients** undergoing surgical resection	5 mg or 1 g daily for one week prior to surgery
Colorectal cancer – ex vivo	pAMPK/AMPK and LC3I/II	Increase in AMPK activation (pAMPK/AMPK ratio) and LC3I/II expression at concentrations of 0.01 and 0.1 μM.	**Ex vivo** treatment of **colorectal cancer tissue** obtained from three different patients undergoing surgery	Ex vivo incubation with concentrations ranging from 0.01 and 10 μM for 2 h
Patel et al. (2010)				
Colorectal cancer	Ki67	Significant reduction (~5%↓) in percentage of Ki67 positive cells when comparing pre and post-dose tumour tissue, for both doses combined.	**Colorectal cancer patients** undergoing surgical resection	0.5 or 1 g daily for 8 days prior to surgery
Howells et al. (2011)				
Metastatic colorectal cancer	Cleaved caspase-3	Significant 39% increase in cleaved caspase-3 in malignant hepatic tissue. Paper also reports no changes in a range of other plasma/tissue biomarkers: IGF-1,	Patients undergoing surgical resection for **metastatic colorectal cancer**	5 g **SRT501** (micronized resveratrol) daily for 14 days

(continued)

Table 2.1 (continued)

Tissue analysed	Biomarkers analysed	Biomarker outcome	Patient or population	Resveratrol dose and duration
		Ki-67, pAkt/Akt, Bcl-2, Bax, pERK/ERK, pGSK3/GSK3, pJNK/JNK, survivin, β-catenin and PARP.		
Kjaer et al. (2015)				
Prostate, serum	Prostate volume, prostate specific antigen (PSA), androstenedione, DHEA and DHEAS	Prostate volume unchanged; No effect on PSA levels; High dose resveratrol decreased androstenedione by 24% ($p = 0.052$), significantly reduced DHEA (41%↓), and DHEAS (50%↓) compared to the control group. Other serum markers including testosterone, and dihydrotestosterone were unchanged by resveratrol.	Middle aged males with **metabolic syndrome**	150 mg or 1 g daily for 4 months
Chow et al. (2014)				
Serum, urine	Systemic hormonal biomarkers linked to breast cancer risk	Significant 10% increase in sex steroid hormone binding globulin; 73% increase in urinary 2-hydroxyestrone levels; No change in serum estradiol, estrone, or testosterone.	**Postmenopausal women** with **high body mass index**	1 g daily for 12 weeks

Biomarkers analysed in each trial are indicated and the key biomarker outcomes described. Trials involving administration of resveratrol as part of a mixture or extract have not been included

Cai et al. 2015; Kundu and Surh 2008). Selected molecular mechanisms underlying these phenotypic responses include inhibition of the constitutive COX-1 and inducible COX-2 enzymes, and nuclear factor κB (NF-κB), a transcription factor that regulates genes driving tumour growth (Kundu and Surh 2008). Resveratrol also supresses Wnt signalling, which is a particularly important pathway in colorectal

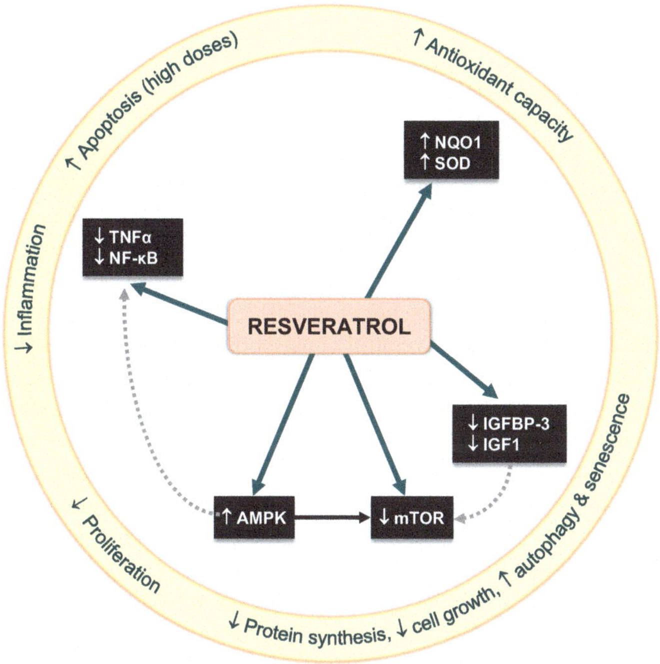

Fig. 2.2 Potential mechanisms of action contributing to the preventive effects of resveratrol in colorectal cancer, based on relevant pathways and targets known to be modulated in human tissue and plasma. Also shown in the outer ring are the phenotypic or functional consequences of these molecular effects

cancer, reducing the expression of Wnt target genes (Chen et al. 2012; Shukla and Singh 2011). Resveratrol activates the cellular energy sensor adenosine monophosphate-activated protein kinase (AMPK) via several routes to shut down anabolic processes required for cell proliferation, and also inhibit the downstream mechanistic target of rapamycin (mTOR), which leads to autophagy (Cai et al. 2015; Gledhill et al. 2007; Park et al. 2012; Dasgupta and Milbrandt 2007) (Fig. 2.2). Detailed accounts of the mechanisms engaged by resveratrol in preclinical models are available (Park and Pezzuto 2015; Shukla and Singh 2011; Varoni et al. 2016) and it is not the purpose of this article to reiterate these reviews, instead the emphasis will be on pathways and endpoints that have been demonstrably modulated in clinical trials or human tissue exposed ex vivo. Moreover, the focus will be on malignancies where clinical trials have been conducted (colorectal, breast, prostate) or there is a significant weight of evidence supporting the design of trials (skin).

2.6 Resveratrol Safety

Our group has previously defined the safety and pharmacokinetics (PK) of resveratrol in phase 1 trials of healthy volunteers (Brown et al. 2010; Boocock et al. 2007) and patients with colorectal cancer (Patel et al. 2010, 2013). We reported a lack of serious adverse reactions, as detected by clinical, biochemical, or haematologic analyses and others have since confirmed that resveratrol is well tolerated at once-daily doses of $\leq$1 g, with the longest published trial in elderly Alzheimer's patients demonstrating an excellent safety profile at doses of up to 1 g taken twice daily for one year (Turner et al. 2015; Gescher et al. 2013; Almeida et al. 2009). The side effect profile associated with resveratrol consists of predominantly gastrointestinal symptoms such as abdominal discomfort, diarrhoea and nausea but these events have generally been reported at doses above 1 g in a variety of healthy populations and patients (Brown et al. 2010; Patel et al. 2010). Furthermore, these symptoms have typically been classed as mild according to the National Cancer Institute Common Terminology Criteria for Adverse Events (CTCAE) and are infrequent, usually self-resolving on cessation of resveratrol. Overall, the current data indicate that resveratrol is a good candidate for further development as a preventive therapy for cancer. It is worth noting that to date it has only been studied in relatively small numbers of people and it is always possible that rarer side effects may come to light as the size and duration of trials increase. Evaluating tolerability and recording adverse events will be an integral component of any future cancer prevention trials, to not only assess the risks associated with intervention but also highlight any issues that could influence compliance. In this respect, it is likely that dividing the dose of resveratrol over the course of a day would help minimise any side effects that may be problematic at higher intakes. However, to date there is little known about the pharmacokinetics (PK) of multiple daily dosing or the effects this would have on PD biomarkers relevant to cancer, which so far have mainly been analysed following a once daily regimen (Cai et al. 2015; Brown et al. 2010; Patel et al. 2010; Howells et al. 2011). A comparison of dosing schedules and how this alters PK-PD relationships, and ultimately efficacy, is certainly warranted as part of ongoing or future clinical trials.

A micronized form of resveratrol SRT501, has been developed in an attempt to improve its bioavailability. Since SRT501 has been proven to generate maximum plasma concentrations around three to four-fold higher than standard resveratrol (Howells et al. 2011) and trials with this formulation have employed a particularly high dose of 5 g per day (Popat et al. 2013; Howells et al. 2011), the safety of SRT501 will be considered separately. SRT501 was initially studied in a phase II trial of patients with multiple myeloma who had relapsed or were refractory to prior therapy (Popat et al. 2013). Patients received SRT501 (5 g) with or without bortezumib daily for 20 days per treatment cycle. The trial was suspended due to safety concerns, as 5 of the 24 patients developed unexpected renal failure. The authors noted that nephrotoxicity was not previously reported in other trials of SRT501 that involved 237 participants (predominantly healthy volunteers and individuals with type two diabetes) in seven studies and that the 5 g dose was safely assessed in these studies (Popat et al. 2013). Moreover, there were no reports of nephrotoxicity from a phase 1 pilot study in patients with metastatic colorectal cancer, where the side effect profile was more akin to that of standard resveratrol at the same high dose (gastrointestinal symptoms) (Popat et al. 2013). Since renal impairment is commonly associated with multiple myeloma and can occur in up to half of patients, it was concluded that this specific group may be at an increased risk of renal failure when taking SRT501 due to their underlying condition.

Another issue that requires further investigation is the possibility of resveratrol-drug interactions, particularly as long-term therapy will be required for cancer prevention. Chow et al. first highlighted the theoretical potential for interactions in a healthy volunteer study in which a 4-week intervention with resveratrol (1 g daily) was shown to modulate the activity of drug metabolising enzymes (Chow et al. 2010). Specifically, resveratrol use was associated with significant inhibition of the phenotypic indices of plasma cytochrome P450 3A4, 2D6 and 2C9, together with induction of 1A2. In addition, in subjects with low baseline values, there was an induction of GST-protein expression and UGT1A1 activity. The authors acknowledged that such enzyme modulation could contribute to the anticancer mechanisms of resveratrol through enhanced detoxification of pro-carcinogenic chemicals and reduced DNA damage. However, since CYP3A4 and 2C9 metabolize a broad range of drugs, inhibition of these P450s in particular could theoretically lead to elevated plasma concentrations and increased likelihood of toxicity, causing the authors to suggest using doses of less than 1 g to minimize adverse drug interactions (Chow et al. 2010). Recent studies have confirmed the potential for pharmacokinetic interactions more directly by co-administering resveratrol with classical drug substrates for the enzymes 2E1, 3A4 and 2C19 (Bedada and Nearati 2015, 2016; Bedada et al. 2016). However, whether such interactions are clinically significant remains to be determined; certainly, there have been no obvious accounts in the literature of adverse events in resveratrol trials attributed to drug interactions. It is also important to recognise that in clinical trials, patients taking certain drugs with narrow therapeutic indices are likely to be excluded as a precaution, so the theoretical potential for interactions should not impact the continued clinical evaluation of resveratrol but may need to be considered if it goes on to be implemented more widely.

2.7 Resveratrol Metabolism and Pharmacokinetics

Like the majority of polyphenolic phytochemicals under investigation for their potential human health benefits, resveratrol has poor systemic bioavailability; since it is relatively well absorbed from the gastrointestinal tract after oral administration (Walle et al. 2004), the low plasma concentrations generated are due to rapid and efficient metabolism. The major routes of metabolism in humans are phase II sulfation and glucuronidation of the three phenolic positions of resveratrol to generate mono-, di- and to a lesser extent, tri-substituted conjugates, together with gut bacteria-mediated biotransformation in the colon (Fig. 2.3).

The plasma pharmacokinetics of resveratrol and its main human conjugates when given as a single agent are well characterised, primarily from trials in healthy volunteers (Boocock et al. 2007; Almeida et al. 2009; Nunes et al. 2009). Key observations from our phase I dose escalation study in which participants took daily resveratrol (0.5, 1.0, 2.5 or 5.0 g) for a month, were that even at the highest intake of

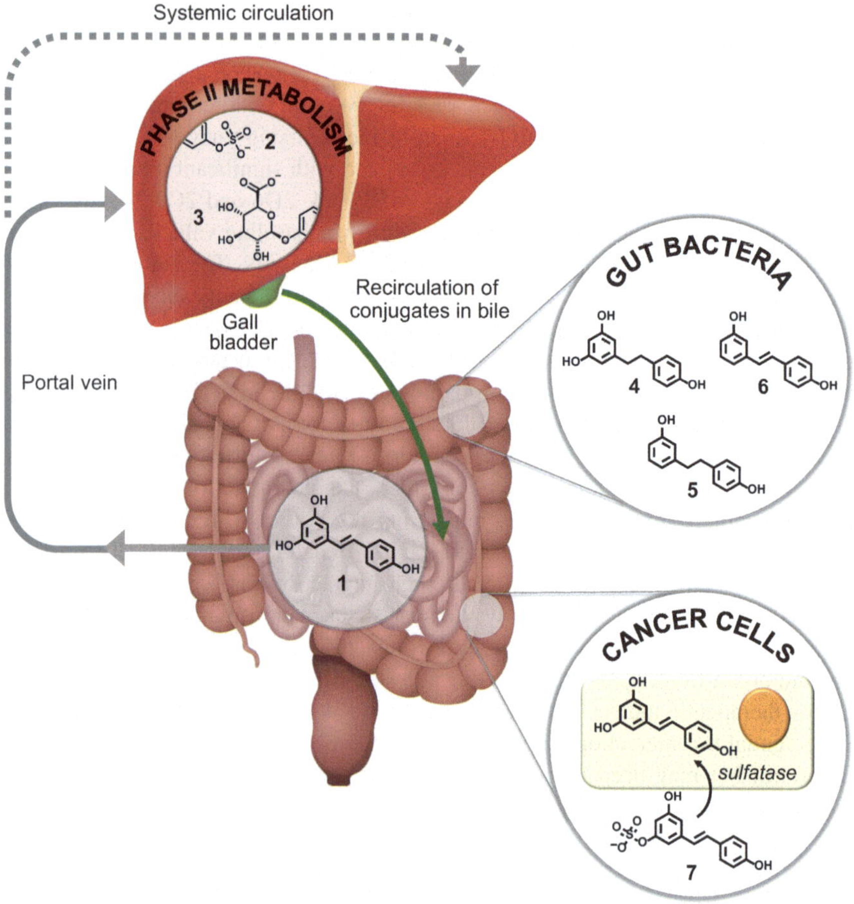

Fig. 2.3 Key features of resveratrol metabolism in humans. Once ingested, resveratrol (**1**) is absorbed in the small intestine and is extensively metabolised (at the three phenolic positions) in the liver by phase II conjugation enzymes to produce sulfate (**2**) and glucuronide derivatives (**3**). Conjugation can generate mono-, di- and tri-substituted metabolites. Resveratrol is also metabolised by the gut microbiota to afford reduced metabolites that include, dihydroresveratrol (**4**) and 3,4′-dihydroxybibenzyl [lunularin (**5**)], plus 3,4′-dihydroxy-*trans*-stilbene (**6**). These metabolites may also be subject to phase II conjugation upon systemic absorption. Resveratrol-3-sulfate (**7**) can act as a reservoir for resveratrol, as it is actively transported into colorectal cancer cells, where it undergoes de-conjugation to afford intracellular resveratrol

5 g, the maximum average peak plasma concentration (C_{max}) of parent resveratrol was only 4.24 μM (Brown et al. 2010). Furthermore, following 0.5 or 1 g per day, which represent two of the most commonly used doses across all the resveratrol clinical trials published to date (Pezzuto 2019), the C_{max} values were 0.2 and 0.6 μM. These findings are important because they define the upper limit for concentrations that should be employed in preclinical experiments to reflect the achievable circulating plasma levels in humans. In reality many published studies have utilised far higher concentrations to elicit responses in vitro, which raises questions as to the clinical relevance of the results (Scott et al. 2012). In comparison, the maximal plasma levels and areas under the concentration versus time curve (AUC) for the main conjugated metabolites resveratrol-3-*O*-sulfate, −3-*O*-glucuronide and -4′-*O*-glucuronide dramatically exceeded those for resveratrol itself, in the case of AUCs, by up to 20-fold (Brown et al. 2010).

It can be difficult to rationalise the potential for resveratrol to exert beneficial biological effects in humans considering its rapid metabolism and low systemic concentrations. Since resveratrol conjugates are present in plasma at higher levels it was long postulated that these metabolites could contribute to any activity in vivo, due to intrinsic activity and/or regeneration of the parent through conjugate hydrolysis. There are few accounts supporting the argument that resveratrol conjugates exert direct activity that could significantly contribute to the anticancer effect of resveratrol in cellular systems; generally they are inactive or less active than the parent (Kenealey et al. 2011; Hoshino et al. 2010). Evidence reinforcing the alternative theory comes from a study demonstrating that resveratrol mono-sulfates reach the systemic circulation in mice after oral administration and are then hydrolysed, liberating detectable concentrations of free resveratrol in plasma and tissues (Patel et al. 2013). The sulfate metabolites were also taken up by human colorectal cancer, but not normal, cells exposed in vitro, with the extent dependent on the expression of specific membrane transporters, including OATP1B3. Once in the cells, the sulfates were converted to the parent in sufficient concentrations to inhibit proliferation, and the treatments also induced autophagy and senescence (Patel et al. 2013; Andreadi et al. 2014). Since these effects were reduced by addition of a sulfatase inhibitor, it was suggested that the parent compound is primarily responsible for causing autophagy and senescence. These findings led to the conclusion that resveratrol sulfates contribute to efficacy, by delivering resveratrol to target tissues in a stable conjugated form enabling gradual regeneration of the parent within selected cell types.

An important feature of resveratrol pharmacokinetics is whether it reaches the proposed sites of action after oral administration in humans and defining the concentrations achieved in potential target tissues. Although the biodistribution of resveratrol has been ascertained in rodents (Böhmdorfer et al. 2017) it undoubtedly presents considerable challenges in humans. It has however proved possible to analyse resveratrol concentrations in colorectal tissue by conducting presurgical window trials, which take advantage of the interval between initial diagnosis of cancer and surgical resection of the tumour, to administer supplements or drugs of interest. The interval differs depending on the specific malignancy and its management but for colorectal cancer the duration is typically 7–8 days, which allowed us to conduct a resveratrol trial in this patient population involving repeated administration of 0.5 and 1 g daily for 1 week (Patel et al. 2010). We found that unlike plasma, parent resveratrol persists in the colorectum and is detectable in normal and cancer tissue, although there was substantial variation between individuals and also different tissue samples from the same patient. Average resveratrol tissue concentrations were ~70-times higher than plasma C_{max} values, supporting the gastrointestinal tract as a target for resveratrol efficacy. Interestingly, levels of resveratrol and its metabolites were consistently higher in tissues taken from the right compared to the left side of the colon. This difference was exemplified by a patient who had two separate tumours resected; the levels of resveratrol-derived species were considerably higher in the cecal (right-sided) tumour than the one excised from the sigmoid colon (left-sided). This may have implications for the preventive efficacy of resveratrol, which could have site-selectivity, as has been reported for aspirin which preferentially reduces the risk of right-sided colorectal adenomas and cancers in humans (Hull et al. 2018; Rothwell et al. 2010).

Less is known about the prevalence of bacterial metabolites and the plasma concentrations achieved in humans but this is a burgeoning area of research given the potential role of the microbiome in a host of pathologies (Wong and Yu 2019; Tilg and Moschen 2014; Tang et al. 2019). The biological activity of bacterial metabolites, which can account for an appreciable fraction of the resveratrol species excreted (Bode et al. 2013), has received limited attention to date (Pallauf et al. 2019). This subject warrants greater clarification since production of metabolites such as dihydroresveratrol or lunularin could either contribute to or abrogate the effects of parent resveratrol in humans, which may be important for personalising therapy; individuals that generate high levels of potentially inactive bacterial metabolites may be less likely to experience a benefit from resveratrol supplementation than those with higher concentrations of resveratrol and human conjugates.

2.8 Colorectal Cancer: Identifying the Optimal Dose for Prevention

On the back of proven anticancer efficacy across a range of preclinical models (Park and Pezzuto 2015; Tessitore et al. 2000; Schneider et al. 2001; Sale et al. 2005) the greatest progress and clinical advances with resveratrol thus far have come in colorectal cancer. Moreover, the fact that relatively high concentrations of resveratrol persist in colorectal tissue after oral ingestion intuitively makes the gastrointestinal tract an ideal target tissue for the protective effects of resveratrol (Patel et al. 2010, 2013). However, significant knowledge gaps, namely the key molecular targets, associated mechanisms of action in humans and identification of the optimal dose, have to date prevented the rational design of trials to assess clinical efficacy. Some of these deficiencies relating to dose were addressed in a recent report by Cai et al. that set out to challenge the assumption that ‘more is better’ in the context of cancer prevention (Cai et al. 2015). The study centred on the conundrum that many dietary constituents being studied for human health benefits first come to our attention as a result of epidemiology data linking dietary consumption with lower rates of certain diseases, as was the case with resveratrol and its association with the French paradox and protection against cardiovascular disease (Bertelli et al. 1995; Renaud and de Lorgeril 1992); this implies that chronic exposure to low doses is required for efficacy, yet such doses are very rarely considered in in the subsequent development of these dietary agents (Scott et al. 2009). Cai et al. aimed to compare the target tissue distribution and activity for a low dietary-achievable dose of resveratrol, equivalent to the amount contained in a couple of glasses of certain red wines (5 mg) and an intake 200-times greater (1 g). The higher dose was considered the maximum that can be taken chronically by healthy populations due to the increased potential for gastrointestinal side-effects at doses exceeding this level.

Firstly, a pre-surgical window trial was conducted in cancer patients to establish the dose response relationship and metabolite profile of [^{14}C]-resveratrol in colorectal tissue. Importantly, the detection of [^{14}C]-resveratrol species in colorectal mucosa from every patient proved that a dietary dose of resveratrol, as well as the higher pharmacological dose, could reach its proposed target tissue; furthermore, both parent compound and conjugated metabolites were present at concentrations in the region of 0.1–0.2 μM after consumption of 5 mg (Cai et al. 2015). Subsequently, equivalent doses of resveratrol were tested for preventive efficacy in a mouse model of human colorectal carcinogenesis. Surprisingly, the low dose was found to be more effective at inhibiting intestinal adenoma development in Apc^{Min} mice than the higher dose, but only in animals fed a high-fat diet (HFD). Use of a HFD was included due to reported observations that resveratrol protects against some age related pathologies and early mortality associated with high-fat intake in mice (Baur et al. 2006; Lagouge et al. 2006); it also provides a model of metabolic dysregulation reflecting certain human populations at elevated risk of colorectal cancer (Aleksandrova et al. 2011; Tsilidis et al. 2015). When the mice were maintained on a standard-fat diet the low dose failed to provide any protection but the high dose retained some activity, albeit the effect was weaker than when combined with a HFD. The differential efficacy across treatment groups correlated with increased protein expression and activation (phosphorylation) of AMPK in intestinal mucosa, and was accompanied by the induction of autophagy and senescence, whilst in adenoma tissue, cell proliferation was significantly reduced.

Further interrogation of the underlying mechanisms using mouse adenoma cells uncovered a bell-shaped dose response for components of the AMPK signalling pathway, leading to mTOR inhibition, autophagy and senescence at low resveratrol concentrations. Interestingly, activation of AMPK was mediated in part by increased generation of reactive oxygen species and a pro-oxidant effect of low dose resveratrol was also apparent in colorectal tissue of patients participating in the window trial. Patients who took 5 mg resveratrol daily had significantly higher levels of oxidative stress markers NQO1 and protein carbonyls, compared to those allocated the 1 g dose and a control group of untreated patients. The combined findings of this study highlight the potential for non-linear dose-responses and illustrate that low dietary exposures of resveratrol not only elicit biological changes in mouse and human tissues germane to colorectal cancer prevention, but have greater potency compared to high doses (Cai et al. 2015). Consequently, it is imperative that a range of doses encompassing the 5 mg used by Cai et al. are included in further clinical trials assessing resveratrol efficacy for colorectal cancer prevention. An overview of the potential mechanisms that might contribute to efficacy in this context, based solely on biological effects detected in human tissue and plasma thus far, is shown in Fig. 2.2.

2.9 Further Clinical Evidence Supporting a Role for Resveratrol in Colorectal Cancer Prevention

Individuals with the inflammatory bowel disease ulcerative colitis (UC) have an increased risk of colorectal cancer. Reducing pro-inflammatory and/or increasing anti-inflammatory mediators is the mainstay of treatment for these patients and resveratrol is being investigated in this setting. Results of a randomized, double-blind, placebo-controlled study in patients with active mild to moderate UC supplemented with resveratrol (500 mg daily) for 6 weeks revealed significant reductions in plasma levels of the inflammatory markers TNF-α and hs-CRP, and the activity of NF-κB in peripheral blood mononuclear cells (Samsami-Kor et al. 2015). There was also evidence that resveratrol significantly improved the antioxidant status, increasing serum superoxide dismutase and total anti-oxidant capacity whilst reducing markers of oxidative stress (malondialdehyde) (Samsamikor et al. 2016). Given the overlapping role of inflammation and oxidative stress in the pathogenesis of both UC and cancer the effects of resveratrol in these patients may have wider relevance for colorectal cancer prevention.

The gastrointestinal tract is densely populated with microorganisms, which constitute the microbiome, a metabolically active biomass in lifelong contact with the colorectal mucosa. These microorganisms interact with host cells to regulate many physiological processes, including energy harvest, metabolism and immune response. In recent years, several species of bacteria have been found to have associations with, and potential roles in, colorectal carcinogenesis (Wong and Yu 2019; Garrett 2019). Sequencing studies have revealed microbial compositional and ecological changes in patients with colorectal cancer. Furthermore, the gut microbiome varies widely between populations at differential risk of colorectal cancer and between individuals within those populations. It is affected by a range of factors but one important contributor is the use of drugs or supplements (Maier et al. 2018). Resveratrol is known to alter the gut microbiome and it has been suggested, based on rodent models, that its beneficial effects across a range of conditions including heart failure, obesity and the metabolic syndrome may be mediated, at least partly through its interaction with gut microbiota (Chaplin et al. 2018; Sung et al. 2017; Bird et al. 2017). It is certainly feasible that resveratrol-induced changes to the gut microbiome is another mechanism that could contribute to its cancer prevention effects, particularly in the colon. Additionally, it appears that bacterial metabolism of resveratrol can differ among individuals; therefore, features of a person's microbiome may influence whether resveratrol is efficacious (Bode et al. 2013).

2.10 Towards a Colorectal Polyp Prevention Trial

There is now a sufficient body of evidence that supports advancing resveratrol to a phase II efficacy trial in which its ability to reduce colorectal polyp recurrence in high-risk patients can be assessed (Fig. 2.1); colorectal polyps are a surrogate endpoint of cancer commonly used in prevention trials (Hull et al. 2018; Higurashi et al. 2016; Cole et al. 2009) and currently represent the best biomarker available for this purpose. The case for resveratrol is underpinned by numerous demonstrations of efficacy in preclinical models of colorectal carcinogenesis, aligned with promising pharmacodynamic biomarker changes in target tissues from pre-surgical window trials (Table 2.1). Crucially, it has an excellent safety profile and good compliance rates have been reported in other long-term trials, which is important because polyp prevention trials typically require an intervention of at least 1 year. Such trials involve recruiting patients who have had prior colorectal polyps detected and removed endoscopically. A significant proportion of these patients (dependent on number, size and histopathology of the original polyps) remain at high-risk for polyp recurrence within a relatively short time frame of 1–3 years, which provides an interval for evaluating potential colorectal cancer preventive therapies. A trial of this nature would provide definitive evidence of whether resveratrol is able to exert preventive efficacy in humans and a positive outcome could lead to further trials comparing resveratrol to other preventive therapies such as aspirin (Hull et al. 2018; Rothwell et al. 2010) and testing combinations in this high-risk population. These steps are vital before resveratrol can ever be evaluated against the ultimate endpoint of colorectal cancer incidence.

2.11 Skin Cancer

Skin cancers can be categorised as melanoma or non-melanoma, the latter being the most frequent type, and can be further subdivided into basal cell carcinoma (BCC) and squamous cell carcinoma (SCC). The vast majority of cases are caused by exposure to ultraviolet (UV) radiation from the sun. Melanoma skin cancers are associated with higher mortality rates and these rates are significantly affected by the stage at which melanomas are diagnosed, with almost 0% mortality at stage I but greater than 70% mortality at stage IV (Cancer Research UK. Available from https://www.cancerresearchuk.org/health-professional/cancer-statistics/statistics-by-cancer-type/melanoma-skin-cancer/mortality n.d.). Following on from the initial discovery of resveratrol as a preventive agent with potent activity against skin cancer (Jang et al. 1997), numerous in vivo studies have reinforced its potential for this indication. These studies have employed a variety of skin cancer models (chemical and UV-induced, genetic and xenografts) with the majority adopting topical administration (Park and Pezzuto 2015). Clearly, direct application to the skin is a viable route that overcomes any concerns around low bioavailability and suggests it is resveratrol, as opposed to a metabolite, that is having the preventive effect. In this context, the development of formulations and delivery systems for dermal administration with a view to exerting local and/or systemic effects is an area of interest, such as hydrogel patches and nanosuspensions to improve transport and solubility of resveratrol (Hung et al. 2008; Kobierski et al. 2009).

In DMBA/TPA models, resveratrol consistently reduces the incidence, multiplicity and volume of tumours resulting from carcinogen exposure and also delays the onset of lesion development, as summarised by Park and Pezzuto (2015). Mechanistically, pre-treatment of CD-1 mice with resveratrol has been shown to protect against the oxidative stress and subsequent gene expression alterations induced by TPA treatment, exemplified by the control of H_2O_2 levels in the skin and down-regulation of c-Fos, c-Jun and TGF-β1 at the transcriptional level (Jang and Pezzuto 1998). Other studies have demonstrated favourable effects on apoptotic pathways and inflammatory biomarkers (Roy et al. 2009; Cichocki et al. 2008).

Given the overwhelming importance of UV radiation in the aetiology of skin cancer, models utilizing this exposure, as opposed to chemical carcinogens, have greater clinical relevance. There are 3 main types of ultraviolet radiation, UVA, UVB, and UVC (in descending wavelength), with varying roles and contributions to carcinogenesis. Most studies have focussed on the impact of resveratrol on the effects of UVB radiation, which is the main cause of skin cancer (Ndiaye et al. 2011). For example, in SKH-1 hairless mice resveratrol has been shown to modulate markers of UVB-mediated skin damage, including decreasing bi-fold skin thickness, hyperplasia, edema, cell proliferation and leukocyte infiltration and enhancing apoptosis, whilst at a molecular level it reduces the ornithine decarboxylase induction caused by UVB, decreases cyclooxygenase and Survivin expression and phosphorylation, as well as H_2O_2 generation and lipid peroxidation (Reagan-Shaw et al. 2004; Aziz et al. 2005a; Afaq et al. 2003).

These cellular and molecular changes appear to correlate with preventive efficacy since in the same mouse model, topical resveratrol delays formation and reduces the incidence of skin tumours caused by UVB exposure (Aziz et al. 2005b). Use of two different protocols for application of resveratrol relative to UVB exposure revealed that post-treatment imparted equal, if not better, protection than pre-treatment, which suggests the observed effects are not through a sunscreen mechanism; rather, resveratrol is absorbed into the skin and activates a protective signalling cascade (Aziz et al. 2005b). It is also of note that in this study UVB caused a variety of tumours in the SKH-1 hairless mice, including SCC, Bowen's disease, invasive carcinomas in situ, and actinic keratoses (AK). However, in the resveratrol group, under both treatment protocols, the majority of lesions were identified as AKs, with or without inflammation. This finding led the authors to hypothesize that resveratrol might be inhibiting the malignant conversion of premalignant conditions such as AK (Aziz et al. 2005b).

Given the wealth of preclinical data on resveratrol and skin cancer it is somewhat surprising that there has been little attempt to translate these findings to the clinic as there are few published trials dedicated to the subject (Aziz et al. 2005a). However, it is intriguing to note that in the trial led by Turner et al. involving elderly patients with Alzheimer's disease and neurological markers as the primary endpoint, there was a significant difference in the number of cancers occurring in the resveratrol versus placebo groups at the end of the 12-month intervention (Turner et al. 2015). There was one case of bladder cancer in the resveratrol group ($n = 64$ patients) and 7 cancers in 6 participants on placebo ($n = 55$ patients); these consisted of three malignant melanomas, two squamous cell carcinomas, one basal cell carcinoma and one malignant glioma. Although these preliminary findings must be interpreted with an appropriate degree of caution, especially given the intervention period was very short to have an effect on cancer outcomes, it is nonetheless encouraging to see a difference in the incidence of malignancies, particularly skin cancers, in this trial. The results add to the weight of evidence supporting clinical testing of resveratrol in an appropriate patient population for skin cancer prevention. Following the general development paradigm laid out for colorectal cancer (Fig. 2.1) and the concept that proof of preventive efficacy is best gained using a high-risk population, a starting point could be establishing the effect of resveratrol on molecular and phenotypic pharmacodynamic biomarkers in human skin from sun-damaged individuals with existing actinic keratosis. Alternatively, it may be possible to advance directly to a phase II pilot study investigating the effect of topical resveratrol on the number of AKs as a surrogate marker of cancer in this same high-risk population (Surjana et al. 2012; Criscione et al. 2009; Gupta et al. 2012).

2.12 Breast Cancer

Early reports using a cell line suggested resveratrol was an estrogenic agonist (Gehm et al. 1997), and this idea was perpetuated by its structural similarity to diethylstibestrol, a synthetic estrogen and endocrine disrupter that causes clear cell adenocarcinoma of the cervix and vagina in the daughters of women who took the drug during pregnancy. However, this claim has not been upheld in subsequent studies (Bhat et al. 2001), whilst others have produced similar effects or suggested it has mixed agonist/antagonist properties for estrogen receptors (ER) depending on the cell types, ER isoform, and the presence of endogenous estrogens (Levenson et al. 2003; Chakraborty et al. 2013; Bowers et al. 2000).

Following on from the initial observation that resveratrol interferes with the development of preneoplastic lesions in a mouse mammary gland culture model it has displayed efficacy in a number of rodent models of breast cancer, particularly those driven by exposure to the chemical carcinogens DMBA and *N*-nitroso-*N*-

methylurea, where it significantly impacts on tumour incidence, multiplicity and the latency period to tumour development (Bhat et al. 2001; Banerjee et al. 2002; Whitsett et al. 2006). In transgenic models resveratrol supplementation delayed the development and reduced the mean number and size of spontaneous mammary tumours whilst diminishing the number of lung metastases in HER-2/*neu* transgenic mice (Provinciali et al. 2005). Downregulation of HER-2/*neu* expression and the induction of apoptosis was cited as a potential mechanism of action. In contrast, resveratrol had no effect on tumour latency in a mouse model of BRCA1-mutated breast cancer ($K14cre;Brca1^{F/F};p53^{F/F}$) that resembles human disease in that the tumours arising are triple-negative, lacking expression of estrogen, progesterone or HER2 growth factor receptors (Zander et al. 2012). The anticancer activity of resveratrol has also been examined in various xenograft models with more conflicting results (Park and Pezzuto 2015; Carter et al. 2014) including cases of enhanced tumourigenesis that may reflect its potential mixed agonist/antagonist properties (Brown et al. 2018); however, overall the majority of in vivo studies are consistent with a protective effect of resveratrol in breast cancer.

In humans, resveratrol species have been shown to reach breast tissue in a pre-surgery window trial involving breast cancer patients. The participants took three capsules daily containing a mixture of fruit and cocoa extracts plus resveratrol for ~6 days (Ávila-Gálvez et al. 2019). Each capsule provided 37 different phenolic compounds including 54 mg of resveratrol (total dose 162 mg per day). Resveratrol-3-*O*-sulfate, 4′-*O*-sulfate, 3-*O*-glucuronide and dihydroresveratrol 3-*O*-glucuronide were all quantifiable in both malignant and normal breast tissue but no free parent resveratrol or the bacterial metabolite dihydroresveratrol were detected. The authors proposed this may be due to the analytical assay having a higher limit of detection for these specific compounds (Ávila-Gálvez et al. 2019) but it could equally be because the unconjugated compounds do not reach or persist in breast tissue, which has implications for the potential direct activity of resveratrol in breast cells.

A pilot study in postmenopausal women with high body mass index (BMI) has sought to determine whether resveratrol (1 g daily) can modulate circulating sex steroid hormones and estrogen metabolites, as potential mechanisms of action for breast cancer prevention (Chow et al. 2014). The rationale underlying this trial was that breast cancer risk increases with increasing concentrations of the following hormones—total estradiol, free estradiol, non-sex hormone binding globulin (SHBG)-bound estradiol, estrone, estrone sulfate, and testosterone (Hormones and Group BCC 2002). In addition, higher SHBG levels are associated with a decrease in breast cancer risk, due to lower concentrations of free non-protein bound sex hormones available for signalling. Furthermore, specific estrogen metabolites vary in their estrogenic potential and ability to cause DNA damage, which could contribute to detrimental effects and cancer risk and some observation studies have demonstrated a correlation between a low urinary 2-hydroxyestrone/16α-hydroxyestrone (2-OHE1/16α-OHE1) ratio and increased breast cancer risk (Chow et al. 2014). Formation of 2-OHE1 and 16α-OHE1 is primarily catalyzed by CYPs 1A2 and 3A4, respectively; since resveratrol has been shown to modulate the activity of these enzymes in humans (Chow et al. 2010) it is possible that supplementation may alter the balance between mitogenic and protective estrogen metabolites. After menopause, adipose tissue is the main source of circulating estrogens, which are formed from androgenic precursors. Resveratrol has been found to inhibit the aromatase enzymes responsible for this conversion in breast cancer cells (Wang et al. 2006). Levels of estrogens therefore correlate with the amount of adipose tissue, which provides a mechanistic basis for the association between high adiposity and increased breast cancer risk and explains why resveratrol was tested in postmenopausal women with high BMI. The results demonstrated that a 12-week resveratrol intervention had no effect on any of the circulating sex steroid hormones but there was a significant 10% increase in SHBG concentrations which may have accounted for a decrease in the levels of bioavailable free testosterone. Furthermore, resveratrol caused a 73% increase in urinary levels of the estrogen receptor antagonist 2-OHE1, which led to a large favourable increase in the urinary 2-OHE1/16α-OHE1 ratio and is consistent with the ability of resveratrol to induce CYP1A2 and inhibit 3A4 activity in humans (Chow et al. 2010). The authors concluded that further research is needed to evaluate whether resveratrol-induced changes in estrogen metabolism could potentially contribute to breast cancer risk modulation (Chow et al. 2014).

Another trial in women at increased risk of breast cancer suggested that resveratrol significantly decreased methylation of the tumour suppressor gene RASSF-1α in mammary tissue after a 12-week intervention with doses of 5 or 50 mg twice daily (Zhu et al. 2012). Whilst there was no simple association between taking resveratrol at either dose and change in RASSF-1α methylation when comparing pre and post-intervention tissue, when the data were analysed with respect to resveratrol serum levels for each patient, higher concentrations correlated with a greater decrease in RASSF-1α methylation. The authors justified this approach based on the inter-individual variability in resveratrol concentrations detected. In addition, the change in the fraction of methylated RASSF-1 α DNA after treatment positively correlated with the change in PGE2 levels in nipple aspirate fluid. Methylation of other genes examined (*p16, APC, CCND2*) was unaffected by the interventions. A limitation of this trial was that they gave patients an extract of *P. cuspidatum* containing resveratrol, rather than the purified single compound, so it is difficult to attribute categorically the effects observed to resveratrol (Zhu et al. 2012).

Considering all the results accrued to date, resveratrol clearly exerts preventive efficacy in preclinical models of breast cancer but the data from human studies are rather limited. More evidence that it can elicit potentially beneficial molecular and cellular changes in human tissue, either through the use of primary explant cultures, other 3D models, or conducting early phase biomarker trials, is needed before attempting to evaluate clinical efficacy.

2.13 Prostate Cancer

In vitro evidence suggests a role for resveratrol in the prevention of prostate cancer where it has growth inhibitory and pro-apoptotic effects in malignant cells without affecting normal prostate epithelial cells (Aziz et al. 2006). However, there are few examples of positive outcomes from in vivo studies. Highlights include the ability of resveratrol to interfere with spontaneous tumour development in two studies employing the transgenic adenocarcinoma of mouse prostate (TRAMP) and analogous rat (TRAP) models (Harper et al. 2007; Seeni et al. 2008). In the former, dietary administration of resveratrol significantly reduced the incidence of poorly differentiated prostatic adenocarcinoma relative to control mice, which may be explained by delayed progression of well-differentiated lesions. There was however, no overall reduction in the total weight or number of tumours per mouse (Harper et al. 2007). A biomarker experiment conducted at an earlier time point revealed decreased cell proliferation within the prostate of resveratrol treated mice compared to animals on control diet. This was accompanied by lower tissue concentrations of IGF-1 and down-regulation of phospho-ERKs 1 and 2, which the authors claimed provide a biochemical basis for resveratrol suppressing prostate cancer development. In the rat TRAP model there was a partial pathologic responses to resveratrol, which significantly albeit weakly suppressed neoplastic lesions in the ventral and lateral lobes (Seeni et al. 2008). The numbers of apoptotic cells in the ventral prostate of resveratrol-treated rats were also significantly increased relative to the controls, and this was accompanied by reduced expression of androgen receptor protein, suggesting a mechanism of action. Furthermore, as was the case in the TRAMP study, resveratrol tended to shift the progression of neoplastic growth by suppressing the number of adenocarcinoma and high grade prostate intraepithelial neoplasia (HG-PIN), with a concomitant increase in low grade-PIN. Similar effects were evident in another genetic model of carcinogenesis, the prostate-specific phosphatase and tensin homolog (PTEN)-knockout mouse in which resveratrol decreased the incidence of HG-PIN lesions (Li et al. 2013).

Resveratrol has also been assessed in various xenograft models of prostate cancer, which are less relevant to the prevention scenario since the cells are fully malignant from the outset. As an example, it had no effect on the growth of tumours or lung metastases arising from transplanted PLS30 cells, possibly because these cells are androgen independent (Seeni et al. 2008). Conflicting results have been described in two separate xenograft studies utilising androgen responsive LNCaP cells in nude mice (Wang et al. 2008). In fact, in one study where resveratrol (0.01 and 0.005% in the diet) failed to inhibit tumour growth or reduce tumour cell proliferation, it was actually associated with reduced apoptosis and increased angiogenesis, which could be detrimental for individuals with prostate cancer. In contrast, LNCaP tumour formation, development, and progression were significantly delayed by resveratrol given by gavage at 50 mg/kg body weight/day on alternate days (Dias et al. 2013). The reasons for this discrepancy are not immediately apparent given that the cell line and mice used are similar and both protocols involved starting resveratrol 2 weeks prior to the injection of cells; perhaps the most likely explanation is that the daily dose was lower in the negative study since it approximates to ~12 and 6 mg/kg body weight.

Overall, the in vivo data, particularly from the genetic models, suggest that resveratrol may have value for the prevention of prostate cancer in humans. However, only one study to date has attempted to investigate this possibility. It was conducted using a population of middle-aged men with metabolic syndrome who participated in a trial with the primary objective of investigating the effects of resveratrol (150 mg or 1 g daily) on bone, through the measurement of bone alkaline phosphatase (Ornstrup et al. 2014). To gain insight into the potential role of resveratrol for the management of benign prostate hyperplasia and prostate cancer, prostate size, prostate specific antigen (PSA), and hormonal markers were examined in these individuals after the 4 month intervention (Kjaer et al. 2015). Resveratrol had no effect on prostate size, serum PSA, or levels of testosterone, free testosterone or dihydrotestosterone. The high dose did however decrease androstenedione and significantly reduce dehydroepiandrosterone (DHEA) by 41%, as well as halving the concentration of dehydroepiandrosterone sulfate (DHEAS) relative to the control group. Overall, the authors concluded that since resveratrol failed to affect prostate volume in healthy middle-aged men there was no evidence to recommend its use for the treatment of benign prostate hyperplasia.

2.14 Concluding Comments

Resveratrol impacts numerous molecular pathways dysregulated in cancer and undoubtedly has the ability to prevent many different cancers in rodent models. The questions that need to be addressed now are whether it can modulate the same pathways in humans in vivo and whether the activity translates to tangible cellular effects, and ultimately clinical efficacy. Research is most advanced in colorectal cancer where there is sufficient evidence from early phase biomarker trials to warrant a phase II efficacy trial in which its ability to reduce colorectal polyp recurrence in high-risk patients can be assessed. Development of a strategy to advance resveratrol for skin cancer prevention in humans is also justified. Although the optimum dose needed for cancer prevention is not yet known, and is likely to differ depending on the tumour site and type, there is reason to expect that the doses required will be well-tolerated and have a good safety profile, which fulfils a key requirement of preventive therapies. Conducting meaningful clinical trials in cancer prevention is particularly challenging, requiring significant funding and the identification of an appropriate high-risk population and endpoints that allow results to be obtained in a reasonable time frame. To maximise the chances of conducting such trials we should take advantage of the knowledge gained from studies of resveratrol in other populations such as individuals with diabetes, metabolic syndrome and inflammatory/immune conditions, given the overlap in aetiology and molecular drivers with cancer. Any evidence of clinical efficacy in humans should help strengthen the case for testing resveratrol in cancer prevention.

References

Afaq F, Adhami VM, Ahmad N (2003) Prevention of short-term ultraviolet B radiation-mediated damages by resveratrol in SKH-1 hairless mice. Toxicol Appl Pharmacol 186(1):28–37

Aleksandrova K, Boeing H, Jenab M, Bas Bueno-de-Mesquita H, Jansen E, van FJB D et al (2011) Metabolic syndrome and risks of colon and rectal cancer: the European Prospective Investigation into Cancer and Nutrition Study. Cancer Prev Res 4(11):1873

Almeida L, Vaz-da-Silva M, Falcao A, Soares E, Costa R, Loureiro AI et al (2009) Pharmacokinetic and safety profile of trans-resveratrol in a rising multiple-dose study in healthy volunteers. Mol Nutr Food Res 53(Suppl 1):S7–S15

Andreadi C, Britton RG, Patel KR, Brown K (2014) Resveratrol-sulfates provide an intracellular reservoir for generation of parent resveratrol, which induces autophagy in cancer cells. Autophagy 10(3):524–525

Ávila-Gálvez MÁ, García-Villalba R, Martínez-Díaz F, Ocaña-Castillo B, Monedero-Saiz T, Torrecillas-Sánchez A et al (2019) Metabolic profiling of dietary polyphenols and methylxanthines in normal and malignant mammary tissues from breast cancer patients. Mol Nutr Food Res 63(9):1801239

Aziz MH, Afaq F, Ahmad N (2005a) Prevention of ultraviolet-B radiation damage by resveratrol in mouse skin is mediated via modulation in survivin. Photochem Photobiol 81(1):25–31

Aziz MH, Reagan-Shaw S, Wu J, Longley BJ, Ahmad N (2005b) Chemoprevention of skin cancer by grape constituent resveratrol: relevance to human disease? FASEB J 19(9):1193–1195

Aziz MH, Nihal M, Fu VX, Jarrard DF, Ahmad N (2006) Resveratrol-caused apoptosis of human prostate carcinoma LNCaP cells is mediated via modulation of phosphatidylinositol 3′-kinase/Akt pathway and Bcl-2 family proteins. Mol Cancer Ther 5(5):1335–1341

Banerjee S, Bueso-Ramos C, Aggarwal BB (2002) Suppression of 7,12-dimethylbenz(a)anthracene-induced mammary carcinogenesis in rats by resveratrol: role of nuclear factor-kappaB, cyclooxygenase 2, and matrix metalloprotease 9. Cancer Res 62(17):4945–4954

Baur JA, Pearson KJ, Price NL, Jamieson HA, Lerin C, Kalra A et al (2006) Resveratrol improves health and survival of mice on a high-calorie diet. Nature 444(7117):337–342

Bedada SK, Nearati P (2015) Effect of resveratrol on the pharmacokinetics of carbamazepine in healthy human volunteers. Phytother Res 29(5):701–706

Bedada SK, Neerati P (2016) Resveratrol pretreatment affects CYP2E1 activity of chlorzoxazone in healthy human volunteers. Phytother Res 30(3):463–468

Bedada SK, Yellu NR, Neerati P (2016) Effect of resveratrol treatment on the pharmacokinetics of diclofenac in healthy human volunteers. Phytother Res 30(3):397–401

Bertelli AA, Giovannini L, Giannessi D, Migliori M, Bernini W, Fregoni M et al (1995) Antiplatelet activity of synthetic and natural resveratrol in red wine. Int J Tissue React 17(1):1–3

Bhat KP, Lantvit D, Christov K, Mehta RG, Moon RC, Pezzuto JM (2001) Estrogenic and antiestrogenic properties of resveratrol in mammary tumor models. Cancer Res 61 (20):7456–7463

Bird JK, Raederstorff D, Weber P, Steinert RE (2017) Cardiovascular and antiobesity effects of resveratrol mediated through the gut microbiota. Adv Nutr 8(6):839–849

Bode LM, Bunzel D, Huch M, Cho GS, Ruhland D, Bunzel M et al (2013) In vivo and in vitro metabolism of trans-resveratrol by human gut microbiota. Am J Clin Nutr 97(2):295–309

Böhmdorfer M, Szakmary A, Schiestl RH, Vaquero J, Riha J, Brenner S et al (2017) Involvement of UDP-glucuronosyltransferases and sulfotransferases in the excretion and tissue distribution of resveratrol in mice. Nutrients 9(12):1347

Boocock DJ, Faust GE, Patel KR, Schinas AM, Brown VA, Ducharme MP et al (2007) Phase I dose escalation pharmacokinetic study in healthy volunteers of resveratrol, a potential cancer chemopreventive agent. Cancer Epidemiol Biomark Prev 16(6):1246–1252

Bowers JL, Tyulmenkov VV, Jernigan SC, Klinge CM (2000) Resveratrol acts as a mixed agonist/antagonist for estrogen receptors alpha and beta. Endocrinology 141(10):3657–3667

Britton RG, Kovoor C, Brown K (2015) Direct molecular targets of resveratrol: identifying key interactions to unlock complex mechanisms. Ann N Y Acad Sci 1348(1):124–133

Brown VA, Patel KR, Viskaduraki M, Crowell JA, Perloff M, Booth TD et al (2010) Repeat dose study of the cancer chemopreventive agent resveratrol in healthy volunteers: safety, pharmacokinetics, and effect on the insulin-like growth factor axis. Cancer Res 70(22):9003–9011

Brown KF, Rumgay H, Dunlop C, Ryan M, Quartly F, Cox A et al (2018) The fraction of cancer attributable to modifiable risk factors in England, Wales, Scotland, Northern Ireland, and the United Kingdom in 2015. Br J Cancer 118(8):1130–1141

Cai H, Scott E, Kholghi A, Andreadi C, Rufini A, Karmokar A et al (2015) Cancer chemoprevention: evidence of a nonlinear dose response for the protective effects of resveratrol in humans and mice. Sci Transl Med 7(298):298ra117

Cancer Research UK. Available from https://www.cancerresearchuk.org/health-professional/cancer-statistics/statistics-by-cancer-type/melanoma-skin-cancer/mortality

Carter LG, D'Orazio JA, Pearson KJ (2014) Resveratrol and cancer: focus on in vivo evidence. Endocr Relat Cancer 21(3):R209–RR25

Chakraborty S, Levenson AS, Biswas PK (2013) Structural insights into Resveratrol's antagonist and partial agonist actions on estrogen receptor alpha. BMC Struct Biol 13:27

Chaplin A, Carpene C, Mercader J (2018) Resveratrol, metabolic syndrome, and gut microbiota. Nutrients 10(11). https://doi.org/10.3390/nu10111651

Chen HJ, Hsu LS, Shia YT, Lin MW, Lin CM (2012) The beta-catenin/TCF complex as a novel target of resveratrol in the Wnt/beta-catenin signaling pathway. Biochem Pharmacol 84 (9):1143–1153

Chow HH, Garland LL, Hsu CH, Vining DR, Chew WM, Miller JA et al (2010) Resveratrol modulates drug- and carcinogen-metabolizing enzymes in a healthy volunteer study. Cancer Prev Res (Phila) 3(9):1168–1175

Chow HH, Garland LL, Heckman-Stoddard BM, Hsu CH, Butler VD, Cordova CA et al (2014) A pilot clinical study of resveratrol in postmenopausal women with high body mass index: effects on systemic sex steroid hormones. J Transl Med 12:223

Cichocki M, Paluszczak J, Szaefer H, Piechowiak A, Rimando AM, Baer-Dubowska W (2008) Pterostilbene is equally potent as resveratrol in inhibiting 12-O-tetradecanoylphorbol-13-acetate activated NFkappaB, AP-1, COX-2, and iNOS in mouse epidermis. Mol Nutr Food Res 52 (Suppl 1):S62–S70

Cole BF, Logan RF, Halabi S, Benamouzig R, Sandler RS, Grainge MJ et al (2009) Aspirin for the chemoprevention of colorectal adenomas: meta-analysis of the randomized trials. J Natl Cancer Inst 101(4):256–266

Criscione VD, Weinstock MA, Naylor MF, Luque C, Eide MJ, Bingham SF et al (2009) Actinic keratoses. Cancer 115(11):2523–2530

Cuzick J, DeCensi A, Arun B, Brown PH, Castiglione M, Dunn B et al (2011) Preventive therapy for breast cancer: a consensus statement. Lancet Oncol 12(5):496–503

Dasgupta B, Milbrandt J (2007) Resveratrol stimulates AMP kinase activity in neurons. Proc Natl Acad Sci USA 104(17):7217–7222

Dias SJ, Li K, Rimando AM, Dhar S, Mizuno CS, Penman AD et al (2013) Trimethoxy-resveratrol and piceatannol administered orally suppress and inhibit tumor formation and growth in prostate cancer xenografts. Prostate 73(11):1135–1146

Evans HM, Howe PR, Wong RH (2016) Clinical evaluation of effects of chronic resveratrol supplementation on cerebrovascular function, cognition, mood, physical function and general well-being in postmenopausal women-rationale and study design. Nutrients 8(3):150

Ferlay J, Soerjomataram I, Ervik M, Dikshit R, Eser S, Mathers C et al. (2013) GLOBOCAN 2012 v1.0, Cancer incidence and mortality worldwide: IARC CancerBase No. 11 Lyon, France, International Agency for Research on Cancer. Available from http://globocan.iarc.fr

Ferlay J, Soerjomataram I, Dikshit R, Eser S, Mathers C, Rebelo M et al (2015) Cancer incidence and mortality worldwide: sources, methods and major patterns in GLOBOCAN 2012. Int J Cancer 136(5):E359–E386

Forman D, Bauld L, Bonanni B, Brenner H, Brown K, Dillner J et al (2018) Time for a European initiative for research to prevent cancer: a manifesto for Cancer Prevention Europe (CPE). J Cancer Policy 17:15–23

Garrett WS (2019) The gut microbiota and colon cancer. Science 364(6446):1133–1135

Gehm BD, McAndrews JM, Chien PY, Jameson JL (1997) Resveratrol, a polyphenolic compound found in grapes and wine, is an agonist for the estrogen receptor. Proc Natl Acad Sci USA 94 (25):14138–14143

Gescher A, Steward WP, Brown K (2013) Resveratrol in the management of human cancer: how strong is the clinical evidence? In: Brown K, Vang O (eds) Resveratrol and health. Ann N Y Acad Sci 1290, pp 12–20

Gledhill JR, Montgomery MG, Leslie AG, Walker JE (2007) Mechanism of inhibition of bovine F1-ATPase by resveratrol and related polyphenols. Proc Natl Acad Sci USA 104 (34):13632–13637

Griswold MG, Fullman N, Hawley C, Arian N, Zimsen SRM, Tymeson HD et al (2018) Alcohol use and burden for 195 countries and territories, 1990–2016: a systematic analysis for the Global Burden of Disease Study 2016. Lancet 392(10152):1015–1035

Gupta AK, Paquet M, Villanueva E, Brintnell W (2012) Interventions for actinic keratoses. Cochrane Database Syst Rev 12:Cd004415

Hait WN, Levine AJ (2014) Genomic complexity: a call to action. Sci Transl Med 6(255):255cm10

Hansson GK (2005) Inflammation, atherosclerosis, and coronary artery disease. N Engl J Med 352 (16):1685–1695

Harper CE, Patel BB, Wang J, Arabshahi A, Eltoum IA, Lamartiniere CA (2007) Resveratrol suppresses prostate cancer progression in transgenic mice. Carcinogenesis 28(9):1946–1953

Higurashi T, Hosono K, Takahashi H, Komiya Y, Umezawa S, Sakai E et al (2016) Metformin for chemoprevention of metachronous colorectal adenoma or polyps in post-polypectomy patients without diabetes: a multicentre double-blind, placebo-controlled, randomised phase 3 trial. Lancet Oncol 17(4):475–483

Hormones TE, Group BCC (2002) Endogenous sex hormones and breast cancer in postmenopausal women: reanalysis of nine prospective studies. J Natl Cancer Inst 94(8):606–616

Hoshino J, Park E-J, Kondratyuk TP, Marler L, Pezzuto JM, van Breemen RB et al (2010) Selective synthesis and biological evaluation of sulfate-conjugated resveratrol metabolites. J Med Chem 53(13):5033–5043

Howells LM, Berry DP, Elliott PJ, Jacobson EW, Hoffmann E, Hegarty B et al (2011) Phase I randomized, double-blind pilot study of micronized resveratrol (SRT501) in patients with hepatic metastases–safety, pharmacokinetics, and pharmacodynamics. Cancer Prev Res (Phila) 4(9):1419–1425

https://www.gov.uk/government/publications/2010-to-2015-government-policy-cancer-research-and-treatment

Hull MA, Sprange K, Hepburn T, Tan W, Shafayat A, Rees CJ et al (2018) Eicosapentaenoic acid and aspirin, alone and in combination, for the prevention of colorectal adenomas (seAFOod polyp prevention trial): a multicentre, randomised, double-blind, placebo-controlled, 2 × 2 factorial trial. Lancet 392(10164):2583–2594

Hung CF, Lin YK, Huang ZR, Fang JY (2008) Delivery of resveratrol, a red wine polyphenol, from solutions and hydrogels via the skin. Biol Pharm Bull 31(5):955–962

Jang M, Pezzuto JM (1998) Effects of resveratrol on 12-O-tetradecanoylphorbol-13-acetate-induced oxidative events and gene expression in mouse skin. Cancer Lett 134(1):81–89

Jang M, Cai L, Udeani GO, Slowing KV, Thomas CF, Beecher CWW et al (1997) Cancer chemopreventive activity of resveratrol, a natural product derived from grapes. Science 275 (5297):218–220

Kenealey JD, Subramanian L, Van Ginkel PR, Darjatmoko S, Lindstrom MJ, Somoza V et al (2011) Resveratrol metabolites do not elicit early pro-apoptotic mechanisms in neuroblastoma cells. J Agric Food Chem 59(9):4979–4986

Kjaer TN, Ornstrup MJ, Poulsen MM, Jorgensen JO, Hougaard DM, Cohen AS et al (2015) Resveratrol reduces the levels of circulating androgen precursors but has no effect on, testosterone, dihydrotestosterone, PSA levels or prostate volume. A 4-month randomised trial in middle-aged men. Prostate 75(12):1255–1263

Kobierski S, Ofori-Kwakye K, Muller RH, Keck CM (2009) Resveratrol nanosuspensions for dermal application--production, characterization, and physical stability. Pharmazie 64 (11):741–747

Kumar A, Park E-J, Pezzuto JM (2018) Resveratrol as an activator or inhibitor of enzymes and proteins. In: Resveratrol: state-of-the-art science and health applications. World Scientific, New York, pp 55–113

Kundu JK, Surh YJ (2008) Cancer chemopreventive and therapeutic potential of resveratrol: mechanistic perspectives. Cancer Lett 269(2):243–261

Lagouge M, Argmann C, Gerhart-Hines Z, Meziane H, Lerin C, Daussin F et al (2006) Resveratrol improves mitochondrial function and protects against metabolic disease by activating SIRT1 and PGC-1α. Cell 127(6):1109–1122

Levenson AS, Gehm BD, Pearce ST, Horiguchi J, Simons LA, Ward JE 3rd et al (2003) Resveratrol acts as an estrogen receptor (ER) agonist in breast cancer cells stably transfected with ER alpha. Int J Cancer 104(5):587–596

Li G, Rivas P, Bedolla R, Thapa D, Reddick RL, Ghosh R et al (2013) Dietary resveratrol prevents development of high-grade prostatic intraepithelial neoplastic lesions: involvement of SIRT1/S6K axis. Cancer Prev Res (Phila) 6(1):27–39

Maier L, Pruteanu M, Kuhn M, Zeller G, Telzerow A, Anderson EE et al (2018) Extensive impact of non-antibiotic drugs on human gut bacteria. Nature 555:623

Ndiaye M, Philippe C, Mukhtar H, Ahmad N (2011) The grape antioxidant resveratrol for skin disorders: promise, prospects, and challenges. Arch Biochem Biophys 508(2):164–170

Nunes T, Almeida L, Rocha JF, Falcao A, Fernandes-Lopes C, Loureiro AI et al (2009) Pharmacokinetics of trans-resveratrol following repeated administration in healthy elderly and young subjects. J Clin Pharmacol 49(12):1477–1482

Ornstrup MJ, Harsløf T, Kjær TN, Langdahl BL, Pedersen SB (2014) Resveratrol increases bone mineral density and bone alkaline phosphatase in obese men: a randomized placebo-controlled trial. J Clin Endocrinol Metabol 99(12):4720–4729

Pallauf K, Chin D, Günther I, Birringer M, Lüersen K, Schultheiß G et al (2019) Resveratrol, lunularin and dihydroresveratrol do not act as caloric restriction mimetics when administered intraperitoneally in mice. Sci Rep 9(1):4445

Park E-J, Pezzuto JM (2015) The pharmacology of resveratrol in animals and humans. Biochim Biophys Acta 1852(6):1071–1113

Park SJ, Ahmad F, Philp A, Baar K, Williams T, Luo H et al (2012) Resveratrol ameliorates aging-related metabolic phenotypes by inhibiting cAMP phosphodiesterases. Cell 148(3):421–433

Patel KR, Brown VA, Jones DJ, Britton RG, Hemingway D, Miller AS et al (2010) Clinical pharmacology of resveratrol and its metabolites in colorectal cancer patients. Cancer Res 70 (19):7392–7399

Patel KR, Andreadi C, Britton RG, Horner-Glister E, Karmokar A, Sale S et al (2013) Sulfate metabolites provide an intracellular pool for resveratrol generation and induce autophagy with senescence. Sci Transl Med 5(205):205ra133

Pezzuto JM (2011) The phenomenon of resveratrol: redefining the virtues of promiscuity. Ann N Y Acad Sci 1215:123–130

Pezzuto JM (2019) Resveratrol: twenty years of growth, development and controversy. Biomol Ther (Seoul) 27(1):1–14

Popat R, Plesner T, Davies F, Cook G, Cook M, Elliott P et al (2013) A phase 2 study of SRT501 (resveratrol) with bortezomib for patients with relapsed and or refractory multiple myeloma. Br J Haematol 160(5):714–717

Provinciali M, Re F, Donnini A, Orlando F, Bartozzi B, Di Stasio G et al (2005) Effect of resveratrol on the development of spontaneous mammary tumors in HER-2/neu transgenic mice. Int J Cancer 115(1):36–45

Reagan-Shaw S, Afaq F, Aziz MH, Ahmad N (2004) Modulations of critical cell cycle regulatory events during chemoprevention of ultraviolet B-mediated responses by resveratrol in SKH-1 hairless mouse skin. Oncogene 23(30):5151–5160

Renaud S, de Lorgeril M (1992) Wine, alcohol, platelets, and the French paradox for coronary heart disease. Lancet 339(8808):1523–1526

Rothwell PM, Wilson M, Elwin C-E, Norrving B, Algra A, Warlow CP et al (2010) Long-term effect of aspirin on colorectal cancer incidence and mortality: 20-year follow-up of five randomised trials. Lancet 376(9754):1741–1750

Roy P, Kalra N, Prasad S, George J, Shukla Y (2009) Chemopreventive potential of resveratrol in mouse skin tumors through regulation of mitochondrial and PI3K/AKT signaling pathways. Pharm Res 26(1):211–217

Sale S, Tunstall RG, Ruparelia KC, Potter GA, Steward WP, Gescher AJ (2005) Comparison of the effects of the chemopreventive agent resveratrol and its synthetic analog trans 3,4,5,4′-tetramethoxystilbene (DMU-212) on adenoma development in the Apc(Min+) mouse and cyclooxygenase-2 in human-derived colon cancer cells. Int J Cancer 115(2):194–201

Samsamikor M, Daryani NE, Asl PR, Hekmatdoost A (2016) Resveratrol supplementation and oxidative/anti-oxidative status in patients with ulcerative colitis: a randomized, double-blind, placebo-controlled pilot study. Arch Med Res 47(4):304–309

Samsami-Kor M, Daryani NE, Asl PR, Hekmatdoost A (2015) Anti-inflammatory effects of resveratrol in patients with ulcerative colitis: a randomized, double-blind, placebo-controlled pilot study. Arch Med Res 46(4):280–285

Schneider Y, Duranton B, Gosse F, Schleiffer R, Seiler N, Raul F (2001) Resveratrol inhibits intestinal tumorigenesis and modulates host-defense-related gene expression in an animal model of human familial adenomatous polyposis. Nutr Cancer 39(1):102–107

Scott EN, Gescher AJ, Steward WP, Brown K (2009) Development of dietary phytochemical chemopreventive agents: biomarkers and choice of dose for early clinical trials. Cancer Prev Res (Phila) 2(6):525–530

Scott E, Steward WP, Gescher AJ, Brown K (2012) Resveratrol in human cancer chemoprevention–choosing the 'right' dose. Mol Nutr Food Res 56(1):7–13

Seeni A, Takahashi S, Takeshita K, Tang M, Sugiura S, Sato SY et al (2008) Suppression of prostate cancer growth by resveratrol in the transgenic rat for adenocarcinoma of prostate (TRAP) model. Asian Pac J Cancer Prev 9(1):7–14

Serrano D, Bonanni B, Brown K (2019) Therapeutic cancer prevention: achievements and ongoing challenges - a focus on breast and colorectal cancer. Mol Oncol 13(3):579–590

Shukla Y, Singh R (2011) Resveratrol and cellular mechanisms of cancer prevention. Ann N Y Acad Sci 1215:1–8

Steward WP, Brown K (2013) Cancer chemoprevention: a rapidly evolving field. Br J Cancer 109 (1):1

Sung MM, Byrne NJ, Robertson IM, Kim TT, Samokhvalov V, Levasseur J et al (2017) Resveratrol improves exercise performance and skeletal muscle oxidative capacity in heart failure. Am J Physiol Heart Circ Physiol 312(4):H842–Hh53

Surjana D, Halliday GM, Martin AJ, Moloney FJ, Damian DL (2012) Oral nicotinamide reduces actinic keratoses in phase II double-blinded randomized controlled trials. J Invest Dermatol 132 (5):1497–1500

Tang WHW, Li DY, Hazen SL (2019) Dietary metabolism, the gut microbiome, and heart failure. Nat Rev Cardiol 16(3):137–154

Tessitore L, Davit A, Sarotto I, Caderni G (2000) Resveratrol depresses the growth of colorectal aberrant crypt foci by affecting bax and p21(CIP) expression. Carcinogenesis 21(8):1619–1622

Tilg H, Moschen AR (2014) Microbiota and diabetes: an evolving relationship. Gut 63 (9):1513–1521

Torre LA, Bray F, Siegel RL, Ferlay J, Lortet-Tieulent J, Jemal A (2015) Global Cancer statistics, 2012. CA Cancer J Clin 65(2):87–108

Tsilidis KK, Kasimis JC, Lopez DS, Ntzani EE, Ioannidis JPA (2015) Type 2 diabetes and cancer: umbrella review of meta-analyses of observational studies. BMJ Br Med J 350:g7607

Turner RS, Thomas RG, Craft S, van Dyck CH, Mintzer J, Reynolds BA et al (2015) A randomized, double-blind, placebo-controlled trial of resveratrol for Alzheimer disease. Neurology 85 (16):1383–1391

Union for International Cancer Control: World Cancer Leader's Summit 2014: the economics of Cancer Prevention & Control Data Digest 2014. World Cancer Leaders Summit 2014. http://www.iccp-portal.org/sites/default/files/resources/WCLS2014_economics_of_cancer_FINAL-2.pdf2014

Varoni EM, Lo Faro AF, Sharifi-Rad J, Iriti M (2016) Anticancer molecular mechanisms of resveratrol. Front Nutr 3:8

Walle T, Hsieh F, DeLegge MH, Oatis JE Jr, Walle UK (2004) High absorption but very low bioavailability of oral resveratrol in humans. Drug Metab Dispos 32(12):1377–1382

Wang Y, Lee KW, Chan FL, Chen S, Leung LK (2006) The red wine polyphenol resveratrol displays bilevel inhibition on aromatase in breast Cancer cells. Toxicol Sci 92(1):71–77

Wang TT, Hudson TS, Wang TC, Remsberg CM, Davies NM, Takahashi Y et al (2008) Differential effects of resveratrol on androgen-responsive LNCaP human prostate cancer cells in vitro and in vivo. Carcinogenesis 29(10):2001–2010

Whitsett T, Carpenter M, Lamartiniere CA (2006) Resveratrol, but not EGCG, in the diet suppresses DMBA-induced mammary cancer in rats. J Carcinog 5:15

Wild CP, Espina C, Bauld L, Bonanni B, Brenner H, Brown K et al (2019) Cancer prevention Europe. Mol Oncol 13(3):528–534

Wong SH, Yu J (2019) Gut microbiota in colorectal cancer: mechanisms of action and clinical applications. Nat Rev Gastroenterol Hepatol 16(11):690–704

Zamora-Ros R, Knaze V, Rothwell JA, Hemon B, Moskal A, Overvad K et al (2016) Dietary polyphenol intake in Europe: the European prospective investigation into cancer and nutrition (EPIC) study. Eur J Nutr 55(4):1359–1375

Zander SA, Kersbergen A, Sol W, Gonggrijp M, van de Wetering K, Jonkers J et al (2012) Lack of ABCG2 shortens latency of BRCA1-deficient mammary tumors and this is not affected by genistein or resveratrol. Cancer Prev Red (Phila) 5(8):1053–1060

Zhu W, Qin W, Zhang K, Rottinghaus GE, Chen Y-C, Kliethermes B et al (2012) Trans-resveratrol alters mammary promoter hypermethylation in women at increased risk for breast cancer. Nutr Cancer 64(3):393–400

Chapter 3
Pterostilbene as a Potent Chemopreventive Agent in Cancer

Anait S. Levenson and Avinash Kumar

Abstract Pterostilbene (Pter, *trans*-3,5-dimethoxy-4′-hydroxystilbene), a natural analog of resveratrol accumulated in grapevine leaves and blueberries, has attracted immense interest in the scientific community due to its potent biological properties, including anti-inflammatory, antioxidative, and anticancer effects. This chapter focuses on summarizing the up-to-date information related to the pharmacological effects and cellular/molecular mechanisms of pterostilbene with an emphasis on cancer. Numerous preclinical studies have reported on the proapoptotic and anticancer properties of pterostilbene against a variety of cancers, both in vitro and in vivo. Pterostilbene, like resveratrol, acts through various mechanisms, targeting specific signaling pathways and affecting epigenetic regulators of cell growth and metastasis. Pterostilbene has also been reported to sensitize cancer cells to standard chemotherapy. Pterostilbene's protective and therapeutic effects have been observed in different cancers, including breast, colorectal, lung, and prostate, among others. Pterostilbene, with improved bioavailability, conferring a superior pharmacokinetic profile and greater anticancer efficacy, may become a stronger candidate than resveratrol for clinical development with potential applications in cancer. Clinical trials examining the chemopreventive and therapeutic potential of pterostilbene are warranted.

Keywords Pterostilbene · Cancer · Chemoprevention · Combination treatment · Cellular mechanisms · Molecular mechanisms · Epigenetics · Signaling pathways · Natural product

A. S. Levenson (✉)
Department of Biomedical Sciences, College of Veterinary Medicine, Long Island University, Brookville, NY, USA
e-mail: anait.levenson@liu.edu

A. Kumar
Division of Pharmaceutical Sciences, Arnold & Marie Schwartz College of Pharmacy and Health Sciences, Long Island University, Brooklyn, NY, USA

J. M. Pezzuto, O. Vang (eds.), *Natural Products for Cancer Chemoprevention*,
https://doi.org/10.1007/978-3-030-39855-2_3

Abbreviations

γ-H2AX	Gamma histone 2A variant X
143B	Human osteosarcoma cell line
22Rv1	Human prostate cancer cell line
4E-BP	Eukaryotic translation initiation factor 4E binding protein
4OHT	4 hydroxy tamoxifen
5-FU	5-fluorouracil
A2058	Human melanoma cell line
A549	Human lung (NSCLC) cancer cells
Ac	Acetylated
ACC	Acetyl-CoA carboxylase
ACF	Aberrant crypt foci
ACTH	Adrenocorticotropic hormone
Ago2	Argonaute 2
AGS	Human gastric cancer cell line
AKT	v-akt murine thymoma viral oncogene (protein kinase B)
AMACR	Alpha-methylacyl-CoA racemase
AMPK	5′ AMP-activated protein kinase
AP1	Jun proto-oncogene
AR	Androgen receptor
ARH77	Human multiple myeloma (MM) cell line
ARP1	Human multiple myeloma (MM) cell line
Arp2	Actin-related protein 2
Arp3	Actin-related protein 3
AsPC1	Human pancreatic cell line
ATF4	Activating transcription factor 4
ATM	Ataxia telangiectasia mutated serine-threonine kinase
B16/F10	Human melanoma cell line
Bad	Bcl2 associated agonist of cell death
Bak	Bcl2 antagonist/killer 1
Bax	Bcl2 associated X
BCL-2	B-cell lymphoma 2
BCL2L14	B-cell lymphoma like 14
BCL-x(L)	B-cell lymphoma like 1
Bid	BH3 interacting domain death agonist
BRCA1	Breast cancer 1
BT20	Breast cancer cell line
BT549	Breast cancer cell line
BxPC3	Human pancreatic cell line
C6	Rat C6 glioblastoma cell line
Ca^{++}/Ca^{2+}	Calcium ion
Caco2	Human colon cancer cell line
CAL27	Head and neck cell line

CAT	Catalase
CCl_4	Carbon tetrachloride
CCSD-18Co	Human colorectal cancer cell line
CD133	Prominin 1 (PROM1)
CD44	Cell-surface glycoprotein, receptor for HA
Cdc25A	Cell division cycle 25A
CDK	Cyclin-dependent kinase
Chk1	Checkpoint kinase 1
Chk2	Checkpoint kinase 2
CHOP	DNA damage inducible transcript 3 (DDIT3)
COX2	Cyclo-oxygenase 2
CpG	Cytosine-phophate-guanine dinucleotide
CRH	Corticotropin releasing hormone
CSCs	Cancer stem cells
CXCR4	C-X-C chemokine receptor type 4
DEN	Diethylnitrosamine
DIABLO	Diablo IAP-binding mitochondrial protein
DLBCL	Diffuse large B-cell lymphoma
DLD-1	Human colon cancer cell line
DMBA	7,12-Dimethylbenzanthracene
DNA	Deoxyribonucleic acid
DNMT	DNA methyltransferase
DR4	Death receptor 4
DR5	Death receptor 5
DU145	Human prostate cancer cell line
E2	17 beta-estradiol, estrogen
EBPα	EBP cholesterol delta-isomerase
EC109	Human esophageal cancer cell line
ECC1	Human endometrial cancer cell line
EGCG	Epigallocatechin gallate
EGF	Epidermal growth factor
EGFR	Epidermal growth factor receptor
Egr1	Early growth response 1
Elf2a	E74-like factor 2a
ELK1	ETS transcription factor ELK1
EMT	Epithelial- to -mesenchymal transition
eNOS	Endothelial nitric oxide synthase
ER	Endoplasmic reticulum
ERK1/2	Extracellular signal-regulated kinase
ERα	Estrogen receptor alpha
ERβ	Estrogen receptor beta
ETS2	ETS protro-oncogene 2, transcription factor
FAK	Focal adhesion kinase
Fas	Fas cell surface death receptor
FasL	Fas ligand

FASN	Fatty acid synthase
FDA	Food and Drug Administration
FLIPS/L	CASP8 and FADD like apoptosis regulator
FOXO1	Forkhead box O1
FOXO3	Forkhead box O3
GADD45G	Growth arrest and DNA damage inducible 45 gamma
GBM	Human glioblastoma cell line
GCR	Glutathione reductase
GPM (GC)	Patient derived glioblastoma cell line
GPx	Glutathione peroxidase
GR	Glucocorticoid receptor
GRIP1	Glutamate receptor interacting protein 1
GRP78	Glucose regulated protein 78
GSG	Germ cell associated 1
GSH	Glutathione
GSK 3β	Glycogen synthase kinase 3β
GSSG	Glutathione disulfide (oxidized glutathione)
GST	Glutathione S-transferase
H1299	Human lung cancer cell line
H_2O_2	Hydrogen peroxide
H3	Histone 3
H4	Histone 4
H441	Human lung cancer cell line
H460	Human lung cancer cell line
H460	Lung cancer cell line
H929	Human multiple myeloma (MM) cell line
H929R	Human multiple myeloma (MM) cell line (bortezomib-resistant)
HAT	Histone acetyltransferase
HBECR	Human bronchial epithelial cells
HCC1806	Breast cancer cell line
HCT-116	Colorectal cancer cell line
HCT116	Human colorectal cell line
HDAC1	Histone deacetylase 1
HDAC2	Histone deacetylase 2
HDM	Histone demethylase
HEC1A	Human endometrial cancer cell line
HeLa	Human cervical cancer cell line
Hep3B	Human liver cancer cell line
HepG2	Human liver cancer cell line
Hes1	Hes family bHLH transcription factor 1
HIF1α	Hypoxia inducible factor 1 alpha
HO1	Heme oxygenase
HOS	Osteosarcoma cell line
HPV	Human papilloma virus
HPV/E6	Human papilloma virus/transforming protein E6

HSP70	Heat shock protein 70
HSP90	Heat shock protein 90
HT1080	Human leukemia cells
HT29	Human colorectal cancer cell line
HT60	Human leukemia cells
HTB111	Human endometrial cancer cell line
Hut-78	Human leukemia/lymphoma cell line
i.p.	Intraperitoneal
i.v.	Intravenous
ICAM1	Intercellular adhesion molecule 1
IGFBP3	Insulin growth factor binding protein 3
IGROV1	Human ovarian cancer cell line
IKK	Inhibitor of nuclear factor kappa B kinase
IL1β	Interleukin 1β
IL6	Interleukin 6
IL8	Interleukin 8
iNOS	Inducible nitric oxide synthase
IRE1	Endoplasmic reticulum to nucleus signaling 1/inositol-requiring enzyme 1
Ishikawa	Endometrial cancer cell line
IκB	Inhibitor of nuclear factor kappa B
IκBα	Inhibitor of nuclear factor kappa B subunit alpha
JAK	Janus kinase
JNK1/2	c-Jun N-terminal kinase
Jurkat	Human leukemia/lymphoma cell line
K562	Human chronic myelogenous leukemia cell line
KITLG	KIT proto-oncogene receptor tyrosine kinase ligand
LC3	Light chain 3 (microtubule associated protein)
LCSC	Human lung cancer stem cells
LDH	L-lactate dehydrogenase
LLC	Human lung cancer cell line
LMP	Lysosomal membrane potential
LNCaP	Human prostate cancer cell line
LNCaP	Prostate cancer cell line
lncRNA	Long non-coding ribonucleic acid
LXR	LexA regulated function
MAML2	Mastermind like transcriptional coactivator 2
MAPK	Mitogen-activated protein kinase
MBD	Methyl-CpG-binding domain
MCF10A	Human immortalized breast epithelial cells
MCF-7	Human breast cancer cell line
MCP1	Monocyte chemotactic protein 1
MDA-MB157	Human breast cancer cell line
MDA-MB231	Human breast cancer cell line
MDA-MB468	Human breast cancer cell line

MDR	Multidrug resistance
MDR1	Multidrug resistance 1
MEK	Mitogen-activated protein kinase kinase
MelJuso	Human melanoma cell line
MeWo	Human melanoma cell line
MG-63	Human osteosarcoma cell line
MIA PaCa2	Human pancreatic cancer cell line
MicroRNA	Micro ribonucleic acid
MiRNA	Micro ribonucleic acid
miR	Micro ribonucleic acid
MKK3	Mitogen activated protein kinase kinase 3
MKK6	Mitogen activated protein kinase kinase 6
MM	Multiple myeloma
MMP	Mitochondrial membrane potential
MMPs	Matrix metalloproteinases
MMP2	Matrix metalloproteinase 2
MMP9	Matrix metalloproteinase 9
MMP26	Matrix metalloproteinase 26
MOLT4	Human leukemia or lymphoma cell line
mnSOD	Mitochondrial superoxide dismutase
mRNA	Messenger ribonucleic acid
MSH	Melanocyte stimulating hormone
MSK1	Mitochondrial lysine-tRNA ligase MSK1
MTA1	Metastasis-associated protein 1
mTOR	Mammalian target of rapamycin
MUC2	Mucin 2
MV4-11	Human leukemia cell line
MYC	Myc protooncogene, bHLH transcription factor
NAD	Nicotinamide adenine dinucleotide
NADPH	Nicotinamide adenine dinucleotide phosphate dehydrogenase
ncRNA	Non-coding ribonucleic acid
NF-κB	Nuclear factor kappa-light-chain-enhancer of activated B cells
NICD	Notch intracellular domain
NSCLC	Non-small cell lung cancer
NO	Nitric oxide
NORA	Noradrenaline
NOX1	NADPH oxidase 1
NOTCH1	Notch transmembrane protein 1
NOTCH2	Notch transmembrane protein 2
NRF2	Nuclear factor erythroid 2-related factor 2
NuRD	Nucleosome remodeling and deacetylase complex
NQO1	NADPH quinone oxidoreductase 1
O_2^-	Superoxide anion
OC1-MY5	Human multiple myeloma (MM) cell line
OCI-LY8	DLBCL (B-cell lymphoma)

OCL	Human leukemia cell line
OH	Hydroxyl radicals
oncomiR	Oncogenic microRNA
OVCAR 4/8	Human ovarian cancer cell line 4 and 8
OV1063	Human ovarian cancer cell line
PAI-1	Plasminogen activator inhibitor 1
PANC1	Human pancreatic cancer cell line
PARP	Poly-(ADP-ribose) polymerase
PC9	Human lung cancer (NSCLC) cell line
PC3	Human prostate cancer cell line
PERK	Protein kinas R (PKR)-like endoplasmic reticulum kinase
PI3K	Phosphatidylinositol 3-kinase/serine/threonine kinase PKB
PIN	Prostatic intraepithelial neoplasia
PKCα	Protein kinase α
PKCβ	Protein kinase β
PKCγ	Protein kinase γ
POMC	Pro-opiomelanocortin
PPARγ	Peroxisome proliferation activated receptor gamma
PTEN	Phosphatase and tensin homolog
Pter	Pterostilbene
PUMA	p53 upregulated modifier of apoptosis
p15	Cyclin-dependent kinase inhibitor 2B
p16	Cyclin-dependent kinase inhibitor 2A
p21	Cyclin-dependent kinase inhibitor 1A
p27	Cyclin-dependent kinase inhibitor 1B
p38	Mitogen-activated protein kinase 14
p53	Tumor suppressor protein 53
p65	Protein 65 (NF-κB subunit)
Ras-GTP	Ras family small GTPase
RAC1	Rac family small GTPase 1
Rb1	Retinoblastoma protein 1
Res	Resveratrol
ROS	Reactive oxygen species
RPMI8226	Human multiple myeloma (MM) cell line
Saos-2	Human osteosarcoma cell line
SAHA	Suberoylanilide hydoxamic acid
SAS	Human oral cancer cell line
s.c.	Subcutaneous
SCC9	human oral cancer cell line
SDK2	Sidekick cell adhesion molecule 2
SDK6	Sidekick cell adhesion molecule 6
SIRT1	Sirtuin 1, silent information regulator 1
SK-BR3	Human breast cancer cell line
SK-MEL2	Human melanoma cell line
SK-MES1	Human lung cancer cell line

SKOV3	Human ovarian cancer cell line
SMAC	Diablo IAP-binding mitochondrial protein
SMAD2	SMAD family member 2/mothers against decapentaplegic homolog 2
SMMC7221	Human liver cancer cell line
SOD	Superoxide dismutase
SOSP9607	Human osteosarcoma cell line
SOX2	SRY (sex determining region Y)-box 2
Sp1	Specificity protein 1
SQSTM1	Sequestosome 1
Src	Src proto-oncogene tyrosine-protein kinase
STAT3	Signal transducer and activator of transcription 3
SUDHL4	Human DLBCL cell line
SW480	Human colon cancer cell line
T98G	Human glioblastoma cell line
TAM	Tumor-associated macrophages
TAP	Tocopherol-associated protein
TCF4	Transcription factor 4
hTERT	Human telomerase reverse transcriptase
TE1	Human esophageal cancer cell line
TGFβ	Transforming growth factor beta
THP1	Human leukemia cell line
TLR4	Toll-like receptor 4
TMD8	Human DLBCL cells
TNBC	Triple-negative breast cancer
TNFα	Tumor necrosis factor alpha
TPA	12-O-tetradecanoylphorbol 13-acetate
TRAIL	TNF-related apoptosis-inducing ligand
TrxR1	Thioredoxin reductase 1
Twist1	Twist family bHLH transcription factor 1
TXNIP	Thioredoxin interacting protein
T24	Human bladder cancer cell line
U2OS	Human osteosarcoma cell line
U266	Human glioblastoma cell line
U937	Human leukemia cell line
VCAM1	Vascular cell adhesion molecule 1
VEGF	Vascular endothelial growth factor
WAVE	WASP family member 1
Wnt	Wnt protein
XBP1	X-box binding protein 1
XIAP	X-linked inhibitor of apoptosis
ZBTB10	Zinc finger and BTB domain containing 10
ZEB1	Zinc finger E-box binding homeobox 1

3.1 Introduction

Cancer is one of the most prevalent diseases affecting men and women worldwide. Although chemotherapeutic medicines have reduced cancer mortality in the last 25 years, their adverse side effects are a major concern. The development of natural chemopreventive drugs that effectively target neoplastic transformation and tumor progression will reduce the incidence and progression of cancer and mortality from this disease.

Naturally occurring polyphenols found in food and plants, particularly stilbenes, have gained increased importance in cancer prevention due to their potent biological properties including anti-inflammatory, antioxidative, antiproliferative and proapoptotic effects. Resveratrol (Res, *trans*-3, 4′, 5-trihydroxystilbene) is the most widely studied stilbene compound with multiple and diverse pharmacological properties including anticarcinogenic effects, which was first reported in 1997 (Jang et al. 1997). Since then, more than three thousand scientific papers on the anticancer activity of resveratrol in vitro, in vivo and in some clinical trials in humans have been reported. However, the potential problem of using resveratrol as an effective chemopreventive agent is that it has a very low systemic bioavailability and rapid metabolism, which lowers its pharmacological efficacy in humans (Wenzel and Somoza 2005; Scott et al. 2012; Gambini et al. 2015). Logically, efforts are being made to find other naturally occurring phytoalexins or to develop resveratrol derivatives with higher systemic bioavailability and more potent anticancer activity than resveratrol.

Aside from resveratrol, another natural stilbenoid, pterostilbene (Pter, *trans*-3,5-dimethoxy-4′-hydroxystilbene), found in grapes and in blueberries, has attracted immense interest from the scientific community due to its more potent biological properties (Estrela et al. 2013; Zhang et al. 2018) and exhibiting no toxicity in humans (Riche et al. 2013). The anti-inflammatory, antioxidant, and anticancer properties of pterostilbene, based on solid preclinical evidence in different cell and animal models of cancer, make pterostilbene among the most promising dietary polyphenols for chemoprevention and therapeutic practices in oncology.

3.2 Pterostilbene: History, Molecular Characteristics and Pharmacology

Pterostilbene is a naturally occurring phytoalexin, which was originally identified in some plant parts such as the leaves of grapevine, *Vitis vinifera* (Langcake et al. 1979), heartwood of sandalwoods, *Pterocarpus santalinus* and *Pterocarpus marsupium* (Seshadri 1972; Maurya et al. 1984), the bark of *Guibourtia tessmanii* (Fuendjiep et al. 2002), and in darakchasava, a traditional Ayurveda medicine prepared from the Indian Kino tree (Paul et al. 1999; Maurya et al. 2004). More relevant to dietary chemoprevention, pterostilbene is present in food sources such as grape berries (Pezet and Pont 1988; Adrian et al. 2000) and blueberries

(Rimando et al. 2004; Rimando and Barney 2005; Rodriguez-Bonilla et al. 2011). It is important to note that there are differences in pterostilbene levels even in *Vaccinium* blueberries and that the levels of pterostilbene vary depending on the time of harvest and environmental and climatic conditions (Table 3.1).

Pterostilbene and resveratrol belong to the stilbene class of polyphenols with ~200–300 g/mol molecular weight. Family members of the stilbenoids have a C6-C2-C6 basic skeleton and consist of two phenol groups linked by an ethene double bond. Pterostilbene is a naturally occurring methoxylated analog of resveratrol. The main difference in the chemical structures of these two stilbenes is the substitution of two hydroxyl groups with methoxy groups (Fig. 3.1).

Various studies have reported on pterostilbene's superior pharmacokinetics compared to resveratrol (Ferrer et al. 2005; Remsberg et al. 2008; Lin et al. 2009; Kapetanovic et al. 2011). The substitution of the hydroxyl group with a methoxy group is believed to make the molecule more stable and more lipophilic, thus increasing its membrane permeability (Cichocki et al. 2008; Lin and Ho 2009). Pterostilbene is less susceptible to phase II metabolism and therefore exhibits much greater bioavailability (95% vs 20%) and a longer half-life (105 vs 14 min) than resveratrol (Estrela et al. 2013). Its superior pharmacokinetic characteristics explain the observed more potent biological activity of pterostilbene over resveratrol both in vitro and in vivo (Paul et al. 2009; Wang et al. 2010; Chiou et al. 2011;

Table 3.1 Pterostilbene content in grapes and blueberries

	Dietary source	Pterostilbene (ng/g)	References
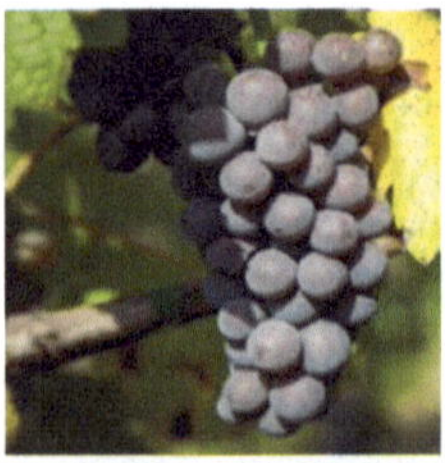	**Grape berries** (*Vitis vinifera*)		
	Fungus-infected var. Chardonnay & Gamay	200–470	Adrian et al. (2000)
	Healthy & immature var. Pinot Noir & Gamay	14–74	Pezet and Pont (1988)
	Fresh grape berries	120–530	Pezet and Pont (1988)
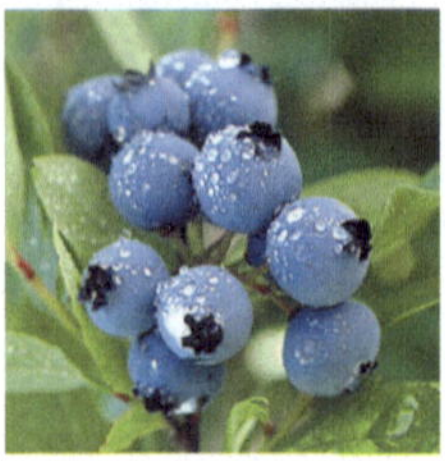	**Blueberries** (*Vaccinium*)		
	V. ashei (rabbit eye)	99–151	Rimando et al. (2004)
	V. stamineum (deerberry)	110	Rodriguez-Bonilla et al. (2011)
	V. corymbosum (high-bush)	520	Rimando et al. (2004)
	V. ovalfolium (oval-leafed)	124–475	Rimando and Barney (2005)
	V. corymbosum x	214	Rimando and Barney (2005)
	V. angustifolium (half-highbush)	142–353	Rimando and Barney (2005)

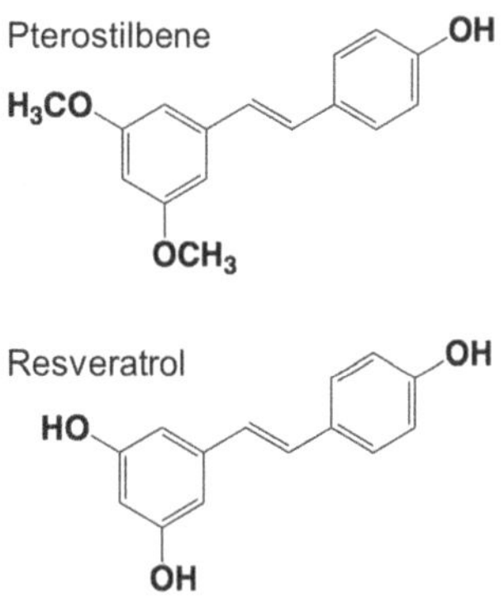

Fig. 3.1 Chemical structures of pterostilbene (*trans*-3,5-dimethoxy-4′-hydroxystilbene) and resveratrol (*trans*-3, 4′, 5-trihydroxystilbene)

Nutakul et al. 2011; Hagiwara et al. 2012; McCormack and McFadden 2012; McCormack et al. 2012; Mena et al. 2012; Tsai et al. 2012; Estrela et al. 2013; Li et al. 2013; Dhar et al. 2015b; Lombardi et al. 2015; Papandreou et al. 2015; Dvorakova and Landa 2017; Zielinska-Przyjemska et al. 2017; Chatterjee et al. 2018; Storniolo and Moreno 2019). Another remarkable property of pterostilbene is its ability to cross the blood-brain barrier and to influence brain activity (Lange and Li 2018). This property of pterostilbene may prove to be vital for favorable effects in glioblastomas (Zielinska-Przyjemska et al. 2017). Finally, although pterostilbene metabolites have been identified in both serum and urine in animal models (Remsberg et al. 2008; Shao et al. 2010), most of the available data indicate that pterostilbene is biologically more active than its metabolites (Asensi et al. 2011).

3.3 Anti-inflammatory Effects of Pterostilbene in Cancer

Inflammation is one of the major precursors of cancer and chronic inflammation is involved in all the major steps of cancer including initiation, progression, and metastasis. The molecular mechanism of inflammation-associated carcinogenesis is the complex crosstalk between inflammatory mediators and oncogenic/tumor suppressor signaling, which can be modulated by natural polyphenols. Pterostilbene has been reported to have anti-inflammatory effects through its reduction of the expression of inflammatory mediators (Ferrer et al. 2007; Paul et al. 2009, 2010; Chiou et al. 2010, 2011; Chen et al. 2012; Mak et al. 2013; Lin et al. 2014; Shen and Rong 2015; Dhar et al. 2016; Huang et al. 2016; Li et al. 2016; Pei et al. 2017; Tsai et al. 2017). Notably, numerous studies have demonstrated pterostilbene-suppressed inflammatory response through downregulation and/or inactivation of the major proinflammatory transcription factor, NF-κB, which regulates various pathways implicated in inflammation and cancer (Pan et al. 2008, 2009; DiDonato et al. 2012; Tsai et al. 2012; Mak et al. 2013; Huang et al. 2016; Zhang and Zhang 2016; Rajagopal et al. 2018). Recent studies have demonstrated strong inhibition of the PI3K/Akt signaling, a pathway upstream of NF-κB that controls cellular functions involved in inflammation and cancer cell survival (Tsai et al. 2012; Erasalo et al. 2018). Erasalo et al. showed that pterostilbene, along with other stilbenes, downregulated Akt phosphorylation in vitro and production of inflammatory mediators IL-6 and MCP1 in mice similar to effects seen with commercial PI3K inhibitor LY294002 (Erasalo et al. 2018). The anti-inflammatory effects of pterostilbene have been demonstrated in endothelial cells through reduction of the production of cytokines including IL-8, ICAM1, MCP1 and decreased expression of endoplasmic reticulum (ER) stress-related proteins (Liu et al. 2016). Pterostilbene also inhibited IL-6 and TNFα secretion and COX-2, iNOS, PAI1, IL-6, TNFα, and MCP1 proinflammatory gene expression during the interaction between adipocytes and macrophages (Hsu et al. 2013). Further, pterostilbene treatment markedly attenuated inflammatory responses through the TLR4/NF-κB signaling (Gao et al. 2018) and TNFα, IL-1β reduction (Yu et al. 2017), protecting against acute renal and myocardial ischemia, respectively. Moreover, pterostilbene showed favorable anti-inflammatory/antitumor effect in a co-culture of tumor-associated inflammatory lung macrophages (TAM) and lung cancer cells through downregulation of MUC1, NF-κB, CD133, β-catenin, and Sox2 expression (Huang et al. 2016). Along the same lines, pterostilbene effectively suppressed the generation of breast cancer stem cells (CSCs) through inhibition of NF-κB and Twist 1 (Mak et al. 2013). Finally, preclinical studies suggested that pterostilbene plays a role in preventing inflammation-associated tumorigenesis in prostate-specific *Pten* heterozygous and *Pten* knockout mouse models through downregulation of proinflammatory IL-1β, TGFβ, Hsp90 and Akt (Dhar et al. 2016). In addition, pterostilbene treatment inhibited 7,12-dimethylbenz(*a*)anthracene/12-*O*-tetradecanoylphorbol-13-acetate (DMBA/TPA)-induced skin tumor formation through suppression of ERK1/2, p38, JNK1/2, and PI3K/Akt (Tsai et al. 2012) and AP-1, COX-2, and iNOS (Cichocki et al. 2008).

3.4 Antioxidative Effects of Pterostilbene in Cancer

Oxidative stress is characterized by an imbalance in the production of reactive oxygen species (ROS) including hydrogen peroxide (H_2O_2), superoxide anion (O_2), hydroxyl radicals (OH) and antioxidant capacity of the cells (Birben et al. 2012). ROS are important for maintaining cellular homeostasis but excessive production of ROS during inflammation, mechanical or chemical stresses, or exposure to radiation can result in irreversible DNA and protein damage and lipid peroxidation that can promote carcinogenesis (Wiseman and Halliwell 1996). ROS-mediated signaling pathways are associated with all stages of cancer development and may result in deregulation of survival/apoptosis signaling, particularly affecting phosphorylation/de-phosphorylation cascades leading to cancer cell proliferation (Lee et al. 2002). Moreover, ROS-mediated increase in angiogenesis plays a critical role in the development of metastasis (Khromova et al. 2009; Kim et al. 2011). Phytochemicals have been shown to modulate ROS-mediated pathways either by inhibiting oxidative stress or by promoting antioxidant defense mechanisms. Interestingly, a number of phytochemicals exhibit both antioxidant and pro-oxidant effects in cancer and that effect depends on the stage of cancer progression, response to chemotherapy, cell environment, concentration used and other factors (Chikara et al. 2018).

The first observation on the anti-oxidant activity of pterostilbene was made in a cell-free system by its inhibition of methyl linoleate oxidation (Charvey-Faury et al. 1998). Further, direct peroxyl-radical scavenging activity of pterostilbene in plant tissue was first evaluated by Rimando et al. (2002), who found that antioxidant activity of pterostilbene was similar to that of resveratrol. The antioxidant potency of pterostilbene has been studied in vitro and in vivo in various cell and animal models. In the context of cancer chemoprevention and treatment, pterostilbene demonstrated a protective effect towards DNA damage by decreasing γH2AX levels in breast cancer cells (Kala et al. 2015) but increasing its expression causing DNA damage and apoptosis in myeloma (Xie et al. 2016; Chen et al. 2017a) and leukemia (Kong et al. 2016). Pterostilbene increased oxidative stress in breast cancer (Chakraborty et al. 2010), ovarian cancer (Dong et al. 2016), multiple myeloma (Xie et al. 2016), leukemia/lymphoma (Kong et al. 2016; Chang et al. 2017), lung cancer (Yang et al. 2013; Ma et al. 2017), and prostate cancer (Chakraborty et al. 2010), consequently inactivating prosurvival pathways by inhibiting PI3K/Akt and MAPKs and promoting ROS-mediated mitochondrial membrane depolarization leading to caspase-dependent or -independent apoptosis.

Pterostilbene's regulation of the antioxidant defense network is related to its modulation of Nrf-2, a transcription factor that plays a significant role in adaptive responses to oxidative stress by triggering transcription of antioxidant enzymes. Several studies have reported on pterostilbene's activation of Nrf2 and its downstream target genes such as MnSOD, HO-1, GR, and GPx (Priego et al. 2008; Chiou et al. 2011; McCormack et al. 2012; Moon et al. 2013) in contrast to reported downregulation of Nrf2 in melanoma and pancreatic cancer (Benlloch et al. 2016). The scientific community recognizes Nrf-2's dual role in cancer, indicating Nrf-2 signaling pathway as a defense mechanism to protect cells against oxidative stress at the early stages but as a contributor to chemoresistance and cancer promotion at the advanced stages (Lau et al. 2008). Therefore, activation of Nrf-2 could be utilized as a cancer prevention strategy, whereas inhibition of Nrf-2 could be effective in cancer treatment (Ma and He 2012; Ma et al. 2012; Kou et al. 2013). Together with the data on pterostilbene activation of ROS and ROS-mediated mitochondrial membrane potential (MMP) loss leading to apoptosis in many cancers (Table 3.2), we can conclude that pterostilbene may possess both antioxidative and pro-oxidative properties depending on the stage of cancer progression and cell environment. It has also been suggested that in addition to pterostilbene's regulation of antioxidant enzymes (indirect antioxidant effects), pterostilbene has an intrinsic antioxidant capacity (direct antioxidant effect) that could be related to its anticancer effects (Kosuru et al. 2016).

Table 3.2 Anticancer effects of pterostilbene on cellular and molecular mechanisms in cancer

Cancer	Model	Dose	Mechanism	Anticancer effect	References
Breast	MCF7	0–100 μM	pAkt, pmTOR, N-cad, Twist, Snail ↓ Slug, Vimentin, ZEB1/2, αSMA, MMP9 ↓ Bax, cl ↓ caspase 3/9, Beclin 1, Atg5/7 ↑ LC3-I/II, spXBP1, GRP78, CHOP ↑ IRE1α, E-cad, ZO1, pp38, pERK1/2 ↑ LINC01121, PTTG3P ↓ MEG3, TUG1, H19, DICER1-AS1 ↑	Cell viability, EMT, migration ↓ ER stress, autophagy, apoptosis ↑	Huang et al. (2018)
	MCF7 MDA-MB-231	0–10 μM	hTERT, telomerase activity, c-Myc ↓	Cell viability ↓ CC arrest G1 (MCF7) CC arrest G2/M (MDA-MB-231) Apoptosis ↑	Daniel and Tollefsbol (2018)
	MDA-MB-231	0–50 μM Combination: α-tocopheryl succinate (0–25 μM)	TAP ↑ CDK2, pAkt, pERK1/2 ↓	Synergistic: Cell viability ↓	Tam et al. (2018)
	MDA-MB-231 xenograft	**40 μg/kg diet** **Combination: α-tocopheryl succinate (42, 99 IU/kg diet)**	**CDK2, pAkt, pERK1/2 ↓**	**Synergistic: Tumor growth and metastasis ↓**	
	BT-20 MDA-MB-468	0–80 μM	cl PARP, DR4, DR5, Bax, tBid ↑ pERK1/2, pJNK1/2, pp38, peIF2α ↑ GRP78, CHOP, ROS ↑ Pro caspase 3/8/9, cFLIPS/L, Bcl-xl ↓ Bcl-2, survivin, XIAP, DcR1/2 ↓	Cell viability, survival ↓ Apoptosis ↑	Hung et al. (2017)

	MCF7 MDA-MB-468 SKBR3	0–100 μM	pERK1/2, p21, Bax ↑ pAkt, pmTOR, Cyclin D1 ↓	Cell proliferation ↓ CC arrest G0/G1 Apoptosis ↑	Wakimoto et al. (2017)
	MDA-MB-468 xenograft	**0.1% w/w diet**		**Tumor growth ↓**	
	Brain metastatic MDA-MB-231 (231BrM) Brain metastatic SKBR3 (SKBrM3)	0–50 μM	c-Met ↓	Endothelial cell binding ↓ Tube formation ↓	Xing et al. (2016)
	231BrM and SKBrM3 xenografts	**30 mg/kg bw**		**Brain metastasis ↓** **Brain metastasis free survival ↑**	
	MCF10CA1h MCF10CA1a	0–15 μM	MAML2, HES1, HEY1, NOTCH1 ↓ DNA methylation ↑	Cell viability, survival, invasion ↓	Lubecka et al. (2016)
	MDA-MB-157 HCC1806	5 μM Combination: Res (15 μM)	ERα, PGR (4-OHT) ↓ HDAC (MDA-MB-157) activity ↓ DNMT activity, DNA metylation ↓ AcH3; AcH3K9; AcH4 ↑ HDAC (HCC1806), HAT activity ↑ PGR (E2) ↑	Sensitization towards E2 and 4OHT treatments	Kala and Tollefsbol (2016)
	MDA-MB-157 HCC1806	0–15 μM Combination: Res (15 μM)	SIRT1, γH2AX, DNMT1/3a/3b ↓ hTERT ↓ SIRT1, DNMT, telomerase activity ↓	Cell viability, survival ↓ CC arrest G2/M (HCC1806) CC arrest S (MDA-MB-157) Apoptosis ↑	Kala et al. (2015)
	MCF7 Hs578t MDA-MB-231	0–10 μM	Snail, Slug, Vimentin, ZEB1, Twist ↓ N-cad, Fibronectin, c-Met, pSrc ↓ pFak, pPaxillin, pAkt, pErk1/2 ↓ pSTAT3 ↓ E-cad, Keratin 18, miR-205 ↑	Migration, invasion, EMT ↓	Su et al. (2015)

(continued)

Table 3.2 (continued)

Cancer	Model	Dose	Mechanism	Anticancer effect	References
	MDA-MB-231 xenograft	**10 mg/kg bw**	**Src, Vimentin, Twist, Slug, ZEB1 ↓**	**Tumor growth ↓**	
	MCF7 BCSCs	0–75 μM	CD44, Hedgehog, pAkt, pGSK3β ↓ c-Myc, Cyclin D1 ↓ β-catenin ↑	Cell viability, BCSC stemness ↓ Mammosphere formation ↓ Sensitivity towards paclitaxel treatment	Wu et al. (2015)
	MCF7 MDA-MB-231 ER-α36 overexpressing MCF7 (MCF7/ER36) ER-α36 silenced MDA-MB-231 (Mb231/Si36)	0–60 μM	ER-α36 ↓ ERα-36-mediated pAkt and pERK1/2 ↓	ER-α36-mediated cell viability ↓ ER-α36-mediated apoptosis ↑	Pan et al. (2014)
	Mb231/Si36 xenografts	**56 mg/kg bw**	**ERα-36 ↓**	**ER-α36-mediated tumor growth ↓**	
	MCF7 MDA-MB-231 T47D	0–60 μM Pter-Isothiocyanate conjugate	PPARγ, PTEN, Bax, cl Caspase 9 ↑ PPARγ, Caspase 3/7/8/9 activity ↑ Bcl-2, survivin ↓	PPARγ-mediated cell viability ↓ PPARγ-mediated differentiation ↓ PPARγ-mediated apoptosis ↑	Nikhil et al. (2014c)
	MDA-MB-231 BT-549	0–80 μM	E-cad, Fas, FasL, β catenin ↑ pGSK3β, LC3-I/II, Beclin 1 ↑ Vimentin, ZEB1, MMP2/9, pERK1/2 ↓ Twist (BT-549) ↓	Fas-mediated cell viability & EMT ↓ Fas-mediated autophagy ↑	Chen et al. (2014)

	MDA-MB-231	0–40 μM	uPA, WAVE2, Arp2/3 ↓ uPA, NF-κB, RAC1 activity ↓	Cell viability, migration, invasion ↓	Ko et al. (2014)
	MCF7 Green gram	0–80 μM 80 μM	Telomerase activity ↓	Cell viability ↓ Mitotic activity ↓	Tippani et al. (2014)
	MCF7 T47D	0–100 μM Pter-Isothiocyanate conjugate	Bcl2, Bcl-xl, survivin, pAkt, pERK ↓ Bax, AIF, cl caspsase 9, pc-Jun ↑ ROS ↑ Cytochrome c release ↑	Cell viability, migration ↓ CC arrest S and G2/M DNA fragmentation Apoptosis ↑	Nikhil et al. (2014a)
	Ehrlich ascitic cell induced tumor bearing mice	**Pter (200 mg/kg bw) Conjugate (20,100mg/kgbw) 5-FU (20 mg/kg bw)**	**VEGF ↓ Bax, cl caspase 3 ↑**	**Tumor growth ↓**	
	MCF-7 + M2 TAMs MDA-MB-231 + M2 TAMs	0–10 μM	miR448, NF-kB, Twist 1, Vimentin ↓ E-cad ↑	CSC generation, migration ↓ Invasion, EMT ↓	Mak et al. (2013)
	MDA-MB-231 + M2 TAMs xenografts	**5 mg/kg bw**	**NF-kB, Twist 1, Vimentin ↓ E-cad ↑**	**Tumor growth ↓**	
	MDA-MB-231	0–100 μM	MMP2, MMP9, Cortactin, MT1-MMP ↓ Src/Tks5 interaction, PDGFRα ↓	Cell viability, migration, invasion ↓ Maturation of invadopodia ↓	Hong et al. (2013)
	MCF7 MDA-MB-231	0–75 μM	Bax ↑ MnSOD activity ↑ Cytochrome c release ↑ mac/DIABLO release ↑ Cytosolic Ca^{2+} ↑	Cell viability ↓	Moon et al. (2013)

(continued)

Table 3.2 (continued)

Cancer	Model	Dose	Mechanism	Anticancer effect	References
Comparison with Res	MCF7	0–100 μM	LC3-I/II, p62/SQSTM1 ↑ Cytosolic cysteine/aspartyl cathepsins activity ↑ LDH release ↑	Cell proliferation, DNA synthesis ↓ CC arrest S Necrosis, autophagy ↑ LMP loss	Mena et al. (2012)
Comparison with Res	MDA-MB-231-luc-D3H2LN	0–100 μM	miR-143, miR-200c, Ago2 ↑		Hagiwara et al. (2012)
	MCF-7 Bcap-37	0–150 μM	Cyclin D1, β-catenin, c-Myc, pAkt ↓ pGSK3 ↓ cl PARP, PTEN, LC3b-I/II ↑	Cell viability ↓ CC arrest G1 Apoptosis, autophagy ↑	Wang et al. (2012)
	MCF7	0–100 μM	TIMP3, c/EBP, Beclin 1, LC3-II, LXR ↑ ORP1L, ABCA1, ABCG1, CHOP ↑ ROS, 7-dehydrocholesterol ↑ DHCR7 ↓ Lipid and triglyceride accumulation	Cell viability, survival ↓ Anchorage-independent growth ↓ Autophagy ↑	Chakraborty et al. (2012)
	MDA-MB-231 ZR-751	0–75 μM	pSTAT3 ↓	Constitutive and leptin-induced cell viability ↓	McCormack et al. (2011)
	MCF7 ZR-751 MDA-MB-231	0–30 μM Combination: Tamoxifen (5 μM)		Cell viability ↓ Apoptosis ↑	Mannal et al. (2010a)
	MCF7	0–30 μM	MMP9, pp38, pAkt ↓	HRGβ1/HER2-mediated cell viability, survival, invasion and motility ↓	Pan et al. (2011)
	MCF7	0–100 μM	Akt, Bcl2, MMP9, AMACR ↓ Glutathione peroxidase ↑ p53, Bax, Caspase 3/9 ↑ ROS, NO, Caspase activity ↑	Cell viability ↓ DNA fragmentation Membrane blebbing Apoptosis ↑	Chakraborty et al. (2010)

	MCF7 MDA-MB-231	0–100 μM	Caspase 3 activity ↑ Superoxide anion ↑	Cell viability, prolifera-tion ↓ CC arrest S (MCF7) Chromatin condensa-tion, MMP loss Apoptosis ↑	Alosi et al. (2010)
Colorectal *Comparison with Res*	Caco-2	0–50 μM		CC arrest S ↑ Cell proliferation ↓ Apoptosis ↑	Storniolo and Moreno (2019)
	HCT116 HT29 CCD-18Co	0–100 μM		Cell viability ↓	Sun et al. (2016)
	HCT116 Caco-2	0–1000 μM Combination: 5-FU (10:1)	pAkt1/2/3, pERK, Bcl2 ↓ ERβ, FOXO1, p27, Bax, cl PARP ↑	Cell viability ↓ Apoptosis ↑	Tolba and Abdel-Rahman 2015
	Caco-2	0–100 μM	LDH release ↑	Cell proliferation ↓ Cell death ↑	Wawszczyk et al. (2014)
	HT29	0–100 μM	GST, GSH, NQO1 ↑		Harun and Ghazali (2012)
	HT29	0–200 μM	LC3-I/II, p62/SQSTM1 ↑	CC arrest G0/G1 Cell proliferation, DNA synthesis ↓ Apoptosis, necrosis ↑ LMP loss	Mena et al. (2012)
Comparison with Res	HCT116 HT29 Caco-2	0–100 μM	cl caspase 3, cl PARP ↑	Cell viability, survival ↓ Apoptosis ↑	Nutakul et al. (2011)

(continued)

Table 3.2 (continued)

Cancer	Model	Dose	Mechanism	Anticancer effect	References
Comparison with Res	**Azoxymethane-treated colon carcinogenesis mouse model**	**50, 250 ppm**	**pPKCβ2, pp65, iNOS, COX2, AR ↓** **NRF2, HO1, GR ↑**	**ACF, LN, tumor formation ↓**	Chiou et al. (2011)
	Azoxymethane-treated colon carcinogenesis mouse model	**50, 250 ppm**	**pGSK3β, β catenin, VEGF, pPI3K ↓** **Cyclin D1, iNOS, COX2, pAkt ↓** **Ras-GTP, EGF, EGFR, Bcl2 ↓** **MMP2/7/9/26, DFF-45 ↓** **E-cad, Bad, Bax, tBid, Fas, FasL ↑** **cl caspase 3/8/9 ↑**	**ACF formation**	Chiou et al. (2010)
	HT29	50 μM	β catenin, cyclin D1, pp65, Myc ↓ pMSK1 ↓		Paul et al. (2010)
	Azoxymethane-treated colon carcinogenesis rat model	**40 ppm**	**β catenin, cyclin D1, iNOS, COX2 ↓** **pp65, PCNA, TNFα, IL1β, IL4 ↓**	**Tumor growth ↓**	
Comparison with Res	HT29	0–100 μM	Myc, Cyclin D1, iNOS, COX2, TNFα ↓ IL1β, pp38, pMKK3/6, pATF2, pElk1 ↓ cl PARP ↑	Cell proliferation ↓ Apoptosis ↑	Paul et al. (2009)
	HT29	40 μM	Bcl2, O_2^- ↓ Bax, Bad, Bak, Bid, SOD, CAT, H_2O_2 ↑ GPx, GR, TrxR1, IκBα, pIκBα, SP1 ↑	Cell proliferation and viability ↓ Apoptosis ↑	Priego et al. (2008)
	HT29 xenografts	**10, 20, 40 mg/kg bw** **Combination: Quercetin (20 μM; 10, 20, 40 mg/kg bw)** **Combination: Quercetin + X rays+FOLFIRI or FOLFOX6**		**Tumor growth ↓**	

	HT29 **Azoxymethane-treated colon carcinogenesis rat model**	1, 10, 30 μM **40 ppm**	iNOS ↓ **PCNA, iNOS ↓** **MUC2 ↑**	**ACF formation, cell proliferation ↓**	Suh et al. (2007)
Lung	PC9 A549	0–60 μM Combination: Thapsigargin (0.5 μM)	Caspase 3 activity, ROS ↑ pPERK; IRE1; ATF4, CHOP ↑ p53, Bax, Caspase 3 ↑ cytosolic Ca^{2+} (PC9) ↑ Bcl2, Glutathione ↓	Cell viability, adhesion ↓ Migration ↓ MMP loss Apoptosis ↑	Ma et al. (2017)
	PC9 xenograft	**50 mg/kg bw Combination: Thapsigargin (1 mg/kg bw)**	**pPERK, CHOP, p53 ↑** **Bax, Caspase 3 ↑** **Bcl2 ↓**	**Tumor growth ↓**	
	H460 H1299	0–100 μM	Telomerase activity ↓ cyclin B, hTERT, cdc25A ↓ H3K9me3 heterochromatin foci ↑ pATM, p-chk2, γH2AX, pNBS1 ↑ Cyclin E/A, pCdk2, p53, p21, p27 ↑	Cell proliferation, survival ↓ Senescence ↑ CC arrest S	Chen et al. (2017b)
	LLC	0–100 μM	Polymeric fibronectin, pERK ↓ pAkt ↑	Adherent cell viability ↓	Wang et al. (2017a)
	Pterostilbene treated LLC iv **LLC-iv**	**50, 100 μM** **5 mg/kg**		**DPP IV binding ↓** **Lung metastasis ↓** **Lung metastasis ↓**	
	A549 + M2-TAMs H441 + M2-TAMs	0–20 μM	CD133, Sox2, β-catenin, Vimentin ↓ MUC1, NF-κB, VEGF ↓	CD133+ cells ↓ Tumor-sphere formation ↓ M2 polarization ↓	Huang et al. (2016)
	A549, HBECR HBECR silenced for p53 (HBECR/p53i)	0–50 μM	pATM, pCHK1/2, pp53, p21 ↑	Cell viability ↓ CC arrest S p53-dependent cell viability and CC arrest ↓ p53-dependent senescence ↑	Lee et al. (2016)

(continued)

Table 3.2 (continued)

Cancer	Model	Dose	Mechanism	Anticancer effect	References
	H460	0–80 μM	Telomerase activity ↓	Cell viability ↓	Tippani et al. (2014)
	A549 A549 resistant to Docetaxel (A549/D16)	0–100 μM	LC3-I/II, Beclin 1, pERK ↑ p62, pPI3K, pAkt, pJNK ↓	Constitutive and docetaxel resistant cell viability ↓ CC arrest G0/G1 Apoptosis, autophagy ↑ AVO formation ↑	Hsieh et al. (2014a)
	A549	0–6 μM Combination: DAPT (10 μM)	NICD, Hes1, Nicastrin, Presenilin 1 ↑ Bax, Cytochrome C, CyclinD1 ↑ Survivin, pAkt, pS6, pmTOR, ↑ DNA-PK, ROS ↑ GSH, GSH/GSSG ↓	Cell viability ↓ MMP loss Apoptosis ↑	Yang et al. (2013)
	A549 xenografts	**100 mg/kg bw** **Combination:**	**NICD, Hes1, pAkt ↑**	**Tumor growth ↓**	
		DAPT (10 mg/kg bw)	**NICD, Hes1, pAkt ↓**	**Tumor growth ↓**	
		LY 294002 (20 mg/kg bw)	**pAkt ↓**	**Tumor growth↓**	
	Urethane-induced lung carcinogenesis mouse model	**50 or 250 mg/kg bw**	**EGFR, pAkt, pmTOR, pERK, PCNA ↓** **Cyclin D1/A, pSTAT3, pIKK, pp65 ↓** **LC3-I/II, cl caspase 3, p53, p21, p27 ↑** **IκBα ↑**	**Tumor number and size ↓** **Apoptosis, autophagy ↑**	Chen et al. (2012)
Comparison with Res	A549	0–100 μM	LC3-I/II, p62/SQSTM1 ↑ Cytosolic cysteine/aspartyl cathepsins activity ↑ LDH release ↑	Cell proliferation, DNA synthesis ↓ CC arrest S Necrosis, autophagy ↑ LMP loss	Mena et al. (2012)

	H460 SK-MES-1	0–100 µM	Caspase 3/7 activity ↑	Cell viability ↓ Chromatin condensation Apoptosis ↑	Schneider et al. (2010)
Prostate	LNCaP PC3M	50 µM	MTA1, HIF1α, VEGFc, IL1β ↓ p27, AcH3 ↑	Cell viability ↓	Butt et al. (2017)
	Prostate-specific *Pten* null mice	**10 mg/kg bw Combination: SAHA (5, 10 µM; 50 mg/kg)**	**Ki67, CD31, MTA1, HIF1α, VEGFc ↓ IL1β ↓ cl caspase 3, p27, AcH3 ↑**	**Tumor growth, angiogenesis ↓ Apoptosis ↑**	
	LNCaP	0–100 µM	AR ↓		Chakraborty et al. (2016)
	Prostate-specific *Pten* heterozygous and *Pten* null mice	**100 mg/kg diet 10 mg/kg bw**	**MTA1, pAkt/Akt, AR, Myc, Cyclin D1 ↓ TGFβ1, Notch 2, Ets2, Hsp90, IL1β ↓ Ki67, VEGFc, CD31 ↓ E-cad, PTEN, Acp53/p53, p21 p27 ↑ Bak, cl caspase 3 ↑**	**Tumor growth, angiogenesis ↓ Inflammation, EMT, survival ↓ Apoptosis ↑**	Dhar et al. (2016)
Comparison with Res	DU145 22Rv1	50 µM	miR-17, −20a, −106a, −106b ↓ PTEN ↑		Dhar et al. (2015b)
	DU145 EV & miR-17/106a Mimic xenografts	**50 mg/kg bw**	**Ki 67, miR-17/106a ↓ cl caspase 3, PTEN, M30 ↑**	**Tumor growth ↓ Apoptosis ↑**	
	LNCaP PC3	0–40 µM Pter-Isothiocyanate conjugate	AR, SRC1, GRIP1, pAkt/Akt ↓ pErk/Erk, Bcl2, Bcl-xL ↓ p53, Bax, Caspase 3/8/9 activity ↑ cl caspase 3 ↑	Cell viability, survival ↓ CC arrest S and G2/M Apoptosis ↑	Nikhil et al. (2014b)
	22Rv1	0–100 µM	AR, AR truncated (80 kDa) ↓	Cell viability ↓	Kumar et al. (2014)
	PC3	20 µM	MnSOD activity ↑	Cell proliferation ↓	Robb and Stuart (2014)

(continued)

Table 3.2 (continued)

Cancer	Model	Dose	Mechanism	Anticancer effect	References
Comparison with Res	LNCaP DU145 PC3M	0–100 μM	MTA1 ↓ Acp53/p53 ↑		Li et al. (2013)
	DU145 EV shMTA1 xenografts	**50 mg/kg bw**	**Ki 67, CD31 ↓** **Acp53/p53, M30 ↑**	**Tumor growth, angiogenesis ↓** **Metastasis ↑** **Apoptosis ↑**	
	LNCaP PC3	0–100 μM	AMPK, p53, p21, cl caspase 3/9 ↑ cl PARP ↑ FASN, pACC, pro-caspase 3/9 ↓	CC arrest G0/G1 (LNCaP) Cell proliferation ↓ Apoptosis ↑	Lin et al. (2012)
	PC3	0–100 μM	Akt, Bcl2, MMP9, AMACR ↓ Glutathione reductase ↓ Glutathione peroxidase ↑ p53, Bax, Caspase 3 ↑ ROS, NO, Glutathione ↑	Cell viability ↓ DNA fragmentation Apoptosis ↑	Chakraborty et al.(2010)
Comparison with Res	LNCaP	0–25 μM	Constitutive and androgen/estrogen-induced PSA ↓ p21, p27 ↑	CC arrest G0/G1 and S Cell proliferation ↓	Wang et al. (2010)
Leukemia & Lymphoma	Jurkat Molt-4	0–180 μM	Fas ↑	Cell viability ↓	Ramezani et al.(2019)
	JeKo-1 Granta-519 Mino Z-138 Rec-1	0–80 μM Combination: Bortezomib (0–18.2 nM) Dexamethasone (0–160 μM)	cl caspase 3/8/9, Bax ↑ Bcl2, Bcl-xl, Cyclin D1, Cdk4/6 ↓ pPI3K, pAkt, pmTOR, pp70S6K ↓	Cell viability ↓ Apoptosis ↑ MMP loss CC arrest G0/G1 Synergistic: Cell viability ↓	Yu et al. (2018)
	JeKo-1 xenografts	**50 mg/kg bw** **Combination: Bortezomib (0.5 mg/kg bw)**	**pmTOR ↓**	**Synergistic: Tumor growth ↓** **Apoptosis ↑**	

	Jurkat Hut-78	0–80 μM	ROS, cl caspase 3/8/9, cl PARP ↑ pERK, Cdc25A, cyclin A2, CDK2 ↓	Cell proliferation ↓ CC arrest S Apoptosis ↑ MMP loss	Chang et al. (2017)
	SUDHL-4 DB NU-DUL-1 TMD8 U2932 OCI-LY8	0–120 μM	ROS, pH2A.X, Chk2, cl PARP ↑ cl caspase 3/8/9, Bax, pp38 ↑ Bcl2, pERK, cdc25A, Cyclin A2 ↓ CDK2 ↓	Cell proliferation ↓ CC arrest S MMP loss Apoptosis ↑	Kong et al. (2016)
	OCI-LY8 xenografts	**30 mg/kg/ 2 days**		**Tumor growth ↓**	
Comparison with Res	HT1080 RCH-ACV 697	0–20 μM Combination: Chloroquine (20 μM)	sp XBP1, CHOP, LC3, GRP78, p62 ↑	Cell viability ↓ ER stress, apoptosis, autophagy ↑ Acidic vesicles ↑	Papandreou et al. (2015)
	HL-60 THP-1 U937 OCI-AML3 MV4-11	0–100 μM	Cyclin D3, CDK 2/6 ↓ cl caspase 3/8/9, cl PARP, ROS ↑ Activated cathepsin B ↑ pERK, pJNK ↑	Cell viability and proliferation ↓ CC arrest G0/G1 Apoptosis ↑ MMP loss Lysosomal permeability ↑	Hsiao et al. (2014)
	HL-60	0–100 μM	LC3-I/II ↑ ROS ↓	Cell viability ↓ AVO formation, autophagy ↑ Apoptosis ↑ DNA fragmentation, MMP loss,	Siedlecka-Kroplewska et al. (2013)
	MOLT4	0–100 μM		Cell viability ↓ DNA fragmentation Apoptosis ↑	Siedlecka-Kroplewska et al. (2012)

(continued)

Table 3.2 (continued)

Cancer	Model	Dose	Mechanism	Anticancer effect	References
	K562	0–100 μM	cl caspase 3/9 ↑	Cell viability ↓ MMP loss Apoptosis, necrosis ↑	Roslie et al. (2012)
	HL-60 K562 Multi drug resistant HL-60 (HL-60R) and K562 (K562-ADR) HUT78 FasL resistant HUT78 (HUT78B1 and HUT78B3)	0–100 μM		Cell proliferation ↓ Apoptosis ↑ MMP loss	Tolomeo (2005)
Liver	SMMC-7221	0–100 μM	MTA1, HDAC1, pAkt/Akt ↓ acPTEN/PTEN ↑	Invasion ↓ Apoptosis ↑	Qian et al. (2018a)
	SMMC-7221 xenografts	**50 mg/kg**		**Tumor growth ↓**	
	SMMC-7221	0–100 μM	miR-19a, pAkt, Akt ↓ PTEN ↑	Cell viability, invasion ↓ CC arrest S Apoptosis ↑	Qian et al. (2018b)
	SMMC-7221	0–100 μM	MTA1, HDAC1, HDAC2 ↓ acp53/p53 ↑	Cell viability, migration, invasion ↓ CC arrest S Apoptosis ↑	Qian et al. (2017)
	HepG2	0–100 μM	SOD2 ↓ p53, ROS, Caspase 3 activity ↑	Cell viability, proliferation ↓ Apoptosis ↑	Guo et al. (2016)
	DEN+CCl_4-treated liver carcinogenesis mouse model	**100, 200 mg/kg bw**	**SOD2 ↓** **Caspase 3 activity, p53, ROS ↑**	**Tumor growth ↓** **Apoptosis ↑**	

Comparison with Res	HepG2	0–250 μM		Cell viability ↓ Antigenotoxic DNA fragmentation MMP loss Apoptosis ↑	Lombardi et al. (2015)
	Hep3B	1 μM Combination: Curcumin and analogs (1 μM)	LOX, pFAK, pSRC, pPaxillin ↓	Migration, invasion ↓ Anchorage-independent growth ↑	Huang et al. (2013)
	HepG2	0–100 μM	MMP9, VEGF, EGF, EGFR, NF-κB ↓ AP1, pErk/Erk, pp38/p38, pJNK/JNK ↓ pPI3K/PI3K, pAkt/Akt, PKCα/β/γ ↓	Migration, invasion, adhesion ↓	Pan et al. (2009)
	HepG2 xenografts	**20, 250 mg/kg bw**	**MMP9, VEGF ↓**	**Lung metastasis ↓**	
Melanoma	B16/F10	0–10 μM	MSH-induced melanin synthesis and tyrosinase activity ↓ MSH-stimulated Melan-A, tyrosinase ↓	Hypopigmentation ↑	Yoon et al. (2016)
	A2058, MeWo and MelJuso xenografts	**20, 30, 40 mg/kg bw**	**Ki67 ↓** **ACTH,CRH, NORA, Corticosterone ↓** **GCLC, GSS, GPX2, GSR, GSTA1 ↓** **TXNRD1, SOD1/2, CAT, G6PD ↓** **ME1, IDH1, Nrf2 ↓**	**Cell proliferation, tumor growth ↓** **Apoptosis ↑**	Benlloch et al. (2016)
	AtT-20	15 μM	ACTH, POMC ↓		
	SK-MEL-2	50 μM Combination: Astragalus (4, 8, 12, 16 g/kg)	Caspase 3/7 activity, Bax ↑ Bcl2 ↓	Synergistic: Cell viability and proliferation ↓ DNA fragmentation Apoptosis ↑	Huang et al. (2014)
	SK-MEL-2 xenografts	**50 μM** **Combination: Astragalus (8, 12 g/kg)**	**Bax ↓** **Bcl2 ↑**	**Tumor growth ↓**	

(continued)

Table 3.2 (continued)

Cancer	Model	Dose	Mechanism	Anticancer effect	References
Comparison with Res	A375	0–100 μM	LC3-I/II, p62/SQSTM1 ↑ Cytosolic cysteine/aspartyl cathepsins activity ↑ LDH release ↑	Cell proliferation ↓ DNA synthesis ↓ CC arrest S Necrosis ↓ LMP loss Autophagy ↑	Mena et al. (2012)
	SK-MEL-2 MeWo	0–100 μM Combination: inositol-6-phosphate (0.25, 0.5, 1 mM)	Caspase 3/7 activity, VEGF ↓	Synergistic: Cell viability ↓ Apoptosis ↑	Schneider et al. (2009)
	B16M-F10	40 μM Combination: Quercetin (20 μM)	NO, H_2O_2, iNOS, Bcl2, pCREB ↓ eNOS, Mg-dependent NSMase ↑ Ceramide ↑	Cell viability, adhesion, invasion ↓ Apoptosis ↑	Ferrer et al. (2007)
	B16M-F10 xenografts	**20 mg/kg bw** **Combination: Quercetin (20 mg/kg bw)** **Res (20 mg/kg bw)**	**Bcl2** ↓	**Liver metastasis** ↓ **Host survival** ↑	Ferrer et al. (2005)
	B16M-F10 HSE	40 μM Combination: Quercetin (20 μM) Res (12 μM)	VCAM 1, Bcl2, Bcl-w, Bcl-xl ↓ Bax, Bad, Bid ↑	Cell viability, adhesion, invasion ↓	

Head & Neck *bis (hydroxymethyl) propionate analogs of pterostilbene*	CAL27 cisplatin-resistant (CAR)	0–100 μM		Cell viability ↓	Hsieh et al. (2018)
	CAL27 cisplatin-resistant xenografts	**25, 50, 100 mg/kg bw**		**Tumor growth ↓**	
	EC109 TE1	0–150 μM	Bcl2, GSH, mitochondrial cyt c, SP1 ↓ GRP78, CHOP, PUMA, ATF6 ↑ pPERK, peIF2α, cytoplasmic cyt c ↑ cl caspase 9/12 ↑ ROS, Caspase 3 activity, Ca^{2+} ↑	Cell viability, adhesion ↓ Migration, Invasion ↓ Apoptosis ↑	Feng et al. (2016)
	EC109 xenografts	**100, 200 mg/kg bw**	**Bcl2 ↓** **GRP78, CHOP, PUMA ↑**	**Tumor growth ↓**	
	SAS OECM1	0–40 μM	pAkt, pErk1/2, pp38, pmTOR ↓ pJNK, pAMPK, pULK, pRaptor ↑ LC3-I/II, Beclin, cl caspase 3, 8, 9 ↑ cl PARP ↑	Cell viability ↓ CC arrest G0/G1 & S Apoptosis, autophagy ↑	Ko et al. (2015)
	SCC-9	0–80 μM	MMP2, uPA, NF-κB, pIκB, CREB ↓ SP1, pAkt, pErk1/2, pJNK1/2 ↓ TIMP2, PAI1 ↑	Cell viability, survival ↓ Migration, invasion ↓	Lin et al. (2014)
ANK-199, a pterostilbene derivative	CAL27 cisplatin-resistant (CAR)	0–100 μM	Rubicon ↓ Atg5/7/12/14, Atg16l1, Beclin 1 ↑ PI3K class III, LC3-I/II ↑	Cell viability ↓ autophagosome, AVO formation ↑ DNA condensation autophagy ↑	Hsieh et al. (2014b)
Pancreatic	**AsPC-1 and BxPC-3 xenograft**	**20, 30, 40 mg/kg bw**	**Ki67, ACTH, corticosterone, Nrf-2 ↓** **GCLC, GSS, GPX2, GSR, GSTA1 ↓** **TXNRD1, SOD1/2, CAT, G6PD ↓** **ME1, IDH1 ↓** **KEAP1 ↑**	**Tumor growth ↓**	Benlloch et al. (2016)

(continued)

Table 3.2 (continued)

Cancer	Model	Dose	Mechanism	Anticancer effect	References
	MIA PaCa-2 PANC1	30 μM Combination: EGCG (20–40 μM)	Cytochrome c activity ↑ Caspase 3/7 activity (PANC1) ↓	Cell viability ↓ CC arrest S (MIA PaCa-2) MMP loss, DNA fragmentation Apoptosis ↑	Kostin et al. (2012)
	MIA PaCa-2 PANC1	0–75 μM	Cytosolic Cytochrome c ↑ Smac/DIABLO, MnSOD activity ↑ pSTAT3 ↓		McCormack et al. (2012)
	MIA PaCa-2 xenografts	**0.1, 0.5, 1 mg/kg bw/day**		**Tumor growth ↓**	
	MIA PaCa-2 PANC1	0–100 μM	Caspase 3/7 activity ↑	Cell viability and proliferation ↓ DNA fragmentation (MIA PaCa-2) MMP loss Apoptosis (MIA PaCa-2) ↑ CC arrest G0/G1 (MIA PaCa-2) CC arrest S (PANC1)	Mannal et al. (2010b)
Cervical	HeLa	0–400 μM	mTOR, pPI3K, pAkt ↓	Cell viability ↓ MMP loss Apoptosis ↑	Hong Bin et al. (2018)
Comparison with Res	HeLa	0–120 μM	HPV E6 oncoprotein ↓ p53 ↑	Cell viability and proliferation ↓ Survival, migration ↓ CC arrest S Apoptosis ↑	Chatterjee et al. (2018)

	HeLa	0–160 μM	GR, GSH, GSH/GSSG ↓ peIF2α, pPERK, pNRF2, GRP78 ↑ CHOP, NQO1, GPX, CAT, ROS ↑	Cell viability ↓ Apoptosis ↑	Zhang et al. (2014)
Glioblastoma	C6 T98G	0–200 μM	cl caspase3, p53 ↑	Cell viability ↓ CC arrest S	Zielinska-Przyjemska et al. (2017)
Comparison with Res				Apoptosis ↑ MMP loss	
	Patient-derived tumor cells	20 μM Combination: Gefitinib (10 μM) Sertraline (7 μM)	pERK1/2, pMEK ↑	Cell viability ↓ CC arrest S DNA synthesis ↓ Gliomasphere formation ↓ Migration ↓	Schmidt et al. (2016)
	GBM8401 U87MG GBM8401 and U87MG CD133$^+$ stem cells	0–5 μM	GRP78, c-Myc, TCF4, GSK3β Vimentin ↓ E-cad, miR-205 ↑	Constitutive and radiation-induced cell viability ↓ Migration, invasion ↓ Gliomasphere formation ↓	Huynh et al. (2015)
	GBM8401 CD133$^+$ xenograft	**2 mg/kg bw Combination: Irradiation (10 Gy)**		**Tumor growth ↓**	
Multiple Myeloma	RPMI8226 ARH77 U266 H929	0–70 μM	pAMPK, pACC, pEIF, cl caspase 3/9 ↑ cl PARP, Beclin1, ATG5, LC3-II ↑ FASN, pmTOR, p4E-BP ↓	Cell viability, metabolism ↓ Apoptosis ↑ AVO formation, autophagy ↑	Mei et al. (2018)
	RPMI8226 xenografts	**50 mg/kg bw**	**pAMPK, cl caspase 3 ↑ FASN, pmTOR ↓**	**Tumor growth ↓ Apoptosis ↑ No toxicity**	

(continued)

Table 3.2 (continued)

Cancer	Model	Dose	Mechanism	Anticancer effect	References
	H929 Bortezomib-resistant H929 (H929R) Patient-derived CD138⁺ multiple myeloma cells	0–50 μM Combination: Panobinostat (25, 30 nM) Vorinostat (0.6, 0.8 μM)	cl caspase 3/8, cl PARP, pp38 ↑ pH2A.X, pChk1 ↑ PI3K, pAkt, cdc25A, CdK2, CyclinA2 ↓	Synergistic: Cell proliferation ↓ MMP loss Apoptosis ↑ CC arrest S DNA damage	Chen et al. (2017a)
	H929 ARP-1 OC1-MY5 RPMI-8226 Patient-derived CD138⁺ multiple myeloma cells	0–50 μM	pERK1/2, pJNK, pChk1/2, p21, ROS ↑ cl caspase3/8/9, γH2AX, pc-Jun ↑ CyclinD1, CDK4/6 ↓	Cell proliferation ↓ Apoptosis ↑ CC arrest GO/G1 DNA damage, MMP loss	Xie et al. (2016)
	H929 xenografts	**50 mg/kg bw**		**Tumor growth ↓**	
Ovarian	OVCAR-8 Caov-3 SKOV3 OVCAR-4 Kuramochi	0–300 μM Combination: Cisplatin (0–50 μM)	pSTAT3, pAkt, pMAPK ↓ MCL1, Bcl2, Cyclin D1 ↓ cl PARP ↑	Synergistic: Cell viability ↓ CC arrest G0/G1 and S Apoptosis ↑ Migration ↓	Wen et al. (2018)
	OVCAR8 OV1063 IGROV-1 SKOV3	0–500 μg/mL	TNFα, NF-κB (p50, p65) ↓ pIKK, pIκB, pAkt, pERK, Egr-1 ↓ NF-κB activity ↓		Pei et al. (2017)
	SKOV3	0–120 μM	ROS, Ca^{2+}, LDH release ↑ lipid peroxidation ↑ caspase 3/9 activity ↑	Cell viability ↓ MMP loss Apoptosis ↑	Dong et al. (2016)

Endometrial	ECC-1 HEC-1A	0–300 μM Combination: Megestrol acetate (0–300 μM)	Bcl-Xl, Bcl2, Cyclin D/B, CDK4 ↓ pSTAT3, pERK, ER66 ↓ cl caspase 3, cl PARP ↑	Cell viability ↓	Wen et al. (2017)
	HEC-1A xenograft	**30 mg/kg bw Combination: Megestrol acetate (10 mg/kg bw)**		**Tumor growth** ↓	
	HTB-111 Ishikawa	0–100 μM	Caspase 3/8/9 activity ↑ miR-663b, miR-221, miR-21 ↓ miR-92, miR-449, miR-1275 ↓ Bcl2l14 ↑	Constitutive and miR-663b-induced cell viability ↓ Constitutive and miR-663b-induced apoptosis ↑	Wang et al. (2017b)
Bladder	T24	0–100 μM	pAkt, pp70S6K, Bcl2, Bcl-xl ↓ cyclin A1/B/D1, pRb ↓ LC3-II, pErk1/2 ↑	Cell viability ↓ CC arrest G0/G1 & S Autophagy, apoptosis ↑ Acidic vesicles ↑	Chen et al. (2010)
Gastric	AGS	0–100 μM	Bcl-xl, pRb, cyclin A/E, Cdk 2/4/6 ↓ Bax, Bad, tBid, GADD45/153, p53 ↑ p21, p27, p16 ↑	Cell viability ↓ CC arrest G1 phase Apoptosis ↑	Pan et al. (2007)
Osteo sarcoma	SOSP-9607	1, 2, 4 μM	Cyclin D1, pJAK2, pSTAT3 ↓ Bcl-xl, MCL1, GSH, GSG/GSSG ↓ p21, p27, Bax, Bak, ROS ↑	Cell viability, migration ↓ Adhesion ↓ CC arrest G1 MMP loss Apoptosis ↑	Liu et al. (2013)

↑, upregulation; ↓, downregulation; in bold, in vivo studies; ac, acetylated; cl, cleaved; p, phosphorylated; sp., spliced; t, truncated; ACF, aberrant crypt foci; AVO, autophagic vacuole; CC, cell cycle; 5-FU, 5-fluorouracil; LN, lymphoid nodules; LMP, lysosomal membrane potential; MMP, mitochondrial membrane potential; Pter, pterostilbene; Res, resveratrol

3.5 Cellular and Molecular Mechanisms of Pterostilbene in Cancer

Until recently there was a paucity of information about the efficacy of pterostilbene to inhibit tumorigenesis and cancer progression. However, five years after the publication of a pivotal article by Jang et al. on the cancer chemopreventive activity of resveratrol (Jang et al. 1997), the role of pterostilbene in cancer prevention was reported by Rimando et al. (2002) using a mouse mammary organ culture model, in which pterostilbene inhibited carcinogen-induced preneoplastic lesions. This finding prompted a reconsideration of the value of pterostilbene as a potential chemopreventive and therapeutic agent in cancer. Subsequent studies in the azoxymethane (AOM)-induced colon carcinogenesis rat models showed that dietary pterostilbene prevented tumorigenesis by decreasing aberrant crypt foci (ACF) formation and mucosal levels of TNFα, IL-1β, and IL-4 (Suh et al. 2007; Paul et al. 2010). Further, pterostilbene inhibited activation of COX2, iNOS, GSK-3β, Ras, PI3K/Akt, EGFR and Wnt/β-catenin signaling and expression of VEGF, MMPs and cyclin D1 (Chiou et al. 2010) and activated the Nrf2-mediated antioxidant pathway (Chiou et al. 2011). In addition, pterostilbene potently inhibited TPA- and DBMA/TPA-induced mouse skin carcinogenesis by suppressing multiple signal transduction pathways including NF-κB, COX2, iNOS, AP1 (Cichocki et al. 2008) and ERK1/2, p38, JNK1/2, PI3K/Akt (Tsai et al. 2012). Preventive effects of pterostilbene has also been shown in urethane-induced lung carcinogenesis in vivo associated with EGFR-mediated signaling and apoptosis (Chen et al. 2012). All this data show pterostilbene's potential in primary chemoprevention. Much more scientific literature exists on the effects of pterostilbene alone and in combination with other natural compounds and/or chemotherapeutic drugs in already established cancers at different stages including progression, drug resistance, and metastasis. Altogether, numerous studies have demonstrated the capacity of pterostilbene to regulate the cell cycle, proliferation, survival, oxidative stress, autophagy, apoptosis, stemness, drug resistance, angiogenesis and other metastatic potential of cancer cells as well as pterostilbene's involvement in regulation of epigenetic network (Fig. 3.2).

Apoptosis is the main mechanism of pterostilbene-induced cell death. Studies have demonstrated that pterostilbene causes activation of both "extrinsic" or death receptor-mediated and "intrinsic" or mitochondrial apoptotic pathways in cancer and can act through caspase- dependent and caspase-independent pathways (Table 3.2, Fig. 3.3). Figure 3.3 summarizes pterostilbene's regulation of molecules involved in multiple signal transduction pathways during cancer development and progression. Treatment with pterostilbene induced apoptosis through the inhibition of the antiapoptotic Bcl family of proteins (Pan et al. 2007; Nikhil et al. 2014a, c; Hung et al. 2017), AR/SRC1/GRIP1 (Nikhil et al. 2014b), and JAK/STAT3 (Wen et al. 2018) and the activation of caspase cascade, TRAIL-induced apoptosis, Fas/FasL, p38MAPK and ROS-induced mitochondrial pathways (Pan et al. 2007; Alosi et al. 2010; Chakraborty et al. 2010; McCormack et al. 2011; Hsiao et al. 2014; Kong et al. 2016; Hung et al. 2017). PI3K/Akt/mTOR signaling is frequently activated in

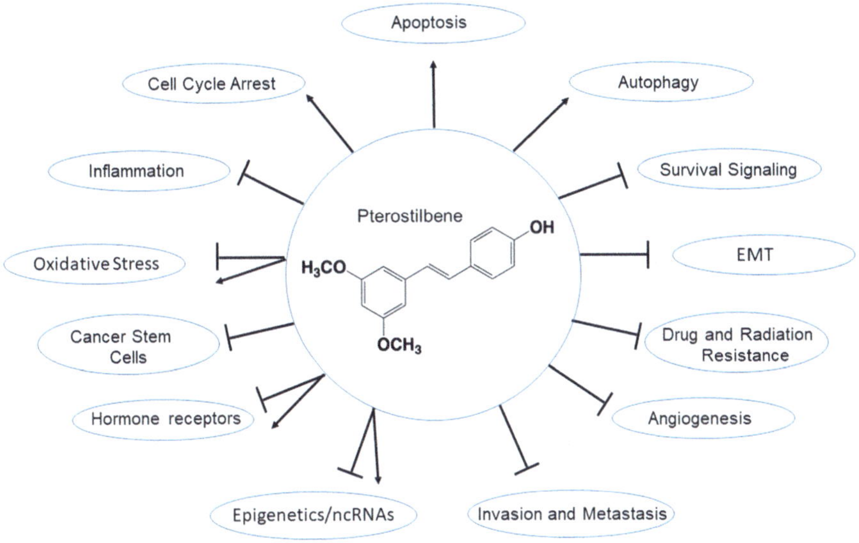

Fig. 3.2 Anticancer mechanisms of pterostilbene

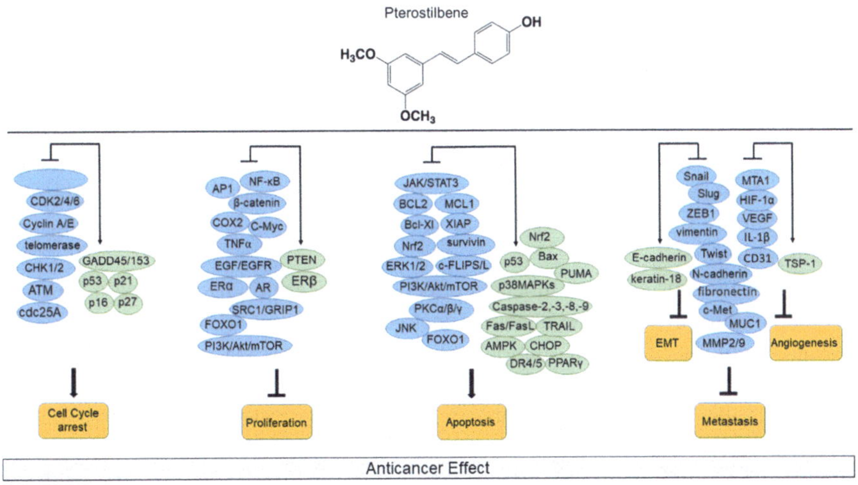

Fig. 3.3 Molecular targets regulated by pterostilbene in cancer

cancer. Studies consistently showed that pterostilbene induced apoptosis through downregulation of PI3K/Akt/mTOR (Yang et al. 2013; Hsieh et al. 2014b; Nikhil et al. 2014a, b; Ko et al. 2015; Tolba and Abdel-Rahman 2015; Chen et al. 2017a; Wakimoto et al. 2017). The MAPK pathway plays a critical role in the pathophysiology of cancer by controlling cell proliferation, differentiation, survival, and apoptosis. MAPKs are composed of several subfamilies, including ERK1/2, JNKs, and p38. The ERK, which is a downstream effector of the pathway, is recognized as a key kinase that controls a large number of cellular processes (Liu et al. 2018) through phosphorylation and the activation of many transcription factors including ELK-1, NF-κB, and c-Myc. The known dual role of ERK1/2 in cancer is reflected in data on pterostilbene's regulation of ERK1/2, which showed both downregulation (Pan et al. 2009, 2014; Chen et al. 2012, 2014; Lin et al. 2014; Nikhil et al. 2014a, b; Ko et al. 2015; Su et al. 2015; Tolba and Abdel-Rahman 2015; Kong et al. 2016; Chang et al. 2017; Pei et al. 2017; Wang et al. 2017a; Wen et al. 2017; Tam et al. 2018) and upregulation (Chen et al. 2010; Hsiao et al. 2014; Hsieh et al. 2014a; Schmidt et al. 2016; Xie et al. 2016; Hung et al. 2017; Wakimoto et al. 2017; Huang et al. 2018) in various cancers. The same kind of discrepancy is present with pterostilbene's effects on p38 (Pan et al. 2009, 2011; Paul et al. 2009; Ko et al. 2015; Kong et al. 2016; Chen et al. 2017a; Hung et al. 2017; Huang et al. 2018).

Several studies have demonstrated that autophagy is involved in pterostilbene-induced apoptosis (Chen et al. 2010, 2012, 2014; Chakraborty et al. 2012; Mena et al. 2012; Wang et al. 2012; Hsieh et al. 2014a, b; Ko et al. 2015; Huang et al. 2018; Mei et al. 2018), which could itself be induced by pterostilbene-promoted escalation of intracellular Ca^{2+} release into the cytoplasm (Moon et al. 2013; Dong et al. 2016) and subsequent ER stress (Siedlecka-Kroplewska et al. 2013; Papandreou et al. 2015; Huang et al. 2018) (Table 3.2).

The antiproliferative mechanisms of pterostilbene involve effects on cell cycle machinery and survival pathways. Similar to other stilbenes, pterostilbene was found to block cell cycle progression by inhibiting cyclin A, E, D1, and D3 and CDK2, -4, -6 (Pan et al. 2007; Hsiao et al. 2014; Wakimoto et al. 2017; Wen et al. 2018) and enhancing the expression of GADD45, GADD 153, and p53, p21, p27, and p16 (Pan et al. 2007) (Table 3.2, Fig. 3.3). As already mentioned, pterostilbene interfered with PI3K/Akt/mTOR, EGFR, MAPK, PKC/AP-1/NF-κB, MTA1/PTEN/Akt, Wnt/β-catenin, JAK/STAT3 and other survival signaling pathways causing cell growth inhibition.

The mechanisms of pterostilbene's effects on cancer progression and metastasis include inhibition of epithelial-to-mesenchymal transition (EMT), cell invasion, migration, colony formation, angiogenesis and metastasis via inhibition of MMPs, uPA, MTA1/HIF1α/VEGF, VCAM1, NO-dependent Bcl2 and upregulation of E-cadherin and TSP1 (Fig. 3.3, Table 3.2). Pterostibene also reduced the stemness of cancer cells. The limited data that are available on regulation of hormone receptors, i.e., androgen and estrogen receptors (AR, ERα/β), by pterostilbene have shown that pterostilbene inhibited AR, ERα and ERα-36 variant but upregulated ERβ (Kumar et al. 2014; Pan et al. 2014; Chakraborty et al. 2016; Dhar et al. 2016; Wen et al. 2017). Pterostilbene's beneficial action was mediated through ERα in breast cancer and through ERβ in prostate and colon cancer (Mannal et al. 2010a; Robb and Stuart 2014; Tolba and Abdel-Rahman 2015). Since hormone therapy in breast and prostate cancers frequently alters the responsiveness of hormone receptors during recurrence, targeting these pathways with pterostilbene may be beneficial for overcoming hormone-resistance. Finally, studies have demonstrated that pterostilbene could effectively inhibit the growth of chemoresistant cells in both solid tumors as well as hematologic malignancies (Tolomeo et al. 2005; Chen et al. 2010; Yang et al. 2013).

To summarize all the above mentioned anticancer effects that pterostilbene offers, we need to remember that while pterostilbene as a single compound can be considered for chemoprevention, it is more likely that combination approaches, which allow concurrent targeting of different signaling pathways, will become therapeutically useful. Combination regimens assume pharmacological interactions, either additive, synergistic, or antagonistic. The combination of pterostilbene with other natural compounds or Food and Drug Administration (FDA)-approved chemotherapeutic drugs has been used in preclinical models and have shown chemosensitizing, additive, or synergistic results that are very promising (Table 3.2). Studies suggest that pterostilbene, when used in combination with other drugs targeting the same pathway or different molecular network, exhibits increased potency, possibly due to a multi-target response or sensitization of tumor cells for more potent response to the drugs. This positive impact from pterostilbene can also be attributed to its anti-inflammatory and antioxidant activity.

3.6 Epigenetic Effects of Pterostilbene in Cancer

Natural bioactive polyphenols present in diet have been studied intensively for the past two decades for their potential as regulators of epigenetic mechanisms driving cancer development and progression (Kai et al. 2010, 2011; Link et al. 2010; Dhar et al. 2011, 2015a, b, 2016; Vanden Berghe 2012; Li et al. 2013; Kumar et al. 2015, 2016, 2017; Butt et al. 2017; Kumar and Levenson 2018; Qian et al. 2018a, b). Epigenetic mechanisms that contribute to the chemopreventive properties of dietary polyphenols are polygonal and include regulation of processes affecting DNA methylation, histone modifications, and modulation of non-coding RNAs (Kai et al. 2010, 2011; Link et al. 2010; Dhar et al. 2011, 2015a, b, 2016; Hardy and Tollefsbol 2011; Huang et al. 2011; Tili and Michaille 2011; Vanden Berghe 2012; Li et al. 2013; Pudenz et al. 2014; Gao and Tollefsbol 2015; Kumar et al. 2015, 2016, 2017; Butt et al. 2017; Kumar and Levenson 2018; Qian et al. 2018a, b). Limited studies have examined the effect of pterostilbene on DNA methylation and histone modifications in cancer. Recent studies from Tollefsbol's group have reported on the inhibition of SIRT1 and showed captivating data on restoration of ERα expression in triple-negative breast cancer (TNBC) cells by combinatorial treatment with resveratrol and pterostilbene via a significant decrease in DNA methylation, DNMT activity, 5-methylcytosine and activation of HATs and HDACs (Kala et al. 2015; Kala and Tollefsbol 2016). In our earliest studies with prostate cancer cell lines, we have demonstrated the anticancer effects of resveratrol mediated through the inhibition of MTA1/NuRD complex-associated deacetylation of p53 followed by the activation of proapoptotic genes Bax and p21 (Kai et al. 2010). MTA1 is a part of the nucleosome remodeling and deacetylase (NuRD) complex, where it functions as an epigenetic reader and transcriptional coactivator/corepressor of downstream signaling (Kumar et al. 2003; Toh and Nicolson 2009). We then showed that pterostilbene more potently inhibited MTA1 in vitro and exerted increased MTA1-dependent p53 acetylation in vivo in prostate cancer (Li et al. 2013). In addition, pterostilbene, like resveratrol in prostate cancer, inhibited the MTA1/HDAC complex leading to p53 and PTEN acetylation in vitro and in vivo in hepatocellular carcinoma (Dhar et al. 2015a; Qian et al. 2017, 2018a).

The epigenetic mechanisms that contribute to the chemopreventive nature of pterostilbene also include modulation of noncoding RNAs (Link et al. 2010; Ross and Davis 2011; Dhar et al. 2015b; Kumar et al. 2015, 2016, 2017; Kumar and Levenson 2018). Noncoding RNAs control gene expression by inducing degradation or inhibiting translation of their target mRNA. MicroRNAs (miRNAs/miRs) are small regulatory RNAs that are implicated as oncogenes or as tumor suppressors in cancer. Moreover, the significance of circulating miRNAs as potential chemopreventive and prognostic/predictive biomarkers for clinical development in cancer has been suggested (Brase et al. 2011; Dhar et al. 2015b; Kumar et al. 2015, 2016, 2017; Kumar and Levenson 2018). In the last decade, numerous studies have examined miRNA profiles under treatment with dietary polyphenols, including resveratrol and pterostilbene (Dhar et al. 2011; Tili and Michaille 2011; Wang et al. 2017b). Pterostilbene significantly downregulated members of oncogenic miR-17~92, miR-106a~363, and miR-106b~25 clusters in prostate cancer cells (Dhar et al. 2015b). Mechanistic studies confirmed the ability of pterostilbene to reverse the direct targeting of PTEN by regulating these miRNAs. Moreover, pterostilbene treatment significantly diminished tumor growth in miR-overexpressing prostate cancer xenografts by downregulating miR-17/106a while simultaneously increasing PTEN levels (Dhar et al. 2015b). Notably, we have detected changes in circulating miR17/106a levels in murine serum after treatment with pterostilbene, signifying the possibility of using miRNAs as predictive biomarkers in prostate cancer (Dhar et al. 2015b). In breast cancer, pterostilbene upregulated tumor suppressive miR-143, miR-200c and Ago-2, a key regulator of miRNA homeostasis and biogenesis (Hagiwara et al. 2012). Pterostilbene inhibited breast cancer EMT and tumor growth and metastasis in xenografts via induction of miRNA-205 expression, which inhibited the Src/Fak signaling (Su et al. 2015). Another study found that pterostilbene-induced modulation of miR448/NF-κB axis resulted in suppression of the generation of breast CSCs and metastatic potential (Mak et al. 2013). Pterostilbene also suppressed the glioblastoma stem cells by upregulating miR-205 and downregulating GRP78 (Huynh et al. 2015). Further, pterostilbene's downregulation of oncogenic miR-663, whose expression is correlated with poor prognosis in endometrial cancer patients, led to induction of proapoptotic BCL2L14 in endometrial cancer cells in vitro (Wang et al. 2017b). Finally, a recent paper by Huang et al. has demonstrated the inhibition of proliferation and induction of autophagy-associated apoptosis in MCF7 cells mediated through the modulation of long noncoding RNAs (lncRNAs) by pterostilbene (Huang et al. 2018). The epigenetic mechanisms of pterostilbene action are summarized in Table 3.2 for corresponding organ-specific cancers.

3.7 Effects of Pterostilbene in Organ-Specific Cancers

A large volume of preclinical evidence shows that pterostilbene produces anticancer responses in a variety of cell lines and animal models of different types of cancer, including breast, prostate, ovarian, colorectal, lung and liver adenocarcinomas, melanomas and glioblastomas among other solid tumors as well as hematological malignancies. Due to the heterogeneity of cancer and uniqueness of the pathophysiology of each organ, in this section we will particularly focus on the anticancer effects of pterostilbene in organ-specific cancers (Table 3.2).

3.7.1 *Breast Cancer*

Breast cancer is the leading and main diet-related cancer in women. Numerous epidemiological studies have shown that phytoestrogen-rich diets are associated with a low incidence of breast cancer (Adlercreutz 2002). In contrast to resveratrol as a known phytoestrogen (Gehm and Levenson 2006), no data are available on pterostilbene binding or affinity to estrogen receptors. Therefore, pterostilbene, at present, is not recognized as a phytoestrogen. However, recent studies have suggested ERα-mediated neuroprotective effects (Song et al. 2015) and ER-β-mediated cell growth inhibition and stress resistance in mouse myoblasts (Robb and Stuart 2014) for pterostilbene. More importantly, two recent intriguing studies have addressed pterostilbene's involvement in estrogen receptor-signaling in breast cancer and found that (1) a combination of resveratrol and pterostilbene epigenetically restored conventional ERα signaling in ERα-negative cells (Kala and Tollefsbol 2016) and (2) pterostilbene-induced apoptosis in ERα-negative breast cancer cells was mediated through high ERα-36 variant expression (Pan et al. 2014). Nevertheless, perhaps not surprisingly, the vast majority of studies with pterostilbene on the tumor biology of breast cancer have been performed with triple-negative models, since this subgroup has highly aggressive features, the worst prognosis, and no targeted therapies. Pterostilbene inhibited the viability of all major breast cancer subtypes, namely MCF7 (ERα-positive); SK-BR-3 (HER2 overexpressing), and MDA-MB-231 (TNBC) in a dose-dependent manner (Table 3.2). Cell viability assays have shown that the IC_{50} for triple-negative cells was generally less than for other subtypes, suggesting more sensitivity to pterostilbene for TNBC cells compared to the ERα-positive MCF7, T47D, or ZR-75-1 cells (Wakimoto et al. 2017). Pterostilbene exerted its anticancer activity in breast cancer by arresting cells in the G0/G1, G2/M or S phase depending on the cell type (Alosi et al. 2010; Wang et al. 2012; Nikhil et al. 2014a; Kala et al. 2015; Wakimoto et al. 2017; Daniel and Tollefsbol 2018). Downregulation of cyclin-dependent kinase CDK2, cyclin D1, and telomerase and upregulation of p21 has been reported in breast cancer cells after treatment with pterostilbene (Wang et al. 2012; Tippani et al. 2014; Wu et al. 2015; Wakimoto et al. 2017; Daniel and

Tollefsbol 2018; Tam et al. 2018). Pterostilbene inhibited PI3K/Akt/mTOR survival signaling pathway (Pan et al. 2011, 2014; Wang et al. 2012; Nikhil et al. 2014a, c; Wu et al. 2015; Wakimoto et al. 2017; Huang et al. 2018; Tam et al. 2018) and downregulated β-catenin and c-Myc (Wang et al. 2012; Wu et al. 2015). The effect of pterostilbene on the phosphorylation state of ERK1/2 in breast cancer is puzzling (Table 3.2) since both activation and downregulation have been reported (Chen et al. 2014; Nikhil et al. 2014a; Pan et al. 2014; Wakimoto et al. 2017; Huang et al. 2018; Tam et al. 2018). Pterostilbene potentiated Fas-mediated and TRAIL-induced apoptosis via ROS-mediated CHOP activation leading to the expression of death receptors DR4 and DR5 (Chen et al. 2014; Hung et al. 2017). However, mitochondrial-dependent apoptosis appears to be the primary mechanism by which pterostilbene exerts its antitumor effects in breast cancer in vitro and in vivo. Pterostilbene caused ROS-associated mitochondrial membrane depolarization (Alosi et al. 2010; Chakraborty et al. 2010; McCormack et al. 2011) resulting in the release of cytochrome c (Moon et al. 2013; Nikhil et al. 2014a) and followed by the activation of effector caspases 3, 3/7, 9 and PARP (Alosi et al. 2010; Chakraborty et al. 2010; Wang et al. 2012; Nikhil et al. 2014a, c; Pan et al. 2014). Pterostilbene upregulated the proapoptotic proteins Bax (Chakraborty et al. 2010; Moon et al. 2013; Nikhil et al. 2014a, c; Hung et al. 2017; Wakimoto et al. 2017), Bid (Hung et al. 2017) while downregulated the antiapoptotic proteins Bcl-2, survivin, (Nikhil et al. 2014a, c; Hung et al. 2017) and XIAP (Hung et al. 2017) in breast cancer cells. Pterostilbene also inhibited EMT through downregulating Snail, Slug, and vimentin (Mak et al. 2013; Chen et al. 2014; Su et al. 2015) and upregulating E-cadherin (Mak et al. 2013). Pterostilbene reduced metastasis by downregulating/inactivating uPA, MMP2 and MMP9 (Pan et al. 2011; Hong et al. 2013; Ko et al. 2014). The potential of pterostilbene or its combinations with resveratrol or tamoxifen for prevention and treatment of human breast cancer, especially triple-negative subtype, is evident from in vivo xenograft mouse models of breast cancer. Data showed that either oral administration or intraperitoneal (i.p.) injections with pterostilbene, in the 10–200 mg/kg dose range, alone or in combination with chemodrugs, significantly suppressed tumor growth in mice (Pan et al. 2014; Su et al. 2015; Wakimoto et al. 2017; Tam et al. 2018).

3.7.2 Colorectal Cancer

Colorectal cancer is "getting younger" and is one of the deadliest cancers in the United States. Fortunately, because of its generally slow progression, close association with inflammation and diet, chemotherapeutic options with the use of natural product drugs seem very promising. The chemopreventive activity of pterostilbene has been shown in studies using azoxymethane (AOM)-induced colon carcinogenesis rat models, in which dietary pterostilbene prevented tumorigenesis by decreasing ACF formation and mucosal levels of TNFα, IL-1β, and IL-4 (Suh et al. 2007; Paul et al. 2010). Mechanisms also involved the reduced expression of inflammatory markers including NF-κB (Paul et al. 2010), inhibition of COX2, iNOS, GSK-3β, Ras, PI3K/Akt, EGFR, VEGF, MMPs, and Cyclin D1 and Wnt/β-catenin signaling activation (Chiou et al. 2010) as well as the activation of Nrf2-mediated antioxidant pathway (Chiou et al. 2011). Activation of defense mechanisms against oxidative stress was also detected in human colon cells in cultures treated with pterostilbene (Chiou et al. 2011; Harun and Ghazali 2012; Mena et al. 2012). In human HT-29 colon carcinoma cells, pterostilbene induced cell cycle arrest, inhibited cell proliferation, and promoted apoptosis via inhibition of multiple signaling pathways including β-catenin, COX2, TNFα, IL4, IL-1β, Myc, Cyclin D1, iNOS and others (Paul et al. 2009, 2010; Chiou et al. 2010). Recent studies using Caco2 and HCT116 cells have also reported on pterostilbene's inhibition of cell proliferation and induction of apoptosis (Wawszczyk et al. 2014; Tolba and Abdel-Rahman 2015; Sun et al. 2016; Storniolo and Moreno 2019). The combination of pterostilbene with quercetin caused inhibition of cell and tumor growth and the induction of apoptosis through activation of antioxidant enzymes (Priego et al. 2008). Finally, pterostilbene was found to sensitize colon cancer cells to 5-fluoroutacil through ERβ-mediated pathways (Tolba and Abdel-Rahman 2015).

3.7.3 Lung Cancer

Lung cancer is the most frequently diagnosed cancer worldwide and the leading cause of cancer-related mortality in men and women. Generally, the major risk factor in lung cancer is attributed to tobacco smoking. However, environmental factors including improper diet are suggested as underlying mechanisms responsible for increasing the incidence of lung cancer among nonsmokers (Akhtar and Bansal 2017). Targeted therapy was suggested as the optimal treatment for lung cancer (Azar et al. 2017). More than 80% of lung cancer cases are classified as non-small-cell lung cancer (NSCLC). Several studies, using NSCLC cell lines such as PC9 and A549, have reported a dose- and time-dependent cytotoxicity by pterostilbene (Lee et al. 2016; Ma et al. 2017). Pterostilbene caused cell cycle arrest and senescence, which were associated with DNA damage response and activation of cell cycle proteins cyclin A/E, p53, p21 and p27 (Chen et al. 2012, 2017b; Tippani et al. 2014). Antimitotic action of pterostilbene resulted in the inhibition of telomerase activity in NCI H-460 lung cancer cells (Tippani et al. 2014; Chen et al. 2017b) apparently due to the binding of pterostilbene to the active site of telomerase (Tippani et al. 2014). Moreover, pterostilbene suppressed the self-renewal ability of lung cancer cells cocultured with M2-TAMs (Huang et al. 2016). Pterostilbene induced apoptosis through ER stress and ROS generation leading to mitochondrial membrane depolarization (Yang et al. 2013; Ma et al. 2017) and changes in lysosomal membrane permeabilization (Mena et al. 2012). Other apoptosis-related cellular changes caused by pterostibene treatment were associated with the release of cytochrome c, the activation of caspase cascade, the accumulation of proapoptotic and downregulation of antiapoptotic proteins, along with the activation of ERK1/2 and Notch 1 pathways and downregulation of PI3K/Akt/JNK and EGFR signaling (Chen et al. 2012; Yang et al. 2013; Hsieh et al. 2014a; Ma et al. 2017). In docetaxel-induced multidrug resistant (MDR) human lung cancer cell lines, pterostilbene has been shown to inhibit cellular growth and induce cell cycle arrest, autophagy, and apoptosis (Hsieh et al. 2014a). The inhibitory effects of pterostilbene on invasive, migratory and metastatic potential were also evaluated in mouse models of lung cancer (Chen et al. 2012; Ma et al. 2017; Wang et al. 2017a). Furthermore, bioavailability and distribution of pterostilbene in plasma and tissues of Lewis lung carcinoma (LLC)-bearing mice revealed that the pharmacokinetic parameters of LLC mice were increased compared to normal mice (Deng et al. 2015).

3.7.4 Prostate Cancer

Prostate cancer is one of the most frequently diagnosed male malignancies and the second leading cause of cancer-related death in the United States. As prostate cancer is typically diagnosed in the elderly population with a relatively slower rate of growth and progression, and diet is a risk factor for prostate cancer (Moyad and Carroll 2004a, b), nutritional chemoprevention is a particularly promising approach for this disease (Kai et al. 2010; Dhar et al. 2011; Kumar et al. 2015, 2016, 2017; Kumar and Levenson 2018). Androgen receptor signaling plays an important role not only in the development and progression but also in manifestation of endocrine/chemo resistance in prostate cancer. The identification of natural phytochemicals as new agents with antiandrogenic activity may offer innovative approaches in chemoprevention and androgen-resistant prostate cancer, in which AR is still present but acts through alternative pathways (Mitchell et al. 1999; Kai and Levenson 2011). Studies have shown that pterostilbene inhibited AR expression (Nikhil et al. 2014b; Chakraborty et al. 2016) and prostate-specific antigen (PSA) (Wang et al. 2010) in LNCaP (T877A AR) cells. Furthermore, the strong antiandrogenic nature of pterostilbene was revealed in integrated experimental and in silico structure-activity studies, in which pterostilbene showed a close resemblance to pure antiandrogen flutamide in AR binding energy and hydrogen bonding interaction patterns (Chakraborty et al. 2016). Notably, pterostilbene dose-dependently inhibited cell growth and, at the high 100 μM dose, AR expression in 22Rv1 castrate-resistant prostate cancer cells that express full length (140/110 kDa) and truncated (80 kDa) AR variants (Kumar et al. 2014). Finally, we have recently demonstrated in vivo that pterostilbene treatment of prostate-specific *Pten*-loss mice had inhibitory effects on AR levels in both prostate luminal cells and reactive stroma (Dhar et al. 2016). Pterostilbene also acted in prostate cancer through various other mechanisms that included the alteration of cell cycle, inhibition of cell growth and promotion of apoptosis (Chakraborty et al. 2010; Wang et al. 2010; Lin et al. 2012; Nikhil et al. 2014b).

Because of the clinical relevance of MTA1 overexpression and its critical mechanistic role in the progression of prostate cancer (Hofer et al. 2004; Kai et al. 2011;

Dias et al. 2013b; Levenson et al. 2014) and our original data on resveratrol's ability to affect MTA1/HDAC (Kai et al. 2010; Dhar et al. 2015a), subsequent studies from our laboratory aimed to discover more potent natural inhibitor(s) of MTA1 and MTA1 signaling. In collaboration with the late Dr. Agnes M. Rimando, who synthesized for us two natural and three synthetic analogs of resveratrol, a comparison of MTA1-inhibitory activities by stilbenes was initiated (Dias et al. 2013a; Li et al. 2013). The results of these studies have demonstrated that pterostilbene downregulated MTA1 in prostate cancer cell lines and blocked MTA-mediated tumor progression through activation of p53/apoptosis and downregulation of angiogenesis in orthotopic prostate cancer mouse models (Li et al. 2013). Importantly, pterostilbene-treated mice developed less metastasis and in fewer organs compared to resveratrol-treated or control mice, who developed the highest incidence of metastasis in the liver, kidneys, and lung/heart (Li et al. 2013). For the first time in a prostate cancer model, we have detected greater serum levels of pterostilbene compared to resveratrol, confirming findings from other groups on the higher bioavailability of pterostilbene (Tolomeo et al. 2005; Lin et al. 2009; Chang et al. 2012; McCormack and McFadden 2012). The encouraging preclinical results with immunocompromised mice prompted us to test pterosrilbene in physiologically and clinically relevant prostate cancer mouse models with carefully designed chemopreventive (dietary supplementation) and therapeutic (i.p. administration) modes. Our results have demonstrated that dietary pterostilbene could restrain prostatic intraepithelial neoplasia (PIN) formation in prostate-specific *Pten* heterozygous mice and reduce tumor development and progression in prostate-specific *Pten*-null mice (Dhar et al. 2016). Mechanistically, pterostilbene inhibited MTA1-associated inflammation, EMT, and angiogenesis and induced caspase-dependent apoptosis (Dhar et al. 2016) (Table 3.2). While the improved bioavailability of pterostilbene and its distribution in various tissues has been reported (Kapetanovic et al. 2011; Azzolini et al. 2014), we were the first to detect accumulation of pterostilbene in the prostate tissues, providing evidence that pterostilbene reached the target organ (Dhar et al. 2016). When prostate-specific *Pten*-null mice were treated with a combination of pterostilbene and HDAC inhibitor, suberoylanilide hydroxamic acid (SAHA), results showed that pterostilbene sensitized tumor cells to SAHA treatment, resulting in the inhibition of tumor growth and an additional decline in tumor progression through the reduction of MTA1-dependent pro-angiogenic factors HIF1α, VEGF, and IL-1β (Butt et al. 2017). Finally, as described in the "Epigenetic effects of pterostilbene in cancer" section, we have demonstrated the miRNA-mediated ability of pterostilbene to rescue the tumor suppressor PTEN expression and induce apoptosis in prostate cancer cells and DU145-xenografts (Dhar et al. 2015b). Notably, we have detected changes in serum circulating miRs after treatment with pterostilbene, signifying responsive miRNA levels as potential prognostic and predictive biomarkers in prostate cancer (Dhar et al. 2015b; Kumar et al. 2015, 2017).

Aside from finasteride (Chau et al. 2015), despite numerous attempts, there is no as yet effective preventive strategy for prostate cancer (Bosland 2016). Based on the comprehensive and meticulous preclinical studies of molecular and cellular anticancer effects of pterostilbene in prostate cancer, described above, we propose pterostilbene as a lead stilbene compound to be tested in human clinical trials for chemoprevention and therapy.

3.7.5 Leukemia and Lymphoma

Hematological malignancies such as leukemia and lymphomas develop and disseminate differently than solid tumors, with shared pathways distinctive to hematological cancers but also have their own unique mechanisms of progression (Curran et al. 2017). Preclinical acute myeloid leukemia (AML) and lymphoma models have suggested that pterostilbene may be a useful candidate as a chemotherapeutic agent for hematological malignancies (Table 3.2). Treatment of various AML cell lines with pterostilbene has resulted in cell cycle arrest accompanied by downregulation of Cyclin D1/D3 and CDK2/4/6 (Hsiao et al. 2014; Yu et al. 2018). Pterostilbene-induced apoptosis has been mediated through MAPKs, ER stress and disruption of mitochondrial and lysosomal membrane potentials followed by caspases and PARP activation (Tolomeo et al. 2005; Roslie et al. 2012; Siedlecka-Kroplewska et al. 2012, 2013; Hsiao et al. 2014; Papandreou et al. 2015; Yu et al. 2018). Caspase-independent apoptosis and involvement of autophagy in the process have been also described (Tolomeo et al. 2005; Siedlecka-Kroplewska et al. 2013; Papandreou et al. 2015; Ramezani et al. 2019). Similar mechanisms of pterostilbene action have been found in diffuse large B-cell lymphoma (DLBCL) and T-cell leukemia/lymphoma cells (Kong et al. 2016; Chang et al. 2017). In MDR leukemia cell lines, pterostilbene induced apoptosis through a caspase-independent mechanism, suggesting its utility in the treatment of resistant hematologic malignancies (Tolomeo et al. 2005).

3.7.6 Liver Cancer

Liver cancer is fatal and death rates in the Unites States are constantly increasing. It has been proposed that dietary natural products may have tangible potential for the prevention and treatment of liver cancer (Zhou et al. 2016). Studies have shown that pterostilbene has caused cell cycle arrest, inhibited viability and proliferation, invasion and migration, and induced apoptosis in human hepatocellular carcinoma cell lines in culture through the regulation of various pathways including MTA1/HDAC, miR-19a/PTEN, EGF/EGFR, PI3K/Akt, MAPK, Fak/Src and MMP9 (Pan et al. 2009; Huang et al. 2013; Lombardi et al. 2015; Qian et al. 2017, 2018a, b). In vivo, pterostilbene inhibited tumor growth and promoted apoptosis in the liver carcinogenesis model (Guo et al. 2016) and in liver cancer xenografts (Pan et al. 2009; Qian et al. 2018a) (Table 3.2).

3.7.7 Melanoma

Although cutaneous melanoma is ranked 15th among most common cancers worldwide, the annual incidence increase is more than any other type of cancer and it remains a lethal cancer, particularly when diagnosed at an advanced stage. UV-A irradiation induces either direct melanocyte-stimulating hormone (MSH)-mediated malignant transformation of normal melanocytes or transformation of melanocytes into benign nevi which can stay indolent or become malignant due to additional genetic mutations. Pterostilbene inhibited melanin biosynthesis, MSH-induced melanin synthesis and MSH-responsive Melan-A expression in B16/F10 murine melanoma cells, which resulted in cell hypopigmentation (Yoon et al. 2016). Others have demonstrated induction of apoptosis and inhibition of metastasis by a combination of pterostilbene with quercetin in a mouse model (Ferrer et al. 2005, 2007). Pterostilbene alone and in combination with the natural compound astragalus (Huang et al. 2014) and inositol-6-phosphate (IPG) (Schneider et al. 2009) inhibited human melanoma growth in vitro and induced apoptosis associated with the activation of proapoptotic proteins and caspases (Schneider et al. 2009; Huang et al. 2014). Furthermore, promising results were obtained in vitro and when pterostilbene was administrated intravenously (i.v.) into human melanoma xenografts causing the inhibition of tumor growth and induction of apoptosis apparently through the modulation of Nrf2 signaling (Benlloch et al. 2016). Finally, topically administered pterostilbene showed full protection against UVB-induced skin carcinogenesis in SKH-1 hairless mice (Estrela and Asensi 2010).

3.7.8 Head and Neck Cancers

Oral squamous cell carcinoma (OSCC) is the most common head and neck cancer. It has a poor prognosis and low survival rate. Oral cancer is the fourth most common cause of cancer-related death in South and Southeast Asian countries where chewing the mixtures of betel leaf and areca nut is a popular custom (Arjungi 1976; Shetty et al. 2013). Moreover, despite a significant reduction in tobacco use in the United States, tongue and oropharyngeal cancer incidence has increased in recent years, particularly in young white men and women (Tota et al. 2017). Pterostilbene treatment of human OSCC cells caused autophagy and apoptosis via activation of JNK1/2 and inhibition of Akt, ERK1/2 and p38 (Ko et al. 2015) and inhibited metastatic potential of cells through regulating MMP2/TIMP2 and uPA/PAI1 axes among others (Lin et al. 2014). A pterostilbene derivative, ANK-199, showed cytotoxic effects in cisplatin-resistant human oral cancer cell line and xenografts (Hsieh et al. 2014b, 2018). Oral cancer patients are known to have a higher risk of second esophageal cancer than the general population. Feng et al. reported that pterostilbene treatment decreased the viability and adhesion of human esophageal cancer cells and increased apoptosis via multiple signal transduction pathways including increased expression of ER stress-related molecules, upregulation of proapoptotic PUMA and downregulation of antiapoptotic Bcl2 together with activation of mitochondria-associated caspase cascade (Feng et al. 2016) (Table 3.2).

3.7.9 Pancreatic Cancer

Pancreatic cancer is an extremely aggressive form of cancer, usually detected in its late stages, making it challenging to treat effectively. As an innovative approach in integrative oncology, natural compounds are considered chemosensitizing and nontoxic agents that may expand current cancer therapies by increasing efficacy and lowering toxicity. Pterostilbene alone and in combination with epigallocatechin gallate (EGCG) showed changes in cytochrome c activity and an additive antiproliferative effects in both MIA PaCa-2 and PANC-1 cells. Interestingly, different cell lines showed a differential response in terms of apoptosis and cell cycle arrest (Kostin et al. 2012). A recent study investigated the effect of the i.v. administration of pterostilbene in AsPC-1 and BxPC-3 xenografts and found that pterostilbene interfered with the growth and defense of cancer cells by downregulating the pituitary gland-dependent ACTH, glucocorticoid receptor and Nrf-2-dependent oxidative stress signaling (Benlloch et al. 2016). Since the inhibition of Nrf-2 was suggested as an effective anticancer pathway during a cancer treatment regimen (Birben et al. 2012; Ma and He 2012; Ma et al. 2012; Kou et al. 2013), the fact that pterostilbene inhibited Nrf-2 signaling in preclinical pancreatic cancer models is very encouraging in terms of known aggressive phenotypes of pancreatic cancer and the necessity for altered Nrf-2 pathway inhibition during chemotherapy.

3.7.10 Cervical Cancer

Although the etiological factor for cervical cancer as human papilloma virus (HPV) infection is recognized and there are approved HPV vaccines and drugs available, it is still one of the most prevalent cancers affecting women worldwide. A compromised cervical microbiome, together with diet, has been suggested as an important risk factor for cervical intraepithelial neoplasia, a precancerous stage of cervical cancer (Seo et al. 2016). Pterostilbene inhibited cervical cancer cell proliferation and induced apoptosis associated with downregulation of HPV E6 protein levels, re-establishment of p53 and activation of caspase 3 more effectively than resveratrol (Chatterjee et al. 2018). Other mechanisms of pterostilbene's effects on HeLa cervical cancer cells such as cell cycle arrest, inhibition of cell viability, cell invasion, and migration as well as induction of autophagy- and mitochondrial membrane depolarization-induced apoptosis were also reported (Zhang et al. 2014; Hong Bin et al. 2018).

3.7.11 Glioblastoma

Glioblastoma (GBM) is the most common malignant primary brain tumor in adults. Pterostilbene is especially relevant and valid for glioblastoma treatment due to its ability to cross the blood-brain barrier and its high brain bioavailability (Joseph et al. 2008; Kapetanovic et al. 2011; Chang et al. 2012). Limited studies in glioblastoma have convincingly showed pterostibene's inhibitory effect on self-renewal, gliomagenesis and irradiation-resistance in vivo (Huynh et al. 2015). Mechanistically, pterostilbene downregulated miR-205-mediated GRP78, c-Myc and other glioma stem-cell (GSC)-related properties simultaneously with inhibiting vimentin and increasing levels of E-cadherin in CD133-positive GSC xenografts (Huynh et al. 2015). Pterostilbene showed great potential for drug synergism in patient-derived glioblastoma cell (GC) cultures: synergistic inhibition of MAPK activity and upregulation of tumor suppressor TXNIP along with an intriguing phosphorylation of ERK1/2 and MEK (Schmidt et al. 2016). In a recent study, pterostilbene induced cell cycle arrest and mitochondrial-mediated apoptosis in ratC6 and humanT98G glioma cell lines (Zielinska-Przyjemska et al. 2017).

3.7.12 Multiple Myeloma

Multiple myeloma (MM) accounts for 13% of hematological malignancies and is characterized by the excessive production of monoclonal immunoglobulins and bone marrow plasmacytosis. The prognosis for MM patients' remains poor due to the disease's resistance to proteasome inhibitor bortezomib, which is a standard of care for newly diagnosed as well as relapsed/refractory MM. Pterostilbene has inhibited proliferation and induced mitochondrial-mediated apoptosis in a panel of MM cell lines and in H929 xenografts (Xie et al. 2016). Importantly, pterostilbene has induced apoptosis associated with the downregulation of PI3K/pAkt, activation of p38 and increased levels of cleaved caspase 3, 8 and PARP in bortezomib-resistant H929R MM cells (Chen et al. 2017a). Notably, combination experiments with pterostilbene and two HDAC inhibitors (panobinostat and vorinostat) currently used in clinic for refractory MM showed synergistic growth inhibitory effects in bortezomib-resistant H929R cells, suggesting potential beneficial usage of pterostilbene together with second-line therapy for synergy and improved safety profiles (Chen et al. 2017a). Recent studies with pterostilbene from a metabolic perspective have demonstrated that its antitumor effects were accompanied with major metabolic changes in a panel of MM cell lines and RPMI-8226 subcutaneous (s.c.) xenografts (Mei et al. 2018). Pterostilbene-induced apoptosis was triggered by activation of AMPK and downregulation of key fatty acid synthesis enzyme FASN 1 (Mei et al. 2018). Interestingly, in contrast to breast cancer cells, pterostilbene-induced autophagy in MM cells had a prosurvival rather than prodeath function (Mei et al. 2018).

3.7.13 Ovarian Cancer

Ovarian cancer is the most lethal gynecological malignancy in women due to the lack of reliable tests for early detection, high rate of recurrence after surgery, and resistance to available therapies. Therefore, there is an urgent need and rationale for novel naturally-occurring chemopreventive agents to reduce the incidence and mortality rates of ovarian cancer, which has been linked to a family history of breast cancer but was also associated with diet as a risk factor (Chang et al. 2007a, b). Pterostilbene in high concentrations (up to 300 μM) repressed cell proliferation via promoting cell cycle arrest in various ovarian cancer cells and showed synergistic antiproliferative effect when used with cisplatin (Wen et al. 2018). Pterostilbene has induced apoptosis through different mechanisms in ovarian cancer cells including the downregulation of antiapoptotic proteins MCL1 and Bcl2 (Wen et al. 2018), deactivation of upstream signaling pathways (Pei et al. 2017), and activation of ROS-mediated mitochondrial apoptosis pathways with activation of caspases 3 and 9 (Dong et al. 2016). Although a number of mouse models for human ovarian cancer have been developed and the preventive effects of genistein, a natural isoflavone, have been shown in clinically relevant spontaneous laying hen model (Sahin et al. 2019), no data is currently available on pterostilbene's effects on the pathogenesis of ovarian cancer in vivo (Table 3.2).

3.7.14 Endometrial Cancer

Endometrial cancer is the most common gynecological cancer. Induction of apoptosis in HTB-111 and Ishikawa cells by pterostilbene was mediated through inhibition of miR-663b, which targeted proapoptotic Bcl2l14 (Wang et al. 2017b). Megestrol acetate is a standard therapy for endometrial cancer patients. Wen et al. reported the potent antiproliferative effect of pterostilbene alone and a synergistic effect using a combination of megestrol acetate and pterostilbene in ECC1 and HEC-1A endometrial cancer cells (Wen et al. 2017). Moreover, oral administration of combined pterostilbene (30 mg/kg) and megestrol acetate (10 mg/kg) resulted in a significant synergistic antitumor effect in s.c. HEC-1A xenograft model (Wen et al. 2017). These data prompted initiation of the first clinical trial with pterostilbene in cancer (www.clinicaltrials.gov).

3.7.15 Other Cancers

Pterostilbene has inhibited growth of cancer cells by inducing cell cycle arrest and apoptosis in gastric cancer (Pan et al. 2007), MMP loss-mediated apoptosis in osteosarcoma (Liu et al. 2013), and autophagy and apoptosis in sensitive and chemoresistant bladder cancer (Chen et al. 2010) (Table 3.2).

3.8 Clinical Trials with Pterostilbene for Cancer Chemoprevention

Pterostilbene as pTeroPure (Chromadex) received GRAS (generally recognized as safe) status from the FDA in 2011. Data from the first human clinical trial with pterostilbene on its effects on cholesterol and blood pressure confirmed the safety of oral doses of twice-daily 125 mg of pTeroPure (Riche et al. 2013). While the available preclinical information so far suggests that pterostilbene-based chemoprevention and combinatorial approaches with chemotherapeutic drugs for therapy may be beneficial for patients, there have been no completed human trials on pterostilbene in cancer. At the time this chapter was submitted, there was only one, the first clinical trial with pterostilbene in cancer recruiting participants for a study on pterostilbene's combination with megestrol acetate in treating patients with endometrial cancer (www.clinicaltrials.gov). Based on the available literature, it appears that trials on prostate, colon, and skin cancer chemoprevention should be a prime focus.

3.9 Conclusions

The presence of significant amounts of pterostilbene in blueberries and in some variety of grapes gives hope for considering dietary pterostilbene as a safe chemoprevention strategy earlier in life in a healthy population. Although pterostilbene's oral bioavailability is higher than resveratrol's, plasma concentrations of dietary pterostilbene might not be sufficient for potent biological effects. Clinical chemoprevention will require the development of natural product drugs for people at high risk and early stage of cancer development and combinatorial treatment strategies for patients at advanced stages. Developing an edible delivery system with enhanced oral bioavailability of pterostilbene is a growing research area. Together with the fact that pterostilbene has a greater tendency to accumulate into tissues due to its much higher lipophilicity compared to resveratrol, the chemopreventive and therapeutic efficacy of pterostilbene seems highly promising.

In vitro data accumulated so far provide substantial support and mechanistic insights into the anticancer potential of pterostilbene in various cancers. More studies using preclinical animal models for particular types of cancer are required for better understanding of the in vivo pharmacokinetic profile and underlying anticancer mechanisms of pterostilbene to provide a strong rationale for clinical trials. There is an evidence that the oral administration of pterostilbene has beneficial effects and no toxicity in humans, however, different optimized pharmaceutical formulations, dosage, delivery systems and combinatorial approaches will be required for particular types and stages of cancer. Future studies are warranted to evaluate the promise of pterostilbene or its derivatives alone and pterostilbene-induced cell sensitization and drug synergism for the efficient management of cancer. The development of pterostilbene as a preventive and therapeutic natural product drug or functional food product may ultimately lead to drastically reduced cancer incidence and better clinical outcomes with improved overall survival rates for patients diagnosed with cancer.

Acknowledgments The writing of this chapter was supported in part by the Department of Defense PCRP under Award W81XWH-13-10370 and the National Cancer Institute of the National Institutes of Health under Award Number R15CA216070 to A.S. Levenson. The content is solely the responsibility of the authors and does not necessarily represent the official views of the Department of Defense or the National Institutes of Health. The authors thank Gabriela Sikorska (LIU Pharmacy) for drawing the chemical structures and Elena V. Levenson for editing the manuscript.

Dedication Dedicated to a dear friend and colleague, the late Dr. Agnes M. Rimando.

This chapter was written ten months after the passing of a dear friend and colleague, Agnes M. Rimando, who died unexpectedly and tragically in the hospital after emergency surgery. She was full of plans for future projects and exciting conferences, and if she were still with us, she would be a co-author of this chapter. In 2002, Agnes M. Rimando was among the first to isolate pterostilbene from blueberries and, in 2004, she was the first to study the antioxidant and chemo-preventive activity of pterostilbene in a cancer model. She understood the potential of pterostilbene as a potent neuromodulator in aging and Alzheimer's, the beneficial effects of pterostilbene in metabolic disorders, including diabetes, and for cancer chemoprevention.

Agnes had a productive career as a medicinal chemist and she understood that in trying to use pterostilbene for disease prevention, including cancer, there needed to be a close collaboration between her and cancer research investigators and clinicians. That is how we began working together in 2010, when I moved from Northwestern University Medical School in Chicago to continue my research in prostate and breast cancer at the newly established Cancer Institute at the University of Mississippi Medical Center, Jackson, MS. Agnes was employed by the United States Department of Agriculture, Agriculture Research Service and was working at the Natural Products Utilization Research Unit, Oxford, MS at the time. We met at a seminar I was giving about my promising studies with resveratrol in cancer, where I pleaded with my audience for collaboration with a medicinal chemist who was interested in anticancer activity of more potent resveratrol analogs. The rest is history.

This book chapter is written testimony to the memory of Dr. Agnes M. Rimando and her dream of using pterostilbene as a chemopreventive agent in cancer.

References

Adlercreutz H (2002) Phyto-oestrogens and cancer. Lancet Oncol 3:364–373

Adrian M, Jeandet P, Douillet-Breuil AC et al (2000) Stilbene content of mature *Vitis vinifera* berries in response to UV-C elicitation. J Agric Food Chem 48:6103–6105

Akhtar N, Bansal JG (2017) Risk factors of lung cancer in nonsmoker. Curr Probl Cancer 41:328–339

Alosi JA, McDonald DE, Schneider JS et al (2010) Pterostilbene inhibits breast cancer in vitro through mitochondrial depolarization and induction of caspase-dependent apoptosis. J Surg Res 161:195–201
Arjungi KN (1976) Areca nut: a review. Arzneimittelforschung 26:951–956
Asensi M, Ortega A, Mena S et al (2011) Natural polyphenols in cancer therapy. Crit Rev Clin Lab Sci 48:197–216
Azar FE, Azami-Aghdash S, Pournaghi-Azar F et al (2017) Cost-effectiveness of lung cancer screening and treatment methods: a systematic review of systematic reviews. BMC Health Serv Res 17:413
Azzolini M, La Spina M, Mattarei A et al (2014) Pharmacokinetics and tissue distribution of pterostilbene in the rat. Mol Nutr Food Res 58:2122–2132
Benlloch M, Obrador E, Valles SL et al (2016) Pterostilbene decreases the antioxidant defenses of aggressive cancer cells in vivo: a physiological glucocorticoids- and Nrf2-dependent mechanism. Antioxid Redox Signal 24:974–990
Birben E, Sahiner UM, Sackesen C et al (2012) Oxidative stress and antioxidant defense. World Allergy Organ J 5:9–19
Bosland MC (2016) Is there a future for chemoprevention of prostate cancer? Cancer Prev Res (Phila) 9:642–647
Brase JC, Johannes M, Schlomm T et al (2011) Circulating miRNAs are correlated with tumor progression in prostate cancer. Int J Cancer 128:608–616
Butt NA, Kumar A, Dhar S et al (2017) Targeting MTA1/HIF-1alpha signaling by pterostilbene in combination with histone deacetylase inhibitor attenuates prostate cancer progression. Cancer Med 6:2673–2685
Chakraborty A, Gupta N, Ghosh K et al (2010) In vitro evaluation of the cytotoxic, anti-proliferative and anti-oxidant properties of pterostilbene isolated from *Pterocarpus marsupium*. Toxicol In Vitro 24:1215–1228
Chakraborty A, Bodipati N, Demonacos MK et al (2012) Long term induction by pterostilbene results in autophagy and cellular differentiation in MCF-7 cells via ROS dependent pathway. Mol Cell Endocrinol 355:25–40
Chakraborty S, Kumar A, Butt NA et al (2016) Molecular insight into the differential anti-androgenic activity of resveratrol and its natural analogs: in silico approach to understand biological actions. Mol BioSyst 12:1702–1709
Chang ET, Canchola AJ, Lee VS et al (2007a) Wine and other alcohol consumption and risk of ovarian cancer in the California Teachers Study cohort. Cancer Causes Control 18:91–103
Chang ET, Lee VS, Canchola AJ et al (2007b) Diet and risk of ovarian cancer in the California Teachers Study cohort. Am J Epidemiol 165:802–813
Chang J, Rimando A, Pallas M et al (2012) Low-dose pterostilbene, but not resveratrol, is a potent neuromodulator in aging and Alzheimer's disease. Neurobiol Aging 33:2062–2071
Chang G, Xiao W, Xu Z et al (2017) Pterostilbene induces cell apoptosis and cell cycle arrest in T-Cell Leukemia/Lymphoma by suppressing the ERK1/2 pathway. Biomed Res Int 2017:9872073
Charvey-Faury S, Derbesy M, Cochini F et al (1998) Sandalwood extract (*Pterocarpus santalinus*): anti-oxidant and anti-UV effects study. Riv Ital EPPOS spec. no.:435–458
Chatterjee K, AlSharif D, Mazza C et al (2018) Resveratrol and pterostilbene exhibit anticancer properties involving the downregulation of HPV Oncoprotein E6 in cervical cancer cells. Nutrients 10(2). https://doi.org/10.3390/nu10020243
Chau CH, Price DK, Till C et al (2015) Finasteride concentrations and prostate cancer risk: results from the prostate cancer prevention trial. PLoS One 10:e0126672
Chen RJ, Ho CT, Wang YJ (2010) Pterostilbene induces autophagy and apoptosis in sensitive and chemoresistant human bladder cancer cells. Mol Nutr Food Res 54:1819–1832
Chen RJ, Tsai SJ, Ho CT et al (2012) Chemopreventive effects of pterostilbene on urethane-induced lung carcinogenesis in mice via the inhibition of EGFR-mediated pathways and the induction of apoptosis and autophagy. J Agric Food Chem 60:11533–11541

Chen WC, Hsu KY, Hung CM et al (2014) The anti-tumor efficiency of pterostilbene is promoted with a combined treatment of Fas signaling or autophagy inhibitors in triple negative breast cancer cells. Food Funct 5:1856–1865
Chen G, Xu Z, Chang G et al (2017a) The blueberry component pterostilbene has potent anti-myeloma activity in bortezomib-resistant cells. Oncol Rep 38:488–496
Chen RJ, Wu PH, Ho CT et al (2017b) P53-dependent downregulation of hTERT protein expression and telomerase activity induces senescence in lung cancer cells as a result of pterostilbene treatment. Cell Death Dis 8:e2985
Chikara S, Nagaprashantha LD, Singhal J et al (2018) Oxidative stress and dietary phytochemicals: Role in cancer chemoprevention and treatment. Cancer Lett 413:122–134
Chiou YS, Tsai ML, Wang YJ et al (2010) Pterostilbene inhibits colorectal aberrant crypt foci (ACF) and colon carcinogenesis via suppression of multiple signal transduction pathways in azoxymethane-treated mice. J Agric Food Chem 58:8833–8841
Chiou YS, Tsai ML, Nagabhushanam K et al (2011) Pterostilbene is more potent than resveratrol in preventing azoxymethane (AOM)-induced colon tumorigenesis via activation of the NF-E2-related factor 2 (Nrf2)-mediated antioxidant signaling pathway. J Agric Food Chem 59:2725–2733
Cichocki M, Paluszczak J, Szaefer H et al (2008) Pterostilbene is equally potent as resveratrol in inhibiting 12-O-tetradecanoylphorbol-13-acetate activated NFkappaB, AP-1, COX-2, and iNOS in mouse epidermis. Mol Nutr Food Res 52(Suppl 1):S62–S70
Curran EK, Godfrey J, Kline J (2017) Mechanisms of immune tolerance in leukemia and lymphoma. Trends Immunol 38:513–525
Daniel M, Tollefsbol TO (2018) Pterostilbene down-regulates hTERT at physiological concentrations in breast cancer cells: potentially through the inhibition of cMyc. J Cell Biochem 119:3326–3337
Deng L, Li Y, Zhang X et al (2015) UPLC-MS method for quantification of pterostilbene and its application to comparative study of bioavailability and tissue distribution in normal and Lewis lung carcinoma bearing mice. J Pharm Biomed Anal 114:200–207
Dhar S, Hicks C, Levenson AS (2011) Resveratrol and prostate cancer: promising role for microRNAs. Mol Nutr Food Res 55:1219–1229
Dhar S, Kumar A, Li K et al (2015a) Resveratrol regulates PTEN/Akt pathway through inhibition of MTA1/HDAC unit of the NuRD complex in prostate cancer. Biochim Biophys Acta 1853:265–275
Dhar S, Kumar A, Rimando AM et al (2015b) Resveratrol and pterostilbene epigenetically restore PTEN expression by targeting oncomiRs of the miR-17 family in prostate cancer. Oncotarget 6 (29):27214–27226
Dhar S, Kumar A, Zhang L et al (2016) Dietary pterostilbene is a novel MTA1-targeted chemopreventive and therapeutic agent in prostate cancer. Oncotarget 7:18469–18484
Dias SJ, Li K, Rimando AM et al (2013a) Trimethoxy-resveratrol and piceatannol administered orally suppress and inhibit tumor formation and growth in prostate cancer xenografts. Prostate 73:1135–1146
Dias SJ, Zhou X, Ivanovic M et al (2013b) Nuclear MTA1 overexpression is associated with aggressive prostate cancer, recurrence and metastasis in African Americans. Sci Rep 3:2331
DiDonato JA, Mercurio F, Karin M (2012) NF-kappaB and the link between inflammation and cancer. Immunol Rev 246:379–400
Dong J, Guo H, Chen Y (2016) Pterostilbene induces apoptosis through caspase activation in ovarian cancer cells. Eur J Gynaecol Oncol 37:342–347
Dvorakova M, Landa P (2017) Anti-inflammatory activity of natural stilbenoids: a review. Pharmacol Res 124:126–145
Erasalo H, Hamalainen M, Leppanen T et al (2018) Natural stilbenoids have anti-inflammatory properties in vivo and down-regulate the production of inflammatory mediators NO, IL6, and MCP1 possibly in a PI3K/Akt-dependent manner. J Nat Prod 81:1131–1142

Estrela JM, Asensi A (2010). Pterostilbene (Pter) for the prevention and/or treatment of skin diseases
Estrela JM, Ortega A, Mena S et al (2013) Pterostilbene: biomedical applications. Crit Rev Clin Lab Sci 50:65–78
Feng Y, Yang Y, Fan C et al (2016) Pterostilbene inhibits the growth of human esophageal cancer cells by regulating endoplasmic reticulum stress. Cell Physiol Biochem 38:1226–1244
Ferrer P, Asensi M, Segarra R et al (2005) Association between pterostilbene and quercetin inhibits metastatic activity of B16 melanoma. Neoplasia 7:37–47
Ferrer P, Asensi M, Priego S et al (2007) Nitric oxide mediates natural polyphenol-induced Bcl-2 down-regulation and activation of cell death in metastatic B16 melanoma. J Biol Chem 282:2880–2890
Fuendjiep V, Wandji J, Tillequin F et al (2002) Chalconoid and stilbenoid glycosides from Guibourtia tessmanii. Phytochemistry 60:803–806
Gambini J, Ingles M, Olaso G et al (2015) Properties of resveratrol: in vitro and in vivo studies about metabolism, bioavailability, and biological effects in animal models and humans. Oxidative Med Cell Longev 2015:837042
Gao Y, Tollefsbol TO (2015) Impact of epigenetic dietary components on cancer through histone modifications. Curr Med Chem 22:2051–2064
Gao D, Jing S, Zhang Q et al (2018) Pterostilbene protects against acute renal ischemia reperfusion injury and inhibits oxidative stress, inducible nitric oxide synthase expression and inflammation in rats via the Toll-like receptor 4/nuclear factor-kappaB signaling pathway. Exp Ther Med 15:1029–1035
Gehm BD, Levenson AS (2006) Resveratrol as a phytoestrogen. In: Aggarwal BB, Shishodia S (eds) Resveratrol in health and disease. Taylor & Francis, Boca Raton, FL, pp 439–464
Guo L, Tan K, Wang H et al (2016) Pterostilbene inhibits hepatocellular carcinoma through p53/SOD2/ROS-mediated mitochondrial apoptosis. Oncol Rep 36:3233–3240
Hagiwara K, Kosaka N, Yoshioka Y et al (2012) Stilbene derivatives promote Ago2-dependent tumour-suppressive microRNA activity. Sci Rep 2:314
Hardy TM, Tollefsbol TO (2011) Epigenetic diet: impact on the epigenome and cancer. Epigenomics 3:503–518
Harun Z, Ghazali AR (2012) Potential chemoprevention activity of pterostilbene by enhancing the detoxifying enzymes in the HT-29 cell line. Asian Pac J Cancer Prev 13:6403–6407
Hofer MD, Kuefer R, Varambally S et al (2004) The role of metastasis-associated protein 1 in prostate cancer progression. Cancer Res 64:825–829
Hong BH, Wu CH, Yeh CT et al (2013) Invadopodia-associated proteins blockade as a novel mechanism for 6-shogaol and pterostilbene to reduce breast cancer cell motility and invasion. Mol Nutr Food Res 57:886–895
Hong Bin W, Da LH, Xue Y et al (2018) Pterostilbene (3′,5′-dimethoxy-resveratrol) exerts potent antitumor effects in HeLa human cervical cancer cells via disruption of mitochondrial membrane potential, apoptosis induction and targeting m-TOR/PI3K/Akt signalling pathway. J BUON 23:1384–1389
Hsiao PC, Chou YE, Tan P et al (2014) Pterostilbene simultaneously induced G0/G1-phase arrest and MAPK-mediated mitochondrial-derived apoptosis in human acute myeloid leukemia cell lines. PLoS One 9:e105342
Hsieh MJ, Lin CW, Yang SF et al (2014a) A combination of pterostilbene with autophagy inhibitors exerts efficient apoptotic characteristics in both chemosensitive and chemoresistant lung cancer cells. Toxicol Sci 137:65–75
Hsieh MT, Chen HP, Lu CC et al (2014b) The novel pterostilbene derivative ANK-199 induces autophagic cell death through regulating PI3 kinase class III/beclin 1/Atgrelated proteins in cisplatinresistant CAR human oral cancer cells. Int J Oncol 45:782–794
Hsieh MT, Huang LJ, Wu TS et al (2018) Synthesis and antitumor activity of bis(hydroxymethyl) propionate analogs of pterostilbene in cisplatin-resistant human oral cancer cells. Bioorg Med Chem 26:3909–3916

Hsu CL, Lin YJ, Ho CT et al (2013) The inhibitory effect of pterostilbene on inflammatory responses during the interaction of 3T3-L1 adipocytes and RAW 264.7 macrophages. J Agric Food Chem 61:602–610
Huang J, Plass C, Gerhauser C (2011) Cancer chemoprevention by targeting the epigenome. Curr Drug Targets 12:1925–1956
Huang CS, Ho CT, Tu SH et al (2013) Long-term ethanol exposure-induced hepatocellular carcinoma cell migration and invasion through lysyl oxidase activation are attenuated by combined treatment with pterostilbene and curcumin analogues. J Agric Food Chem 61:4326–4335
Huang XY, Zhang SZ, Wang WX (2014) Enhanced antitumor efficacy with combined administration of astragalus and pterostilbene for melanoma. Asian Pac J Cancer Prev 15:1163–1169
Huang WC, Chan ML, Chen MJ et al (2016) Modulation of macrophage polarization and lung cancer cell stemness by MUC1 and development of a related small-molecule inhibitor pterostilbene. Oncotarget 7:39363–39375
Huang Y, Du J, Mi Y et al (2018) Long Non-coding RNAs contribute to the inhibition of proliferation and EMT by pterostilbene in human breast cancer. Front Oncol 8:629
Hung CM, Liu LC, Ho CT et al (2017) Pterostilbene enhances TRAIL-induced apoptosis through the induction of death receptors and downregulation of cell survival proteins in TRAIL-resistance triple negative breast cancer cells. J Agric Food Chem 65:11179–11191
Huynh TT, Lin CM, Lee WH et al (2015) Pterostilbene suppressed irradiation-resistant glioma stem cells by modulating GRP78/miR-205 axis. J Nutr Biochem 26:466–475
Jang M, Cai L, Udeani GO et al (1997) Cancer chemopreventive activity of resveratrol, a natural product derived from grapes. Science 275:218–220
Joseph JA, Fisher DR, Cheng V et al (2008) Cellular and behavioral effects of stilbene resveratrol analogues: implications for reducing the deleterious effects of aging. J Agric Food Chem 56:10544–10551
Kai L, Levenson AS (2011) Combination of resveratrol and antiandrogen flutamide has synergistic effect on androgen receptor inhibition in prostate cancer cells. Anticancer Res 31:3323–3330
Kai L, Samuel SK, Levenson AS (2010) Resveratrol enhances p53 acetylation and apoptosis in prostate cancer by inhibiting MTA1/NuRD complex. Int J Cancer 126:1538–1548
Kai L, Wang J, Ivanovic M et al (2011) Targeting prostate cancer angiogenesis through metastasis-associated protein 1 (MTA1). Prostate 71:268–280
Kala R, Tollefsbol TO (2016) A novel combinatorial epigenetic therapy using resveratrol and pterostilbene for restoring estrogen receptor-alpha (ERalpha) expression in ERalpha-negative breast cancer cells. PLoS One 11:e0155057
Kala R, Shah HN, Martin SL et al (2015) Epigenetic-based combinatorial resveratrol and pterostilbene alters DNA damage response by affecting SIRT1 and DNMT enzyme expression, including SIRT1-dependent gamma-H2AX and telomerase regulation in triple-negative breast cancer. BMC Cancer 15:672
Kapetanovic IM, Muzzio M, Huang Z et al (2011) Pharmacokinetics, oral bioavailability, and metabolic profile of resveratrol and its dimethylether analog, pterostilbene, in rats. Cancer Chemother Pharmacol 68:593–601
Khromova NV, Kopnin PB, Stepanova EV et al (2009) p53 hot-spot mutants increase tumor vascularization via ROS-mediated activation of the HIF1/VEGF-A pathway. Cancer Lett 276:143–151
Kim J, Koyanagi T, Mochly-Rosen D (2011) PKCdelta activation mediates angiogenesis via NADPH oxidase activity in PC-3 prostate cancer cells. Prostate 71:946–954
Ko HS, Kim JS, Cho SM et al (2014) Urokinase-type plasminogen activator expression and Rac1/WAVE-2/Arp2/3 pathway are blocked by pterostilbene to suppress cell migration and invasion in MDA-MB-231 cells. Bioorg Med Chem Lett 24:1176–1179
Ko CP, Lin CW, Chen MK et al (2015) Pterostilbene induce autophagy on human oral cancer cells through modulation of Akt and mitogen-activated protein kinase pathway. Oral Oncol 51:593–601

Kong Y, Chen G, Xu Z et al (2016) Pterostilbene induces apoptosis and cell cycle arrest in diffuse large B-cell lymphoma cells. Sci Rep 6:37417

Kostin SF, McDonald DE, McFadden DW (2012) Inhibitory effects of (-)-epigallocatechin-3-gallate and pterostilbene on pancreatic cancer growth in vitro. J Surg Res 177:255–262

Kosuru R, Rai U, Prakash S et al (2016) Promising therapeutic potential of pterostilbene and its mechanistic insight based on preclinical evidence. Eur J Pharmacol 789:229–243

Kou X, Kirberger M, Yang Y et al (2013) Natural products for cancer prevention associated with Nrf2–ARE pathway. Food Sci Hum Wellness 2:22–28

Kumar A, Levenson AS (2018) Epigenetic mechanisms of resveratrol and its analogs in cancer prevention and treatment. In: Bishayee A, Bhatia D (eds) Epigenetics of cancer prevention. Academic, London, pp 169–186

Kumar R, Wang RA, Bagheri-Yarmand R (2003) Emerging roles of MTA family members in human cancers. Semin Oncol 30:30–37

Kumar A, Lin SY, Dhar S et al (2014) Stilbenes inhibit androgen receptor expression in 22Rv1 castrate-resistant prostate cancer cells. J Med Active Plants 3:1–8

Kumar A, Dhar S, Rimando AM et al (2015) Epigenetic potential of resveratrol and analogs in preclinical models of prostate cancer. Ann N Y Acad Sci 1348:1–9

Kumar A, Butt NA, Levenson AS (2016) Natural epigenetic-modifying molecules in medical therapy. In: Tollefsbol T (ed) Medical epigenetics. Elsevier, London, pp 747–798

Kumar A, Rimando AM, Levenson AS (2017) Resveratrol and pterostilbene as a microRNA-mediated chemopreventive and therapeutic strategy in prostate cancer. Ann N Y Acad Sci 1403:15–26

Langcake P, Cornford CA, Pryce RJ (1979) Identification of pterostilbene as a phytoalexin from *Vitis vinifera* leaves. Phytochemistry 18:1025–1027

Lange KW, Li S (2018) Resveratrol, pterostilbene, and dementia. Biofactors 44:83–90

Lau A, Villeneuve NF, Sun Z et al (2008) Dual roles of Nrf2 in cancer. Pharmacol Res 58:262–270

Lee SR, Yang KS, Kwon J et al (2002) Reversible inactivation of the tumor suppressor PTEN by H2O2. J Biol Chem 277:20336–20342

Lee H, Kim Y, Jeong JH et al (2016) ATM/CHK/p53 pathway dependent chemopreventive and therapeutic activity on lung cancer by pterostilbene. PLoS One 11:e0162335

Levenson AS, Kumar A, Zhang X (2014) MTA family of proteins in prostate cancer: biology, significance, and therapeutic opportunities. Cancer Metastasis Rev 33:929–942

Li K, Dias SJ, Rimando AM et al (2013) Pterostilbene acts through metastasis-associated protein 1 to inhibit tumor growth, progression and metastasis in prostate cancer. PLoS One 8:e57542

Li J, Ruzhi D, Hua X et al (2016) Blueberry component pterostilbene protects corneal epithelial cells from inflammation via anti-oxidative pathway. Sci Rep 6:19408

Lin HS, Ho PC (2009) A rapid HPLC method for the quantification of 3,5,4′-trimethoxy-trans-stilbene (TMS) in rat plasma and its application in pharmacokinetic study. J Pharm Biomed Anal 49:387–392

Lin HS, Yue BD, Ho PC (2009) Determination of pterostilbene in rat plasma by a simple HPLC-UV method and its application in pre-clinical pharmacokinetic study. Biomed Chromatogr 23:1308–1315

Lin VC, Tsai YC, Lin JN et al (2012) Activation of AMPK by pterostilbene suppresses lipogenesis and cell-cycle progression in p53 positive and negative human prostate cancer cells. J Agric Food Chem 60:6399–6407

Lin CW, Chou YE, Chiou HL et al (2014) Pterostilbene suppresses oral cancer cell invasion by inhibiting MMP-2 expression. Expert Opin Ther Targets 18:1109–1120

Link A, Balaguer F, Goel A (2010) Cancer chemoprevention by dietary polyphenols: promising role for epigenetics. Biochem Pharmacol 80:1771–1792

Liu Y, Wang L, Wu Y et al (2013) Pterostilbene exerts antitumor activity against human osteosarcoma cells by inhibiting the JAK2/STAT3 signaling pathway. Toxicology 304:120–131

Liu J, Fan C, Yu L et al (2016) Pterostilbene exerts an anti-inflammatory effect via regulating endoplasmic reticulum stress in endothelial cells. Cytokine 77:88–97

Liu F, Yang X, Geng M et al (2018) Targeting ERK, an Achilles' Heel of the MAPK pathway, in cancer therapy. Acta Pharm Sin B 8:552–562

Lombardi G, Vannini S, Blasi F et al (2015) In vitro safety/protection assessment of resveratrol and pterostilbene in a Human Hepatoma Cell Line (HepG2). Nat Prod Commun 10:1403–1408

Ma Q, He X (2012) Molecular basis of electrophilic and oxidative defense: promises and perils of Nrf2. Pharmacol Rev 64:1055–1081

Ma X, Zhang J, Liu S et al (2012) Nrf2 knockdown by shRNA inhibits tumor growth and increases efficacy of chemotherapy in cervical cancer. Cancer Chemother Pharmacol 69:485–494

Ma Z, Yang Y, Di S et al (2017) Pterostilbene exerts anticancer activity on non-small-cell lung cancer via activating endoplasmic reticulum stress. Sci Rep 7:8091

Mak KK, Wu AT, Lee WH et al (2013) Pterostilbene, a bioactive component of blueberries, suppresses the generation of breast cancer stem cells within tumor microenvironment and metastasis via modulating NF-kappaB/microRNA 448 circuit. Mol Nutr Food Res 57:1123–1134

Mannal P, McDonald D, McFadden D (2010a) Pterostilbene and tamoxifen show an additive effect against breast cancer in vitro. Am J Surg 200:577–580

Mannal PW, Alosi JA, Schneider JG, McDonald DE, McFadden DW (2010b) Pterostilbene inhibits pancreatic cancer in vitro. J Gastrointest Surg 14(5):873–879

Maurya R, Ray AB, Duah FK et al (1984) Constituents of *Pterocarpus marsupium*. J Nat Prod 47:179–181

Maurya R, Singh R, Deepak M et al (2004) Constituents of *Pterocarpus marsupium*: an ayurvedic crude drug. Phytochemistry 65:915–920

McCormack D, McFadden D (2012) Pterostilbene and cancer: current review. J Surg Res 173: e53–e61

McCormack D, Schneider J, McDonald D et al (2011) The antiproliferative effects of pterostilbene on breast cancer in vitro are via inhibition of constitutive and leptin-induced Janus kinase/signal transducer and activator of transcription activation. Am J Surg 202:541–544

McCormack DE, Mannal P, McDonald D et al (2012) Genomic analysis of pterostilbene predicts its antiproliferative effects against pancreatic cancer in vitro and in vivo. J Gastrointest Surg 16:1136–1143

Mei H, Xiang Y, Mei H et al (2018) Pterostilbene inhibits nutrient metabolism and induces apoptosis through AMPK activation in multiple myeloma cells. Int J Mol Med 42:2676–2688

Mena S, Rodriguez ML, Ponsoda X et al (2012) Pterostilbene-induced tumor cytotoxicity: a lysosomal membrane permeabilization-dependent mechanism. PLoS One 7:e44524

Mitchell SH, Zhu W, Young CY (1999) Resveratrol inhibits the expression and function of the androgen receptor in LNCaP prostate cancer cells. Cancer Res 59:5892–5895

Moon D, McCormack D, McDonald D et al (2013) Pterostilbene induces mitochondrially derived apoptosis in breast cancer cells in vitro. J Surg Res 180:208–215

Moyad MA, Carroll PR (2004a) Lifestyle recommendations to prevent prostate cancer, part I: time to redirect our attention? Urol Clin North Am 31:289–300

Moyad MA, Carroll PR (2004b) Lifestyle recommendations to prevent prostate cancer, part II: time to redirect our attention? Urol Clin North Am 31:301–311

Nikhil K, Sharan S, Chakraborty A et al (2014a) Role of isothiocyanate conjugate of pterostilbene on the inhibition of MCF-7 cell proliferation and tumor growth in Ehrlich ascitic cell induced tumor bearing mice. Exp Cell Res 320:311–328

Nikhil K, Sharan S, Chakraborty A et al (2014b) Pterostilbene-isothiocyanate conjugate suppresses growth of prostate cancer cells irrespective of androgen receptor status. PLoS One 9:e93335

Nikhil K, Sharan S, Singh AK et al (2014c) Anticancer activities of pterostilbene-isothiocyanate conjugate in breast cancer cells: involvement of PPARgamma. PLoS One 9:e104592

Nutakul W, Sobers HS, Qiu P et al (2011) Inhibitory effects of resveratrol and pterostilbene on human colon cancer cells: a side-by-side comparison. J Agric Food Chem 59:10964–10970

Pan MH, Chang YH, Badmaev V et al (2007) Pterostilbene induces apoptosis and cell cycle arrest in human gastric carcinoma cells. J Agric Food Chem 55:7777–7785

Pan MH, Chang YH, Tsai ML et al (2008) Pterostilbene suppressed lipopolysaccharide-induced up-expression of iNOS and COX-2 in murine macrophages. J Agric Food Chem 56:7502–7509

Pan MH, Chiou YS, Chen WJ et al (2009) Pterostilbene inhibited tumor invasion via suppressing multiple signal transduction pathways in human hepatocellular carcinoma cells. Carcinogenesis 30:1234–1242

Pan MH, Lin YT, Lin CL et al (2011) Suppression of Heregulin-beta1/HER2-Modulated Invasive and Aggressive Phenotype of Breast Carcinoma by Pterostilbene via Inhibition of Matrix Metalloproteinase-9, p38 Kinase Cascade and Akt Activation. Evid Based Complement Alternat Med 2011:562187

Pan C, Hu Y, Li J et al (2014) Estrogen receptor-alpha36 is involved in pterostilbene-induced apoptosis and anti-proliferation in in vitro and in vivo breast cancer. PLoS One 9:e104459

Papandreou I, Verras M, McNeil B et al (2015) Plant stilbenes induce endoplasmic reticulum stress and their anti-cancer activity can be enhanced by inhibitors of autophagy. Exp Cell Res 339:147–153

Paul B, Masih I, Deopujari J et al (1999) Occurrence of resveratrol and pterostilbene in age-old darakchasava, an ayurvedic medicine from India. J Ethnopharmacol 68:71–76

Paul S, Rimando AM, Lee HJ et al (2009) Anti-inflammatory action of pterostilbene is mediated through the p38 mitogen-activated protein kinase pathway in colon cancer cells. Cancer Prev Res (Phila) 2:650–657

Paul S, DeCastro AJ, Lee HJ et al (2010) Dietary intake of pterostilbene, a constituent of blueberries, inhibits the beta-catenin/p65 downstream signaling pathway and colon carcinogenesis in rats. Carcinogenesis 31:1272–1278

Pei HL, Mu DM, Zhang B (2017) Anticancer activity of pterostilbene in human ovarian cancer cell lines. Med Sci Monit 23:3192–3199

Pezet R, Pont V (1988) Demonstration of pterostilbene in clusters of *Vitis vinifera*. Plant Physiol Biochem (Paris) 26:603–607

Priego S, Feddi F, Ferrer P et al (2008) Natural polyphenols facilitate elimination of HT-29 colorectal cancer xenografts by chemoradiotherapy: a Bcl-2- and superoxide dismutase 2-dependent mechanism. Mol Cancer Ther 7:3330–3342

Pudenz M, Roth K, Gerhauser C (2014) Impact of soy isoflavones on the epigenome in cancer prevention. Nutrients 6:4218–4272

Qian YY, Liu ZS, Pan DY et al (2017) Tumoricidal activities of pterostilbene depend upon destabilizing the MTA1-NuRD complex and enhancing P53 acetylation in hepatocellular carcinoma. Exp Ther Med 14:3098–3104

Qian YY, Liu ZS, Yan HJ et al (2018a) Pterostilbene inhibits MTA1/HDAC1 complex leading to PTEN acetylation in hepatocellular carcinoma. Biomed Pharmacother 101:852–859

Qian YY, Liu ZS, Zhang Z et al (2018b) Pterostilbene increases PTEN expression through the targeted downregulation of microRNA-19a in hepatocellular carcinoma. Mol Med Rep 17:5193–5201

Rajagopal C, Lankadasari MB, Aranjani JM et al (2018) Targeting oncogenic transcription factors by polyphenols: a novel approach for cancer therapy. Pharmacol Res 130:273–291

Ramezani G, Pourgheysari B, Shirzad H et al (2019) Pterostilbene increases Fas expression in T-lymphoblastic leukemia cell lines. Res Pharm Sci 14:55–63

Remsberg CM, Yanez JA, Ohgami Y et al (2008) Pharmacometrics of pterostilbene: preclinical pharmacokinetics and metabolism, anticancer, antiinflammatory, antioxidant and analgesic activity. Phytother Res 22:169–179

Riche DM, McEwen CL, Riche KD et al (2013) Analysis of safety from a human clinical trial with pterostilbene. J Toxicol 2013:463595

Rimando AM, Barney DL (2005) Resveratrol and naturally occurring analogues in *Vaccinium* species. Acta Hort 680:137–143

Rimando AM, Cuendet M, Desmarchelier C et al (2002) Cancer chemopreventive and antioxidant activities of pterostilbene, a naturally occurring analogue of resveratrol. J Agric Food Chem 50:3453–3457

Rimando AM, Kalt W, Magee JB et al (2004) Resveratrol, pterostilbene, and piceatannol in vaccinium berries. J Agric Food Chem 52:4713–4719
Robb EL, Stuart JA (2014) The stilbenes resveratrol, pterostilbene and piceid affect growth and stress resistance in mammalian cells via a mechanism requiring estrogen receptor beta and the induction of Mn-superoxide dismutase. Phytochemistry 98:164–173
Rodriguez-Bonilla P, Lopez-Nicolas JM, Mendez-Cazorla L et al (2011) Development of a reversed phase high performance liquid chromatography method based on the use of cyclodextrins as mobile phase additives to determine pterostilbene in blueberries. J Chromatogr B Analyt Technol Biomed Life Sci 879:1091–1097
Roslie H, Chan KM, Rajab NF et al (2012) 3,5-dibenzyloxy-4′-hydroxystilbene induces early caspase-9 activation during apoptosis in human K562 chronic myelogenous leukemia cells. J Toxicol Sci 37:13–21
Ross SA, Davis CD (2011) MicroRNA, nutrition, and cancer prevention. Adv Nutr 2:472–485
Sahin K, Yenice E, Bilir B et al (2019) Genistein prevents development of spontaneous ovarian cancer and inhibits tumor growth in hen model. Cancer Prev Res (Phila) 12:135–146
Schmidt L, Baskaran S, Johansson P et al (2016) Case-specific potentiation of glioblastoma drugs by pterostilbene. Oncotarget 7:73200–73215
Schneider JG, Alosi JA, McDonald DE et al (2009) Effects of pterostilbene on melanoma alone and in synergy with inositol hexaphosphate. Am J Surg 198:679–684
Schneider JG, Alosi JA, McDonald DE, McFadden DW (2010) Pterostilbene inhibits lung cancer through induction of apoptosis. J Surg Res 161(1):18–22
Scott E, Steward WP, Gescher AJ et al (2012) Resveratrol in human cancer chemoprevention-choosing the 'right' dose. Mol Nutr Food Res 56:7–13
Seo SS, Oh HY, Lee JK et al (2016) Combined effect of diet and cervical microbiome on the risk of cervical intraepithelial neoplasia. Clin Nutr 35:1434–1441
Seshadri TR (1972) Polyphenols of Pterocarpus and Dalbergia woods. Phytochemistry 11:881–898
Shao X, Chen X, Badmaev V et al (2010) Structural identification of mouse urinary metabolites of pterostilbene using liquid chromatography/tandem mass spectrometry. Rapid Commun Mass Spectrom 24:1770–1778
Shen H, Rong H (2015) Pterostilbene impact on retinal endothelial cells under high glucose environment. Int J Clin Exp Pathol 8:12589–12594
Shetty SR, Babu S, Kumari S et al (2013) Salivary ascorbic acid levels in betel quid chewers: a biochemical study. South Asian J Cancer 2:142–144
Siedlecka-Kroplewska K, Jozwik A, Kaszubowska L et al (2012) Pterostilbene induces cell cycle arrest and apoptosis in MOLT4 human leukemia cells. Folia Histochem Cytobiol 50:574–580
Siedlecka-Kroplewska K, Jozwik A, Boguslawski W et al (2013) Pterostilbene induces accumulation of autophagic vacuoles followed by cell death in HL60 human leukemia cells. J Physiol Pharmacol 64:545–556
Song Z, Han S, Pan X et al (2015) Pterostilbene mediates neuroprotection against oxidative toxicity via oestrogen receptor alpha signalling pathways. J Pharm Pharmacol 67:720–730
Storniolo CE, Moreno JJ (2019) Resveratrol analogs with antioxidant activity inhibit intestinal epithelial cancer Caco-2 cell growth by modulating arachidonic acid cascade. J Agric Food Chem 67:819–828
Su CM, Lee WH, Wu AT et al (2015) Pterostilbene inhibits triple-negative breast cancer metastasis via inducing microRNA-205 expression and negatively modulates epithelial-to-mesenchymal transition. J Nutr Biochem 26:675–685
Suh N, Paul S, Hao X et al (2007) Pterostilbene, an active constituent of blueberries, suppresses aberrant crypt foci formation in the azoxymethane-induced colon carcinogenesis model in rats. Clin Cancer Res 13:350–355
Sun Y, Wu X, Cai X et al (2016) Identification of pinostilbene as a major colonic metabolite of pterostilbene and its inhibitory effects on colon cancer cells. Mol Nutr Food Res 60:1924–1932
Tam KW, Ho CT, Tu SH et al (2018) alpha-Tocopherol succinate enhances pterostilbene anti-tumor activity in human breast cancer cells in vivo and in vitro. Oncotarget 9:4593–4606

Tili E, Michaille JJ (2011) Resveratrol, MicroRNAs, inflammation, and cancer. J Nucleic Acids 2011:102431
Tippani R, Prakhya LJ, Porika M et al (2014) Pterostilbene as a potential novel telomerase inhibitor: molecular docking studies and its in vitro evaluation. Curr Pharm Biotechnol 14:1027–1035
Toh Y, Nicolson GL (2009) The role of the MTA family and their encoded proteins in human cancers: molecular functions and clinical implications. Clin Exp Metastasis 26:215–227
Tolba MF, Abdel-Rahman SZ (2015) Pterostilbine, an active component of blueberries, sensitizes colon cancer cells to 5-fluorouracil cytotoxicity. Sci Rep 5:15239
Tolomeo M, Grimaudo S, Di Cristina A et al (2005) Pterostilbene and 3′-hydroxypterostilbene are effective apoptosis-inducing agents in MDR and BCR-ABL-expressing leukemia cells. Int J Biochem Cell Biol 37:1709–1726
Tota JE, Anderson WF, Coffey C et al (2017) Rising incidence of oral tongue cancer among white men and women in the United States, 1973–2012. Oral Oncol 67:146–152
Tsai ML, Lai CS, Chang YH et al (2012) Pterostilbene, a natural analogue of resveratrol, potently inhibits 7,12-dimethylbenz[a]anthracene (DMBA)/12-O-tetradecanoylphorbol-13-acetate (TPA)-induced mouse skin carcinogenesis. Food Funct 3:1185–1194
Tsai HY, Ho CT, Chen YK (2017) Biological actions and molecular effects of resveratrol, pterostilbene, and 3′-hydroxypterostilbene. J Food Drug Anal 25:134–147
Vanden Berghe W (2012) Epigenetic impact of dietary polyphenols in cancer chemoprevention: lifelong remodeling of our epigenomes. Pharmacol Res 65:565–576
Wakimoto R, Ono M, Takeshima M et al (2017) Differential Anticancer Activity of Pterostilbene Against Three Subtypes of Human Breast Cancer Cells. Anticancer Res 37:6153–6159
Wang TT, Schoene NW, Kim YS et al (2010) Differential effects of resveratrol and its naturally occurring methylether analogs on cell cycle and apoptosis in human androgen-responsive LNCaP cancer cells. Mol Nutr Food Res 54:335–344
Wang Y, Ding L, Wang X et al (2012) Pterostilbene simultaneously induces apoptosis, cell cycle arrest and cyto-protective autophagy in breast cancer cells. Am J Transl Res 4:44–51
Wang YJ, Lin JF, Cheng LH et al (2017a) Pterostilbene prevents AKT-ERK axis-mediated polymerization of surface fibronectin on suspended lung cancer cells independently of apoptosis and suppresses metastasis. J Hematol Oncol 10:72
Wang YL, Shen Y, Xu JP et al (2017b) Pterostilbene suppresses human endometrial cancer cells in vitro by down-regulating miR-663b. Acta Pharmacol Sin 38:1394–1400
Wawszczyk J, Kapral M, Hollek A et al (2014) In vitro evaluation of antiproliferative and cytotoxic properties of pterostilbene against human colon cancer cells. Acta Pol Pharm 71:1051–1055
Wen W, Lowe G, Roberts CM et al (2017) Pterostilbene, a natural phenolic compound, synergizes the antineoplastic effects of megestrol acetate in endometrial cancer. Sci Rep 7:12754
Wen W, Lowe G, Roberts CM et al (2018) Pterostilbene suppresses ovarian cancer growth via induction of apoptosis and blockade of cell cycle progression involving inhibition of the STAT3 pathway. Int J Mol Sci 19(7). https://doi.org/10.3390/ijms19071983
Wenzel E, Somoza V (2005) Metabolism and bioavailability of trans-resveratrol. Mol Nutr Food Res 49:472–481
Wiseman H, Halliwell B (1996) Damage to DNA by reactive oxygen and nitrogen species: role in inflammatory disease and progression to cancer. Biochem J 313(Pt 1):17–29
Wu CH, Hong BH, Ho CT et al (2015) Targeting cancer stem cells in breast cancer: potential anticancer properties of 6-shogaol and pterostilbene. J Agric Food Chem 63:2432–2441
Xie B, Xu Z, Hu L et al (2016) Pterostilbene inhibits human multiple myeloma cells via ERK1/2 and JNK pathway in vitro and in vivo. Int J Mol Sci 17
Xing F, Liu Y, Sharma S, Wu K, Chan MD, Lo H-W, Carpenter RL, Metheny-Barlow LJ, Zhou X, Qasem SA, Pasche B, Watabe K (2016) Activation of the c-Met pathway mobilizes an inflammatory network in the brain microenvironment to promote brain metastasis of breast cancer. Cancer Res 76(17):4970–4980
Yang Y, Yan X, Duan W et al (2013) Pterostilbene exerts antitumor activity via the Notch1 signaling pathway in human lung adenocarcinoma cells. PLoS One 8:e62652

Yoon HS, Hyun CG, Lee NH et al (2016) Comparative depigmentation effects of resveratrol and its two methyl analogues in alpha-melanocyte stimulating hormone-triggered B16/F10 murine melanoma cells. Prev Nutr Food Sci 21:155–159

Yu Z, Wang S, Zhang X et al (2017) Pterostilbene protects against myocardial ischemia/reperfusion injury via suppressing oxidative/nitrative stress and inflammatory response. Int Immunopharmacol 43:7–15

Yu D, Zhang Y, Chen G et al (2018) Targeting the PI3K/Akt/mTOR signaling pathway by pterostilbene attenuates mantle cell lymphoma progression. Acta Biochim Biophys Sin Shanghai 50:782–792

Zhang Y, Zhang Y (2016) Pterostilbene, a novel natural plant conduct, inhibits high fat-induced atherosclerosis inflammation via NF-kappaB signaling pathway in Toll-like receptor 5 (TLR5) deficient mice. Biomed Pharmacother 81:345–355

Zhang B, Wang XQ, Chen HY et al (2014) Involvement of the Nrf2 pathway in the regulation of pterostilbene-induced apoptosis in HeLa cells via ER stress. J Pharmacol Sci 126:216–229

Zhang X, Zhang J, Xu L et al (2018) Emerging actions of pterostilebene on cancer research. Zhongguo Fei Ai Za Zhi 21:931–936

Zhou Y, Li Y, Zhou T et al (2016) Dietary natural products for prevention and treatment of liver cancer. Nutrients 8:156

Zielinska-Przyjemska M, Kaczmarek M, Krajka-Kuzniak V et al (2017) The effect of resveratrol, its naturally occurring derivatives and tannic acid on the induction of cell cycle arrest and apoptosis in rat C6 and human T98G glioma cell lines. Toxicol In Vitro 43:69–75

Chapter 4
Pharmacokinetics and Bioavailability Enhancement of Natural Products

Palak S. Phansalkar, Zhenxian Zhang, Svetlana Verenich, and Phillip M. Gerk

Abstract Many natural products show promising activities in in vitro studies and preclinical in vivo studies, including cancer chemoprevention agents. However, results of human clinical trials with some of these natural products often vary. One of the major reasons for the unsuccessful translation of in vitro and animal studies to human studies is the poor bioavailability associated with natural products. Recent research has progressed much in the way of isolating individual active natural products and investigating their potential, leading to exciting treatment possibilities. The continued characterization of the mechanisms of their pharmacokinetic dispositions yields helpful information about issues that need to be managed to realize successful clinical utility. This chapter gives an introduction to the pharmacokinetics of six selected natural product chemopreventive agents. We discuss their absorption, distribution, metabolism, and elimination (ADME), based on in vitro and in vivo experimental models. Next, we discuss approaches to improve oral bioavailability of natural compounds. A few of the novel approaches undertaken to make formulations of natural compounds with improved pharmacokinetic profiles and higher oral bioavailability are described. Finally, we present select natural compounds which have been or may be used as bioavailability enhancers in in vivo studies. Some mechanisms for bioenhancement include inhibition of metabolic enzymes (enzyme inhibition) and inhibition of the transporters involved in the elimination of molecules. Natural products have a wide range of promising biological effects, but their pharmacokinetic properties need to be understood in order to better address biopharmaceutical challenges. Addressing these challenges will allow us to better explore the pharmacological potential of these compounds, either as single agents or in bioenhancing combinations.

Keywords Bioavailability · Bioenhancement · Curcumin · Enzyme inhibition · Metabolism · Natural compounds · Pharmacokinetics · Pterostilbene · Quercetin · Resveratrol

---

P. S. Phansalkar · Z. Zhang · S. Verenich · P. M. Gerk (✉)
Department of Pharmaceutics, School of Pharmacy, Virginia Commonwealth University, Richmond, VA, USA
e-mail: pmgerk@vcu.edu

J. M. Pezzuto, O. Vang (eds.), *Natural Products for Cancer Chemoprevention*,
https://doi.org/10.1007/978-3-030-39855-2_4

4.1 Introduction

Conventional medications are commonly designed to include considerations of favorable oral bioavailability and pharmacokinetics. However, many natural products show promising activities in in vitro studies and preclinical in vivo studies, but results of human clinical trials often vary. Meanwhile, scientists may neglect oral bioavailability and pharmacokinetics as links between oral dosing and desired tissue concentrations. Often, such determinations are difficult due to the inherent challenges involved in characterizing the pharmacokinetic disposition of complex mixtures found in herbal extracts. Recent research has progressed much in the way of isolating individual active natural products and investigating their potential, leading to exciting treatment possibilities. The continued characterization of the mechanisms of their pharmacokinetic dispositions yields helpful information about issues that need to be overcome to realize successful clinical utility. Particularly, formulation approaches and combinations of natural products to inhibit their typically extensive pre-systemic metabolism should result in more informative and successful clinical trials.

This chapter will discuss the pharmacokinetics of selected natural compounds, covering a range of structural scaffolds, with a focus on oral dosing as is usually the case with natural compounds taken as dietary supplements. Next, we will discuss approaches to improve oral bioavailability of natural compounds. Finally, we will discuss selected natural compounds which have been or may be used as bioavailability enhancers (bioenhancers) in in vivo studies (*N.B.* The advanced reader may wish to skip to Sect. 4.2).

To get started, a few basics are in order. Regarding oral drug absorption, several steps are involved in getting a molecule from a dosage form into blood circulation. First, the compound needs to be released from the dosage form. In the case of dietary supplements containing natural products, this could involve dissolution of the capsule shell, and digestion of the plant matter therein (such as ground roots or leaves). Next would be dissolution of the molecule into the gastrointestinal fluids, typically in the stomach but also in the duodenum. After that, the molecule needs to survive the gut environment long enough to be absorbed; this involves stability to strong acid environment (stomach) and resistance to gut microbiota (which often cleave glycosides). Permeability across the intestinal cell membrane is the next barrier. A molecule needs to be sufficiently lipophilic to pass through the membrane lipid environment. Following that, the molecule is exposed to enzymes in the intestine which may convert the structure into one or more metabolites, which often lack the intended activity. If the molecule manages to overcome these obstacles and reach the blood in the hepatic portal vein, the last challenge is hepatic extraction. Commonly, natural molecules suffer from serious issues with one or more of these processes, depending on the molecule.

Solubility, stability, and permeability problems may be addressed by one or more formulation strategies. Depending on the molecule, particle size reduction, lipid-based delivery systems, enteric coating, permeability enhancers, and nanoformulations may be utilized. However, for issues with presystemic metabolism, knowledge of the enzymes involved, their location, and their selectivity for substrates and inhibitors must be gained.

Xenobiotic metabolism processes are generally grouped into Phase I and Phase II. Phase I metabolism can involve several types of reactions, but most commonly involves cytochrome P450 (CYP)-mediated oxidation. The levels of expression of CYPs are highest in the liver, although appreciable activity of one particular CYP isoform (CYP3A4) is also found in the intestinal epithelium (Michaels and Wang 2014). CYP3A4 is also known to metabolize approximately 50% of marketed drug molecules, and is rife with drug interaction possibilities (Zhang et al. 2009). However, the extent to which it metabolizes natural compounds overall has not been established; but generally speaking, it metabolizes large lipophilic molecules (Pearson and Wienkers 2009).

Phase II metabolism includes what is known as conjugation reactions. In general, the conjugation reactions with endogenous substrates occur on the metabolites of a parent compound after Phase I metabolism; however, in some cases, the parent compound itself can be subject to Phase II metabolism. Typical conjugation reactions of Phase II metabolism include glucuronidation, sulfonation, glutathione-conjugation, *N*-acetylation, methylation, and conjugation with amino acids (amidation). The enzymes that are involved in these reactions are, respectively, uridine diphosphate-glucuronosyltransferases (UGTs), sulfotransferases, *N*-acetyltransferases, glutathione *S*-transferases, methyltransferase, and amidotransferases (Pearson and Wienkers 2009).

Glucuronidation is quantitatively the most important conjugation reaction of xenobiotics/drugs. It is generally considered to be a low-affinity and high-capacity reaction in which glucuronic acid is conjugated to alcohols, phenols, amines, amides, carboxylic acids, and thiols. By addition of glucuronic acid, the conjugates become more polar, are ionized at physiological pH ($pK_a \sim 4.0$) and increase their molecular weight by 176 Da (Remmel et al. 2008). These modifications result in excretion of glucuronides via the kidney either by glomerular filtration, or active secretion, or both. Glucuronide formation is generally considered to be the final metabolic step. However, recent evidence suggests that monoglucuronides of non-steroidal anti-inflammatory agents might also be substrates for CYP2C9-mediated oxidation, and monoglucuronides of polyphenolic compounds like quercetin can undergo further glucuronidation, sulfation, or methylation (Remmel et al. 2008; O'Leary et al. 2003). There are more than 60 UGTs identified in mammalian species, and 16 functional UGTs were found in humans (McCarver and Hines 2002). Since most natural compounds contain hydroxyl or amine groups, they may be susceptible to glucuronidation during "first-pass" (presystemic) metabolism and/or clearance from the circulation.

Natural compounds may interact with enzymes in multiple ways. First, they may be substrates which are metabolized, resulting in a chemical transformation. Second, they may increase the expression level of the enzyme in a tissue such as the liver or intestine; these compounds are known as enzyme inducers. Third, they may inhibit the metabolic activity of an enzyme; these are known as enzyme inhibitors. Enzyme inhibition may comprise several different mechanisms: competitive, noncompetitive, uncompetitive, or mixed. Of these, competitive is the most common inhibition mechanism. Furthermore, the inhibition may comprise two different modes: reversible or irreversible (mechanism-based inhibition, or suicide inactivation). One may consult other references for further details on the kinetic nature of these types of inhibition and their clinical implications (Pearson and Wienkers 2009).

4.2 Pharmacokinetics of Selected Natural Compounds

4.2.1 Anthocyanins

Anthocyanins comprise a class of compounds containing three aromatic rings including a flavylium cation (positively charged triple-bonded oxygen atom), conjugated to a sugar as a glycoside. As such, they tend to be reasonably water soluble, but have low passive diffusional permeability through biological membranes. However, the glucosides have higher permeability across the rat hepatocyte membranes and the Caco-2 human intestinal epithelial cell culture model compared to galactosides or their aglycones (Vanzo et al. 2011; Yi et al. 2006). Furthermore, human clinical studies have shown that cyanidin 3-glucoside and cyanidin 3-sambubioside are rapidly absorbed from elderberry extract (Milbury et al. 2002). Similarly, quercetin 3-glucoside is more rapidly absorbed than quercetin in humans (Hollman et al. 1995). These data suggest that a biological membrane transporter, such as an endogenous glucose transporter, may be involved in their absorption from the intestine.

4.2.2 Curcumin

The absorption and pharmacokinetics of curcumin have been thoroughly reviewed (Anand et al. 2007). Briefly, curcumin suffers from poor aqueous solubility, poor permeability, rapid presystemic metabolism, and rapid systemic clearance. These factors lead to low oral bioavailability (F_{oral}), short half-life ($t_{1/2}$), and minimal systemic exposure. Cheng et al. gave escalating oral doses of curcumin of up to 12 g daily for 3 months to cancer patients; although this highest dosage regimen was not tolerated by the subjects (due to its high bulk), the peak serum concentrations of curcumin at 8 g/day were only 1.77 ± 1.87 μM (Cheng et al. 2001). Several formulation efforts have been made to enhance the oral bioavailability of curcumin, especially nanoparticle formulations, lipid-based drug delivery systems, and coformulation with enzyme inhibitors such as piperine (which are discussed below).

4.2.3 Pterostilbene

Stilbenes are small, naturally occurring compounds found in a wide range of plant sources, aromatherapy products, and dietary supplements. Naturally occurring stilbenes overwhelmingly exist in the *trans* form. Additional research has shown *trans*-stilbene compounds to be significantly more potent in their ability to inhibit cyclooxygenase I (COX-I) activity compared to *cis*-stilbene compounds (Roupe et al. 2006).

Pterostilbene (PT), or 3,5-dimethoxy-4′-hydroxystilbene (molecular weight: 256.3), is a lipid soluble compound that exists in *cis* and *trans* forms, with the *trans* form being most abundant. It was first isolated in 1940 from heartwood of red sandalwood (*Pterocarpus santalinus*) and later identified in grapevines (*Vitis vinifera*) and blueberries (Kosuru et al. 2016).

Based on the structure of pterostilbene (Fig. 4.1), we can see that it has few hydrogen bond donors and acceptors, and few rotatable bonds (Remsberg et al. 2008). PT has a cLogP value of 4.1 indicating moderate lipophilicity (Perecko et al. 2008). However, it has a low aqueous solubility (approximately 21 μg/ml) (Bethune et al. 2011) which would hinder its absorption from the GIT.

The pharmacokinetic profile of PT has been extensively studied in species like rat, mouse, etc. (Remsberg et al. 2008; Azzolini et al. 2014; Kapetanovic et al. 2011; Yeo et al. 2013). PT was found to possess dose–dependent pharmacokinetics (Kapetanovic et al. 2011; Yeo et al. 2013). The comparative pharmacokinetic profile of PT and resveratrol in rats following oral administration after single and multiple dose was studied (Azzolini et al. 2014; Kapetanovic et al. 2011; Yeo et al. 2013). PT demonstrated markedly higher peak serum concentration and area under curve (AUC) values, and had a higher F_{oral} compared to resveratrol (66.9% vs 29.8%). Following intravenous dosing, total body clearance of resveratrol (11 L/h/kg) exceeded that of pterostilbene (2.7 L/h/kg). Pterostilbene exhibited a steady state volume of distribution (V_{ss}) value (5.3 L/kg) that was greater than total body water (~0.7 L/kg), suggesting extensive tissue distribution (Kapetanovic et al. 2011). A trend of increasing F with increasing dose was observed in animals exposed to PT (Kapetanovic et al. 2011). Evidence suggests that phase II metabolism, particularly glucuronidation and sulfation, is the chief clearance pathway of PT with the contribution of sulfation being greater than glucuronidation (Azzolini et al. 2014; Kapetanovic et al. 2011). Plasma concentrations of phase II metabolites were much higher than the parent compound. However, the sulfation pathway was found to be saturable and AUC sulfate/glucuronide decreased at higher doses of PT (Kapetanovic et al. 2011). Higher doses may saturate/partially saturate the phase II metabolism of PT leading to an increased F_{oral} (Kapetanovic et al. 2011; Yeo et al. 2013).

Dellinger et al. found that UGT1A1 had the most metabolic activity towards PT (Dellinger et al. 2014). It was also observed that female human liver microsomes (HLMs) are more efficient than male HLMs in the glucuronidation of pterostilbene. Kinetic data revealed that although male and female K_ms were similar, female HLMs had a significantly higher V_{max} indicating they were capable of much higher catalytic turnover than male HLMs (Dellinger et al. 2014).

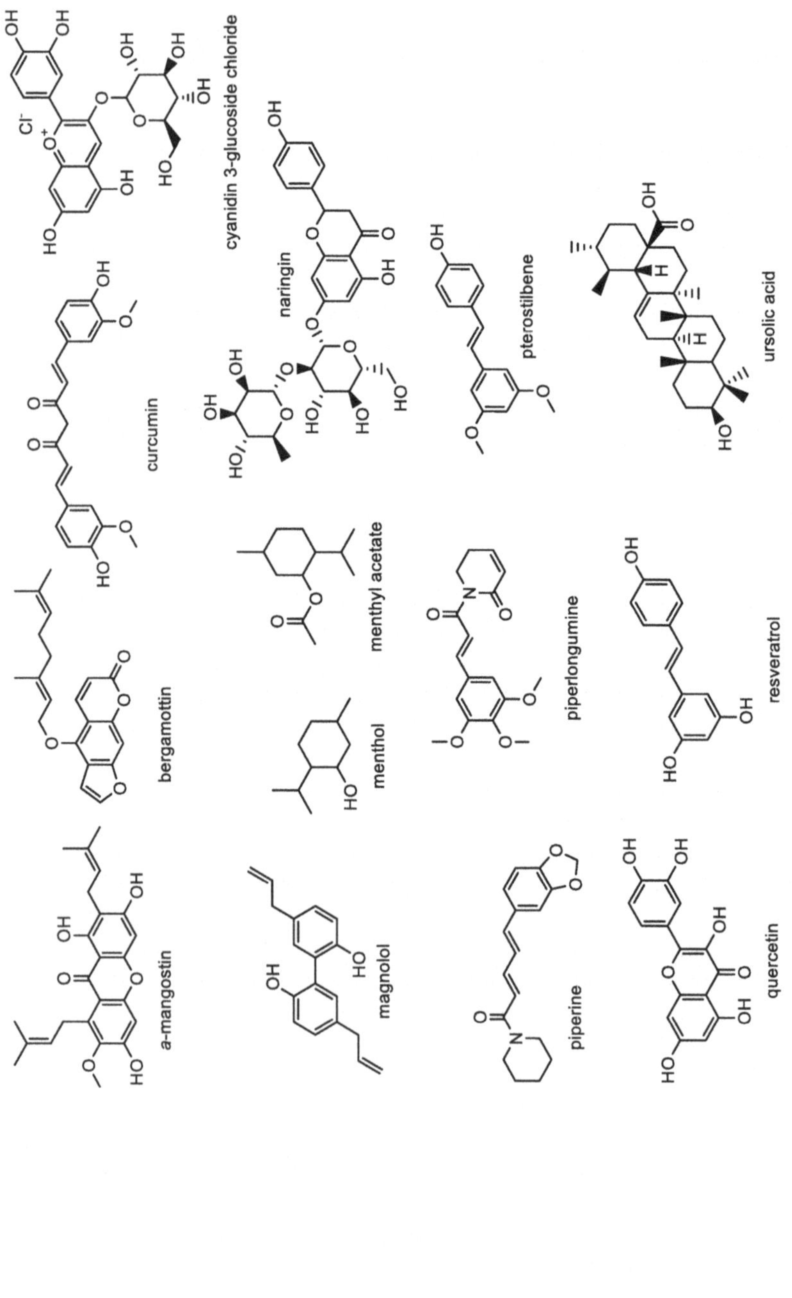

Fig. 4.1 Structures of selected natural compounds

There was normal appearance of vital organs, including kidney, in the macroscopic examinations after necropsy, as well as no effect on the final body weight or the mean growth rate after oral administration up to 3000 mg PT/kg/day for 28 days suggesting that PT is nontoxic even at very high doses (Ruiz et al. 2009).

4.2.4 *Quercetin*

Quercetin is a major representative of dietary flavonol, a subgroup of flavonoids. This compound is found ubiquitously in foods of plant origin such as onion, lettuce, broccoli, cranberry, apple skin, olive, red wine, and tea. The exact amount of quercetin in food is not known but it was roughly estimated to be 2–250 mg/kg of fruits, 0–100 mg/kg of vegetables, 4–16 mg/l in red wine, and 10–25 mg/l in tea (Manach et al. 1998).

Little is known about absorption and distribution of quercetin or quercetin aglycone in the body, but several experiments have been conducted to establish the extent of oral absorption and bioavailability of quercetin glucosides, a typical form of quercetin present in food. Studies on healthy volunteers have established that the peak plasma concentration (C_{max}) was achieved after about 3 h of food ingestion containing 60–90 mg of quercetin with $t_{1/2}$ being 0.87 h, 3.8 h, and 16.8 h for absorption, distribution, and elimination phases, respectively (Manach et al. 1998; Hollman et al. 1996). C_{max} for quercetin aglycone (in a pure form, not in food) was achieved with some delay, after 1.9 to 4.8 h, for doses between 8 and 50 mg (Erlund et al. 2000). Bioavailability of quercetin glucosides can be as high as 52%, whereas quercetin aglycone had a bioavailability of only 24% (Hollman et al. 1995).

Once quercetin is absorbed, it undergoes extensive metabolism. Due to the presence of five hydroxyl groups (Fig. 4.1), it forms methylated, glucuronidated, and/or sulfated conjugates (Manach et al. 1998; Erlund et al. 2000). Analysis of plasma from volunteers fed with a quercetin-supplemented diet shows that quercetin mainly circulates as quercetin glucuronides (Yang et al. 2006). The major sites for quercetin metabolism are 7-, 3-, 3′-, and 4′-hydroxyl moieties with UGT1A1, UGT1A3, UGT1A8, and UGT1A9 being the most active UGT isoforms (Boersma et al. 2002; Chen et al. 2005). The apparent K_m for the formation of 7-, 4′-, and 3′-glucuronides determined with liver cell-free extract were found to be 6.5 ± 0.9 μM, 0.6 ± 0.2 μM, and 0.8 ± 0.2 μM, respectively (Day et al. 2000). However, incubations with recombinant UGTs resulted in values which were about ten-fold higher (Chen et al. 2005). 3′- and 4′-hydroxyl groups are the first moieties attacked by UGTs, and interestingly these groups are primarily responsible for the pro-oxidant properties of this flavonoid (Boersma et al. 2002; Day et al. 2000).

Once absorbed through the intestine wall, quercetin forms glucuronide conjugates which tend to be excreted back into the gut via active transport. It was established that quercetin glucuronides, especially 7-*O*-glucuronosyl quercetin, are likely to be transported via MRPs and are capable of inhibiting MRP1/ABCC1 and to the lesser degree MRP2/ABCC2 (van Zanden et al. 2007). Additionally, quercetin is an inhibitor for MDR1/ABCB1, MRP1/ABCC1, and BCRP/ABCG2 transporters (Choiprasert et al. 2010; Wang et al. 2004; Yoshikawa et al. 2004). K_i values were determined to be 0.33 μM, 1 μM, and 0.28 μM for MDR1/ABCB1, MRP1/ABCC1, and BCRP/ABCG2, respectively (Choiprasert et al. 2010; Yoshikawa et al. 2004). Meanwhile, the plasma concentrations in humans are likely to be in the low nanomolar range, thus the likelihood of systemic herb-drug interactions is doubtful.

4.2.5 Resveratrol

Resveratrol (3, 4′, 5-trihydroxystilbene) is composed of two aromatic rings connected by a styrene double bond. Resveratrol has two isoforms: *trans*-resveratrol (t-RES) and *cis*-resveratrol; t-RES is generally considered more active or more potent than *cis*-resveratrol (Orallo 2006). t-RES can be converted to *cis*-resveratrol by exposure to sunlight (Chen et al. 2007). t-RES is well absorbed when given orally but it is extensively metabolized, especially via phase II sulfation and glucuronidation. Due to its extensive presystemic metabolism, t-RES has poor F_{oral} (Walle et al. 2004). This review will discuss the absorption, distribution, metabolism, transport, and bioavailability studies conducted for resveratrol by in vitro and in vivo models.

4.2.5.1 Absorption of Resveratrol

Several studies such as Caco-2 cell model and rat intestine perfusion model have assessed the absorption of t-RES. t-RES was found to be highly absorbed in the GI tract with enterohepatic circulation. The permeability of t-RES was determined as 7×10^{-6} cm/s independent of the direction of transport in Caco-2 monolayer experiment (Kaldas et al. 2003). These high values indicated t-RES had high permeability through the Caco-2 cells.

When 25 μM t-RES was perfused through the rat jejunum, around 72.1% of intact t-RES was absorbed 30 min (Juan et al. 2010a). The amount of t-RES absorbed was proportional to the initial concentration of t-RES in the range up to 100 μM (Juan et al. 2010a). Some of the absorbed t-RES was metabolized while crossing the jejunum and predominantly glucuronide metabolite with some sulfated t-RES (Juan et al. 2010a). Enterohepatic circulation of resveratrol was observed in mice (van de Wetering et al. 2009).

4.2.5.2 Plasma Protein Binding

t-RES was highly plasma protein-bound and the plasma protein binding was a fast process. It can be bound to serum albumin, hemoglobin, and lipoprotein. t-RES metabolites also bind to plasma protein but to a lower extent as compared with the parent compound. In ex vivo model experiments using human plasma samples, 93.6% t-RES was bound to human plasma proteins immediately without incubation; however after incubation for 24 h, 91.0% t-RES was found bound to plasma proteins (Burkon and Somoza 2008). 87.2% t-RES (10 μM) was bound to bovine serum albumin (100 μM) after incubation for 24 h. Under the same conditions, after increasing the concentrations of t-RES and bovine serum albumin to 100 μM and 1000 μM respectively, 95.1% t-RES was bound to bovine serum albumin (Burkon and Somoza 2008). After administration of t-RES (85.5 mg per 70 kg of body weight), the plasma protein binding was determined as 33.9, 43.6, and 46% for *trans*-resveratrol-3-sulfate, *trans*-resveratrol-disulfate, and *trans*-resveratrol-diglucuronide, respectively (Burkon and Somoza 2008).

4.2.5.3 Distribution of Resveratrol and Its Metabolites

The distribution of resveratrol and its metabolites after intravenous dose were investigated in rats by Juan et al. (2010b). t-RES was mainly distributed in the kidney (1.45 ± 0.35 nmol/g) and lung (1.13 ± 0.34 nmol/g) after an intravenous dose of 15 mg/kg. t-RES can also be found in brain (0.17 ± 0.04 nmol/g) and testes (0.05 ± 0.01 nmol/g). The highest amount of *trans*-resveratrol glucuronide was found in kidney (2.91 ± 0.19 nmol/g), followed by testes (0.70 ± 0.03 nmol/g), liver (0.58 ± 0.09 nmol/g), and lungs (0.28 ± 0.02 nmol/g). *trans*-Resveratrol sulfate was eliminated rapidly from plasma and thus was below LLOQ after 90 min. Compared with the parent compound and glucuronide, the levels of sulfate in tissues were much lower, with highest amount in lungs (0.42 ± 0.10 nmol/g), followed by testes (0.23 ± 0.01 nmol/g), liver (0.11 ± 0.02 nmol/g), and brain (0.04 ± 0.10 nmol/g) (Juan et al. 2010b). The authors did not specify where the glucuronide or sulfate moieties were attached.

In the study by Vitrac et al., a single oral administration of 5 mg/kg ^{14}C-labeled t-RES was given to male Balb/c mice (Vitrac et al. 2003). The radioactivity in the blood was relatively low during the entire experiment for 6 h after the dose. The radioactivity in urine and bile was much higher than that in the blood. After 3 h, the highest radioactivity was detected in duodenum, followed by kidney, lung, and liver. The radioactivity was also detected in other organs such as colon, spleen, heart, testes, and brain (Vitrac et al. 2003). After a 10-fold higher oral dose of 50 mg/kg, mice were sacrificed at 1.5, 3, and 6 h post-dose. At 1.5 h, there was no radioactivity in intestine and the highest concentration of radioactivity was found in stomach. At 3 and 6 h, the highest radioactivity was observed in intestine. Liver and kidney had lower radioactivity from 1.5 to 6 h (Vitrac et al. 2003). The major radioactive compound was found to be unchanged t-RES in kidney. Unchanged t-RES as well as glucuronide and/or sulfate conjugates were found in liver extract. But 3-*O*-β-glucuronide was not observed during the experiment period (Vitrac et al. 2003).

4.2.5.4 Metabolism of Resveratrol

Due to species differences, the metabolism of t-RES in animals is different from that in humans. The LLOQ for t-RES and its metabolites differed in each analytical method for various studies. Therefore, the metabolites detected in each study were not the same even though using the same models. In vitro models used for the metabolism study included recombinant enzymes, fresh hepatocytes, GI contents, cytosolic fractions, and microsomes. Ex vivo model used was isolated rat intestine perfusion model. Both animals and humans were involved in in vivo models.

t-RES was found to be quickly metabolized when incubated with isolated rat parenchymal liver cells (Asensi et al. 2002). It was converted to monoglucuronide or monosulfate form when incubated with primary rat hepatocytes (Williams et al. 2009). In the study by Yu et al., monosulfate was identified as *trans*-resveratrol-3-sulfate after incubation with rat hepatocytes for 4 h. Monoglucuronide was also found and was speculated to be *trans*-resveratrol-3-glucuronide. The formation of resveratrol sulfate was more than glucuronide (Yu et al. 2002). There were no Phase I metabolites found during the incubation with rat hepatocytes (Williams et al. 2009).

t-RES metabolism occurred immediately when perfused through the rat jejunum with an initial concentration of 25 μM. The metabolites were formed in the enterocytes and effluxed back into the lumen. 5.2 and 0.9% of the initial *trans*-resveratrol effluxed as glucuronides and sulfates, respectively, at 3 min (Juan et al. 2010a). The efflux of glucuronides and sulfates were proportional to time up to 45 min (Juan et al. 2010a). Compared with sulfate, *trans*-resveratrol-3-glucuronide was the major metabolite in the rat jejunum and ileum (Juan et al. 2010a).

Resveratrol-3-glucuronide and resveratrol-3-sulfate were the major metabolites found in the circulation after t-RES was orally administered in mice (van de Wetering et al. 2009). Resveratrol-di-sulfate can only be detected in urine at a very low level (van de Wetering et al. 2009). After male Sprague–Dawley rats were orally administered a dose of 20 mg/kg t-RES, resveratrol monoglucuronide, dihydroresveratrol monosulfate, resveratrol monosulfate, and dihydroresveratrol were found in the urine (Wang et al. 2005). In another study by Williams et al. after oral administration of t-RES in rats, the two major metabolites in the urine were resveratrol monoglucuronide and dihydroresveratrol monoglucuronide. Conjugates accounted for more than 90% of the metabolites in the urine (Williams et al. 2009).

After intravenous (i.v.) administration of 15 mg/kg of t-RES to male Sprague–Dawley rats, resveratrol glucuronides and sulfates were detected in plasma. The metabolites were formed rapidly. Only 1 min after administration, 33 and 8% of the total amount of t-RES was converted to glucuronides and sulfates, respectively. Glucuronide was the major conjugate observed in plasma. Dihydroresveratrol was detected in intestinal content but not in plasma (Juan et al. 2010b).

When t-RES (20 mg/kg) was administered by the intraperitoneal route to female Sprague–Dawley rats, only resveratrol monoglucuronide was detected in rat urine, which was speculated to be *trans*-resveratrol-3-glucuronide (Yu et al. 2002).

Resveratrol glucuronides and sulfates were observed in mouse serum after both intraperitoneal and intragastric administration. Resveratrol sulfate had a higher level than glucuronide (Yu et al. 2002).

Two *trans*-resveratrol monoglucuronides and one *cis*-resveratrol monoglucuronide were detected after incubation with human hepatocytes for 4 h. They were speculated as *trans*-resveratrol-4′-glucuronide, *trans*-resveratrol-3-glucuronide, and *cis*-resveratrol-3-glucuronide. Sulfation played a minor role in the incubation with human hepatocytes (Yu et al. 2002). When t-RES was incubated in HepG2 cells, monosulfate and disulfate were observed as the main metabolites (Lancon et al. 2007). The sulfation was the major pathway in Caco-2 cells and glucuronidation played a minor role (Kaldas et al. 2003). *trans*-Resveratrol-4-′-glucuronide and *trans*-resveratrol-3-glucuronide were detected in another study with the Caco-2 cell model. UGT1A1 was involved in the formation of glucuronide metabolites (Henry-Vitrac et al. 2006).

t-RES was metabolized in HLM with cofactor NADPH. Two major metabolites were piceatannol and unconfirmed tetrahydroxystilbene. The metabolism followed Michaelis-Menten kinetics, showing V_{max} and K_m values of 86 pmol/min/mg protein and 21 μM for piceatannol, and 130 pmol/min/mg protein and 31 μM for the tetrahydroxystilbene, respectively (Piver et al. 2004). CYP1A2 played a major role in catalyzing the metabolism. CYP1A1, CYP1B1, and CYP2E1 played a minor role in biotransforming t-RES into piceatannol and the tetrahydroxystilbene. CYP2C8, CYP2C9, CYP3A4, and CYP4A11 did not contribute in t-RES metabolism (Piver et al. 2004). The Phase I metabolites of t-RES were formed by aromatic hydroxylation after incubating with human lymphoblast expressed CYP1B1 microsomes. CYP1B1 protein is highly expressed in tumors of various organs such as brain, breast, colon, lung, and ovary, but not detected under normal conditions. One major metabolite was confirmed by authentic standards as piceatannol (3,4,3′,5-′-tetrahydroxystilbene). The other major metabolite was proposed to be probably 3,4,5,4′-tetrahydroxystilbene. The minor one was 3,4,5,3′,4′-pentahydroxystilbene (Potter et al. 2002).

Using human liver and duodenum cytosolic fractions, the rates of t-RES (2 μM) sulfation were 90 $\pm$ 21 pmol/min/mg and 74 $\pm$ 60 pmol/min/mg, respectively (De Santi et al. 2000a). These results were consistent with the rates found in a similar study as 80 $\pm$ 22 pmol/min/mg in the liver and 83 $\pm$ 32 pmol/min/mg in the duodenum (De Santi et al. 2000b). The kinetics of sulfation fit the Michaelis-Menten model with K_m as 0.63 $\pm$ 0.03 μM and 0.50 $\pm$ 0.26 μM in human liver and duodenum cytosolic fractions, respectively. The corresponding V_{max} values were 125 $\pm$ 31 pmol/min/mg in the liver and 129 $\pm$ 85 pmol/min/mg in the duodenum (De Santi et al. 2000a).

t-RES glucuronidation was investigated with HLM. The rate of resveratrol glucuronidation was 0.69 $\pm$ 0.34 nmol/min/mg. The kinetics of glucuronidation fit the Michaelis-Menten model with a K_m of 0.15 $\pm$ 0.09 mM and V_{max} of 1.3 $\pm$ 0.3 nmol/min/mg (De Santi et al. 2000c).

4.2.5.5 Pharmacokinetics of Resveratrol in Humans

Several studies were conducted to determine the pharmacokinetic characteristics of t-RES in humans. Bioavailability and metabolism of t-RES were investigated by oral and i.v. administration using pure t-RES, a moderate amount of wine, or grape juice. The effect of matrices such as white wine, grape juice, and vegetable juice on absorption of t-RES was also tested. Dose escalation and multiple-dose pharmacokinetic studies further investigated bioavailability, metabolism, and safety of t-RES.

Walle et al. administered ^{14}C labeled t-RES after an overnight fast both orally and by i.v. to six and five healthy subjects, respectively, at least a week apart. The diet was low in polyphenols both 4 days before and during the study. A dose of 25 mg t-RES was chosen to represent a typical dose range of 20–50 mg of t-RES as a dietary supplement. A much smaller dose of 0.2 mg t-RES was also administered by i.v. route. The same amount of radioactivity of 50 μCi was applied for both 25 mg oral dose and 0.2 mg i.v. dose. Serial blood and feces samples were collected over 72 h. Urine samples were only collected for 12 h. Considering the elimination $t_{1/2}$ of t-RES (7–14 h), it seems the duration of urine sample collection was inadequate for a complete collection. This may underestimate the contribution of renal elimination of t-RES and its metabolites. After an oral dose of 25 mg ^{14}C labeled t-RES, an early peak of resveratrol equivalent of 491 ± 90 ng/ml in plasma was reached around 1 h. At about 6 h after dosing, there was a second peak of 290 ± 68 ng/ml, which could be consistent with the enterohepatic recirculation. The plasma concentration of resveratrol equivalent then declined. After i.v. dose of 0.2 mg ^{14}C labeled t-RES, there was a rapid fall of plasma concentrations of resveratrol equivalent over the first hour. Then the plasma concentration of resveratrol equivalent declined in parallel with the oral dose curve. The oral dose was 150-times higher than the i.v. dose, which makes AUC comparisons between the two routes difficult if t-RES shows non-linear pharmacokinetics at such a high oral dose. This study was based on the total radioactivity of resveratrol equivalent that cannot tell resveratrol from its metabolites. There were no significant differences between the elimination half-lives for oral dose (9.2 ± 0.6 h) and i.v. dose (11.4 ± 1.1 h). The interindividual variability in AUC was very small for both oral (6240 ± 680 μg·h/l) and i.v. (66.6 ± 11.8 μg·h/l) administration. Most of the total radioactivity of resveratrol equivalent was recovered in urine after both the oral (70.5 ± 4.3%) and i.v. (64.1 ± 7.7%) doses, indicating most of the resveratrol equivalent was eliminated by kidney. Some of the total radioactivity was recovered in feces. The recovery in feces was highly variable. The mass balance was less than 90% after adding up the recovery in both urine and feces. The possible reason is the short collection period for urine. In order to quantify metabolites in urine, 25 mg ^{14}C labeled t-RES were administered orally. The sulfates in the urine accounted for 24 ± 3% of the oral dose and the glucuronides for 13 ± 1%. In order to detect resveratrol metabolites in plasma, 0.2 mg ^{14}C labeled t-RES was infused in three healthy subjects. Plasma samples were collected at 10 min. Unchanged t-RES (3.7–16.4 ng/ml) was found in all three subjects. Two of them showed sulfate conjugates peaks. At 30 min only one subject demonstrated unchanged t-RES. Beyond 30 min there was no unchanged t-RES detected in any of them.(Walle et al. 2004)

Meng et al. also determined plasma and urinary levels of t-RES in humans after ingestion of t-RES and grape juice (Meng et al. 2004). Two subjects were administered a single oral dose of t-RES (0.5 or 1 mg/kg) after overnight fasting. After 3 days, one of the two subjects received an oral dose of t-RES at 0.03 mg/kg. Only one subject was involved in the administration of t-RES by grape juice with 0.16 mg resveratrol per 100 ml. The grape juice was given at dose levels of 200, 400, 600, 1200 ml with a 2-week washout period. Unlike the dose of pure t-RES, the dose of resveratrol by grape juice was not balanced by body weight. Urine samples were collected and analyzed by HPLC. After an oral dose of pure t-RES or high doses of grape juice (600 and 1200 ml), the peak identical to t-RES standard was detected in urine by simultaneous enzymatic hydrolysis with β-glucuronidase and sulfatase. If the hydrolysis with β-glucuronidase was treated separately from that with sulfatase, the glucuronide conjugates could have been distinguished from sulfate conjugates but that was unfortunately not performed. With the lowest dose of 0.03 mg/kg, most of the resveratrol equivalent was excreted by urine in the first 2 or 3 h. When increasing the dose to 1 mg/kg in the same subject, it took more than 7–10 h to excrete most of the resveratrol equivalent in urine. 52 and 26% of the administered doses 0.03 mg/kg and 1 mg/kg, respectively, in the subject were excreted by urine. Another subject given 0.5 mg/kg t-RES showed 34% of the administered dose was excreted by urine. Only at higher dose levels of 600 and 1200 ml grape juice, t-RES can be detected after enzymatic hydrolysis of urine samples. At the highest dose level of 1 mg/kg pure compounds, t-RES was detectable in plasma samples after enzymatic hydrolysis (Meng et al. 2004).

The level of free t-RES is low in grape juice or wine which contains mainly resveratrol derivatives. This may cause the lower bioavailability of t-RES in grape juice or wine. Vitaglione studied the bioavailability of t-RES from red wine and the effect of meal composition on the absorption of t-RES in humans. Ten healthy males were involved in the first experiment. A standard meal was served with 300 ml red wine (Lambrusco, 0.82 ± 0.27 mg/l t-RES). Unchanged t-RES was never detected in serum samples collected over 4 h. Four subjects showed t-RES after hydrolysis in serum samples with β-glucuronidase. The amounts of glucuronide conjugates were highly variable from less than 30–160 ng/l. Five healthy volunteers participated in the second experiment and drank 600 ml red wine (Cabernet Franc 3.2 mg/l) before breakfast. Glucuronide conjugates were detected in three subjects as 3-monoglucuronide and 4′-monoglucuronide. Unchanged t-RES was found in two subjects but the amount was below LLOQ. In the third experiment, ten healthy volunteers drank red wine (Aglianico, 0.8 mg/l resveratrol) with a "fat meal" (1321 kcal and 69 g lipid content) or a "lean meal" (1200 kcal and 3.3 g lipid content). Unchanged t-RES (1.1–6.2 ng/ml) was found in serum samples of four subjects receiving either meal after 30 min. Glucuronide conjugates were found only in two of them. It seemed the bioavailability of t-RES with red wine consumption was associated with neither the presence of the meal nor the lipid content of the meal (Vitaglione et al. 2005).

4.2.6 *Ursolic Acid*

Ursolic acid is a very hydrophobic molecule with a pKa of 4.7, cLogP value of 8.7, and a melting point of 284 °C (SciFinder database). Thus, it has negligible aqueous solubility. Ursolic acid has a low apparent permeability of 2.7×10^{-6} cm/sec in Caco-2 cell monolayers, and does not appear to be conjugated by Caco-2 cells (Qiang et al. 2011). Ursolic acid is glucuronidated by HLM and HIM; it is a high-affinity substrate for UGT1A3 (Km = 2.6 μM) & UGT1A4 (Km = 4.7 μM), forming a hydroxyl glucuronide rather than acid glucuronide, as shown by lack of mild alkaline hydrolysis (Gao et al. 2016). It inhibits the OATP1B1 and OATP1B3 hepatic uptake transporters (Roth et al. 2011; Gui et al. 2010), and also inhibits CYP2C19 and CYP3A4 in vitro (Kim et al. 2004; Kim et al. 2011). Curiously, it also is an inhibitor of PXR- and CAR- mediated induction (Chang et al. 2017).

The absolute F_{oral} of ursolic acid in humans is unknown, but expected to be extremely low due to its very poor aqueous solubility, low membrane permeability, and extensive metabolism. To overcome some of these aspects, a nanoliposome formulation (particle size 200 nm) was prepared and given to cancer patients by a 4 h i.v. infusion. The results show that this product displays fairly linear pharmacokinetics over a dosing range from 37 to 98 mg/m^2, and a plasma $t_{1/2}$ of 4.00 ± 1.27 h, with minimal accumulation after 14 days of daily dosing (Zhu et al. 2013). Meanwhile, several dietary supplements are currently marketed containing varying amounts of ursolic acid powder in capsules for oral consumption; the utility of these preparations is dubious.

4.3 Approaches to Improve Oral Bioavailability

4.3.1 *Formulation Approaches*

In order to improve oral bioavailability, there are several common approaches in the literature such as modified formulations, pro-drugs, and inhibiting pre-systemic metabolism by co-administration of enzyme inhibitors. Examples of these are discussed briefly below.

4.3.1.1 Curcumin (Jaisamut et al. 2018)

There are factors that limits oral delivery of curcumin including its low water solubility and its ease of degradation at a high pH value. These characteristics restrict its oral absorption from the small intestine and results in its low bioavailability after oral administration. The SMEDDS are defined as isotropic mixtures of oils, surfactants, or alternatively, co-surfactants and co-solvent. A drug is partitioned within an oil in water (o/w) microemulsion upon dilution with an aqueous medium under gentle agitation in the GI tract.

Recently, supersaturable SMEDDS (S-SMEDDS) containing low surfactant levels have been developed to minimize the toxic effect of the normally high quantity of surfactants used. In addition, the S-SMEDDS can achieve an enhanced aqueous solubility and a rapid and complete absorption of lipophilic drugs. Furthermore, a small amount of hydrophilic polymers such as polyvinylpyrrolidone (PVP) and hydroxypropyl methylcellulose (HPMC) have been added into the S-SMEDDS formulation as a polymer precipitation inhibitor (PPI) in order to prevent drug precipitation and maintain the supersaturation state during the absorption phase. These PPIs in the S-SMEDDS can be utilized to increase the drug solubility either for the entrapped drug in the microemulsions or the free drug. The curcumin S-SMEDDS formulations were prepared using a mixture of surfactants (Cremophor® EL: Labrasol®) together with incorporation of the Eudragit® E PO.

The P_{app} of the unformulated curcumin in the absorptive and secretory directions was 1.002 and 1.11 × 10^{-5} cm/s, respectively. The $P_{app\ (AP\text{-}BL)}$ and $P_{app\ (BL\text{-}AP)}$ of curcumin in the S-SMEDDS was 4.99 and 6.79 × 10^{-5} cm/s, respectively, which was 5-fold higher than those of the unformulated curcumin. Curcumin permeated across the Caco-2 monolayers without interactions with the cellular efflux pump systems. Based on these findings, the increase of the curcumin permeability could be explained by the permeation enhancing properties of the surfactants used in the S-SMEDDS formulation.

There was no change in the appearance and no visible precipitates of both formulations after 6 months under both storage conditions (30C, 65% relative humidity and 45C, 75% relative humidity). The curcumin content of the S-SMEDDS was still high (>90%) until up to 6 months of storage under both storage conditions. The precipitation rate of the curcumin in the S-SMEDDS in a non-sink dissolution medium was also improved when compared with the SMEDDS in both storage conditions up to 6 months storage. The decrease of the precipitation behavior of curcumin in the S-SMEDDS was from the increased ionic interactions between the cationic group of Eudragit® E PO and the phenolic group of curcumin.

The curcumin S-SMEDDS gave a 31-fold greater amount in the C_{max} (5.84 ± 0.19 μg/ml) than that obtained from an aqueous suspension (0.19 ± 0.10 μg/ml) at the same administered dose of curcumin (50 mg/kg). Moreover, a 1.14- and 1.22-fold increase in the C_{max} and $AUC_{0\text{–}6\ h}$ of curcumin from the S-SMEDDS compared to the conventional SMEDDS was achieved. Meanwhile, the T_{max} (60 min) of the curcumin S-SMEDDS was the same as that observed in the conventional SMEDDS and the aqueous suspension after oral treatment in the rabbits. The enhanced in vitro absorption of the curcumin from the S-SMEDDS indicated improved bioavailability of the drug by oral administration of the supersaturable formulations contained lower surfactant amounts and PPI.

4.3.1.2 Pterostilbene (Schultheiss et al. 2010)

Cocrystals are multi-component crystals in which the individual, neutral molecules are held together by freely reversible, noncovalent interactions, typically hydrogen bonds. Cocrystals have been reported to alter aqueous solubility and/or dissolution rates, increase stability with respect to relative humidity, and improve bioavailability of APIs.

Cocrystal 1 (pterostilbene:caffeine 1:1 molar ratio) showed remarkable physical stability displaying no dissociation at 75, 94, or 98% relative humidity after 4 weeks by XRPD. This concentration at approximately 5 h for cocrystal 1 was 33 times lower compared to the solubility of caffeine hydrate but was 27 times higher than pterostilbene's aqueous solubility.

4.3.1.3 Quercetin (Tran et al. 2014)

Clinical applications of quercetin for chemoprotection are limited due to its hydrophobicity, poor gastrointestinal absorption, and extensive xenobiotic metabolism in intestine and liver, which collectively contribute to its low oral bioavailability. To overcome the low oral bioavailability, a novel formulation approach called Self-nanoemulsifying drug delivery systems (SNEDDS) was utilized. SNEDDS are anhydrous homogeneous liquid mixtures of oil, surfactant, cosurfactant, and lipophilic drug, which spontaneously form transparent nanoemulsions upon aqueous dilution with gentle agitation. Quercetin-containing SNEDDS (Q-SNEDDS) have also been reported to improve quercetin bioavailability, but this formulation requires a large amount of ethanol (20%), which may limit the clinical application.

Q-SNEDDS nanoemulsions exhibited slow quercetin release at both pH 1.2 and pH 6.8 with about 8% release within 24 h. Q-SNEDDS in both media showed no sign of precipitation, cloudiness, or separation within 24 h. The results indicated that Q-SNEDDS formulation improved quercetin solubility but retained quercetin within the nanoemulsions for an extended period of time.

To visualize quercetin absorption in rat intestines in response to Q-SNEDDS, the hydrophobic fluorescent dye (nile red) was incorporated into Q-SNEDDS and quercetin suspended in CMC-Na (control). After 40 min, the red fluorescent signal originating from nile red was minimally visible in intestinal segments of rats treated with the control, whereas a strong red signal appeared in all intestinal segments of rats treated with the Q-SNEDDS. Moreover, stronger red signals were visible outside than inside the intestine villi, which may be attributed to the fact that the Q-SNEDDS remained intact and became attached to the intestine villi. The red signal of the Q-SNEDDS outside the intestine villi decreased and no red signal was visible inside the villi after 1 and 2 h, indicating that the dye/quercetin were absorbed rapidly from the intestinal lumen. The intensity of the red signal was not significantly different in duodenum, jejunum, and ileum, suggesting that these three sites of the rat intestine were all important for Q-SNEDDS absorption. Q-SNEDDS increased quercetin C_{max} (3-fold) and $AUC_{0–24\ h}$ (2-fold) without affecting its elimination kinetics, suggesting that Q-SNEDDS improved quercetin bioavailability by enhancing its absorption. Like quercetin, plasma isorhamnetin and tamarixetin (methylated metabolites of quercetin) increased after ingestion of Q-SNEDDS and returned to baseline levels by 24 h. These findings indicate that the extent and rate of methylation of quercetin increased in response to Q-SNEDDS administration, approximately in proportion to the increase in quercetin bioavailability. Collectively, these findings demonstrate that Q-SNEDDS increases quercetin absorption, thereby enhancing its bioavailability.

Poor absorption of quercetin is partly attributed to its limited water solubility. The optimal SNEDDS formulation used in this study increases the apparent water solubility of quercetin and maintains quercetin at supersaturated concentrations in gastrointestinal tract, thereby the large surface area provided by the fine droplets of the nanoemulsion increases dissolution, which is one of the rate limiting factors for quercetin absorption. The presence of surfactants in the SNEDDS formulation may increase intestinal epithelial permeability by disturbing the cell membrane and partitioning into the cell membrane where they can form polar defects in the lipid bilayer. SNEDDS formulation may also produce an increased reversible effect on the opening of tight junction thus improving the permeability. Because quercetin is transported by chylomicrons, Q-SNEDDS may increase lymphatic transport of quercetin in small intestine. Tween®80 also enhances chylomicron secretion in Caco-2 cells. Thus, administration of Q-SNEDDS is expected to increase chylomicron-dependent transport of quercetin into the lymphatic system. Cremorphor®RH 40 was reported to decrease the efflux activity of MRP2. This suggests that SNEDDS formulation may reduce intestinal excretion of quercetin in the presence of Cremorphor®RH 40 to favor its absorption.

4.3.1.4 Resveratrol (Lu et al. 2015)

SNEDDS is a transparent, thermodynamically stable system, usually composed of oil, surfactant, and co-solvent. It rapidly forms oil in water (o/w) nanoemulsions when diluted with gastrointestinal fluid. As SNEDDS has nanometer particle size and much larger surface area, it is able to notably enhance the dispersion of drug. High surface area of nanoemulsions also provides better interaction between drug and GI fluid, resulting in improved absorption as well as bioavailability.

Pomegranate seed oil (PSO) or isopropyl palmitate (IP), Cremophor EL, and polyethylene glycol 400 (PEG 400) were selected as oil phase, surfactant, and co-solvent in t-RES SNEDDS-PSO or t-RES SNEDDS-IP, respectively. It was observed that compared with control solution, both SNEDDS exhibited remarkable sustained release property. t-RES solubilities in nanoemulsions formed by SNEDDS-PSO was 25.56 ± 1.17 and 25.91 ± 1.08 mg/ml, respectively. The actual water solubility of t-RES was 1.67 ± 0.17 mg/ml, manifesting that the nanoemulsions dramatically improved t-RES dissolution.

It was seen that RES SNEDDS-PSO blocked the proliferation of MCF-7 cells more efficiently than t-RES SNEDDS-IP, especially at low dosages. At concentrations of 12.5 and 25 μg/ml, MCF-7 cells incubated with t-RES SNEDDS-IP remained 55 and 27% viability while cancer cells with RES SNEDDS-PSO were only 8.7 and 9.2% alive. Viabilities of MCF-7 cells co-cultured with blank SNEDDS-IP and SNEDDS-PSO were 58.3 and 34.8%, respectively.

The SNEDDS-PSO nanoemulsions substantially enhanced water solubility of t-RES by 20 times, significantly improved the stability of t-RES in intestinal fluid, and slowed down t-RES degradation in water. Moreover, the anti-inflammation activity and cytotoxicity against MCF-7 cancer cells of t-RES SNEDDS-PSO were much more potent than those of t-RES SNEDDS-IP.

4.3.1.5 Silybin

Another approach that has been increasingly used in the natural products dietary supplement industry is the use of phosphatidylcholine complexes, called "phytosomes" (Gnananath et al. 2017; Angelico et al. 2014). A phytosome product containing silybin ("Siliphos") has been clinically demonstrated to cause a 4.6-fold increase in the relative F_{oral} of silybin-related compounds (Kidd and Head 2005). A phase 1 clinical trial in cancer patients giving increasing oral doses of silybin phytosomes showed C_{max} approximating 100 μM (Flaig et al. 2007). Thus, the phytosome approach has some supporting clinical data for silybin. However, regarding other natural compounds, our impression is that the phytosome approach has not been clinically tested as widely as it has been implemented in marketed products, and that more clinical research establishing its utility is needed.

4.3.2 Chemical and Pharmacokinetic Properties of Potential Bioenhancers

Modified formulations with chitosan microsphere or cyclodextrin complex can only increase the solubility of poorly soluble compounds, but cannot inhibit the presystemic metabolism of the compound (Peng et al. 2010; Lu et al. 2009). So, when the compound is absorbed in the intestine and goes through the portal vein into the liver, it is still metabolized, which lowers the oral bioavailability. These new formulations could not solve the problem of low F_{oral} due to extensive presystemic metabolism. Prodrugs can be synthesized to protect groups on the molecule which are easily metabolized by first-pass metabolism. But, since the prodrug would be a new chemical entity, the toxicity would be unknown and would need extensive and expensive investigation. Stability studies must be done to prove it is an effective prodrug, which is stable in the gastric fluid and can be converted to the active drug in plasma. Efforts must also be put into synthesizing the prodrug. In contrast oral co-administration of enzyme inhibitors with the compound orally can inhibit presystemic metabolism of the compound and thus, increase its F_{oral}. Ritonavir is used as an inhibitor of presystemic metabolism of lopinavir (Kumar et al. 2004).

Among these approaches, co-administration of the inhibitors for presystemic metabolism is the most appropriate one for compounds with extensive presystemic metabolism, which will be discussed in the next section.

Considering safety concerns, phenolic compounds from FDA's "GRAS" list, substances added to food (SAF), or dietary supplements are the first choice of potential inhibitors. GRAS substances are compounds generally recognized as safe. Experts have already evaluated the safety of these compounds from many aspects such as systemic exposure, metabolism, pharmacokinetics, and toxicology. Many toxicologic aspects are considered such as carcinogenicity, genotoxicity, reproductive toxicity, and the median lethal dose in animals. Adequate scientific information is available to prove their safety as food additives. SAF lists the substances used as food additives, some of which are included in FDA's "GRAS" list. The substances listed in SAF can be directly added to food. Dietary supplements are basically vitamins, minerals, botanicals, herbs, herbal extracts, amino acids, and various other natural compounds, most of which have been used for many years without reported safety issues. Many successful examples of applying dietary compounds to inhibit metabolism and finally improve the oral bioavailability can be found in the literature: when 2 g curcumin was orally administered alone to human subjects, the plasma concentration of the parent compound was very low or even below LLOQ (Shoba et al. 1998). But when orally co-administered with 20 mg piperine, the plasma concentration of curcumin was significantly increased between 0.25 and 1 h. The F_{oral} was increased by 20-fold after co-administration with piperine (Shoba et al. 1998). Piperine is used as a feasible absorption/bioavailability enhancer for some compounds probably by improving absorption and decreasing metabolism (Atal et al. 1985). Piperine was also found to enhance the plasma concentration and the oral bioavailability of resveratrol (Johnson et al. 2011). Co-administration of biochanin A with quercetin and (−)-epigallocatechin-3-gallate lead to an increase in the F_{oral} of biochanin A in rats (Moon and Morris 2007).

The chemical and PK properties of potential inhibitors are shown in Tables 4.1 and 4.2, respectively. This list of potential inhibitors does not have any amines, which could be typical monoamine oxidase substrates. The molecular weights are calculated with the 1997 IUPAC atomic weights. The values of logD, molar solubility, logP, and pKa were predicted by Advanced Chemistry Development/Labs software. These predicted values are determined based on the database of accurate experimental values of a large number of compounds. Most phenolic dietary compounds are unionized at the physiological pH, like intestinal pH and plasma pH, except naringin and quercetin. Most phenolic dietary compounds probably cross the cell membrane by passive diffusion based on their chemical properties. As seen in the tables, potential inhibitors are small molecules, most of which are substrates for SULTs. In Table 4.2, the fraction of the oral dose absorbed (F_a) for most potential inhibitors were determined by the percentage of the dose recovered in urine in animals or humans in the literature. According to the available data, potential inhibitors have moderate to high F_a. The data of F_{oral} for potential inhibitors are limited and predictions were not performed. The enzymes responsible for metabolism of these phenolic compounds are also listed in Table 4.2.

Table 4.1 Chemical properties of selected natural compounds as potential inhibitors (SciFinder 2012)

Compound	logD (25 °C, pH 7)	Solubility (25 °C, pH 7)	logP (25 °C)	Molecular weight	pKa (25 °C)	
Curcumin	3.02	1.4^{E-4} mol/L	3.071 ± 0.444	368.38	Most acidic	8.11 ± 0.46
Ethylvanillin	1.67	0.011 mol/L	1.718 ± 0.272	166.17	Most acidic	7.91 ± 0.18
Eugenol	2.4	0.011 mol/L	2.403 ± 0.236	164.2	Most acidic	10.29 ± 0.18
Guaiacol	1.34	0.086 mol/L	1.341 ± 0.220	124.14	Most acidic	9.97 ± 0.10
Isoeugenol	3.08	$7.3E^{-3}$ mol/L	3.081 ± 0.248	164.2	Most acidic	10.10 ± 0.31
Naringin	−0.42	$1.9E^{-4}$ mol/L	−0.198 ± 0.791	580.53	Most acidic	7.17 ± 0.40
Pterostilbene	4.06	$2.7E^{-4}$ mol/L	4.056 ± 0.261	256.3	Most acidic	9.96 ± 0.26
Quercetin	1.08	$6.3E^{-3}$ mol/L	1.989 ± 1.075	302.24	Most acidic	6.31 ± 0.40
trans-Resveratrol	3.02	$9.4E^{-5}$ mol/L	3.024 ± 0.267	228.24	Most acidic	9.22 ± 0.10
Vanillin	1.14	0.028 mol/L	1.208 ± 0.272	152.15	Most acidic	7.78 ± 0.18
Zingerone	1.17	0.024 mol/L	1.168 ± 0.237	194.23	Most acidic	10.03 ± 0.20

Table 4.2 Pharmacokinetic properties of selected natural compounds as potential inhibitors

Compounds	F_{oral}	F_a	Metabolite	Metabolizing enzyme	Dose range
Curcumin		60%* (Ravindranath and Chandrasekhara 1980)	Glucuronide, sulfate (Garcea et al. 2005; Ireson et al. 2001, 2002), tetrahydrocurcumin (Ireson et al. 2002), hexahydrocurcumin, hexahydrocurcuminol (Ireson et al. 2001, 2002)	SULT1A1, SULT1A3, alcohol dehydrogenase (Ireson et al. 2002)	0–1.0 mg/kg body weight/day (Evaluation of Certain Food Additives 2000), not toxic in humans at 8.0 g/day oral dose for 3 months (Cheng et al. 2001), 4.0 g, 6.0 g, 8.0 g (Cheng et al. 2001), 450–800 mg (dietary supplement)
Ethylvanillin			3-ethoxy-4-hydroxybenzoic acid, 3-ethoxy-4-hydroxymandelic acid (Mamer et al. 1985)		0.143 mg (Mamer et al. 1985)
Eugenol		95% (Fischer et al. 1990)	Conjugates of eugenol, 4-hydroxy-3-methoxyphenyl-propane, cir- and trans-isoeugenol, 3-(4-hydroxy-3-methoxyphenyl)-propylene-1,2-oxide, 3-(4-hydroxy-3-methoxyphenyl)-propane-1,2-diol, 3-(4-hydroxy-3-methoxy-phenyl)-propionic acid (Fischer et al. 1990)		
Guaiacol		45% (Ogata et al. 1995)	Glucuronide, sulfate (Ogata et al. 1995)		54 mg (Ogata et al. 1995; Kuge et al. 2003)
Isoeugenol		85%* (Badger et al. 2002)	Glucuronide*, sulfate* (Badger et al. 2002)		
Naringin			Naringenin (human intestinal bacteria) (Yu et al. 1997),		16.2 mg/kg (Sharma et al. 2011)

(continued)

Table 4.2 (continued)

Compounds	F_{oral}	F_a	Metabolite	Metabolizing enzyme	Dose range
			naringenin glucuronide, naringenin sulfate		
Pterostilbene	12.5%* (Lin et al. 2009), 80%* (Kapetanovic et al. 2011)		Glucuronide* (Remsberg et al. 2008; Kapetanovic et al. 2011), sulfate* (Kapetanovic et al. 2011)		50–250 mg (dietary supplement)
Quercetin		36–53% (Walle et al. 2001), 65–81% (Walle et al. 2000)	3-glucuronide, 3′-sulfate (Manach et al. 1998; Moon et al. 2000; Day et al. 2001), 3′-methylquercetin-3-glucuronide (Day et al. 2001)	Catechol-O-methyltransferase (Caccia 2005)	8 mg, 20 mg, 50 mg (Erlund et al. 2000), 100 mg (i.v.) (Graefe et al. 1999), 100–1575 mg (i.v.) (Ferry et al. 1996), 500 mg (dietary supplement)
trans-Resveratrol		71% (Walle et al. 2004)	3-glucuronide, 4′-glucuronide (Vitaglione et al. 2005; Aumont et al. 2001), 3-sulfate (Boocock et al. 2007; Miksits et al. 2005), 4′-sulfate, 3,4′-disulfate (Miksits et al. 2005)	SULT1A1, SULT1A2, SULT1A3, SULT1E1 (Miksits et al. 2005), UGT1A1, UGT1A6, UGT 1A7, UGT 1A9, UGT1A10 (Aumont et al. 2001)	25 mg, 50 mg, 100 mg, 150 mg (Almeida et al. 2009), 0.5 g, 1.0 g, 2.5 g, 5.0 g (Boocock et al. 2007), 100–700 mg (dietary supplement)
Vanillin		94%* (Strand and Scheline 1975)	Vanillin, vanillyl alcohol, vanillic acid, vanilloylglycine, catechol, 4-methylcatechol, guaiacol, 4-methylguaiacol, protocatechuic acid (free and conjugated forms)* (Strand and Scheline 1975), sulfate (Bamforth et al. 1993; Dajani et al. 1998)	SULT1A3 (Bamforth et al. 1993; Dajani et al. 1998)	10 mg/kg/day
Zingerone		95%* (Monge et al. 1976)	Glucuronide*, sulfate* (Monge et al. 1976)		10 mg (dietary supplement)

F_{oral}: oral bioavailability; F_a: fraction of the oral dose absorbed; SULT: sulfotransferase; UGT: uridine 5′-diphospho-glucuronosyltransferase. The asterisks (*) indicate data from animal studies

4.4 Effects of Bioenhancers on Enzymes and Transporters

4.4.1 General Concepts

The concept of pharmacoenhancement has been clinically implemented in several cases. First, probenecid was used during World War II to decrease the urinary secretion of penicillin, thus stretching the limited supply of this life-saving drug. More recently, probenecid was proposed to stretch the supply of oseltamivir for the treatment of avian flu (Butler 2005). In the treatment of HIV infected patients, ritonavir is commonly used in combination with HIV protease inhibitors like lopinavir to inhibit the CYP3A4-mediated metabolism and the P-glycoprotein-mediated efflux transport of lopinavir (van Heeswijk et al. 2001; Holmstock et al. 2012). For organ transplant patients, diltiazem is used to decrease the dosages of cyclosporine (Ingsathit et al. 2006), thus decreasing the cost of therapy. Another recent example is cobicistat which is used to enhance the pharmacokinetics of elvitegravir (Temesgen 2012). However, many attempts to achieve pharmacoenhancement by targeting P-glycoprotein have failed (Robey et al. 2018). Additionally, UGT-mediated interactions resulting in AUC ratios >2 are rare, for several reasons: low affinities of substrates and inhibitors, multiple pathways for elimination, and common involvement of multiple UGT isoforms (Williams et al. 2004). As a result, attempts to create a strategy to enhance the bioavailability and pharmacokinetics of any natural compound must consider all the pathways of its elimination (both excretion and metabolism), the affinities of the natural compound and the proposed inhibitor(s), and the biopharmaceutical properties of both compounds.

4.4.2 α-Mangostin

Coming from the mangosteen fruit pulp, α-mangostin is a major xanthone found in commercially available mangosteen juice products. Chitchumroonchokchai et al. (2012) studied the disposition of xanthones in mangosteen juice in healthy adults. They analyzed the juice, and found that the vast majority of xanthone masses were found in the pericarp portion of the juice rather than the liquid portion; furthermore, α-mangostin comprised 60% of the total xanthones, at a concentration of 3.2 mM. After administering a 60 ml dose of the juice to the subjects with a high-fat meal (to stimulate chylomicron incorporation), they found peak plasma concentrations of α-mangostin ranging from 66 ± 49 nM in males to 159 ± 165 nM in females. Despite the use of a high-fat meal, the apparent absorption of α-mangostin (total urinary excretion free and conjugated) was only 1.7 ± 1.0% in males and 1.9 ± 1.2% in females (Chitchumroonchokchai et al. 2012). These data demonstrate very low and highly variable total exposure of xanthones from mangosteen juice. Additionally, Foti et al. (2009) analyzed the effects of individual xanthones on various CYP isoforms. α-Mangostin had K_i values for CYPs 2B6, 2C8, 2C9, and 3A4 of 1.91,

0.64, 0.60, and 2.79 μM, respectively, while β-mangostin was the most potent inhibitor over all xanthones with a K_i for CYP2C9 of 0.34 μM (Foti et al. 2009). However, considering the very low plasma concentrations of α-mangostin and unmeasurable concentrations of β-mangostin, these compounds are not likely to have any effects on systemic pharmacokinetics of xenobiotics as a result of mangosteen juice ingestion. Nonetheless, they may exert effects locally during absorption for compounds highly metabolized by these enzymes in the intestinal epithelium, especially if given in more concentrated dosage forms. In addition to inhibiting CYP isoforms, α-mangostin significantly inhibits the glucuronidation of buprenorphine, with an IC_{50} of 5.6 ± 1.0 μM and 2.0 ± 0.1 μM in pooled human intestinal and hepatic microsomes, respectively (Maharao et al. 2019).

4.4.3 Grapefruit Juice

The effects of grapefruit juice (GFJ) on the oral bioavailability and pharmacokinetics of many drugs have been extensively reviewed (Hanley et al. 2011). Briefly, GFJ contains varying concentrations of the flavanone glycoside naringin ranging from 200 to 2000 μM, as well as the furanocoumarins bergamottin (1–37 μM) and dihydroxybergamottin (0.2–52.5 μM) (Hanley et al. 2011). The structures of naringin and bergamottin are shown in Fig. 4.1. Hanley et al. (2011) reviewed many clinical studies of interactions between GFJ and a long list of drugs. The effects are variable amongst the studies, with AUC ratios ranging from 0.37 to 5.95, depending on the drug, the study, and the GFJ regimen used. Several mechanisms have been invoked for these effects: inhibition (or induction) of CYP enzymes (especially CYP3A), esterases, sulfotransferases, and transporters including P-glycoprotein and the OATPs. Notably, the strongest clinical evidence for GFJ effects exists on CYP3A and OATPs. Although widely invoked, the inhibition of P-glycoprotein by GFJ has limited clinical evidence. It is also important to note that the GFJ shows irreversible (mechanism-based) inhibition of CYP3A, so that the maximum effect may not be seen until several days after dosing. Interestingly, the number of drugs showing strong CYP3A inhibition (AUC ratio $\geq$5) is not large, although there are many drugs showing more modest effects (Hanley et al. 2011). Amongst the OATPs, the clinical effects were originally attributed to intestinal OATP1A2, but since the expression of OATP1A2 is extremely low, it should apparently be more correctly attributed to OATP2B1 (Muller et al. 2016).

4.4.4 Magnolol

Magnolol is a substrate for UGT2B7 and UGT1A10 in HIM and UGT2B7 in HLM (Zhu et al. 2012). This neolignan compound, found in from magnolia tree bark extract, inhibits several UGT isoforms in HIM and HLM, and abolished propofol glucuronidation activity in vitro, but failed to significantly inhibit CYP isoforms (Sarrica et al. 2018). Thus, its utility as a bioavailability enhancer would be limited to compounds which are exclusively eliminated by UGT isoforms which are strongly inhibited by concentrations of magnolol which are clinically achievable.

4.4.5 Peppermint Oil

In a study by Dresser et al. (2002) in healthy volunteers, 600 mg peppermint oil taken orally increased the AUC of felodipine 10 mg (orally) to 140%, and inhibition of CYP3A4 was noted. However, two main components of peppermint oil (menthol and menthyl acetate) demonstrated low affinities for CYP3A4 (87 and 124 μM, respectively). Meanwhile, grapefruit juice (300 ml) taken orally increased the AUC of felodipine to 173%. Furthermore, ascorbyl palmitate (500 mg orally) did not alter felodipine AUC, despite its higher potency against CYP3A4 (12.3 μM) (Dresser et al. 2002). In a study with recombinant human CYP isoforms, Unger showed that peppermint oil inhibited >50% of activities of CYPs 2C8, 2C9, 2C19 at 100 μg/ml, while it also inhibited CYPs 1A2 and 2D6 at 500 μg/ml, but showed little inhibition of CYP3A4 (Unger and Frank 2004).

4.4.6 Piperine

Piperine is widely used as a "bioenhancer" for many herbal products marketed in the USA, at a typical single oral dose of 5 mg. Piperine inhibits both CYP3A4 and P-glycoprotein (Bhardwaj et al. 2002), thus shows the potential for reducing the presystemic metabolism of some drugs and natural compounds. Assuming a gastro-intestinal fluid volume of 250 ml and rapid dissolution, a 5 mg dose of piperine would result in a maximum concentration of 70 μM. Piperine has an aromatic methylenedioxyphenyl functional group, similar to known mechanism-based CYP inhibitors like methylenedioxymethamphetamine (MDMA, "ecstasy") (Heydari et al. 2004) and tadalafil (Ring et al. 2005). Piperine also exhibits time-dependent inhibition of some SULTs and UGTs (Zeng et al. 2017). Piperine inhibits P-glycoprotein alone and synergistically with capsaicin (Okura et al. 2010). In combination with piperlongumine (which contains a Michael acceptor group), piperine synergistically inhibits CYP3A4 (Nayak et al. 2012). The structures of piperine and piperlongumine are shown in Fig. 4.1. Clinically, piperine (20 mg daily for 7 days) has been shown to enhance the F_{oral} of propranolol or theophylline by approximately 2-fold (Bano et al. 1991). Furthermore, Shoba et al. gave healthy volunteers 2 g of curcumin alone or with 20 mg piperine orally with water, and found a 20-fold increase in relative F_{oral} of curcumin (Shoba et al. 1998). However, the absolute F_{oral} of curcumin with or without piperine remains unknown. Finally, there are many marketed products combining piperine with t-RES. Meanwhile, a clinical study giving a single dose of t-RES (2.5 g) alone or with piperine 5 mg or 25 mg was completed in 2012 (ClinicalTrials.gov Identifier: NCT01324089), but unfortunately the results have not been published to date. Such a study would help to establish whether piperine does improve the F_{oral} of t-RES, which is extremely low (<1%) (Walle 2011). Additionally, in rats, piperine enhances the F_{oral} of several pharmaceutical compounds (Ajazuddin et al. 2014); however, the numerous differences between rodents and humans in terms of drug transport and metabolism make these results difficult to extrapolate to humans, especially for compounds with low absolute F_{oral}.

4.5 Conclusions and Future Directions

Although natural products possess a wide array of promising biologic activities, the challenge of getting these molecules from their sources to the desired sites of action in the body has often been neglected or at least underestimated. In clinical trials with cancer patients, gram-level doses of compounds like curcumin, resveratrol, and quercetin have been given. In some of these studies, the pharmacokinetic performance of these dosage regimens have been analyzed, and challenges remain. The challenges include problems with release from the biomass matrix, dissolution into gastrointestinal fluids, permeability across the intestinal epithelium, and presystemic ("first-pass") metabolism. These factors lead to very low absolute oral bioavailability. In the case of conventional drug development, many of these problems can be solved through modifications to the chemical structure, and indeed, many natural compounds have served as scaffolds for the discovery of new drugs. However, from the regulatory perspective, these changes in chemical structures render a molecule no longer a natural product, thus it becomes a "new chemical entity" and requires greater pre-clinical data before it can be administered in human clinical trials.

To address these biopharmaceutical challenges, many creative approaches have been used, including nanoparticle formulations, phytosomes, and the use of bioenhancers. The effects of these approaches have been shown effective for some molecules, then applied to other molecules and assumed to be effective in humans (without being studied). We hope that future dietary supplement product development will include an increased level of attention to the biopharmaceutical issues challenging effective use of natural molecules. It has been said that the lack of scientific methods used in herbal medicine product development is "a disaster waiting to happen." (Talalay and Talalay 2001) Meanwhile, the natural products market in the USA has been reported as $8.8 billion in 2018, and the trend shows that growth in this market continues to accelerate (Smith et al. 2018). However, such a potential disaster could be avoided if the industry is willing to put more resources from increasing sales into the development, testing, and post-market surveillance of natural products, especially for cancer chemoprevention.

References

Ajazuddin, Alexander A, Qureshi A, Kumari L, Vaishnav P, Sharma M, Saraf S, Saraf S (2014) Role of herbal bioactives as a potential bioavailability enhancer for active pharmaceutical ingredients. Fitoterapia 97:1–14

Almeida L, Vaz-da-Silva M, Falcao A, Soares E, Costa R, Loureiro AI, Fernandes-Lopes C, Rocha JF, Nunes T, Wright L, Soares-da-Silva P (2009) Pharmacokinetic and safety profile of trans-resveratrol in a rising multiple-dose study in healthy volunteers. Mol Nutr Food Res 53(Suppl 1):S7–S15

Anand P, Kunnumakkara AB, Newman RA, Aggarwal BB (2007) Bioavailability of curcumin: problems and promises. Mol Pharm 4:807–818

Angelico R, Ceglie A, Sacco P, Colafemmina G, Ripoli M, Mangia A (2014) Phyto-liposomes as nanoshuttles for water-insoluble silybin-phospholipid complex. Int J Pharm 471:173–181

Asensi M, Medina I, Ortega A, Carretero J, Bano MC, Obrador E, Estrela JM (2002) Inhibition of cancer growth by resveratrol is related to its low bioavailability. Free Radic Biol Med 33:387–398

Atal C, Dubey R, Singh J (1985) Biochemical basis of enhanced drug bioavailability by piperine: evidence that piperine is a potent inhibitor of drug metabolism. J Pharmacol Exp Ther 232:258–262

Aumont V, Krisa S, Battaglia E, Netter P, Richard T, Merillon JM, Magdalou J, Sabolovic N (2001) Regioselective and stereospecific glucuronidation of trans- and cis-resveratrol in human. Arch Biochem Biophys 393:281–289

Azzolini M, La Spina M, Mattarei A, Paradisi C, Zoratti M, Biasutto L (2014) Pharmacokinetics and tissue distribution of pterostilbene in the rat. Mol Nutr Food Res 58:2122–2132

Badger DA, Smith RL, Bao J, Kuester RK, Sipes IG (2002) Disposition and metabolism of isoeugenol in the male Fischer 344 rat. Food Chem Toxicol 40:1757–1765

Bamforth KJ, Jones AL, Roberts RC, Coughtrie MW (1993) Common food additives are potent inhibitors of human liver 17 alpha-ethinyloestradiol and dopamine sulphotransferases. Biochem Pharmacol 46:1713–1720

Bano G, Raina RK, Zutshi U, Bedi KL, Johri RK, Sharma SC (1991) Effect of piperine on bioavailability and pharmacokinetics of propranolol and theophylline in healthy volunteers. Eur J Clin Pharmacol 41:615–617

Bethune SJ, Schultheiss N, Henck JO (2011) Improving the poor aqueous solubility of nutraceutical compound Pterostilbene through Cocrystal formation. Cryst Growth Des 11:2817–2823

Bhardwaj RK, Glaeser H, Becquemont L, Klotz U, Gupta SK, Fromm MF (2002) Piperine, a major constituent of black pepper, inhibits human P-glycoprotein and CYP3A4. J Pharmacol Exp Ther 302:645–650

Boersma MG, van der Woude H, Bogaards J, Boeren S, Vervoort J, Cnubben NH, van Iersel ML, van Bladeren PJ, Rietjens IM (2002) Regioselectivity of phase II metabolism of luteolin and quercetin by UDP-glucuronosyl transferases. Chem Res Toxicol 15:662–670

Boocock DJ, Faust GE, Patel KR, Schinas AM, Brown VA, Ducharme MP, Booth TD, Crowell JA, Perloff M, Gescher AJ, Steward WP, Brenner DE (2007) Phase I dose escalation pharmacokinetic study in healthy volunteers of resveratrol, a potential cancer chemopreventive agent. Cancer Epidemiol Biomark Prev 16:1246–1252

Burkon A, Somoza V (2008) Quantification of free and protein-bound trans-resveratrol metabolites and identification of trans-resveratrol-C/O-conjugated diglucuronides – two novel resveratrol metabolites in human plasma. Mol Nutr Food Res 52:549–557

Butler D (2005) Wartime tactic doubles power of scarce bird-flu drug. Nature 438:6–6

Caccia S (2005) Antidepressant-like components of *Hypericum perforatum* extracts: an overview of their pharmacokinetics and metabolism. Curr Drug Metab 6:531–543

Chang HY, Chen CJ, Ma WC, Cheng WK, Lin YN, Lee YR, Chen JJ, Lim YP (2017) Modulation of pregnane X receptor (PXR) and constitutive androstane receptor (CAR) activation by ursolic acid (UA) attenuates rifampin-isoniazid cytotoxicity. Phytomedicine 36:37–49

Chen YK, Chen SQ, Li X, Zeng S (2005) Quantitative regioselectivity of glucuronidation of quercetin by recombinant UDP-glucuronosyltransferases 1A9 and 1A3 using enzymatic kinetic parameters. Xenobiotica 35:943–954

Chen X, He H, Wang G, Yang B, Ren W, Ma L, Yu Q (2007) Stereospecific determination of cis- and trans-resveratrol in rat plasma by HPLC: application to pharmacokinetic studies. Biomed Chromatogr 21:257–265

Cheng AL, Hsu CH, Lin JK, Hsu MM, Ho YF, Shen TS, Ko JY, Lin JT, Lin BR, Ming-Shiang W, Yu HS, Jee SH, Chen GS, Chen TM, Chen CA, Lai MK, Pu YS, Pan MH, Wang YJ, Tsai CC, Hsieh CY (2001) Phase I clinical trial of curcumin, a chemopreventive agent, in patients with high-risk or pre-malignant lesions. Anticancer Res 21:2895–2900

Chitchumroonchokchai C, Riedl KM, Suksumrarn S, Clinton SK, Kinghorn AD, Failla ML (2012) Xanthones in mangosteen juice are absorbed and partially conjugated by healthy adults. J Nutr 142:675–680

Choiprasert W, Dechsupa N, Kothan S, Garrigos M, Mankhetkorn S (2010) Quercetin, Quercetrin except Rutin potentially increased Pirarubicin cytotoxicity by non-competitively inhibiting the P-glycoprotein-and MRP1 function in living K562/adr and GLC4/adr cells. Am J Pharmacol Toxicol 5:24–33

Dajani R, Hood AM, Coughtrie MW (1998) A single amino acid, glu146, governs the substrate specificity of a human dopamine sulfotransferase, SULT1A3. Mol Pharmacol 54:942–948

Day AJ, Bao Y, Morgan MR, Williamson G (2000) Conjugation position of quercetin glucuronides and effect on biological activity. Free Radic Biol Med 29:1234–1243

Day AJ, Mellon F, Barron D, Sarrazin G, Morgan MR, Williamson G (2001) Human metabolism of dietary flavonoids: identification of plasma metabolites of quercetin. Free Radic Res 35:941–952

De Santi C, Pietrabissa A, Spisni R, Mosca F, Pacifici GM (2000a) Sulphation of resveratrol, a natural product present in grapes and wine, in the human liver and duodenum. Xenobiotica 30:609–617

De Santi C, Pietrabissa A, Spisni R, Mosca F, Pacifici GM (2000b) Sulphation of resveratrol, a natural compound present in wine, and its inhibition by natural flavonoids. Xenobiotica 30:857–866

De Santi C, Pietrabissa A, Mosca F, Pacifici GM (2000c) Glucuronidation of resveratrol, a natural product present in grape and wine, in the human liver. Xenobiotica 30:1047–1054

Dellinger RW, Garcia AM, Meyskens FL Jr (2014) Differences in the glucuronidation of resveratrol and pterostilbene: altered enzyme specificity and potential gender differences. Drug Metab Pharmacokinet 29:112–119

Dresser GK, Wacher V, Wong S, Wong HT, Bailey DG (2002) Evaluation of peppermint oil and ascorbyl palmitate as inhibitors of cytochrome P4503A4 activity in vitro and in vivo. Clin Pharmacol Ther 72:247–255

Erlund I, Kosonen T, Alfthan G, Maenpaa J, Perttunen K, Kenraali J, Parantainen J, Aro A (2000) Pharmacokinetics of quercetin from quercetin aglycone and rutin in healthy volunteers. Eur J Clin Pharmacol 56:545–553

Evaluation of Certain Food Additives (2000) Fifty-first report of the Joint FAO/WHO Expert Committee on Food Additives. World Health Organ Tech Rep Ser 891(i-viii):1–168

Ferry DR, Smith A, Malkhandi J, Fyfe DW, deTakats PG, Anderson D, Baker J, Kerr DJ (1996) Phase I clinical trial of the flavonoid quercetin: pharmacokinetics and evidence for in vivo tyrosine kinase inhibition. Clin Cancer Res 2:659–668

Fischer IU, von Unruh GE, Dengler HJ (1990) The metabolism of eugenol in man. Xenobiotica 20:209–222

Flaig T, Gustafson D, Su L-J, Zirrolli J, Crighton F, Harrison G, Pierson AS, Agarwal R, Glodé LM (2007) A phase I and pharmacokinetic study of silybin-phytosome in prostate cancer patients. Investig New Drugs 25:139–146

Foti RS, Pearson JT, Rock DA, Wahlstrom JL, Wienkers LC (2009) In vitro inhibition of multiple cytochrome P450 isoforms by xanthone derivatives from mangosteen extract. Drug Metab Dispos 37:1848–1855

Gao R, Liu M, Chen Y, Xia C, Zhang H, Xiong Y, Huang S (2016) Identification and characterization of human UDP-glucuronosyltransferases responsible for the in vitro glucuronidation of ursolic acid. Drug Metab Pharmacokinet 31:261–268

Garcea G, Berry DP, Jones DJ, Singh R, Dennison AR, Farmer PB, Sharma RA, Steward WP, Gescher AJ (2005) Consumption of the putative chemopreventive agent curcumin by cancer patients: assessment of curcumin levels in the colorectum and their pharmacodynamic consequences. Cancer Epidemiol Biomark Prev 14:120–125

Gnananath K, Sri Nataraj K, Ganga Rao B (2017) Phospholipid complex technique for superior bioavailability of phytoconstituents. Adv Pharm Bull 7:35–42

Graefe EU, Derendorf H, Veit M (1999) Pharmacokinetics and bioavailability of the flavonol quercetin in humans. Int J Clin Pharmacol Ther 37:219–233

Gui C, Obaidat A, Chaguturu R, Hagenbuch B (2010) Development of a cell-based high-throughput assay to screen for inhibitors of organic anion transporting polypeptides 1B1 and 1B3. Current Chemical Genomics 4:1–8

Hanley MJ, Cancalon P, Widmer WW, Greenblatt DJ (2011) The effect of grapefruit juice on drug disposition. Expert Opin Drug Metab Toxicol 7:267–286

Henry-Vitrac C, Desmouliere A, Girard D, Merillon JM, Krisa S (2006) Transport, deglycosylation, and metabolism of trans-piceid by small intestinal epithelial cells. Eur J Nutr 45:376–382

Heydari A, Yeo KR, Lennard MS, Ellis SW, Tucker GT, Rostami-Hodjegan A (2004) Mechanism-based inactivation of CYP2D6 by methylenedioxymethamphetamine. Drug Metab Dispos 32:1213–1217

Hollman PC, de Vries JH, van Leeuwen SD, Mengelers MJ, Katan MB (1995) Absorption of dietary quercetin glycosides and quercetin in healthy ileostomy volunteers. Am J Clin Nutr 62:1276–1282

Hollman PC, vd Gaag M, Mengelers MJ, van Trijp JM, de Vries JH, Katan MB (1996) Absorption and disposition kinetics of the dietary antioxidant quercetin in man. Free Radic Biol Med 21:703–707

Holmstock N, Annaert P, Augustijns P (2012) Boosting of HIV protease inhibitors by ritonavir in the intestine: the relative role of cytochrome P450 and P-glycoprotein inhibition based on Caco-2 monolayers versus in situ intestinal perfusion in mice. Drug Metab Dispos 40:1473–1477

Ingsathit A, Sumethkul V, Chalermsanyakorn P, Jirasiritham S (2006) Co-administration of diltiazem and cyclosporine for kidney transplant recipients: a four year follow-up study. J Med Assoc Thail 89(Suppl 2):S235–S241

Ireson C, Orr S, Jones DJ, Verschoyle R, Lim CK, Luo JL, Howells L, Plummer S, Jukes R, Williams M, Steward WP, Gescher A (2001) Characterization of metabolites of the chemopreventive agent curcumin in human and rat hepatocytes and in the rat in vivo, and evaluation of their ability to inhibit phorbol ester-induced prostaglandin E2 production. Cancer Res 61:1058–1064

Ireson CR, Jones DJ, Orr S, Coughtrie MW, Boocock DJ, Williams ML, Farmer PB, Steward WP, Gescher AJ (2002) Metabolism of the cancer chemopreventive agent curcumin in human and rat intestine. Cancer Epidemiol Biomark Prev 11:105–111

Jaisamut P, Wiwattanawongsa K, Graidist P, Sangsen Y, Wiwattanapatapee R (2018) Enhanced Oral bioavailability of curcumin using a Supersaturatable self-microemulsifying system incorporating a hydrophilic polymer; in vitro and in vivo investigations. AAPS PharmSciTech 19:730–740

Johnson JJ, Nihal M, Siddiqui IA, Scarlett CO, Bailey HH, Mukhtar H, Ahmad N (2011) Enhancing the bioavailability of resveratrol by combining it with piperine. Mol Nutr Food Res 55:1169–1176

Juan ME, Gonzalez-Pons E, Planas JM (2010a) Multidrug resistance proteins restrain the intestinal absorption of trans-resveratrol in rats. J Nutr 140:489–495

Juan ME, Maijo M, Planas JM (2010b) Quantification of trans-resveratrol and its metabolites in rat plasma and tissues by HPLC. J Pharm Biomed Anal 51:391–398
Kaldas MI, Walle UK, Walle T (2003) Resveratrol transport and metabolism by human intestinal Caco-2 cells. J Pharm Pharmacol 55:307–312
Kapetanovic IM, Muzzio M, Huang Z, Thompson TN, McCormick DL (2011) Pharmacokinetics, oral bioavailability, and metabolic profile of resveratrol and its dimethylether analog, pterostilbene, in rats. Cancer Chemother Pharmacol 68:593–601
Kidd P, Head K (2005) A review of the bioavailability and clinical efficacy of milk thistle phytosome: a silybin-phosphatidylcholine complex (Siliphos). Altern Med Rev 10:193–203
Kim KA, Lee JS, Park HJ, Kim JW, Kim CJ, Shim IS, Kim NJ, Han SM, Lim S (2004) Inhibition of cytochrome P450 activities by oleanolic acid and ursolic acid in human liver microsomes. Life Sci 74:2769–2779
Kim E, Sy-Cordero A, Graf TN, Brantley SJ, Paine MF, Oberlies NH (2011) Isolation and identification of intestinal CYP3A inhibitors from cranberry (*Vaccinium macrocarpon*) using human intestinal microsomes. Planta Med 77:265–270
Kosuru R, Rai U, Prakash S, Singh A, Singh S (2016) Promising therapeutic potential of pterostilbene and its mechanistic insight based on preclinical evidence. Eur J Pharmacol 789:229–243
Kuge T, Shibata T, Willett MS (2003) Wood creosote, the principal active ingredient of seirogan, an herbal antidiarrheal medicine: a single-dose, dose-escalation safety and pharmacokinetic study. Pharmacotherapy 23:1391–1400
Kumar GN, Jayanti VK, Johnson MK, Uchic J, Thomas S, Lee RD, Grabowski BA, Sham HL, Kempf DJ, Denissen JF (2004) Metabolism and disposition of the HIV-1 protease inhibitor lopinavir (ABT-378) given in combination with ritonavir in rats, dogs, and humans. Pharm Res 21:1622–1630
Lancon A, Hanet N, Jannin B, Delmas D, Heydel JM, Lizard G, Chagnon MC, Artur Y, Latruffe N (2007) Resveratrol in human hepatoma HepG2 cells: metabolism and inducibility of detoxifying enzymes. Drug Metab Dispos 35:699–703
Lin HS, Yue BD, Ho PC (2009) Determination of pterostilbene in rat plasma by a simple HPLC-UV method and its application in pre-clinical pharmacokinetic study. Biomed Chromatogr 23:1308–1315
Lu Z, Cheng B, Hu Y, Zhang Y, Zou G (2009) Complexation of resveratrol with cyclodextrins: solubility and antioxidant activity. Food Chem 113:17–20
Lu LY, Liu Y, Zhang ZF, Gou XJ, Jiang JH, Zhang JZ, Yao Q (2015) Pomegranate seed oil exerts synergistic effects with trans-resveratrol in a self-nanoemulsifying drug delivery system. Biol Pharm Bull 38:1658–1662
Maharao N, Venitz J, Gerk PM (2019) Use of generally recognized as safe or dietary compounds to inhibit buprenorphine metabolism: potential to improve buprenorphine oral bioavailability. Biopharm Drug Dispos 40:18–31
Mamer OA, Montgomery JA, Deckelbaum RJ, Granot E (1985) Identification of urinary 3-ethoxy-4-hydroxybenzoic and 3-ethoxy-4-hydroxymandelic acids after dietary intake of ethyl vanillin. Biomed Mass Spectrom 12:163–169
Manach C, Morand C, Crespy V, Demigne C, Texier O, Regerat F, Remesy C (1998) Quercetin is recovered in human plasma as conjugated derivatives which retain antioxidant properties. FEBS Lett 426:331–336
McCarver DG, Hines RN (2002) The ontogeny of human drug-metabolizing enzymes: phase II conjugation enzymes and regulatory mechanisms. J Pharmacol Exp Ther 300:361–366
Meng X, Maliakal P, Lu H, Lee MJ, Yang CS (2004) Urinary and plasma levels of resveratrol and quercetin in humans, mice, and rats after ingestion of pure compounds and grape juice. J Agric Food Chem 52:935–942
Michaels S, Wang MZ (2014) The revised human liver cytochrome P450 "pie": absolute protein quantification of CYP4F and CYP3A enzymes using targeted quantitative proteomics. Drug Metab Dispos 42:1241–1251

Miksits M, Maier-Salamon A, Aust S, Thalhammer T, Reznicek G, Kunert O, Haslinger E, Szekeres T, Jaeger W (2005) Sulfation of resveratrol in human liver: evidence of a major role for the sulfotransferases SULT1A1 and SULT1E1. Xenobiotica 35:1101–1119

Milbury PE, Cao G, Prior RL, Blumberg J (2002) Bioavailability of elderberry anthocyanins. Mech Ageing Dev 123:997–1006

Monge P, Scheline R, Solheim E (1976) The metabolism of zingerone, a pungent principle of ginger. Xenobiotica 6:411–423

Moon YJ, Morris ME (2007) Pharmacokinetics and bioavailability of the bioflavonoid biochanin A: effects of quercetin and EGCG on biochanin A disposition in rats. Mol Pharm 4:865–872

Moon JH, Nakata R, Oshima S, Inakuma T, Terao J (2000) Accumulation of quercetin conjugates in blood plasma after the short-term ingestion of onion by women. Am J Phys Regul Integr Comp Phys 279:R461–R467

Muller J, Keiser M, Drozdzik M, Oswald S (2016) Expression, regulation and function of intestinal drug transporters: an update. Biol Chem 398(2):175–192

Nayak A, Nayak T, Bhatt C (2012) Synergetic inhibitory activity of piperine and piperlongumine on CYP3A4. J Pharm Res 5:2244

O'Leary KA, Day AJ, Needs PW, Mellon FA, O'Brien NM, Williamson G (2003) Metabolism of quercetin-7- and quercetin-3-glucuronides by an in vitro hepatic model: the role of human beta-glucuronidase, sulfotransferase, catechol-O-methyltransferase and multi-resistant protein 2 (MRP2) in flavonoid metabolism. Biochem Pharmacol 65:479–491

Ogata N, Matsushima N, Shibata T (1995) Pharmacokinetics of wood creosote: glucuronic acid and sulfate conjugation of phenolic compounds. Pharmacology 51:195–204

Okura T, Ibe M, Umegaki K, Shinozuka K, Yamada S (2010) Effects of dietary ingredients on function and expression of P-glycoprotein in human intestinal epithelial cells. Biol Pharm Bull 33:255–259

Orallo F (2006) Comparative studies of the antioxidant effects of Cis- and trans- resveratrol. Curr Med Chem 13:87–98

Pearson PG, Wienkers LC (2009) Handbook of drug metabolism, vol 186, 2nd edn. Informa Healthcare, New York, p 694

Peng H, Xiong H, Li J, Xie M, Liu Y, Bai C, Chen L (2010) Vanillin cross-linked chitosan microspheres for controlled release of resveratrol. Food Chem 121:23–28

Perecko T, Jancinova V, Drabikova K, Nosal R, Harmatha J (2008) Structure-efficiency relationship in derivatives of stilbene. Comparison of resveratrol, pinosylvin and pterostilbene. Neuro Endocrinol Lett 29:802–805

Piver B, Fer M, Vitrac X, Merillon JM, Dreano Y, Berthou F, Lucas D (2004) Involvement of cytochrome P450 1A2 in the biotransformation of trans-resveratrol in human liver microsomes. Biochem Pharmacol 68:773–782

Potter GA, Patterson LH, Wanogho E, Perry PJ, Butler PC, Ijaz T, Ruparelia KC, Lamb JH, Farmer PB, Stanley LA, Burke MD (2002) The cancer preventative agent resveratrol is converted to the anticancer agent piceatannol by the cytochrome P450 enzyme CYP1B1. Br J Cancer 86:774–778

Qiang Z, Ye Z, Hauck C, Murphy PA, McCoy JA, Widrlechner MP, Reddy MB, Hendrich S (2011) Permeability of rosmarinic acid in Prunella vulgaris and ursolic acid in *Salvia officinalis* extracts across Caco-2 cell monolayers. J Ethnopharmacol 137:1107–1112

Ravindranath V, Chandrasekhara N (1980) Absorption and tissue distribution of curcumin in rats. Toxicology 16:259–265

Remmel RP, Nagar S, Argikar U (2008) Conjugative metabolism of drugs. In: Zhang D, Zhu M, Humphreys WG (eds) Drug metabolism in drug design and development. Wiley, Hoboken, NJ

Remsberg CM, Yanez JA, Ohgami Y, Vega-Villa KR, Rimando AM, Davies NM (2008) Pharmacometrics of pterostilbene: preclinical pharmacokinetics and metabolism, anticancer, antiinflammatory, antioxidant and analgesic activity. Phytother Res 22:169–179

Ring BJ, Patterson BE, Mitchell MI, Vandenbranden M, Gillespie J, Bedding AW, Jewell H, Payne CD, Forgue ST, Eckstein J, Wrighton SA, Phillips DL (2005) Effect of tadalafil on cytochrome P450 3A4-mediated clearance: studies in vitro and in vivo. Clin Pharmacol Ther 77:63–75

Robey RW, Pluchino KM, Hall MD, Fojo AT, Bates SE, Gottesman MM (2018) Revisiting the role of ABC transporters in multidrug-resistant cancer. Nat Rev Cancer 18:452–464

Roth M, Araya JJ, Timmermann BN, Hagenbuch B (2011) Isolation of modulators of the liver-specific organic anion-transporting polypeptides (OATPs) 1B1 and 1B3 from Rollinia emarginata Schlecht (Annonaceae). J Pharmacol Exp Ther 339:624–632

Roupe KA, Remsberg CM, Yanez JA, Davies NM (2006) Pharmacometrics of stilbenes: seguing towards the clinic. Curr Clin Pharmacol 1:81–101

Ruiz MJ, Fernandez M, Pico Y, Manes J, Asensi M, Carda C, Asensio G, Estrela JM (2009) Dietary administration of high doses of pterostilbene and quercetin to mice is not toxic. J Agric Food Chem 57:3180–3186

Sarrica A, Kirika N, Romeo M, Salmona M, Diomede L (2018) Safety and toxicology of magnolol and honokiol. Planta Med 84(16):1151–1164

Schultheiss N, Bethune S, Henck JO (2010) Nutraceutical cocrystals: utilizing pterostilbene as a cocrystal former. CrystEngComm 12:2436–2442

SciFinder (2012) Chemical abstracts service: 2012

Sharma AK, Bharti S, Ojha S, Bhatia J, Kumar N, Ray R, Kumari S, Arya DS (2011) Up-regulation of PPARgamma, heat shock protein-27 and -72 by naringin attenuates insulin resistance, beta-cell dysfunction, hepatic steatosis and kidney damage in a rat model of type 2 diabetes. Br J Nutr 106:1713–1723

Shoba G, Joy D, Joseph T, Majeed M, Rajendran R, Srinivas PS (1998) Influence of piperine on the pharmacokinetics of curcumin in animals and human volunteers. Planta Med 64:353–356

Smith T, Gillespie M, Eckl V, Knepper J, Morton Reynolds C (2018) Herbal supplement sales in US increase by 9.4% in. Herbal Gram 2019(2019):62–73

Strand LP, Scheline RR (1975) The metabolism of vanillin and isovanillin in the rat. Xenobiotica 5:49–63

Talalay P, Talalay P (2001) The importance of using scientific principles in the development of medicinal agents from plants. Acad Med 76:238–247

Temesgen Z (2012) Cobicistat-boosted elvitegravir-based fixed-dose combination antiretroviral therapy for HIV infection. Drugs of Today 48:765–771

Tran TH, Guo Y, Song D, Bruno RS, Lu X (2014) Quercetin-containing self-nanoemulsifying drug delivery system for improving oral bioavailability. J Pharm Sci 103:840–852

Unger M, Frank A (2004) Simultaneous determination of the inhibitory potency of herbal extracts on the activity of six major cytochrome P450 enzymes using liquid chromatography/mass spectrometry and automated online extraction. Rapid Commun Mass Spectrom 18:2273–2281

van de Wetering K, Burkon A, Feddema W, Bot A, de Jonge H, Somoza V, Borst P (2009) Intestinal breast cancer resistance protein (BCRP)/Bcrp1 and multidrug resistance protein 3 (MRP3)/Mrp3 are involved in the pharmacokinetics of resveratrol. Mol Pharmacol 75:876–885

van Heeswijk RP, Veldkamp A, Mulder JW, Meenhorst PL, Lange JM, Beijnen JH, Hoetelmans RM (2001) Combination of protease inhibitors for the treatment of HIV-1-infected patients: a review of pharmacokinetics and clinical experience. Antivir Ther 6:201–229

van Zanden JJ, van der Woude H, Vaessen J, Usta M, Wortelboer HM, Cnubben NH, Rietjens IM (2007) The effect of quercetin phase II metabolism on its MRP1 and MRP2 inhibiting potential. Biochem Pharmacol 74:345–351

Vanzo A, Vrhovsek U, Tramer F, Mattivi F, Passamonti S (2011) Exceptionally fast uptake and metabolism of Cyanidin 3-glucoside by rat kidneys and liver. J Nat Prod 74:1049–1054

Vitaglione P, Sforza S, Galaverna G, Ghidini C, Caporaso N, Vescovi PP, Fogliano V, Marchelli R (2005) Bioavailability of trans-resveratrol from red wine in humans. Mol Nutr Food Res 49:495–504

Vitrac X, Desmouliere A, Brouillaud B, Krisa S, Deffieux G, Barthe N, Rosenbaum J, Merillon JM (2003) Distribution of [14C]-trans-resveratrol, a cancer chemopreventive polyphenol, in mouse tissues after oral administration. Life Sci 72:2219–2233

Walle T (2011) Bioavailability of resveratrol. Ann N Y Acad Sci 1215:9–15

Walle T, Otake Y, Walle UK, Wilson FA (2000) Quercetin glucosides are completely hydrolyzed in ileostomy patients before absorption. J Nutr 130:2658–2661

Walle T, Walle UK, Halushka PV (2001) Carbon dioxide is the major metabolite of quercetin in humans. J Nutr 131:2648–2652

Walle T, Hsieh F, DeLegge MH, Oatis JE Jr, Walle UK (2004) High absorption but very low bioavailability of oral resveratrol in humans. Drug Metab Dispos 32:1377–1382

Wang YH, Chao PD, Hsiu SL, Wen KC, Hou YC (2004) Lethal quercetin-digoxin interaction in pigs. Life Sci 74:1191–1197

Wang D, Hang T, Wu C, Liu W (2005) Identification of the major metabolites of resveratrol in rat urine by HPLC-MS/MS. J Chromatogr B Anal Technol Biomed Life Sci 829:97–106

Williams JA, Hyland R, Jones BC, Smith DA, Hurst S, Goosen TC, Peterkin V, Koup JR, Ball SE (2004) Drug-drug interactions for UDP-glucuronosyltransferase substrates: a pharmacokinetic explanation for typically observed low exposure (AUCi/AUC) ratios. Drug Metab Dispos 32:1201–1208

Williams LD, Burdock GA, Edwards JA, Beck M, Bausch J (2009) Safety studies conducted on high-purity trans-resveratrol in experimental animals. Food Chem Toxicol 47:2170–2182

Yang JH, Hsia TC, Kuo HM, Chao PD, Chou CC, Wei YH, Chung JG (2006) Inhibition of lung cancer cell growth by quercetin glucuronides via G2/M arrest and induction of apoptosis. Drug Metab Dispos 34:296–304

Yeo SC, Ho PC, Lin HS (2013) Pharmacokinetics of pterostilbene in Sprague-Dawley rats: the impacts of aqueous solubility, fasting, dose escalation, and dosing route on bioavailability. Mol Nutr Food Res 57:1015–1025

Yi W, Akoh CC, Fischer J, Krewer G (2006) Absorption of anthocyanins from blueberry extracts by caco-2 human intestinal cell monolayers. J Agric Food Chem 54:5651–5658

Yoshikawa M, Ikegami Y, Sano K, Yoshida H, Mitomo H, Sawada S, Ishikawa T (2004) Transport of SN-38 by the wild type of human ABC transporter ABCG2 and its inhibition by quercetin, a natural flavonoid. J Exp Ther Oncol 4:25–35

Yu KU, Jang IS, Kang KH, Sung CK, Kim DH (1997) Metabolism of saikosaponin c and naringin by human intestinal bacteria. Arch Pharm Res 20:420–424

Yu C, Shin YG, Chow A, Li Y, Kosmeder JW, Lee YS, Hirschelman WH, Pezzuto JM, Mehta RG, van Breemen RB (2002) Human, rat, and mouse metabolism of resveratrol. Pharm Res 19:1907–1914

Zeng X, Cai D, Zeng Q, Chen Z, Zhong G, Zhuo J, Gan H, Huang X, Zhao Z, Yao N, Huang D, Zhang C, Sun D, Chen Y (2017) Selective reduction in the expression of UGTs and SULTs, a novel mechanism by which piperine enhances the bioavailability of curcumin in rat. Biopharm Drug Dispos 38:3–19

Zhang L, Zhang YD, Zhao P, Huang SM (2009) Predicting drug-drug interactions: an FDA perspective. AAPS J 11:300–306

Zhu L, Ge G, Zhang H, Liu H, He G, Liang S, Zhang Y, Fang Z, Dong P, Finel M, Yang L (2012) Characterization of hepatic and intestinal glucuronidation of magnolol: application of the relative activity factor approach to decipher the contributions of multiple UDP-glucuronosyltransferase isoforms. Drug Metab Dispos 40:529–538

Zhu Z, Qian Z, Yan Z, Zhao C, Wang H, Ying G (2013) A phase I pharmacokinetic study of ursolic acid nanoliposomes in healthy volunteers and patients with advanced solid tumors. Int J Nanomedicine 8:129–136

Chapter 5
Vitamin D Compounds and Cancer Stem Cells in Cancer Prevention

Nanjoo Suh, Hubert Maehr, and David Augeri

Abstract Cancer is a disease process comprising distinct stages, from initiation to promotion and progression to metastasis, where multiple factors can enhance or delay each stage during the development. Cancer stem cells, a small subpopulation of cancer cells with self-renewal and differentiating capacity, have been suggested to be involved in initiation, progression, and recurrence of tumors. Thus, targeting cancer stem cells may be important for cancer prevention. Natural products, hormones, nutritional and dietary factors have the ability to change the fate of cancer stem cells. Revealing the effect of compounds on the regulation of self-renewal or differentiation of cancer stem cells in malignancies, including breast, colorectal, prostate, and pancreatic cancers, could be useful for implementing novel cancer preventive approaches. Vitamin D compounds are known to induce hematopoietic stem cells to become more functionally differentiated cells, and differentiation therapy has been well established in blood cancers. Based on the differentiating and anti-proliferating effects, targeting cancer stem cells by vitamin D compounds may potentially contribute to the inhibition of solid tumors. In this chapter, we review the role of vitamin D compounds in regulation of cancer stem cell markers such as CD44, ALDH1, CD24, CD133, EpCAM, CD49f, as well as cancer stem cell signaling pathways including Notch, Wnt or Hedgehog in cancer. Further, diverse

N. Suh (✉)
Department of Chemical Biology and Medicinal Chemistry, Ernest Mario School of Pharmacy, Rutgers, The State University of New Jersey, Piscataway, NJ, USA

Rutgers Cancer Institute of New Jersey, New Brunswick, NJ, USA
e-mail: nsuh@pharmacy.rutgers.edu

H. Maehr
Department of Chemical Biology and Medicinal Chemistry, Ernest Mario School of Pharmacy, Rutgers, The State University of New Jersey, Piscataway, NJ, USA

D. Augeri
Department of Chemical Biology and Medicinal Chemistry, Ernest Mario School of Pharmacy, Rutgers, The State University of New Jersey, Piscataway, NJ, USA

Department of Medicinal Chemistry, Ernest Mario School of Pharmacy, Rutgers, The State University of New Jersey, Piscataway, NJ, USA

J. M. Pezzuto, O. Vang (eds.), *Natural Products for Cancer Chemoprevention*,
https://doi.org/10.1007/978-3-030-39855-2_5

structures of vitamin D compounds as well as combination strategies are considered for improving differentiating activities and cancer preventive effects. Understanding the role of vitamin D compounds targeting cancer stem cells may support their potential use as cancer preventive and therapeutic agents.

Keywords Vitamin D · Cancer stem cells · Differentiation · Self-renewal · Cancer prevention

5.1 Introduction

Vitamin D has been well established as an important fat-soluble vitamin for maintaining calcium homeostasis and bone metabolism (Christakos et al. 2016). Due to anti-inflammatory, anti-proliferative, differentiating and immune-modulating properties, epidemiologic studies have suggested inverse relationships between low vitamin D levels and increased incidence and mortality of chronic diseases such as cancer, autoimmune and cardiovascular diseases (Cianferotti et al. 2017; Grant 2006; Pludowski et al. 2013; Stechschulte et al. 2009). For potential preventive measure, vitamin D supplementation has been often consumed as health-promoting supplements, and biological benefits of vitamin D supplementation as well as related natural or synthetic vitamin D compounds have been tested for prevention or treatment of chronic diseases including cancer (Cianferotti et al. 2017; Feldman et al. 2014; Grant 2006; Pludowski et al. 2013; Stechschulte et al. 2009). However, data from randomized controlled trials of vitamin D supplementation in cancer prevention provide conflicting results (Hossein-nezhad and Holick 2013; Manson et al. 2019; Narvaez et al. 2014; Rosas-Peralta et al. 2017; Scragg et al. 2018). This chapter discusses the recent findings with vitamin D and its related compounds targeting cancer stem cells in solid tumors, possibly contributing to their role in cancer prevention.

5.2 Vitamin D for Health Benefit and Cancer Prevention in Humans

Vitamin D has been suggested to decrease cell proliferation and tumor growth in numerous preclinical studies, in vitro experimental models as well as in epidemiological studies, providing a strong foundation for human intervention trials (Feldman et al. 2014; Mondul et al. 2017). However, several recent clinical studies with vitamin D supplementation concluded that the overall results of the most recent vitamin D trials in cancer prevention seem to be either negative or inconclusive (Manson et al. 2019; Scragg et al. 2018). The Vitamin D, Diet and Activity (ViDA) randomized controlled trial is a prevention study to determine effects of vitamin D supplementation on cardiovascular and respiratory disease, fractures and cancer (Khaw et al. 2017; Malihi et al. 2019; Scragg et al. 2016, 2018; Wu et al. 2019). It was designed to test whether vitamin D supplementation may affect weight loss achieved by diet and exercise, and/or other breast cancer risk factors in overweight and obese postmenopausal women (Scragg et al. 2016, 2018). In the ViDA study with 5108 participants average age of 65 years old, high dose of vitamin D3 supplementation (initial 200,000 IU oral capsule at baseline followed by 100,000 IU oral capsule monthly) for a median of over 3 years provided no benefits, which was based on the post hoc analysis of the primary invasive and in situ malignant neoplasms as primary outcomes (Scragg et al. 2018). The overall 4-year ViDA study concluded that high-dose vitamin D supplementation given monthly without calcium may not prevent cancer, and further suggested that more frequent (daily or weekly dosing) for a longer period should be tested in the future trial (Trial # ACTRN12611000402943).

In VITamin D and OmegA-3 TriaL (VITAL) study, the trial evaluated whether vitamin D supplementation could reduce the risk of cancer or any major cardiovascular diseases (Bassuk et al. 2016; Manson et al. 2012, 2019). It is a randomized, placebo-controlled trial, with a two-by-two factorial design, with 2000 IU per day of vitamin D3 (cholecalciferol) and 1 g per day of marine n-3 (also called omega-3) fatty acids for the prevention of cancer and cardiovascular disease among 25,871 participants in the United States. This large-scale randomized trial was well designed to include both men (over 50 years of age) and women (over 55 years of age) as well as over 5000 black participants. The results of the primary endpoint showed that after median follow-up of over 5 years, vitamin D supplementation did not lower the risk of invasive cancer of any type or major cardiovascular events such as myocardial infarction, stroke, or death from cardiovascular causes (Manson et al. 2019). Overall, supplementation with vitamin D did not result in a lower incidence of invasive cancer or cardiovascular events than placebo, and secondary end points with site-specific cancers, death from cancer did not provide any major differences from the placebo group. Additionally, there were no adverse events including excess risks of hypercalcemia (VITAL ClinicalTrials.gov number, NCT01169259).

From two recent large-scale cancer trials with vitamin D supplementation, it is concluded that vitamin D supplementation may not have any major beneficial effects in cancer prevention. Interestingly, although this 5-year study with 2000 IU of vitamin D per day suggests that there is no significant benefit of the use for reducing the risk for developing colon cancer, the intriguing data indicates statistically significant 25% reduced risk of dying from colon cancer in patients with vitamin D supplementation (Manson et al. 2019). In the Nurses' Health Study II, adolescent vitamin D intake has been shown to be associated with a lower risk of benign breast disease. In 6593 adolescent girls with ages ranging from 9 to 15 years old in the prospective Growing Up Today Study cohort, the inverse association was suggested between dietary vitamin D and biopsy-confirmed benign breast disease (Boeke et al. 2015). Additionally, in a recent meta-analysis of 68 studies published between 1998–2018 with breast cancer and vitamin D exposure, it is concluded that no significant association was found for vitamin D intake but there was a strong protective relationship between circulating vitamin D (measured as 25(OH)D) and breast cancer development in premenopausal women (Estebanez et al. 2018). These data warrant further studies to understand the mechanisms and the effects of natural vitamin D supplementation as well as analogs related to vitamin D structure in cancer prevention.

5.3 Targeting Cancer Stem Cells for Cancer Prevention with Vitamin D Compounds: Balance Between Self-Renewal or Differentiation

Cancer is a developmental process where cellular changes, such as sustaining proliferative signaling, evading growth suppressors, resisting cell death, enabling replicative immortality, inducing angiogenesis, and activating invasion and metastasis, constitute an organizing principle for rationalizing the complexities of neoplastic disease (Hanahan and Weinberg 2011). While significant progress has been made in the early detection of cancer and cancer treatment options, cancer recurrence and metastasis remain to be challenging problems. Tumors comprise from heterogeneous populations of cells with varying degrees of tumorigenic potentials, and biologically unique population of cancer stem cells (also known as tumor-initiating cells) exists in most neoplasms and may be responsible for tumor initiation, progression, metastasis, and recurrence (Beck and Blanpain 2013; Lytle et al. 2018; Nguyen et al. 2012; Shibue and Weinberg 2017). Numerous studies suggest that cancer stem cells possess the capacity to self-renew or differentiate and to cause the heterogeneous lineages of cancer cells that consist of the tumor (Frank et al. 2010; Jones and Watt 1993; Nguyen et al. 2012; Reya et al. 2001; Shackleton et al. 2009; Wicha 2014). Therefore, the better understanding of cancer stem cells in cancer development could provide a key to cancer prevention, and inhibitors of cancer stem cells may be attractive potential therapeutics (Shibue and Weinberg 2017; Wicha 2014).

The first evidence of cancer stem cells was shown in acute myeloid leukemia where only a small fraction of primary leukemia cells was capable of initiating and sustaining leukemia when transplanted into mice (Bonnet and Dick 1997; Lapidot et al. 1994). More recently, a small subset of cells from solid tumors including breast, brain, prostate, colon and rectum, pancreas, and liver have also shown capability to initiate tumors in vivo (Al-Hajj et al. 2003; Hermann et al. 2010; Visvader and Lindeman 2008). More complex than leukemia or other blood cell tumors, the genetic basis of most solid tumors involves cooperation of multiple oncogenic pathways (Vogelstein et al. 2013). Cancer stem cells are present in recurring tumors and distant metastases of various cancers, including those of the breast, pancreas, and colon, suggesting that targeting cancer stem cells with selective agents could be important for cancer prevention and treatment (Clevers 2011; Sampieri and Fodde 2012; Shibue and Weinberg 2017).

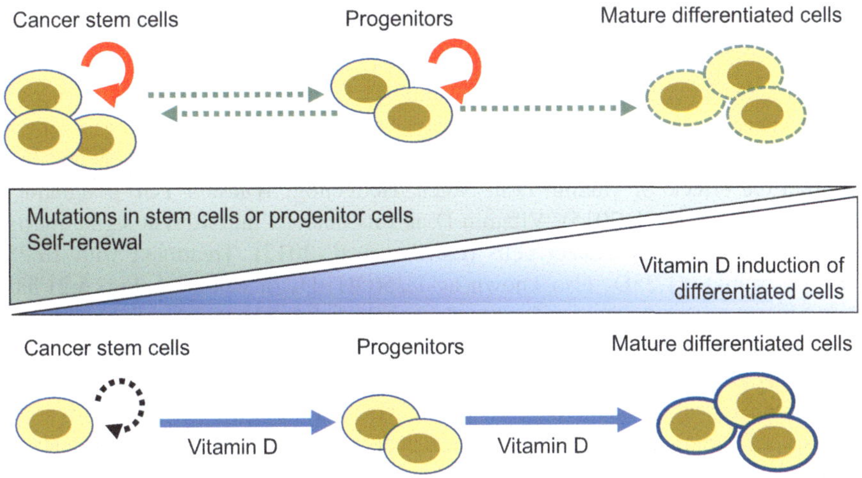

Fig. 5.1 Targeting cells with stem cell characteristics in hematopoietic cancers and solid tumors with vitamin D compounds for cancer prevention

Cancer cells treated with agents with differentiating activities could reduce tumorigenic capacity (de The 2018; Yan and Liu 2016). Differentiated cells losing stem-like characteristics and reduced tumorigenic potential could be important. Therefore, targeting stem like cells with differentiating agents to elicit a more differentiated and less proliferative state could be an attractive approach to control or manage cancer (Fig. 5.1). The loss of self-renewal along with induction of differentiation by compounds could provide a critical way to inhibit tumor growth, and vitamin D compounds may potentially contribute in this process (de The 2018). Vitamin D has been well established as an inducer of the terminal differentiation of human myeloid leukemia cells into monocytes and macrophages, possibly via mechanisms of regulating leukemic cancer stem cells/progenitors (Gocek and Studzinski 2009). Studies in primary acute myeloid leukemia (AML) blasts have revealed that vitamin D3 may promote differentiation, delaying AML progression (Hughes et al. 2010; Paubelle et al. 2013). Vitamin D has also been shown to play an important role in the regulation of stem cells of the prostate and the skin (Cianferotti et al. 2007; Luderer and Demay 2010; Maund et al. 2011). Vitamin D and its related compounds have been shown to decrease cancer stem cells in breast cancer (So et al. 2011), further supporting their potential as cancer stem cell targeting agents. The diverse effects of vitamin D on the stem cell-associated signaling pathways suggest that vitamin D may regulate and target cancer stem cells (Li et al. 2011; So and Suh 2015; Srivastava et al. 2018). In many cases, vitamin D and its analogs exert inhibitory effects on the cancer stem cell signaling pathways, which may be due to aberrant and highly activated status of these signaling pathways in cancer cells. These cancer stem cell signaling pathways include Notch, Wnt, Hedgehog, and others (Takebe et al. 2015).

5.4 Vitamin D and Cancer Stem Cell Signaling Pathways

Increasing evidence has demonstrated inhibitory effects of vitamin D and its analogs on the cancer stem cell signaling pathways, suggesting vitamin D as a potential preventive and therapeutic agent against cancer stem cells. A recent review has reported the effects of vitamin D in Notch, Hedgehog, Wnt and TGF-β signaling pathways (So and Suh 2015). Vitamin D and its analogs inhibit Wnt signaling by several mechanisms in cancer cells (Larriba et al. 2013). Treatment with 1α,25 $(OH)_2$vitaminD_3 (1,25D_3 also known as 1,25$(OH)_2D_3$ or calcitriol, Fig. 5.2) has been shown to inhibit the self-renewal capacity, the sphere formation rate and mRNA expression levels of CD44, NANOG, OCT4, SOX2, Krüppel-like factor 4 (KLF-4) and adenosine triphosphate binding cassette subfamily G member 2 in ovarian cancer, suggesting a role for vitamin D in restraining the stemness of ovarian cancer via the vitamin D receptor (VDR) (Ji et al. 2019). Further, vitamin D3 delayed the onset of tumor formation in vivo when given with ovarian cancer stem cells (Ji et al. 2019). In glioma cells where acidic microenvironment elevated stem cell-like glioma cells, 1,25D_3 has been shown to attenuate acidosis-induced self-renewal and mitochondrial respiration, indicating the acidosis-CYP24A1 pathway as an important axis in regulating cancer stem cell phenotype in malignant glioma (Hu et al. 2019).

Zheng et al. reported that vitamin D treatment reduces tamoxifen resistance in CD133+ cancer stem cells by inhibiting Wnt/β-catenin signaling in MCF-7 breast cancer (Zheng et al. 2018). In a study using subcutaneous xenograft tumor model with human ovarian cancer cells, active form of vitamin D, 1,25D_3, delayed tumor growth, depleted the ovarian cancer stem cell population characterized by ALDH+ and CD44+ CD117+, decreased tumorsphere formation, and reduced tumor initiating frequency in vivo. Its mechanism studies with 1,25D_3 reveals its role in the inhibition of Wnt signaling in cancer stem cells (Srivastava et al. 2018). In a recent study by Chen et al. demonstrated that deficiency of 1,25D_3 increases tumor initiation and growth via inducing oxidative stress and DNA damage and stimulating malignant cell proliferation while inhibiting cell senescence, and supplementation with 1,25D_3 prevented spontaneous tumor development (Chen et al. 2018). A study by Jeong et al. demonstrated the inhibitory effect of dietary vitamin D and 1,25D_3 on cancer stem cells from MMTV-Wnt1 mammary tumors (Jeong et al. 2015). In their report with MMTV-Wnt1 tumors where express functional VDR and estrogen receptors (ER), it is shown that vitamin D-supplemented diet or 1,25D_3 treatment significantly delayed in tumor appearance and growth, while a vitamin D-deficient diet could accelerate tumor appearance and growth. Further in the MMTV-Wnt1 tumor model, 1,25D_3 significantly decreased tumorsphere formation and forming frequency in in vivo limiting dilution analyses. The mechanistic investigation explained that the Wnt/β-catenin pathway is an important mechanism mediating the inhibitory activity of 1,25D_3 on tumor initiating cells (Jeong et al. 2015).

VDR can directly bind to β-catenin in the presence of 1,25D_3, and compete with a T cell transcription factor (TCF)-4 and repress the β-catenin/TCF-4 transcriptional

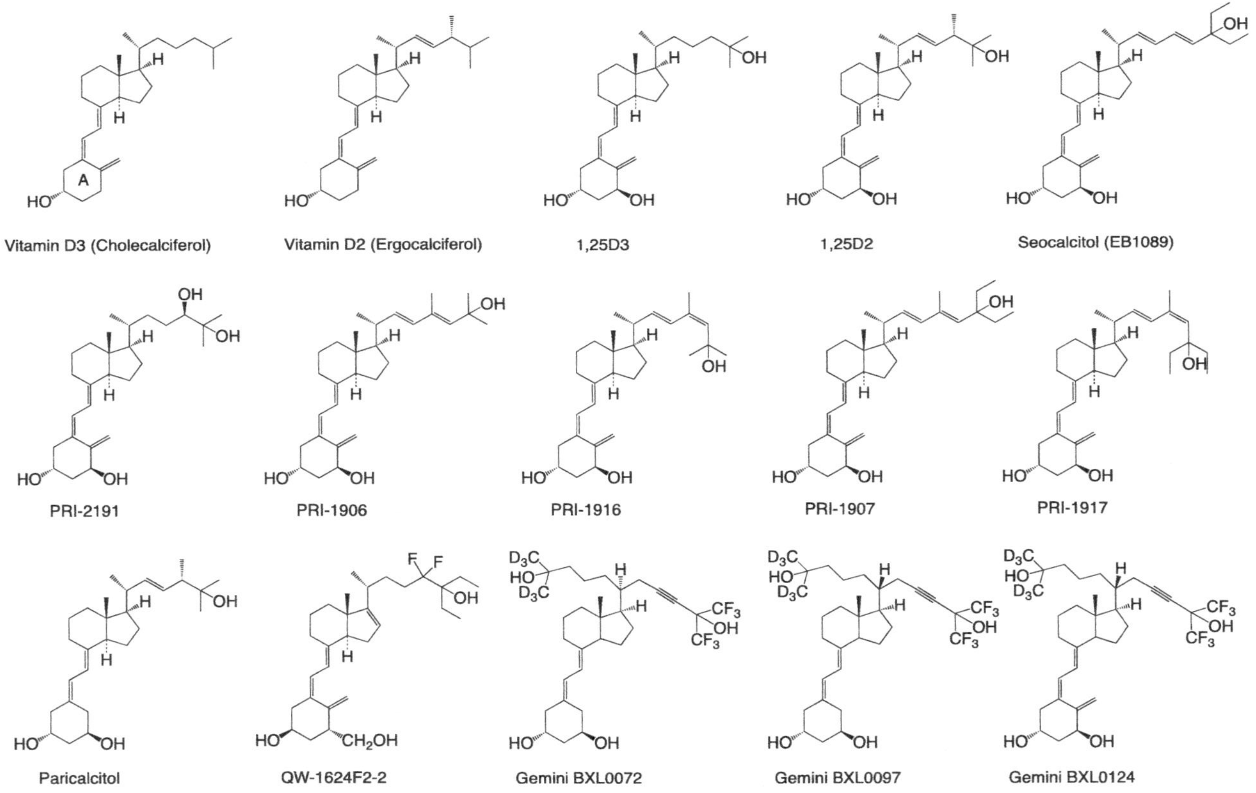

Fig. 5.2 Vitamin D compounds have shown to increase differentiating activities and/or inhibit cancer stem cell activities. Structures of vitamin D compounds are based on published literature (Belorusova et al. 2017; Guyton et al. 2003; Kotlarz et al. 2016; Lee et al. 2010; Maehr et al. 2013; Neska et al. 2016; Pickholtz et al. 2014; Xun et al. 2017)

activity (Jiang et al. 2013; Palmer et al. 2001; Shah et al. 2006). 1,25D_3 suppresses Wnt signaling by inducing the expression of DKK-1, which antagonizes Wnt signaling by binding to LRP5/6 (Aguilera et al. 2007). Treatment with 1,25D_3 or its analogs decreased tumor burden in an animal model of intestinal cancer of $Apc^{min/+}$ mice with dysregulated Wnt signaling by inducing E-cadherin expression and reducing nuclear β-catenin (Huerta et al. 2002; Xu et al. 2010). In colon cancer cells, 1,25D_3 inhibits Wnt signaling by the induction of E-cadherin (Palmer et al. 2001). However, vitamin D seems to have opposite effects on stem cell signaling between normal and malignant cells. While treatment with a vitamin D analog inhibited β-catenin induced-hair follicle tumors in mice (Pálmer et al. 2008), VDR was required for the activation of Wnt signaling in normal keratinocytes to form the hair follicle (Cianferotti et al. 2007), suggesting that the role of vitamin D and VDR on Wnt signaling may differ in cancer cells where aberrant activation of β-catenin is sustained.

In the Hedgehog signaling pathway, it is reported that vitamin D_3 or 3-β-hydroxysteroid (pro-) vitamin D_3 inhibits activation of the Hedgehog signaling by directly binding to SMO in zebrafish, yeast, and mouse fibroblast cells (Bijlsma et al. 2006). In basal cell carcinoma, vitamin D_3 or 1,25D_3 exerted anti-proliferative effects in vitro and in vivo, and inhibited Hedgehog signaling by repressing GLI1 mRNA (Tang et al. 2011; Uhmann et al. 2011). Vitamin D_3 is also shown to inhibit Hedgehog signaling by repressing GLI2 expression and tumor growth of renal carcinoma xenografts (Dormoy et al. 2012). Vitamin D_3 antagonizes the Hedgehog signaling pathway as shown with Gli-reporter activation and reduced hematopoietic stem and progenitor cells, and interestingly the effect was specific with vitamin D3, but not with 1,25D_3, acting on the extracellular sterol-binding domain of Smoothened (Cortes et al. 2015). The expression of the several Hedgehog signaling molecules was inhibited by treatment with 1,25D_3 in mouse skin cells in a VDR-dependent manner (Bikle et al. 2013), suggesting the important role of the receptor. In the VDR knockout mice, the mRNA levels of *Shh*, *Gli1* and *Gli2*, were increased in chemically induced epidermal tumors when compared to those in tumors of wild-type mice (Teichert et al. 2011), providing the role of VDR as a negative regulator in the Hedgehog signaling pathway.

Several studies have reported the effects of vitamin D on Notch signaling pathways in different cancer cells. In HepG2 liver cancer cells, treatment with 1,25D_3 inhibited proliferation, migration and invasion, and it also inactivated key Notch signaling molecules such as Notch1, Notch2, Jagged1 and Jagged2 (Cai et al. 2018). In an immortalized, non-tumorigenic prostate epithelial cell line RWPE1 cells, 1,25D_3 treatment induced growth arrest and suppressed WNT, Notch, NF-κB, and IGF1 signaling (Kovalenko et al. 2010). However, similar studies with 1,25D_3 treatment had negative results in different cancer cell types. Five glioblastoma (GBM) cell lines (Tx3095, Tx3868, U87, U118, and U373) were tested for changes in several components of Notch signaling pathways (Notch-1, Notch-2, Notch-3, Notch-4, Delta-like 1, Delta-like 3, Delta-like 4, Jagged-1, Jagged-2), and in vitro treatment of GBM cells with 1,25D_3 did not result in a modulation of the expression of key components of Notch signaling (Reichrath et al. 2010). Additionally, two important molecules in the Notch signaling pathway (Notch-1 and Jagged-1) were examined with 1,25D_3 in immortalized HaCaT and malignant SCL-1 human keratinocytes, and negative results have been reported (Reichrath and Reichrath 2012). The role of vitamin D in the regulation of the Notch signaling pathway remains to be further investigated in cancer.

5.5 Potential Development Improving Differentiating Properties of Vitamin D Related Compounds and Their Use in Combination for Cancer Prevention

Since cancer stem cells have been recognized as a key player in cancer development and treatment resistance, understanding the role of vitamin D compounds, either natural or synthetic, in regulation of cancer stem cells, especially for its potential ability to regulate cells to self-renew, differentiate or proliferate, could lead to the establishment of a novel strategy to prevent cancer (So and Suh 2015). Vitamin D has been often consumed as health-promoting supplements, and for this reason, it would be important to understand potential biological benefit and mechanisms of vitamin D supplementation as well as related natural or synthetic vitamin D compounds for prevention of chronic diseases including cancer (Cianferotti et al. 2017; Feldman et al. 2014; Hossein-nezhad and Holick 2013; Krishnan et al. 2012). The clinical use of naturally active vitamin D metabolites, such as 1,25D_3, for cancer prevention and treatment in solid tumors has not been feasible due to hypercalcemic toxicity, modest efficacy and poor bioavailability (Deeb et al. 2007; Gravellone et al. 2011; Trump et al. 2006, 2010). The naturally occurring active metabolite 1,25D_3, or currently effective vitamin D analogs frequently cause hypercalcemia at pharmacologic doses and therefore, the development of safer and effective molecules for clinical chemopreventive use is critical (Rossdeutscher et al. 2015). Numerous analogs have been synthesized to develop molecules with a clear dissociation between the beneficial anti-proliferative effects and the adverse calcemic side effects of naturally occurring vitamin D metabolites (Christakos et al. 2016; Deeb et al. 2007; Leyssens et al. 2014). While many vitamin D analogs have been clinically approved for the treatment of hyperproliferative skin disease, osteoporosis and secondary hyperparathyroidism, none have yet proven efficacious for cancer prevention (Christakos et al. 2016; Leyssens et al. 2014).

Earlier syntheses of vitamin D analogs were based on trial and error approaches, which include several key modifications, such as 19-nor, 16-ene, 23-yne, and 20-epi. However, the seminal work by Moras and Rochel on the VDR crystal structure in 2000 opened up more rational design of new generations of vitamin D analogs (Rochel et al. 2000). The crystal structures of VDR-ligand binding domain (LBD) bound to vitamin D analogs showed each anchored to the same residues in the LBD via the hydroxyl groups of the A-ring and one side chain (Leyssens et al. 2014). New insights were gathered by the synthesis of the Gemini analogs, such as Gemini

BXL0072, BXL0097 and BXL0124 (Fig. 5.2), which have two identical side chains branching at carbon 20 and are characterized by less VDR affinity but more transactivation potency and better biological activities (Belorusova et al. 2017; Huet et al. 2011; Lee et al. 2006, 2008; Maehr et al. 2009; Norman et al. 2000). A study with a novel Gemini vitamin D analog, 1α,25-dihydroxy-20R-21(3-hydroxy-3-deuteromethyl-4,4,4-trideuterobutyl)-23-yne-26,27-hexafluoro-cholecalciferol (BXL0124), has shown the superior activities to 1,25D_3 in inhibiting CD44 expression and mammosphere formation in breast cancer (So et al. 2011; Wahler et al. 2015). Further, a Gemini vitamin D analog BXL0124 reduced a stem-like cell subpopulation, $CD44^+/CD24^{-/low}$ cells, Notch signaling, Notch1 receptor and Notch ligands, Jagged-1, Jagged-2 and DLL1 in MCF10DCIS basal-like breast cancer cells (So et al. 2015; Wahler et al. 2015). Gemini vitamin D analog, BXL0124, represses the tumor-initiating subpopulation by HES1-mediated inhibition of Notch1 signaling as well as repression of c-Myc, a key downstream target of Notch signaling in basal-like breast cancer (So et al. 2015). In triple negative breast cancer, vitamin D and its Gemini analog BXL0124 have been shown as agents inducing differentiating markers, while decreasing cancer stem cell markers and cancer stem-like phenotype (Shan et al. 2017).

In BRCA1 expressing cells, it has been shown that BRCA1 associates with VDR and the complex co-occupies vitamin D responsive elements (VDRE) at the CDKN1A (p21waf1) promoter and enhances acetylation of histone H3 and H4 at these sites in the presence of VDR agonists. Two non-calcemic analogs of 1,25D_3, seocalcitol (EB1089) and QW-1624F2-2, collaborate with BRCA1 in mediating growth inhibition of breast cancer cells and breast cancer stem-like cells, suggesting BRCA1 expression is important for action of vitamin D3 in breast tumor cells (Pickholtz et al. 2014). In a mechanistic study in pancreatic cancer, inverse association was found between VDR levels and FOXM1 expression in human pancreatic ductal adenocarcinoma (PDAC) cells and tissues. Further, treatment with 1,25D_3, its synthetic analogue EB1089 (EB), and VDR transgenics inhibited FOXM1 signaling as well as cancer stemness, growth and metastasis in human pancreatic ductal adenocarcinoma cells (Li et al. 2015), suggesting the critical role of vitamin D and VDR signaling in PDAC stemness, invasion and metastasis.

In colon cancer, combination of targeting cancer stem cells with vitamin D and inhibition of the bulk tumor cells with 5-fluorouracil (5-FU) treatment was tested with a focus using different hypocalcemic analogs of vitamin D2 and vitamin D3, analogs of 1,25-dihydroxyvitamin D_2 (PRI-1906) and 1,25-dihydroxyvitamin D_3 (PRI-2191 and PRI-2205) (Kotlarz et al. 2016). PRI-1906 and PRI-1906 decreased genes involved in invasion, renewal growth and survival whereas PRI-2205 upregulated differentiation genes. Overall, PRI-2191 may be a good vitamin D analog in reducing the renewal of both moderately and poorly differentiated colon cancer cells following conventional 5-FU treatment (Kotlarz et al. 2016). Additionally, analogs of 1,25D_2 decreased the clonogenicity and the proliferative activity of HT-29 cells after 5-FU treatment. Several stemness markers, such as NANOG, OCT3/4, PROM1, SOX2, ALDHA1, CXCR4, were reduced by 1,25D_2 and analogues (PRI-1907 and PRI-1917), as well as 1,25D_3 and analog PRI-2191 in HT-29 colon cancer cells after 5-FU treatment (Neska et al. 2016). Side-chain branched analogs of 1,25D_2 (PRI-1907 and PRI-1917) and the analog of 1,25D_3 (PRI-2191) have been shown to inhibit cancer cells with stem-like phenotypes after surviving chemotherapy while upregulated genes with more epithelial characteristics such as E-cadherin (Neska et al. 2016). Moreover, a combination of imatinib with PRI-2191 downregulated stemness-related genes in HCT-116/5-FU cells more efficiently than imatinib alone, suggesting that imatinib could also be combined with vitamin D PRI-2191 to prevent recurrence more efficiently than imatinib alone (Kotlarz et al. 2019).

Treatment with an agonist of VDR, paricalcitol, suppresses expression of Oct4, a transcription factor recognized to drive cancer stemness, while induces JMJD3, a histone H3K27 demethylase, to decease stem cell-like characteristics of breast cancer (Xun et al. 2017). Regulation of inflammation, epithelial mesenchymal transition (EMT) and cancer stem cells has been considered as potential mechanisms of vitamin D compounds in the prevention of inflammatory bowel disease and colitis-associated colorectal cancer (Luan et al. 2017). Additionally, vitamin D have been involved in regulating cancer stem cells and related signaling pathways in esophagus, stomach and pancreas, and liver cancer (Li et al. 2017). In a study by Li et al., use of 1,25D_3 in combination with suberoylanilide hydroxamic acid (SAHA) in lung adenocarcinoma cells has contributed to reduced expression of Oct4 and Nanog, two key transcription factors known to involved in stem cell programming, and inhibited tumor growth in vivo. These effects may be due to regulation of p63 and FOXJ1 losing stem cell characteristics (Li et al. 2016). On the contrary, high dose of vitamin D3 in combination with docetaxel or other chemotherapeutic drugs increased the cancer stem cell properties and the probability of drug resistance in glioma cells in vitro, cautioning the combined use of vitamin D3 in drug resistance (Maleklou et al. 2016). In triple negative breast cancer cells, use of 1,25D_3 in combination with an androgen receptor agonist, dihydrotestosterone (DHT), induced cell cycle arrest and apoptosis, and further induced differentiation and inhibited cancer stem cells measured by reduction in tumorsphere formation efficiency, high aldehyde dehydrogenase (ALDH) activity, and cancer stem cell markers (Thakkar et al. 2016). Using thyrospheres, 1,25D_3 is shown to inhibit stem cell-derived sphere formation and decrease the size, exerting differentiating effects in thyroid cancer stem cells (Peng et al. 2016).

Among cancer stem cell signaling pathways, vitamin D compounds and related secosteroids have shown their potential to regulate the hedgehog signaling, which is involved in maintaining stem cell population in adult tissues and possibly important for human development and diseases (Hadden 2016). In addition, treatment with vitamin D and 1,25D_3 decreased insulin resistance, inhibited leptin and overall reduction in local estrogen synthesis in the obese mice, suggesting that beneficial effects of vitamin D compounds in obesity-enhanced breast cancer development (Swami et al. 2016). Estrogen has been involved in expansion of cancer stem-like cells (Bak et al. 2018). Thus, the potential inhibitory role of vitamin D compounds is suggested in obesity or estrogen-mediated carcinogenesis via targeting cancer stem cells in breast cancer. Taken together, the recent investigation of targeting caner stem cells with vitamin D and its related compounds, or in combination, warrant further studies in vitro and in vivo.

5.6 Conclusions

Vitamin D and related compounds have been extensively studied for their health benefits as nutritional factors as well as pharmacological agents in the treatment and prevention of numerous diseases including cancer. Recently, vitamin D and its relevant analogs have shown inhibitory effects and mechanisms targeting cancer stem cell signaling in various types of cancers. Since activation of cancer stem cell programs can lead to cancer progression, resistance and metastasis, better understanding of vitamin D-mediated mechanisms targeting cancer stem cells would provide valuable direction of the future vitamin D studies, and their use as potential cancer preventive and therapeutic agents.

Acknowledgements The content is solely the responsibility of the authors and does not necessarily represent the official views of the National Institutes of Health.

Conflict of Interest Statement None declared.

Funding This work was supported by the National Institute of Environmental Health Sciences grant [ES005022]; Busch Biomedical Grant at Rutgers University.

References

Aguilera O, Pena C, Garcia JM, Larriba MJ, Ordonez-Moran P, Navarro D, Barbachano A, Lopez de Silanes I, Ballestar E, Fraga MF et al (2007) The Wnt antagonist DICKKOPF-1 gene is induced by 1alpha,25-dihydroxyvitamin D3 associated to the differentiation of human colon cancer cells. Carcinogenesis 28:1877–1884

Al-Hajj M, Wicha MS, Benito-Hernandez A, Morrison SJ, Clarke MF (2003) Prospective identification of tumorigenic breast cancer cells. Proc Natl Acad Sci U S A 100:3983–3988

Bak MJ, Furmanski P, Shan NL, Lee HJ, Bao C, Lin Y, Shih WJ, Yang CS, Suh N (2018) Tocopherols inhibit estrogen-induced cancer stemness and OCT4 signaling in breast cancer. Carcinogenesis 39(8):1045–1055

Bassuk SS, Manson JE, Lee IM, Cook NR, Christen WG, Bubes VY, Gordon DS, Copeland T, Friedenberg G, D'Agostino DM et al (2016) Baseline characteristics of participants in the VITamin D and OmegA-3 TriaL (VITAL). Contemp Clin Trials 47:235–243

Beck B, Blanpain C (2013) Unravelling cancer stem cell potential. Nat Rev Cancer 13:727–738

Belorusova AY, Suh N, Lee HJ, So JY, Maehr H, Rochel N (2017) Structural analysis and biological activities of BXL0124, a gemini analog of vitamin D. J Steroid Biochem Mol Biol 173:69–74

Bijlsma MF, Spek CA, Zivkovic D, van de Water S, Rezaee F, Peppelenbosch MP (2006) Repression of smoothened by patched-dependent (pro-)vitamin D3 secretion. PLoS Biol 4:e232

Bikle DD, Elalieh H, Welsh J, Oh D, Cleaver J, Teichert A (2013) Protective role of vitamin D signaling in skin cancer formation. J Steroid Biochem Mol Biol 136:271–279

Boeke CE, Tamimi RM, Berkey CS, Colditz GA, Giovannucci E, Malspeis S, Willett WC, Frazier AL (2015) Adolescent dietary vitamin D and sun exposure in relation to benign breast disease. Cancer Causes Control 26:1181–1187

Bonnet D, Dick JE (1997) Human acute myeloid leukemia is organized as a hierarchy that originates from a primitive hematopoietic cell. Nat Med 3:730–737

Cai L, Luo L, Tang Z, Meng X (2018) Combined antitumor effects of 1,25dihydroxy vitamin D3 and Notch inhibitor in liver cancer. Oncol Rep 40:1515–1524

Chen L, Yang R, Qiao W, Yuan X, Wang S, Goltzman D, Miao D (2018) 1,25-Dihydroxy vitamin D prevents tumorigenesis by inhibiting oxidative stress and inducing tumor cellular senescence in mice. Int J Cancer 143:368–382

Christakos S, Dhawan P, Verstuyf A, Verlinden L, Carmeliet G (2016) Vitamin D: metabolism, molecular mechanism of action, and pleiotropic effects. Physiol Rev 96:365–408

Cianferotti L, Cox M, Skorija K, Demay MB (2007) Vitamin D receptor is essential for normal keratinocyte stem cell function. Proc Natl Acad Sci U S A 104:9428–9433

Cianferotti L, Bertoldo F, Bischoff-Ferrari HA, Bruyere O, Cooper C, Cutolo M, Kanis JA, Kaufman JM, Reginster JY, Rizzoli R et al (2017) Vitamin D supplementation in the prevention and management of major chronic diseases not related to mineral homeostasis in adults: research for evidence and a scientific statement from the European society for clinical and economic aspects of osteoporosis and osteoarthritis (ESCEO). Endocrine 56:245–261

Clevers H (2011) The cancer stem cell: premises, promises and challenges. Nat Med 17:313–319

Cortes M, Liu SY, Kwan W, Alexa K, Goessling W, North TE (2015) Accumulation of the vitamin D precursor cholecalciferol antagonizes Hedgehog signaling to impair hemogenic endothelium formation. Stem Cell Reports 5:471–479

de The H (2018) Differentiation therapy revisited. Nat Rev Cancer 18:117–127

Deeb KK, Trump DL, Johnson CS (2007) Vitamin D signalling pathways in cancer: potential for anticancer therapeutics. Nat Rev Cancer 7:684–700

Dormoy V, Beraud C, Lindner V, Coquard C, Barthelmebs M, Brasse D, Jacqmin D, Lang H, Massfelder T (2012) Vitamin D3 triggers antitumor activity through targeting hedgehog signaling in human renal cell carcinoma. Carcinogenesis 33:2084–2093

Estebanez N, Gomez-Acebo I, Palazuelos C, Llorca J, Dierssen-Sotos T (2018) Vitamin D exposure and risk of breast cancer: a meta-analysis. Sci Rep 8:9039

Feldman D, Krishnan AV, Swami S, Giovannucci E, Feldman BJ (2014) The role of vitamin D in reducing cancer risk and progression. Nat Rev Cancer 14:342–357

Frank NY, Schatton T, Frank MH (2010) The therapeutic promise of the cancer stem cell concept. J Clin Invest 120:41–50

Gocek E, Studzinski GP (2009) Vitamin D and differentiation in cancer. Crit Rev Clin Lab Sci 46:190–209

Grant WB (2006) Epidemiology of disease risks in relation to vitamin D insufficiency. Prog Biophys Mol Biol 92:65–79

Gravellone L, Rizzo MA, Martina V, Mezzina N, Regalia A, Gallieni M (2011) Vitamin D receptor activators and clinical outcomes in chronic kidney disease. Int J Nephrol 2011:419524. https://doi.org/10.4061/2011/419524

Guyton KZ, Kensler TW, Posner GH (2003) Vitamin D and vitamin D analogs as cancer chemopreventive agents. Nutr Rev 61:227–238

Hadden MK (2016) Hedgehog and vitamin D signaling pathways in development and disease. Vitam Horm 100:231–253

Hanahan D, Weinberg RA (2011) Hallmarks of cancer: the next generation. Cell 144:646–674

Hermann PC, Bhaskar S, Cioffi M, Heeschen C (2010) Cancer stem cells in solid tumors. Semin Cancer Biol 20:77–84

Hossein-nezhad A, Holick MF (2013) Vitamin D for health: a global perspective. Mayo Clin Proc 88:720–755

Hu P, Li S, Tian N, Wu F, Hu Y, Li D, Qi Y, Wei Z, Wei Q, Li Y et al (2019) Acidosis enhances the self-renewal and mitochondrial respiration of stem cell-like glioma cells through CYP24A1-mediated reduction of vitamin D. Cell Death Dis 10:25

Huerta S, Irwin RW, Heber D, Go VL, Koeffler HP, Uskokovic MR, Harris DM (2002) 1alpha,25-(OH)(2)-D(3) and its synthetic analogue decrease tumor load in the Apc(min) Mouse. Cancer Res 62:741–746

Huet T, Maehr H, Lee HJ, Uskokovic MR, Suh N, Moras D, Rochel N (2011) Structure-function study of gemini derivatives with two different side chains at C-20, Gemini-0072 and Gemini-0097. Medchemcomm 2:424–429

Hughes PJ, Marcinkowska E, Gocek E, Studzinski GP, Brown G (2010) Vitamin D3-driven signals for myeloid cell differentiation-implications for differentiation therapy. Leuk Res 34:553–565
Jeong Y, Swami S, Krishnan AV, Williams JD, Martin S, Horst RL, Albertelli MA, Feldman BJ, Feldman D, Diehn M (2015) Inhibition of mouse breast tumor-initiating cells by calcitriol and dietary vitamin D. Mol Cancer Ther 14:1951–1961
Ji M, Liu L, Hou Y, Li B (2019) 1alpha,25Dihydroxyvitamin D3 restrains stem celllike properties of ovarian cancer cells by enhancing vitamin D receptor and suppressing CD44. Oncol Rep 41:3393–3403
Jiang YJ, Teichert AE, Fong F, Oda Y, Bikle DD (2013) 1alpha,25(OH)2-dihydroxyvitamin D3/VDR protects the skin from UVB-induced tumor formation by interacting with the beta-catenin pathway. J Steroid Biochem Mol Biol 136:229–232
Jones PH, Watt FM (1993) Separation of human epidermal stem cells from transit amplifying cells on the basis of differences in integrin function and expression. Cell 73:713–724
Khaw KT, Stewart AW, Waayer D, Lawes CMM, Toop L, Camargo CA Jr, Scragg R (2017) Effect of monthly high-dose vitamin D supplementation on falls and non-vertebral fractures: secondary and post-hoc outcomes from the randomised, double-blind, placebo-controlled ViDA trial. Lancet Diabetes Endocrinol 5:438–447
Kotlarz A, Przybyszewska M, Swoboda P, Miloszewska J, Grygorowicz MA, Kutner A, Markowicz S (2016) Differential interference of vitamin D analogs PRI-1906, PRI-2191, and PRI-2205 with the renewal of human colon cancer cells refractory to treatment with 5-fluorouracil. Tumour Biol 37:4699–4709
Kotlarz A, Przybyszewska M, Swoboda P, Neska J, Miloszewska J, Grygorowicz MA, Kutner A, Markowicz S (2019) Imatinib inhibits the regrowth of human colon cancer cells after treatment with 5-FU and cooperates with vitamin D analogue PRI-2191 in the downregulation of expression of stemness-related genes in 5-FU refractory cells. J Steroid Biochem Mol Biol 189:48–62
Kovalenko PL, Zhang Z, Cui M, Clinton SK, Fleet JC (2010) 1,25 dihydroxyvitamin D-mediated orchestration of anticancer, transcript-level effects in the immortalized, non-transformed prostate epithelial cell line, RWPE1. BMC Genomics 11:26
Krishnan AV, Trump DL, Johnson CS, Feldman D (2012) The role of vitamin D in cancer prevention and treatment. Rheum Dis Clin N Am 38:161–178
Lapidot T, Sirard C, Vormoor J, Murdoch B, Hoang T, Caceres-Cortes J, Minden M, Paterson B, Caligiuri MA, Dick JE (1994) A cell initiating human acute myeloid leukaemia after transplantation into SCID mice. Nature 367:645–648
Larriba MJ, Gonzalez-Sancho JM, Barbachano A, Niell N, Ferrer-Mayorga G, Munoz A (2013) Vitamin D Is a multilevel repressor of Wnt/b-catenin signaling in cancer cells. Cancers (Basel) 5:1242–1260
Lee HJ, Wislocki A, Goodman C, Ji Y, Ge R, Maehr H, Uskokovic M, Reiss M, Suh N (2006) A novel vitamin D derivative activates bone morphogenetic protein signaling in MCF10 breast epithelial cells. Mol Pharmacol 69:1840–1848
Lee HJ, Paul S, Atalla N, Thomas PE, Lin X, Yang I, Buckley B, Lu G, Zheng X, Lou YR et al (2008) Gemini vitamin D analogues inhibit estrogen receptor-positive and estrogen receptor-negative mammary tumorigenesis without hypercalcemic toxicity. Cancer Prev Res (Phila) 1:476–484
Lee HJ, So JY, DeCastro A, Smolarek A, Paul S, Maehr H, Uskokovic M, Suh N (2010) Gemini vitamin D analog suppresses ErbB2-positive mammary tumor growth via inhibition of ErbB2/AKT/ERK signaling. J Steroid Biochem Mol Biol 121:408–412
Leyssens C, Verlinden L, Verstuyf A (2014) The future of vitamin D analogs. Front Physiol 5:122
Li Y, Wicha MS, Schwartz SJ, Sun D (2011) Implications of cancer stem cell theory for cancer chemoprevention by natural dietary compounds. J Nutr Biochem 22:799–806
Li Z, Jia Z, Gao Y, Xie D, Wei D, Cui J, Mishra L, Huang S, Zhang Y, Xie K (2015) Activation of vitamin D receptor signaling downregulates the expression of nuclear FOXM1 protein and suppresses pancreatic cancer cell stemness. Clin Cancer Res 21:844–853

Li R, Huang J, Ma M, Lou Y, Zhang Y, Wu L, Chang DW, Zhao P, Dong Q, Wu X et al (2016) Two-stage induced differentiation of OCT4+/Nanog+ stem-like cells in lung adenocarcinoma. Oncotarget *7*:68360–68370

Li MX, Li LF, Zhang L, Xiao ZG, Shen J, Hu W, Zeng Q, Cho CH (2017) Vitamin D and cancer stem cells in the gastrointestinal tract. Curr Med Chem 24:918–927

Luan Z, Ma Y, Xin Y, Qian J, Wang H (2017) Possible molecular mechanisms by which vitamin D prevents inflammatory bowel disease and colitis-associated colorectal cancer. Curr Med Chem *24*:911–917

Luderer HF, Demay MB (2010) The vitamin D receptor, the skin and stem cells. J Steroid Biochem Mol Biol 121:314–316

Lytle NK, Barber AG, Reya T (2018) Stem cell fate in cancer growth, progression and therapy resistance. Nat Rev Cancer 18:669–680

Maehr H, Lee HJ, Perry B, Suh N, Uskokovic MR (2009) Calcitriol derivatives with two different side chains at C-20. V. Potent inhibitors of mammary carcinogenesis and inducers of leukemia differentiation. J Med Chem 52:5505–5519

Maehr H, Rochel N, Lee HJ, Suh N, Uskokovic MR (2013) Diastereotopic and deuterium effects in gemini. J Med Chem 56:3878–3888

Maleklou N, Allameh A, Kazemi B (2016) Targeted delivery of vitamin D3-loaded nanoparticles to C6 glioma cell line increased resistance to doxorubicin, epirubicin, and docetaxel in vitro. In Vitro Cell Dev Biol Anim 52:989–1000

Malihi Z, Lawes CMM, Wu Z, Huang Y, Waayer D, Toop L, Khaw KT, Camargo CA, Scragg R (2019) Monthly high-dose vitamin D supplementation does not increase kidney stone risk or serum calcium: results from a randomized controlled trial. Am J Clin Nutr 109(6):1578–1587

Manson JE, Bassuk SS, Lee IM, Cook NR, Albert MA, Gordon D, Zaharris E, Macfadyen JG, Danielson E, Lin J et al (2012) The VITamin D and OmegA-3 TriaL (VITAL): rationale and design of a large randomized controlled trial of vitamin D and marine omega-3 fatty acid supplements for the primary prevention of cancer and cardiovascular disease. Contemp Clin Trials 33:159–171

Manson JE, Cook NR, Lee IM, Christen W, Bassuk SS, Mora S, Gibson H, Gordon D, Copeland T, D'Agostino D et al (2019) Vitamin D supplements and prevention of cancer and cardiovascular disease. N Engl J Med 380:33–44

Maund SL, Barclay WW, Hover LD, Axanova LS, Sui G, Hipp JD, Fleet JC, Thorburn A, Cramer SD (2011) Interleukin-1alpha mediates the antiproliferative effects of 1,25-dihydroxyvitamin D3 in prostate progenitor/stem cells. Cancer Res 71:5276–5286

Mondul AM, Weinstein SJ, Layne TM, Albanes D (2017) Vitamin D and cancer risk and mortality: state of the science, gaps, and challenges. Epidemiol Rev 39:28–48

Narvaez CJ, Matthews D, LaPorta E, Simmons KM, Beaudin S, Welsh J (2014) The impact of vitamin D in breast cancer: genomics, pathways, metabolism. Front Physiol 5:213

Neska J, Swoboda P, Przybyszewska M, Kotlarz A, Bolla NR, Miloszewska J, Grygorowicz MA, Kutner A, Markowicz S (2016) The effect of analogues of 1alpha,25-Dihydroxyvitamin D(2) on the regrowth and gene expression of human colon cancer cells refractory to 5-Fluorouracil. Int J Mol Sci 17:903

Nguyen LV, Vanner R, Dirks P, Eaves CJ (2012) Cancer stem cells: an evolving concept. Nat Rev Cancer 12:133–143

Norman AW, Manchand PS, Uskokovic MR, Okamura WH, Takeuchi JA, Bishop JE, Hisatake JI, Koeffler HP, Peleg S (2000) Characterization of a novel analogue of 1 alpha,25(OH)(2)-vitamin D-3 with two side chains: interaction with its nuclear receptor and cellular actions. J Med Chem 43:2719–2730

Palmer HG, Gonzalez-Sancho JM, Espada J, Berciano MT, Puig I, Baulida J, Quintanilla M, Cano A, de Herreros AG, Lafarga M et al (2001) Vitamin D(3) promotes the differentiation of colon carcinoma cells by the induction of E-cadherin and the inhibition of beta-catenin signaling. J Cell Biol 154:369–387

Pálmer HG, Anjos-Afonso F, Carmeliet G, Takeda H, Watt FM (2008) The vitamin D receptor is a Wnt effector that controls hair follicle differentiation and specifies tumor type in adult epidermis. PLoS One *3*:e1483

Paubelle E, Zylbersztejn F, Alkhaeir S, Suarez F, Callens C, Dussiot M, Isnard F, Rubio MT, Damaj G, Gorin NC et al (2013) Deferasirox and vitamin D improves overall survival in elderly patients with acute myeloid leukemia after demethylating agents failure. PLoS One 8:e65998
Peng W, Wang K, Zheng R, Derwahl M (2016) 1,25 dihydroxyvitamin D3 inhibits the proliferation of thyroid cancer stem-like cells via cell cycle arrest. Endocr Res 41:71–80
Pickholtz I, Saadyan S, Keshet GI, Wang VS, Cohen R, Bouwman P, Jonkers J, Byers SW, Papa MZ, Yarden RI (2014) Cooperation between BRCA1 and vitamin D is critical for histone acetylation of the p21waf1 promoter and growth inhibition of breast cancer cells and cancer stem-like cells. Oncotarget 5:11827–11846
Pludowski P, Holick MF, Pilz S, Wagner CL, Hollis BW, Grant WB, Shoenfeld Y, Lerchbaum E, Llewellyn DJ, Kienreich K et al (2013) Vitamin D effects on musculoskeletal health, immunity, autoimmunity, cardiovascular disease, cancer, fertility, pregnancy, dementia and mortality-a review of recent evidence. Autoimmun Rev 12:976–989
Reichrath S, Reichrath J (2012) No evidence for induction of key components of the Notch signaling pathway (Notch-1, Jagged-1) by treatment with UV-B, 1,25(OH)(2)D(3), and/or epigenetic drugs (TSA, 5-Aza) in human keratinocytes in vitro. Dermatoendocrinol 4:44–52
Reichrath S, Muller CS, Gleissner B, Pfreundschuh M, Vogt T, Reichrath J (2010) Notch- and vitamin D signaling in 1,25(OH)2D3-resistant glioblastoma multiforme (GBM) cell lines. J Steroid Biochem Mol Biol 121:420–424
Reya T, Morrison SJ, Clarke MF, Weissman IL (2001) Stem cells, cancer, and cancer stem cells. Nature 414:105–111
Rochel N, Wurtz JM, Mitschler A, Klaholz B, Moras D (2000) The crystal structure of the nuclear receptor for vitamin D bound to its natural ligand. Mol Cell 5:173–179
Rosas-Peralta M, Holick MF, Borrayo-Sanchez G, Madrid-Miller A, Ramirez-Arias E, Arizmendi-Uribe E (2017) Dysfunctional immunometabolic effects of vitamin D deficiency, increased cardiometabolic risk. Potential epidemiological alert in America? Endocrinol Diabetes Nutr 64:162–173
Rossdeutscher L, Li J, Luco AL, Fadhil I, Ochietti B, Camirand A, Huang DC, Reinhardt TA, Muller W, Kremer R (2015) Chemoprevention activity of 25-hydroxyvitamin D in the MMTV-PyMT mouse model of breast cancer. Cancer Prev Res (Phila) 8:120–128
Sampieri K, Fodde R (2012) Cancer stem cells and metastasis. Semin Cancer Biol 22:187–193
Scragg R, Waayer D, Stewart AW, Lawes CMM, Toop L, Murphy J, Khaw KT, Camargo CA Jr (2016) The Vitamin D Assessment (ViDA) study: design of a randomized controlled trial of vitamin D supplementation for the prevention of cardiovascular disease, acute respiratory infection, falls and non-vertebral fractures. J Steroid Biochem Mol Biol 164:318–325
Scragg R, Khaw KT, Toop L, Sluyter J, Lawes CMM, Waayer D, Giovannucci E, Camargo CA Jr (2018) Monthly high-dose Vitamin D supplementation and cancer risk: a post hoc analysis of the Vitamin D assessment randomized clinical trial. JAMA Oncol 4:e182178
Shackleton M, Quintana E, Fearon ER, Morrison SJ (2009) Heterogeneity in cancer: cancer stem cells versus clonal evolution. Cell 138:822–829
Shah S, Islam MN, Dakshanamurthy S, Rizvi I, Rao M, Herrell R, Zinser G, Valrance M, Aranda A, Moras D et al (2006) The molecular basis of vitamin D receptor and beta-catenin crossregulation. Mol Cell 21:799–809
Shan NL, Wahler J, Lee HJ, Bak MJ, Gupta SD, Maehr H, Suh N (2017) Vitamin D compounds inhibit cancer stem-like cells and induce differentiation in triple negative breast cancer. J Steroid Biochem Mol Biol 173:122–129
Shibue T, Weinberg RA (2017) EMT, CSCs, and drug resistance: the mechanistic link and clinical implications. Nat Rev Clin Oncol 14:611–629
So JY, Suh N (2015) Targeting cancer stem cells in solid tumors by vitamin D. J Steroid Biochem Mol Biol 148:79–85
So JY, Lee HJ, Smolarek AK, Paul S, Wang CX, Maehr H, Uskokovic M, Zheng X, Conney AH, Cai L et al (2011) A novel Gemini vitamin D analog represses the expression of a stem cell marker CD44 in breast cancer. Mol Pharmacol 79:360–367

So JY, Wahler J, Das Gupta S, Salerno DM, Maehr H, Uskokovic M, Suh N (2015) HES1-mediated inhibition of Notch1 signaling by a Gemini vitamin D analog leads to decreased CD44(+)/CD24 (−/low) tumor-initiating subpopulation in basal-like breast cancer. J Steroid Biochem Mol Biol 148:111–121

Srivastava AK, Rizvi A, Cui T, Han C, Banerjee A, Naseem I, Zheng Y, Wani AA, Wang QE (2018) Depleting ovarian cancer stem cells with calcitriol. Oncotarget 9:14481–14491

Stechschulte SA, Kirsner RS, Federman DG (2009) Vitamin D: bone and beyond, rationale and recommendations for supplementation. Am J Med 122:793–802

Swami S, Krishnan AV, Williams J, Aggarwal A, Albertelli MA, Horst RL, Feldman BJ, Feldman D (2016) Vitamin D mitigates the adverse effects of obesity on breast cancer in mice. Endocr Relat Cancer 23:251–264

Takebe N, Miele L, Harris PJ, Jeong W, Bando H, Kahn M, Yang SX, Ivy SP (2015) Targeting notch, hedgehog, and Wnt pathways in cancer stem cells: clinical update. Nat Rev Clin Oncol 12:445–464

Tang JY, Xiao TZ, Oda Y, Chang KS, Shpall E, Wu A, So PL, Hebert J, Bikle D, Epstein EH Jr (2011) Vitamin D3 inhibits hedgehog signaling and proliferation in murine Basal cell carcinomas. Cancer Prev Res (Phila) 4:744–751

Teichert AE, Elalieh H, Elias PM, Welsh J, Bikle DD (2011) Overexpression of hedgehog signaling is associated with epidermal tumor formation in vitamin D receptor-null mice. J Invest Dermatol 131:2289–2297

Thakkar A, Wang B, Picon-Ruiz M, Buchwald P, Ince TA (2016) Vitamin D and androgen receptor-targeted therapy for triple-negative breast cancer. Breast Cancer Res Treat 157:77–90

Trump DL, Muindi J, Fakih M, Yu WD, Johnson CS (2006) Vitamin D compounds: clinical development as cancer therapy and prevention agents. Anticancer Res *26*:2551–2556

Trump DL, Deeb KK, Johnson CS (2010) Vitamin D: considerations in the continued development as an agent for cancer prevention and therapy. Cancer J 16:1–9

Uhmann A, Niemann H, Lammering B, Henkel C, Hess I, Nitzki F, Fritsch A, Prufer N, Rosenberger A, Dullin C et al (2011) Antitumoral effects of calcitriol in basal cell carcinomas involve inhibition of hedgehog signaling and induction of vitamin D receptor signaling and differentiation. Mol Cancer Ther 10:2179–2188

Visvader JE, Lindeman GJ (2008) Cancer stem cells in solid tumours: accumulating evidence and unresolved questions. Nat Rev Cancer 8:755–768

Vogelstein B, Papadopoulos N, Velculescu VE, Zhou S, Diaz LA Jr, Kinzler KW (2013) Cancer genome landscapes. Science 339:1546–1558

Wahler J, So JY, Cheng LC, Maehr H, Uskokovic M, Suh N (2015) Vitamin D compounds reduce mammosphere formation and decrease expression of putative stem cell markers in breast cancer. J Steroid Biochem Mol Biol 148:148–155

Wicha MS (2014) Targeting self-renewal, an Achilles' heel of cancer stem cells. Nat Med 20:14–15

Wu Z, Camargo CA Jr, Sluyter JD, Khaw KT, Malihi Z, Waayer D, Toop L, Lawes CMM, Scragg R (2019) Association between serum 25-hydroxyvitamin D levels and self-reported chronic pain in older adults: a cross-sectional analysis from the ViDA study. J Steroid Biochem Mol Biol 188:17–22

Xu H, Posner GH, Stevenson M, Campbell FC (2010) Apc(MIN) modulation of vitamin D secosteroid growth control. Carcinogenesis 31:1434–1441

Xun J, Wang D, Shen L, Gong J, Gao R, Du L, Chang A, Song X, Xiang R, Tan X (2017) JMJD3 suppresses stem cell-like characteristics in breast cancer cells by downregulation of Oct4 independently of its demethylase activity. Oncotarget 8:21918–21929

Yan M, Liu Q (2016) Differentiation therapy: a promising strategy for cancer treatment. Chin J Cancer 35:3

Zheng W, Duan B, Zhang Q, Ouyang L, Peng W, Qian F, Wang Y, Huang S (2018) Vitamin D-induced vitamin D receptor expression induces tamoxifen sensitivity in MCF-7 stem cells via the suppression of Wnt/beta-catenin signaling. Biosci Rep 38(6). https://doi.org/10.1042/BSR20180595

Chapter 6
Anti-cancer Effects of Silibinin: The Current Status in Cancer Chemoprevention

Dominique Reed, Komal Raina, and Rajesh Agarwal

Abstract The naturally occurring flavonolignan Silibinin (also known as Silybin) is a bioactive constituent of silymarin isolated from the seeds of the milk thistle plant (*Silybum marianum* L. Gaernt.), a member of the Asteraceae family. The milk thistle plant is a part of the native vegetation in Southern Europe, Southern Russia, Asia Minor and Northern Africa. This multi-functional flavonolignan possesses strong hepatoprotective, cardioprotective, neuroprotective, immune-modulatory, antidotal and anti-neoplastic properties. To date, over 600 peer-reviewed research reports and limited clinical trials have evaluated the anti-oncogenic efficacy of silibinin to combat tumor growth, angiogenesis, and metastasis. As a promising agent, silibinin mediates a wide-range of potent chemopreventive and anti-cancer activities in several frequently diagnosed epithelial malignancies, including skin, colon, prostate and lung. In addition, several combinatorial anti-cancer strategies of silibinin with other therapeutics exhibit synergistic interactions to suppress drug-induced toxic effects and chemoresistance. In this chapter, the pre-clinical and clinical efficacy of silibinin and/or silymarin derivatives against several cancers will be reviewed. Moreover, the chapter will summarize silibinin effects on key signaling pathways, such as: transforming Growth Factor beta (TGFβ), epidermal growth factor receptor (EGFR), insulin-like growth factor-1 receptor (IGF-1R), and NF-κB (nuclear factor-kappa B), which are crucial to the anti-cancer activity of silibinin in cancer prevention, disease progression/recurrence and reversal of drug resistance.

D. Reed
Department of Pharmaceutical Sciences, Skaggs School of Pharmacy and Pharmaceutical Sciences, University of Colorado Anschutz Medical Campus, Aurora, CO, USA

K. Raina
Department of Pharmaceutical Sciences, South Dakota State University, Brookings, SD, USA

R. Agarwal (✉)
Department of Pharmaceutical Sciences, Skaggs School of Pharmacy and Pharmaceutical Sciences, University of Colorado Anschutz Medical Campus, Aurora, CO, USA

University of Colorado Cancer Center, University of Colorado Denver-Anschutz Medical Campus, Aurora, CO, USA
e-mail: Rajesh.Agarwal@UCDenver.edu

J. M. Pezzuto, O. Vang (eds.), *Natural Products for Cancer Chemoprevention*,
https://doi.org/10.1007/978-3-030-39855-2_6

Keywords Silibinin · Skin cancer · Bladder cancer · Colorectal cancer · Prostate cancer · Non-small lung cancer · Cancer stem cells

6.1 Introduction

Globally, extensive and cutting edge research on oncological diseases has led to the development of potent adjuvant and neo-adjuvant agents for use in therapeutic combinatorial strategies to address the biological complexities accompanying tumorigenesis and drug resistance in various tumor types. Life expectancies for cancer survivors has greatly improved due to research advancements in cancer screening and treatments; the cancer survivorship is estimated to grow to 26 million by 2040 in the United States (U.S.) (Shapiro 2018). Despite these efforts (Kumar et al. 2015; Martinez Rodriguez et al. 2017; Mateen et al. 2013; Raina et al. 2016; Reed et al. 2018; Ting et al. 2013, 2014), short- and long-term exposure to treatment strategies such as chemo- and radio-therapies have resulted in the onset of intricate medical issues associated with systemic toxicity that diminish the quality of life and heighten mortality risk among cancer survivors (Miller et al. 2016). Standard cancer treatment regimens include chemotherapy with or without radiation, a most common treatment strategy for advanced malignancies at stage III and higher, whereas, surgical procedures are more likely utilized to treat localized and/or organ bound disease. However, these therapies are often associated with cardiovascular complications, hepatic injury, pneumonitis, urinary or bowel dysfunction, neurological, nephrological, gastrointestinal toxicities and other unintended side effects in patients (Klee et al. 2017; Miller et al. 2016; Vietor and George 2012).

In recent years, natural product-based cancer chemoprevention/ intervention strategies have garnered attention in regard to their strong preventive efficacy, synergism with anti-cancer agents against multiple tumor types, and minimization of systemic toxicities associated with cancer treatment modalities (Zhang et al. 2018). Several classes of natural products such as flavonoids, alkaloids, phenylpropanoids, polyketides, and terpenoids have been shown to function as effective chemopreventive agents under in vitro and in vivo scenario including clinical studies (Raffa et al. 2017; Reed et al. 2018; Salehi et al. 2018). This chapter focuses on one such beneficial agent—silibinin.

6.1.1 Silibinin

One of the most promising anti-cancer natural products is the flavonolignan silibinin, extracted from the seeds of *Silybum marianum* (also known as "milk thistle"), a member of the Asteraceae family. Silibinin, a 1:1 ratio of silibin A and silibin B isomers, functions as a weak acid in aqueous conditions and is very stable in acidic environment but becomes unstable in the presence of bases as well as Lewis acids

(Abenavoli et al. 2018). For more than 2000 years, medicinal use of silibinin has included the treatment of gout, mushroom poisoning, hydrophobia, organ toxicities (kidney, spleen, liver and gallbladder), and most recently cancer, diabetes and neurological disorders (Abenavoli et al. 2018; Post-White et al. 2007). Several studies have also demonstrated beneficial effects of silibinin against toxicities associated with short- and long-term exposure to chemotherapy and radiation treatments (Raffa et al. 2017; Redondo-Blanco et al. 2017).

Notably, silibinin is a multi-facet nutraceutical that targets several features of cancer development and progression such as oxidative stress, inflammation, proliferation, apoptosis, angiogenesis, metastasis, etc. (Deep and Agarwal 2010; Kumar et al. 2015; Ramasamy and Agarwal 2008). In this chapter, the current state of progress regarding silibinin potential and efficacy against hallmarks of cancer will be discussed in regard to its effects alone and/or in combination therapies against epithelial malignancies. Furthermore, mechanisms associated with silibinin effects to curtail toxic side effects and overcome drug resistance associated with clinical chemotherapeutic agents will also be discussed. In addition, new literature detailing the minimizing effects of silibinin on systemic toxicity and cancer survivorship that further support the promise of silibinin as a strong candidate for combination therapy regimens will be examined.

6.1.2 Bioavailability and Metabolism of Silibinin

Absorption of silibinin after oral administration is rapid and has half-life time of 6 h with gastrointestinal re-absorption between 20 and 40% (Bijak 2017; Saller et al. 2008). Post-1 hour oral administration, silibinin or its conjugates are in the following organs (in decreasing order): stomach, liver, pancreas, lung, prostate and skin. Silibinin undergoes hepatic metabolism and extensive biotransformation by phase I and II enzymes (Bijak 2017; Javed et al. 2011; Zhao and Agarwal 1999). Several reports have shown silibinin exerts modulatory effect against several cytochrome P450 enzymes, which are the predominate species of enzymes involved in hepatic and other types of metabolism in various cell types. The cytochrome P450 isoforms affected by silibinin include CYP450 2D6, CYP450 2E1, CYP450 3A4, CYP450 2C9, CYP450 2C8 (Bijak 2017), but has little to no effect on CYP450 1A2, CYP450 2C9, CYP450 2D6 and CYP450 3A4/5 (Bijak 2017).

Though silibinin's bioavailability remains a limiting factor in clinical studies focused on oral delivery, this issue has been addressed by the development of various silibinin complexes (with phosphatidylcholine, such as silipide and siliphos) and formulations (such as i.v. Legalon), which have significantly improved its bioavailability in pre-clinical and clinical trials (Bijak 2017; Flaig et al. 2007a; Hoh et al. 2006). Silipide, a silibinin-phosphatidylcholine formulation, showed safe consumption and achieved high levels of silibinin concentration in the colorectal mucosa of colorectal cancer patients with no adverse effects. However, oral administration of silibinin to three advanced liver cancer patients resulted in high mortality rates between 23 and 69 days (Siegel et al. 2014). Patient mortality was partially attributed to liver failure, severe disease state and silibinin intervention was not implemented at an optimal time during disease progression to improve liver dysfunction. Contrary to this, a successful injectable formulation of silibinin, Legalon^{R}, has shown efficacy against acute liver toxicity in patients (Bijak 2017; Mengs et al. 2012). Various formulations and delivery methods (Bijak 2017) of silibinin have been investigated in cell-based, pre-clinical and limited clinical trials (NCT03440164, NCT02633696) (Bijak 2017; Jeter et al. 2019).

6.2 Skin Cancer

Epidermis is the most dominant organ in the integumentary system that serves as a protective barrier against pathogens and environmental insults. Accumulation of chronic DNA damage to the epidermis can trigger molecular changes that favor development of skin carcinogenesis due to several factors. Etiological factors of skin cancer include high exposure to solar ultraviolet radiation (UVR), outdoor activities, indoor tanning, heightened sun sensitivity, and environmental and/or chemical agents (arsenic, petroleum by-products) (Rajput et al. 2018; Society 2019). Chronic UVR exposure accounts for 90% of skin cancer. As epithelia derived neoplasms, skin cancers are classified as cutaneous melanoma (MSC) or non-melanoma (NMSC) [basal cell, squamous cell, Merkel cell, lymphoma, Kaposi sarcoma]. Global skin cancer incidence and mortality estimates show over 348,000 and approximately 1.1 million people were affected by melanoma and non-melanoma in 2018, respectively (Bray et al. 2018; Ferlay et al. 2019). Among North American men and women, melanoma is fifth most frequently diagnosed cancer and has a 22% 5-year survival rate for metastatic disease in the U.S. (Ferlay et al. 2019).

Solar radiation consists of several types of UVRs, which include UVA (320–400 nm), UVB (280–320 nm) and UVC (200–280 nm). Of these types, solar UVR on earth's surface consists of 90–99% UVA and 1–10% UVB radiation. Skin carcinogenic murine studies have revealed that only high doses of UVA were sufficient to initiate delayed skin tumor development, but UVB triggered skin carcinogenesis within a time interval more relevant to clinical conditions. Relative to NMSC, MSC is more aggressive and accounts for up to 75% of deaths related to skin carcinogenesis (Kumar et al. 2015; Society 2019). Two of the most common subtypes of NMSC are basal (BCC) and squamous cell carcinomas (SCC). SCC is most common in African-Americans; whereas, European-Americans, Asians and Latinos are most frequently diagnosed with BCC (Higgins et al. 2018).

6.2.1 *Targeting of UV Radiation-Regulated Signaling in Skin Carcinogenesis by Silibinin*

Epidermal carcinoma cell lines based in vitro experiments and in vivo studies in the SKH-1 mice model aid in identifying major signaling mechanisms involved in the initiation and disease progression in skin carcinogenesis (SCC) (Kumar et al. 2015). Genetic mutations in *PTCH1* and tumor suppressor *TP53 (p53)* genes are critical to UV radiation-induced skin cancer (Kumar et al. 2015). Specifically this type of radiation can cause cyclobutane/thymine dimers leading to CC/TT and C/T mutations due to replication of unrepaired DNA damage (Kumar et al. 2015). These UV-associated mutations occur in 60% of SCCs and 50% of sporadic BCCs (Kumar et al. 2015). UVB radiation absorbed by epidermal DNA can produce photoproducts (CPDs, 6–4 photoproducts), DNA/protein crosslinks, genomic instability, and reactive oxygen species in the skin.

The anti-cancer properties of silibinin has been shown to alter tumor suppressor p53, cell cycle, serine/threonine protein kinase, and survival signaling proteins in skin carcinogenesis (Dheeraj et al. 2017; Kumar et al. 2015; Tilley et al. 2015, 2016). Pre- and post- silibinin treatment in respect to UVB exposure exerted some opposite effects in human epidermoid tumor A431 cells. Pre-treatment with silibinin sensitized A431 cells to apoptosis (cleaved caspases 3 and 7), and stimulated the activation of mitogen-activated protein kinases (MAPKs) such as pERK1/2 and pJNK (Mohan et al. 2004). In contrast, these effects were reversed and/or comparable to UVB alone. In HaCaT cells, silibinin alone inhibited pERK1/2 signaling and increased levels of transcription factor AP-1 and mitochondrial Bclx(L) expression (Dhanalakshmi et al. 2004a). At low dosages of UVB exposure, silibinin had a stimulatory effect on MAPK signaling and continue to activate apoptotic signaling (survivin, Bcl-2, caspase-9), but maintained protection of HaCaT cells against apoptosis via prolonged S phase allowing for sufficient DNA repair in cells. However, higher UVB exposure mitigated this protective effect and silibinin induced apoptosis via increased cleaved PARP and this effect was reversed by a pan caspase inhibitor C1 (Dhanalakshmi et al. 2004a). This study suggested silibinin plays a dual role and can either be protective against or promote cell death cell dependent on dosage of UVB exposure. Moreover, silibinin supplementation has exerted its anti-neoplastic effects on cell cycle molecules and DNA repair mechanisms in response to UVB caused DNA damage in UVB-induced skin carcinogenesis initiation. Pre-treatment of the JB6 cell line with silibinin promoted p53 signaling and the activation of DNA repair machinery (DNA-PK, ATM) in response to UVB exposure, but also induced pERK, pAKT and pro-apoptotic signaling (Dhanalakshmi et al. 2005). Interestingly, inhibition of MAPK and DNA repair signaling via MEK1/2 inhibitor PD98059, DNA-PK inhibitor LY294002, ATM/ATR inhibitor caffeine did not impede silibinin activation of p53 signaling. The consistent activation of p53 signaling by silibinin could suggests silibinin anti-cancer activity does not require the down-regulation of MAPK and DNA repair mechanisms alone. Cyclin dependent kinase inhibitors (p21, p27) and p53 signaling were induced by silibinin dietary feeding in SKH-1 hairless mice as well as concurrent down-regulation of proliferation, cyclins (A, B1, D1), cyclin dependent kinases, CDK2/4, kinase cascade signaling (pERK1/2, pJNK1/2, p38, pAKT) and inhibition of tumorigenesis (Dhanalakshmi et al. 2004b; Gu et al. 2005a, b, 2006; Mallikarjuna et al. 2004). UVB-induced activation of [nuclear factor-kappa B (NF- κB)] and AP-1 as well as epidermal growth factor (EGF)-mediated ERK1/2, JNK1/2, MAPK/p38 and protein kinase B (AKT) phosphorylation in keratinocytes were strongly suppressed by silibinin (Dhanalakshmi et al. 2004a; Mallikarjuna et al. 2004; Singh et al. 2006b). Chronic UVB exposure of SKH-1 mice activated the anti-apoptotic effects of transcription factor, E2F1; but topical and dietary silibinin reduced E2F1 levels with no effect on E2F2/3 to induce apoptosis and tumor suppressor p53 in tumors (Gu et al. 2006). However, opposite effects were observed in the epidermis, UVB down-regulated E2F1 and p53 accompanied by reduced cyclin-dependent kinase inhibitors and upregulation of E2F2/3 transcription factors, cyclin-dependent kinases, cyclins, CDC25C, MAPK and Akt signaling; importantly, these effects were reversed by silibinin (Gu et al. 2006).

Tumor suppressor p53 signaling also plays a critical role in silibinin efficacy against skin cancer-its dependency on this tumor suppressor has been evaluated in several studies. Silibinin treatment of actinic keratosis, a potential precursor to NMSC, in mixed actinic keratosis and SCC specimens, exhibited moderate (10–50%) to strong expression of key proteins in skin cancer such as COX-2, EZH-2 (Enhancer Of Zeste 2 Polycomb Repressive Complex 2 Subunit) and p53 (Athanassiadou et al. 2013). In BCC murine tumor cell lines (p53 mutant ASZ and p53 null BSZ), cell growth, clonogenicity and expression of proliferative markers (PCNA and cyclin D1) in ASZ allografts were strongly inhibited by silibinin and its derivative-2,3-dehydrosilibinin; additionally, both exhibited pro-apoptotic signaling in ASZ and BSZ cells (Tilley et al. 2016).

Hedgehog/Gli signaling pathway has been shown to negatively regulate and override p53-mediated anti-tumorigenic effects. Inhibition of Hedgehog signaling has been shown to demonstrate anti-cancer effects, but resistant disease develops following such therapies (Dheeraj et al. 2017; Tilley et al. 2016). Silibinin treatment has been shown to overcome disease resistance to hedgehog signaling inhibition via reduction of phosphorylated and total levels of ERK1/2, AKT, EGF receptor (EGFR) and STAT3 (Tilley et al. 2016). Also, tumor growth, and DNA binding activity of transcription factors, NF-κB and AP-1, were reduced by both silibinin and its derivative in ASZ allografts as well (Tilley et al. 2016). Moreover, silibinin improved the sensitivity of BCC cells resistant to hedgehog inhibitors (Sant-1, GDC-0449) by targeting molecules associated with this resistance. Silibinin significantly reduced phosphorylated Akt and ERK1/2, cyclin D1 and hedgehog signaling molecule-Gli levels, and increased protein levels of cleaved caspase-3, cleaved PARP, tumor suppressor SUFU in ASZ001-Sant1 resistant cells (Dheeraj et al. 2017).

Modulation of immune and angiogenesis mechanisms is another silibinin effect directed towards skin cancer. Pre- and post-silibinin topical application (9 mg in acetone) and dietary (1% silibinin) treatments in response to chronic UVB exposure delayed tumor growth and reduced pro-angiogenic proteins (HIF-1α, iNOS), NF-κB and STAT3 inflammatory signaling and associated mediator (COX-2) (Tilley et al. 2015). Immunosuppression and suppression of contact hypersensitivity in C3H/HeN photo- carcinogenic mouse model by UVB was also minimized by silibinin (Meeran et al. 2006). Our lab has also shown IL-12 elevation by silibinin in UVB exposed JB6 and SKH-1 model as well as rapid repair of DNA damage (cyclobutane-pyrimidine dimers) by silibinin alone and/or in a synergistic combination with exogenous recombinant exogenous IL-12 via its reduction of cleaved caspase-3 and cleaved PARP protein levels (Narayanapillai et al. 2014). Skin pre-treatment or immediate treatment with silibinin after UV exposure also upregulates GADD45α, a downstream target of p53, and anti-autophagy effect mediated by p53-activation to protect against UVB-caused DNA damage (Singh et al. 2006b; Wang et al. 2013). However, the protection exerted by silibinin against UVB-induced DNA damage and carcinogenesis are p53-dependent and become compromised in heterozygous (p53+/−) and knockout (p53−/−) in vivo models (Rigby et al. 2017).

Furthermore, Sati and co-workers (2016) have shown that tumor incidence, growth and burden were reduced by silibinin in chemically induced [7, 12-dimethylbenz(*a*)anthracene (DMBA) and 12-*O*-tetradecanoylphorbol-13-acetate (TPA)] skin tumorigenesis model. This anti-cancer effect was mediated via its pro-oxidative activity, altered choline metabolism and induction of apoptosis by elevated lipid peroxidation levels during later stages of disease (Sati et al. 2016). Also, the chemopreventive effects of silibinin in chemically-induced kin cancer in Swiss albino mice resulted in the down-regulation of pro-inflammatory cytokines (TNF-α, IL-6, IL-1β, NO), COX-2 and restoration of anti-oxidant enzyme levels (Khan et al. 2014). In human keratinocytes, silibinin effectively sensitized HaCaT cells to UVA irradiation-induced apoptosis and ER oxidative stress via up-regulation of CHOP protein levels (Narayanapillai et al. 2014).

6.2.2 Silibinin-Associated Combination Therapies Against Skin Cancer

For skin carcinogenesis, the efficacy of therapeutic strategies have been capitulated by disease resistance and adverse side effects of clinically accepted therapies. Clinical evidence does show a supportive role of silibinin to treat hepatoxicity and other associated adverse effects in the treatment of cancer (Greenlee et al. 2007). Surgery is the primary treatment strategy for melanoma, but more recent strategies have included immunotherapies for more advanced disease (Miller et al. 2016). While immunotherapies such as ipilimumab, pembrolizumab, nivolumab, BRAF and MEK inhibitors greatly improve melanoma survival, these agents can further increase risk of SCC, disease resistance, and their autoimmune-related side effects (Hwang and Fernandez-Penas 2018) can result in mortality (Drysdale et al. 2019; Hodi et al. 2010; Mackiewicz and Mackiewicz 2018; Randhawa et al. 2019). The anti-oxidant properties and anti-cancer activity of natural products such as silibinin can minimize the onset of adverse side effects induced by both immuno- and chemotherapies and other aggressive regimens against carcinogenesis. Notably, silibinin has strong efficacy against Hedgehog inhibitor resistant disease in skin cancer. In a study investigating the effects of silibinin on mouse basal cell carcinoma cell line ASZ001-resistant to hedgehog inhibitors (Sant-1, GDC-0449), silibinin improved cytotoxic response in these resistant cells to these inhibitors [via suppression of EGFR phosphorylation (Tyr-1173), total EGFR, pAkt (Ser 473), cyclin D1 expression, and induction of a high bax/bcl-2 ratio and cleaved caspase 3 levels (Dheeraj et al. 2017)]. Together, hedgehog inhibitor drugs and silibinin decreased cell proliferation, colony formation and induced substantial apoptosis in ASZ001 resistant cells. Silibinin showed a dose-dependent inhibition of cell growth in Sant-1 and GDC-0449 resistant ASZ001 cells. Although recent clinical studies have not fully evaluated silibinin and its effects against therapy-related toxicities in skin cancer, our silibinin-based topical drug formulation, Difinsa53, has been investigated as a preventive strategy against radiation-associated dermatitis in breast cancer patients (NCT02534129). Difinsa53 is a skin protectant lotion formulated with dimethicone 1%, silibinin, aloe vera and niacinamide, and hyaluronic acid. Unfortunately, this Phase I study was terminated due to control subjects having insufficient dermatitis.

6.3 Bladder Cancer

Over 500,000 incidences and approximately 200,000 deaths are attributed to bladder carcinoma-the seventh most prevalent malignancy worldwide (Bray et al. 2018; Ferlay et al. 2019). For 2018, bladder cancer incidences were at its highest in Northern African, Western Asian and Southern European countries. Male populations in these countries as well as in the U.S. are predominantly affected by this malignancy. American men are 4 times at higher risk than women in developing urinary bladder cancer. Also, European American men are twice more likely to be diagnosed with this disease relative to African American men (Society 2019). Patients 65 years of age or older diagnosed with stage IV bladder cancer treated with systemic chemotherapy were linked to a fourfold increase in overall survival relative to untreated individuals (Flannery et al. 2018). Increasing chemotherapy access to high-grade bladder cancer patients may improve the follow-up per patient per month (PPPM) health care cost in this population. Unfortunately, major health institutions and organization have not yet come to a consensus on a standard screening test for bladder cancer detection or whether early screening improves bladder cancer mortality (DeGeorge et al. 2017). High-risk of bladder cancer development is strongly linked to family history of bladder cancer/infections, endemic schistosomiasis infection tobacco-use, genetic changes, consumption of Chinese herb *Aristolochia fangchi*, exposure to chemo- or radiation therapies, occupational use of paints/dyes, metal, petroleum to arsenic and chlorine in drinking water. Bladder carcinoma is classified into urothelial and non-urothelial subtypes.

Approximately 90% of bladder cancer cases are classified as urothelial carcinoma in situ and invasive (Kaseb and Aeddula 2019). Non-urothelial bladder malignancy is uncommon and largely composed of squamous cell and adenocarcinoma intermixed tumors, but other cancer types include squamous cell, and adenocarcinoma (Grignon 2009). Non-muscle invasive disease, which is associated with a more favorable prognosis compared to muscle invasive disease, is between 70 and 80% of bladder cancers (DeGeorge et al. 2017). Primary treatment for non-muscle invasive bladder cancer includes transurethral resection of bladder tumor (TURBT) followed by Bacillus Calmette-Guerin (BCG) or intravesical chemotherapy. Superficial recurrent disease has a 50% incidence rate in high-risk non-muscle patients that only receive TURBT.

6.3.1 Modulation of Signaling Mechanisms in Bladder Cancer by Silibinin

Silymarin and its components, such as silibinin, have been evaluated in regard to their efficacy against bladder cancer by Vinh et al. (2002) and various labs including ours (Agarwal et al. 2013; Polachi et al. 2016). In *N*-butyl-N-(4-hydroxybutyl) nitrosamine (OHBBN)–induced urinary bladder carcinogenesis models, silibinin significantly minimizes tumor phenotypes associated with bladder cancer by modulating several biological pathways including cell survival, apoptotic and epithelial mesenchymal transition (EMT) signaling (Polachi et al. 2016; Vinh et al. 2002). One of the earliest studies on the OHBBN-induced bladder cancer model was by Vinh and associates (2002). During and post-cancer initiation, dietary feeding of silymarin (1000 ppm) showed a protective effect against the development of bladder tumors, pre-malignant lesions and decreased the proliferative capacity of lesions via cyclin D1 positive cell ratio and 5-bromodeoxyuridine (BrdU) levels (Vinh et al. 2002). Initial pre-clinical efficacy studies in our lab identified important p53-dependent and independent anti-tumorigenic signaling mechanisms associated with silibinin as a pre-treatment option against the development of dyplasia and progression to tumorigenesis in bladder carcinoma models (Singh et al. 2008). Pre-treatment with silymarin or its major bioactive constituent silibinin (200 mg/kg per bodyweight) for 6 weeks significantly suppressed the prevalence of urothelial lesions and the progression of tumorigenesis (development of mucosa and papillary nodular dyplasia and invasive disease) (Tyagi et al. 2007). Interestingly, the protective effect of both silymarin and silibinin pre-treatments in ICR mice remain effective against 12 months of OHBBN exposure. In addition, the apoptotic index was elevated and proliferation was decreased by more than 40% in bladder specimens, together with down-regulation in MAPK1/2, cyclin D1, survivin and nuclear phospho-p65 protein levels in both silymarin and silibinin treatment groups (Tyagi et al. 2007). Daily oral administration of silibinin (100, 200 mg/kg) suppressed RT4 xenograft tumor cell proliferation, microvasculature, growth and induced apoptosis via a significant decrease in p53-independent nuclear localization and protein levels of survivin and concurrent up-regulation of p53 and cleaved caspase-3 (Singh et al. 2008).

Silibinin treatment of high-risk superficial bladder carcinoma cells, 5637, led to inhibition of tumor cell growth and caspase-dependent and independent apoptotic cell death via disruption of the mitochondria potential (Zeng et al. 2011). In vitro and xenograft studies with 5637 tumor cells revealed suppression of survivin, activation of caspase-3 and translocation of apoptosis inducing factor (AIF) due to silibinin treatment. Furthermore, silibinin reduced the incidence rates linked to superficial and invasive bladder lesion development in intravesical *N*-methyl-*N*-nitrosourea (MNU)-induced bladder carcinogenesis. Recently, Li et al. (2018) demonstrated that silibinin inhibits TGF β1 signaling and induction of cell migration, invasion and epithelial mesenchymal transition (EMT) via down-regulation of COX-2 in bladder transitional cell carcinoma (Li et al. 2018). This EMT reversal effect of silibinin was also observed by Wu and associates (2013) in the highly metastatic model, T24-L (Wu et al. 2013). Silibinin caused reduction of glycogen synthase kinase-3β (GSK-3β) phosphorylation, β-catenin nuclear translocation, vimentin, MMP-2 and cytokeratins 18 and 19 expression in T24-L tumor cells (Wu et al. 2013). Also, a dual role of silibinin against EMT and stem-like properties were shown via its down-regulation of both cancer stem cell marker CD44 and ZEB1, a regulator of MMP-2, expression levels.

Bladder cancer cell lines, T24 and J82, resistant to chemotherapy agent cisplatin have shown enhanced proliferative capacity, migration, and invasion via activation of NF-κB signaling, up-regulation of EMT markers (N-cadherin, Vimentin, MMP-2, MMP-9) and multiple drug resistant gene, ABCB1 (Sun et al. 2017). These effects were reversed by silibinin (100 μM) treatment not only in cisplatin-resistant, but parental bladder tumor cell lines as well. Expression of E-cadherin, a marker for epithelial cells, was also induced by silibinin in both cisplatin resistant cell lines. Interestingly, silibinin cytotoxic activity evoked epigenetic changes in bladder tumor cells associated with its ant-cancer effects. Silibinin treatment reduced levels of histone H3 lysine4 trimethylation (H3K4me3), DNA methyltransferase 1 (DNMT1), and H3 acetylation (AcH3) in T24, UM-UC-3 and/or RT4 bladder tumor cells (DE Oliveira et al. 2017; Imai-Sumida et al. 2017). Silibinin treatment induced early apoptosis in p53 mutated T24 cells; however, p53 wildtype RT4 cells underwent late apoptosis and necrosis (DE Oliveira et al. 2017). Also, FRAP/mTOR signaling is an important component of PI3K/AKT pathway and associated miRNAs, miR-100 and miR-203, were significantly modulated by silibinin (DE Oliveira et al. 2017).

NF-κB signaling is a potent stimulator of tumor initiation, development, and metastasis. Inhibition of NF-κB signaling utilizing NF-κB inhibitor, pyrrolidine dithiocarbamate (PDTC) did not affect proliferation, migration, invasion, and expression of EMT markers and ABCB1 in parental T24 and J82 cell lines. However, silibinin exposure alone had a potent anti-cancer activity against these cells, which indicated that its effect was independent of NF-κB pathway (Sun et al. 2017). In addition, PI3K/Akt signaling associated molecules (EGFR, KRAS, PI3K p85/p110, SOS1, pAKT), actin cytoskeleton proteins, Rac Family Small GTPase 1 (RAC1), p21 (RAC1) activated kinase 1 (PAK1), discoid in domain receptor

1 (DDR1), and oncogenic long non-coding RNAs, HOX Transcript Antisense RNA (HOTAIR) and ZNFX1 Antisense RNA 1 (ZFAS1) were significantly down-regulated by silibinin in UM-UC-3 and T24 cell lines (Imai-Sumida et al. 2017). Additionally, wound healing, migration and invasion of bladder cell lines, T24 and UM-UC-3 were impaired after exposure to silibinin.

6.3.2 *Enhancement of Gold-Standard Therapies Against Bladder Cancer by Silibinin*

For 90% of bladder cancers, cystectomy alone or in combination with BCG immunotherapy or intravesical chemotherapy is the primary treatment option, followed by watchful surveillance (Society 2019). More advanced tumors receive neoadjuvant chemotherapy prior to cystectomy, and chemotherapy and radiation combination. Resistant bladder cancer-unresponsive to chemotherapy or radiotherapy are treated with immune checkpoint inhibitor based immunotherapy. Alternatively, studies have shown silibinin plays a critical role in the improvement of standard therapies' efficacy against aggressive bladder cancer. Sensitivity of invasive bladder cancer tumor cells, MB49-I, to radiation was dramatically enhanced by silibinin (80 μM), which was evident by a decrease in clonogenicity and S phase cellular arrest (Prack Mc Cormick et al. 2018). Silibinin alone or in combination with radiation caused an inhibition of NF-κB activation, reduced levels of survivin, cleaved PARP, phosphorylation of Akt and increased reactive oxidative species generation in MB49-I cells. Partial inhibition of MB49-I tumor growth was observed with radiation alone, however, on combination with silibinin, it significantly reduced tumor size and improved overall survival of C57BL/6J mice (Prack Mc Cormick et al. 2018).

Non-invasive strategies such as hyperthermia and photodynamic (PDT) therapies have garnered attention as enhancing complimentary approaches for chemotherapy and radiation for bladder cancer (Gandara et al. 2014; Longo et al. 2016). In fact, PDT is anti-cancer treatment strategy that utilizes photosensitizer, Protoporphyrin IX, in combination with 5-aminolevulinic acid (ALA). Gandara and co-workers (2014) showed silibinin enhances the cytotoxicity of PDT in MB49 and T24 bladder tumor cells (Gandara et al. 2014). Under the Chou-Talalay model, PDI-AIA LD_{75} with silibinin was synergic; whereas, LD_{50} had an additive effect in the MB49 cell line. Furthermore, this combination treatment also strongly induced apoptosis and reduced cell viability and migratory capacity in MB49 and T24 bladder cancer cells (Gandara et al. 2014).

6.4 Colorectal Cancer

Over 60% of colorectal cancer cases are identified in developed countries with high human development indexes (Arnold et al. 2017). Colorectal cancer death rates globally (Bray et al. 2018; Ferlay et al. 2019) and projected cost of care in U.S. for 2020 are the second highest compared to other cancers (Mariotto et al. 2011). In recent decades, colorectal cancer preventive strategies and lifestyle changes have effectively reduced disease incidence and mortality burden worldwide (Bray et al. 2017; Derry et al. 2013). Despite preventive strategies and declining mortality rates, historically low incidence and mortality rates for this malignancy in certain geographic regions have slightly risen due to Western life-style influences (Arnold et al. 2017). Major risk factors such as tobacco smoke, obesity, low fiber/high fat diet, sedentary lifestyle, high alcohol and red meat consumption are strongly linked to colorectal cancer development (Derry et al. 2013). Other risk factors are age, genomic instability-chromosomal instability (CIN), microsatellite instability (MSI) and CpG island methylator phenotype (CIMP), family history or personal history of inflammatory bowel disease and/or colorectal cancer. Chronic inflammation in inflammatory bowel disease can promote non-malignant dysplasia which can further develop into cancer Colorectal malignancies are classified according to their mutation of origin (sporadic, inherited and familial). Of these colorectal cancer cases, 70% are sporadic, 5% are inherited and 25% are familial (Marmol et al. 2017). Sporadic colorectal cancer is heterogeneous and initiated by a point mutation in tumor suppressor adenomatous polyposis coli (*APC*), which triggers the development of non-malignant adenomas called polyps. Only 15% of these adenomas progress into carcinoma by accumulating point mutations in *KRAS*, *TP53* and *DCC* (Marmol et al. 2017). Inherited mutations can develop into polyposis and non-polyposis inherited colorectal cancers, such as: familial adenomatous polyposis (FAP) characterized by multiple malignant polyps in the colon due to *APC* mutation, and hereditary non-polyposis colorectal cancer (HNPCC) or Lynch syndrome-characterized by fewer polyps (which can become cancerous more quickly) due to the inheritance of mutations in DNA mismatch repair mechanisms (*MSH2*, *MLH1*, *MLH6*, *PMS1*, *PMS2*) (Marmol et al. 2017).

6.4.1 Modulation of Signaling Mechanisms in Colorectal Cancer by Silibinin

In colorectal cancer, an array of molecular signaling in prostanoid biosynthesis, and cell division are targeted by flavonoid silibinin (Raina et al. 2016; Zheng et al. 2018). Studies in several different rodent strains have shown the versatility of silibinin anti-cancer activity against colon tumorigenesis (Raina et al. 2016). In the spontaneous intestinal tumorigenesis $APC^{min/+}$ murine model, silibinin has shown efficacy against tumor development (Rajamanickam et al. 2010). Size and number of polyps formed throughout the middle and distal sections of the small intestine were decreased by dietary silibinin (750 mg/kg body weight) in $APC^{min/+}$ mice. In the intestinal polyps of silibinin-treated mice the anti-proliferative, anti-inflammatory and anti-angiogenic effects were associated with decreased expression of cell growth (PCNA, cyclin D1), Wnt marker (β-catenin), inflammatory mediators (COX-2, PGE-2) and angiogenesis-related molecules (nestin, HIF-1α, VEGF and its downstream target eNOS) (Rajamanickam et al. 2010). Importantly, aberrant crypt foci formation in azoxymethane (AOM) initiated-colorectal tumorigenesis in male Fisher 344 rats were suppressed by silibinin treatment (pre- and post-initiation of AOM) (Velmurugan et al. 2008). The inhibitory effects of dietary silibinin increased cleaved PARP, as well as decreased levels of proliferative (PCNA, cyclin D1) and pro-inflammatory markers (iNOS, COX-2) in colonic tissue. In addition to these markers, silibinin also suppressed cell cycle progression, angiogenesis (VEGF), survival (pAkt), insulin growth factor signaling, and elevated levels of pro-apoptotic protein, cleaved caspase-3 in AOM-induced colon cancer in A/J mice (Ravichandran et al. 2010). Moreover, other studies have shown silibinin pro-apoptotic and anti-inflammatory properties in colorectal cancer as well (Nafees et al. 2018; Raina et al. 2016; Zheng et al. 2018). Loss of APC, a major hallmark of colorectal tumorigenesis, is strongly associated with Wnt signaling enhancement; interestingly, silibinin shows inactivation of this pathway via down-regulation of pGSK-3β, nuclear and cytoplasmic β-catenin protein levels (Ravichandran et al. 2010). Similar effects by silibinin were also observed against SW480 xenograft tumorigenesis as well (Velmurugan et al. 2010). Under in vitro conditions, silibinin has shown dual targeting of both apoptotic and autophagic mediated pathways in colorectal cancer cells (Raina et al. 2016).

Several published reports on 1,2-dimethylhydrazine (DMH)-induced colon tumorigenesis models demonstrated that the anti-inflammatory properties of dietary silibinin administration (50 mg/kg) reduced aberrant crypt foci pre-neoplastic lesions or macroscopic polyps incidences, gastrointestinal enzymatic activity (β-glucosidase and β-galactosidase), tissue lipid peroxidation, suppressed Wnt signaling (caudal-type homeobox transcription factor (CDX2) and its downstream target, guanylyl cyclase C (GCC) as well as normalized oxidative stress marker levels and intestinal homeostasis (Sangeetha et al. 2009, 2010, 2012). Xenobiotic metabolism is also a target of silibinin efficacy-shown previously by its modulation of select CYP450s (Bijak 2017). Expression patters of colonic and hepatic levels of phase I enzymes (CYP450, CYP4502E1, CYP450B5, CYP450 reductase, cytochrome b5 reductase, were elevated and Phase II enzymes UDPGT, GST and DTD) directed by DMH-induced colon cancer were reversed by silibinin (Sangeetha et al. 2012).

Recent research focuses on the development of anti-cancer agents that employ immune response machinery to target critical mechanisms to block and terminate tumorigenesis. In further support of this effort, considerable attention has been given to the diverse cytotoxic and physiological effects of nutraceuticals on tumor biology. Natural products such as silibinin possess immunomodulatory functions that target proteins essential to colon tumor cellular processes (Raina et al. 2016; Woo et al. 2014). Cytokine profiling in intestinal polyp tissue of silibinin-treated $APC^{min/+}$ mice revealed that silibinin suppressive effects targeted pro-inflammatory cytokines, angiogenesis and immunoevasion (Rajamanickam et al. 2010). Specifically, cytokine-associated signaling processes modulated by silibinin were pro-inflammatory cytokines (TNF-α, IL-1α, IL-1β, IL-4), apoptosis (Fas ligand), cell adhesion molecules (VCAM-1, P-selectin), adipocytokine (leptin, leptin receptor), chemotaxis (eotoxin-2/CCL24, MCP-1/CCL2, MCP-5/CCL12), angiogenesis (VEGF), extracellular matrix regulator (TIMP), hematopoietic growth factor (M-CSF), and immunoevasion (IFN-γ) (Raina et al. 2016). Synergistic interaction between silibinin and a member of the TNF superfamily, tumor necrosis factor-related apoptosis-inducing ligand (TRAIL), triggered the activation of the death receptor pathway (Kauntz et al. 2012b). Silibinin stimulated the early growth response (EGR) signaling cascade, which in turn elevates the promoter activity of non-steroidal anti-inflammatory drug-activated gene-1 (NAG-1), a pleiotropic member of the cytokine TGF β family in both p53 wild-type and p53 null colon cancer cell models (Woo et al. 2014). This study suggests silibinin may exert its anti-cancer activity independent of p53 signaling in colon cancer.

Cancer stem cells (CSC) serve as critical challenges for therapeutic strategies against recurrent and resistance disease. Colorectal-CSCs exploit inflammatory signaling and associated mechanisms to support tumor growth and progression (Kumar et al. 2014; Patel et al. 2018; Wang et al. 2012). Colorectal-CSCs maintenance was disrupted by silibinin suppression of PP2Ac and AKT/mTOR signaling as evident by a decrease in CD133 enrichment, and capacity to form spheres (Wang et al. 2012). Treatment of colon CSC populations with silibinin lead to a loss of their self-renewal capacity and reduction in the number and size of spheroids via inhibition of survival mechanisms mediated by pro-inflammatory IL-4/IL-6 signaling (Kumar et al. 2014). Inhibition of proliferation, migration and sphere formation in HCT116 $CD44^+$ cells by silibinin was further enhanced by first line chemotherapeutic agent 5FU (Patel et al. 2018). This treatment also induced G0/G1 arrest via both intrinsic apoptosis and autophagy as well as cleaved PARP. Silibinin reduced levels of CSC-associated factors, Nanog, CTNNB1 and CDKN2A and up-regulated epithelial marker E-cadherin (Patel et al. 2018), which indicated the suppressive effect of silibinin on tumor cell stemness potential and a possible promotion of mesenchymal-epithelial transition (MET) in colorectal cancer.

6.4.2 Silibinin-Based Combinatorial Treatments Against Colorectal Cancer

Chemotherapy is the primary treatment combined with colectomy for colon cancer (stage III or higher), and for rectal cancer (stage II or higher) the treatment regimen consists of neoadjuvant chemotherapy, radiation followed by proctocolectomy (Society 2016). Disease recurrence and resistance along with systemic toxicities are major barriers for aggressive chemotherapy. Although multiple toxicities are induced by first-line colorectal cancer chemotherapeutic agents, both pre-clinical and clinical evidence has shown that combining silibinin with these chemotherapeutic agents enhances their cytotoxicity and reduces the associated lethal side effects (Belli et al. 2017; Tsai et al. 2015; Yan et al. 2012). Also, silibinin when administered alone has shown no adverse effects in colorectal cancer patients (Hoh et al. 2006). Other chemopreventive agents have also shown a potent inhibitory effect against tumor cells when given in supplementation with silibinin. In a recent study by Tsai and associates (2015), the combined anti-tumor activity of metformin and silibinin strongly induced apoptosis, inhibited pAkt-driven cell survival, promoted the activation of metabolic regulator, AMPK, and tumor suppressor PTEN in COLO 205 tumor cells without adverse side effects (Tsai et al. 2015). Furthermore, this treatment had no toxic effect on non-malignant HCoEpiC colon epithelial cells. The investigation of Regorafenib, a potent pan-kinase inhibitor, in combination with silibinin resulted in higher median progression-free, overall survival of metastatic colorectal cancer patients (Belli et al. 2017). In addition, silibinin also exhibited a protective effect against Regorafenib-induced hepatoxicity as evident by the normalization of Aspartate transaminase (AST), Alanine transaminase (ALT) and bilirubin levels.

Elevation of TNF-α signaling is frequently observed in highly inflamed intestinal epithelium and colon tumor cells. Pro-inflammatory signaling elicited by TNF-α activation and associated Snail1/2 transcription factors had a suppressive effect on vitamin D receptor (VDR) expression. Down-regulation of VDR in colon tumor cells resulted in the loss of 1,25-dihydroxyvitamin D (1,25D) protective effects against accelerated migration and proliferation. In HT-29 colon carcinoma cells resistant to 1,25D, silibinin reduced TNF-α-induction of Snail 1/2 as well as Snail 1 overexpression in the 1,25D-resistant human colon carcinoma cells HT-29 (Bhatia and Falzon 2015). Both vitamin D-response element (VDRE) promoter activity, VDR levels, and 1,25D protective and sensitivity effects were restored in resistant colon tumor cells. Also, co-treatment of silibinin and 1,25D suppressed proliferative and migratory capacities of colon cancer cells (Bhatia and Falzon 2015). Vanadium—a transition metal element—exerts anti-cancer activity through its derivatives and complexes (Leon et al. 2015). Specifically, oxovanadium(IV) complexes with silibinin have demonstrated several anti-tumor effects in colon cancer cells. Oxovanadium(IV) complexes with silibinin (VOsil) decreased cell viability, mitochondrial and lysosomal activities and induced early apoptotic death marked by elevated phosphatidylserine externalization, activation of caspase-3 and inactivation of NF-κB signaling in the HT-29 tumor cell line (Leon et al. 2015). VOsil showed more cytotoxicity in colon tumor cells compared to cisplatin alone. Moreover, VOsil showed an inhibitory effect on pAKT, total AKT, intracellular PI3K/AKT/mTOR signaling effectors, ribosomal S6 kinase (p70-S6K) and 4EBP1 protein (p4EB-P1) in HT-29 colon tumor cells (Leon et al. 2015). Silibinin even affects the enzymatic activity of topoisomerases, which regulate the helical structure of DNA by severing and reconnecting strands. VOsil suppressed topoisomerase IB relaxation activity in a dose dependent manner in HT-29 colon cancer cells (Leon et al. 2015). A combination treatment with another flavonoid, Rutin, also showed a synergistic effect with silibinin via induction of pro-apoptotic and suppression of NF-κB signaling (Nafees et al. 2018). Currently, silibinin is under evaluation as an adjuvant treatment to FOLFIRI for metastatic colorectal cancer in a Phase 4 study (NCT03130634).

6.5 Prostate Cancer

According to cancer diagnoses-statistics in men worldwide, prostate cancer accounts for 13.5% of these cancer cases and is the second leading cause of cancer-related deaths (Bray et al. 2018; Ferlay et al. 2019). Prostate cancer prevalence is highest in developed countries (Ferlay et al. 2019), and high risk of prostate cancer development is associated with African ancestry, family history, genomic alterations, obesity and smoking (Society 2019). This disease has an apparent health disparity as evident by African- and Caribbean-Americans being twice as more likely to die from prostate cancer compared to European Americans. Localized prostate cancer are frequently classified as E26 transformation-specific (ETS) positive and/or negative (Arora and Barbieri 2018). The ETS family is the largest gene family of transcription factors in the Animalia kingdom. Fusion of ETS transcription factors occur commonly with androgen receptor (AR)-regulated and prostate-specific transcripts such as transmembrane serine protease 2 (TMPRSS2). (Arora and Barbieri 2018). Approximately 40–50% of prostate cancer tumors express the TMPRSS2-ETS fusion gene (Arora and Barbieri 2018). Primary treatments for localized disease are radiation and surgery. In advanced prostate cancer, fusion-positive disease are frequently associated with mutations in tumor suppressor genes, *PTEN* and *p53*, and DNA repair-molecule, ATM. However, mutations in Chromodomain Helicase DNA Binding Protein 1 (CHD1) and serine peptidase inhibitor, Kazal type 1 (SPINK1) as well as ATM have been linked to ETS negative prostate cancer (Arora and Barbieri 2018). More progressive disease is further classified as castration resistant prostate cancer and develop an insensitivity to AR. Consequently, androgen deprivation and/or chemo-therapies are directed toward the treatment of metastatic and castration resistant prostate cancer (Arora and Barbieri 2018).

6.5.1 Modulation of Signaling Mechanisms by Silibinin in Its Efficacy Against Prostate Cancer

Initial preclinical anti-cancer efficacy studies using silibinin conducted by our group have shown its strong inhibitory effect against inflammation, DNA synthesis/cycle cell, growth factor, retinoblastoma protein (Rb) transcription factors, androgen receptor (AR), EGFR and MAPK signaling to induce an anti-neoplastic effect in both androgen-dependent and independent prostate cancer cells (Reed et al. 2018; Ting et al. 2013, 2014). Silibinin mediated G1 cell arrest in androgen-independent (DU145) and -dependent (22Rv1) prostate carcinoma via p21 and p27 induction (Roy et al.

2007). Other than its anti-proliferative effects, silibinin also impaired cell motility, wound healing and invasion of prostate tumor cells (Deep et al. 2014; Ting et al. 2013, 2014). Fibronectin is one of the major ligands of integrins that interact with the extracellular matrix components involved in tumor progression; silibinin caused inhibition of fibronectin-induced events in tumor progression (i.e., motility, invasion, survival) (Deep et al. 2014). In the transgenic adenocarcinoma mouse prostate (TRAMP) model, dietary silibinin feeding (0.1–1% w/w) attenuated early stages of prostate cancer development at PIN stage and progression to late stage metastasis via its down-regulation of cyclins A, B1, and E, protective effect against angiogenesis, decreased proliferative and EMT signaling (Raina et al. 2007). On another front, a combination of JAK-1 inhibitor, piceatannol, and silibinin triggered a strong pro-apoptotic signaling via blocking Stat3 phosphorylation, activation of caspases-3/9 and up-regulation of cleaved PARP in DU145 cells (Agarwal et al. 2007).

EMT is a critical mechanism and entry to the advanced cancer phenotype prior to progressive disease. Expression of E-cadherin, an epithelial maker, was elevated by silibinin; whereas, pAkt, pro-EMT markers, Slug and Snail, were decreased in aggressive prostate cancer cell models (PC-3, PC-3MM2 and C4-2B) (Deep et al. 2011). Thioredoxin (TRX) system plays a critical role in regulating redox signaling pathways and is regulated by silibinin. As a result of reduced reactive oxygen species production to prevent TRX oxidation due to silibinin treatment, this flavonoid induced an inhibitory effect on cell growth on prostate tumor cells (Rodriguez-Garcia et al. 2017). Silibinin derivatives also possess anti-cancer properties in prostate cancer (Manivannan et al. 2017; Vue et al. 2017). More potent anti-proliferative effects have been attributed to derivatives 5- or/and 20-*O*-alkyl-2,3-dehydrosilybins compared to silibinin (Vue et al. 2017). A 2-Br substituent modification in the chemical structure of silibinin dramatically enhanced its cytotoxic activity against prostate carcinoma DU-145 cells (Manivannan et al. 2017). Other constituents of silymarin-isosilybin A and isosilybin B also exhibited anti-growth effect on prostate tumor cells. Both compounds attenuated cell-cycle signaling mediated by cyclins (D1, D3, E and A) and cyclin-dependent kinases (Cdk2/4 and Cdc25A), but elevated levels of p27 and p53 in LNCaP and 22Rv1 cell lines (Deep et al. 2007). Based on the aforementioned silibinin efficacy studies in prostate cancer, p53 activation is not essential to silibinin anti-tumor function in this malignancy.

This nutraceutical agent has also modulated both pro-inflammatory and pro-angiogenic signaling in prostate tumorigenesis. Hypoxia-inducible factor-1 (HIF-1) is an important key regulator of tumor progression in oxygen sensitive environments and potent stimulator of VEGF expression. Oxygen depletion and oxygen-independent signaling (i.e. cytokines) induces the accumulation of HIF-1α, a positive mediator of vascular endothelial growth factor (VEGF) levels (Deep et al. 2012; Jung et al. 2009). Silibinin has been reported to down-regulate HIF-1α expression in androgen-regulated LNCaP cells and -independent PC-3 cells via elevated phosphorylation of the translation initiation factor 2a (eIF-2a) and decreased eIF-4f complex formation) (Jung et al. 2009).These cellular events ultimately lead to the suppression of global protein synthesis including de novo synthesis of HIF-1α protein. Phospholipase A2 (sPLA2) enzymes are also implicated in inflammation and carcinogenesis. Elevated serum levels of secreted phospholipase A2 (sPLA2) enzymes are strongly associated and considered a prognostic maker in different malignancies (Hagelgans et al. 2014). Down-regulation of group IIA, IB, III and V phospholipase A2 (sPLA2) enzymes were caused by silibinin in unstimulated and cytokine-primed HepG2 and PC-3 cells (Hagelgans et al. 2014).

Dysregulation of androgen receptor (AR) signaling has been associated with refractory prostate cancer; importantly, silibinin exerts an inhibitory effect on androgen-regulated genes and proteins in prostate cancer. In AR-sensitive prostate tumor cells, silibinin exposure negatively regulates AR signaling in LNCaP cells. The localization of the AR to the nucleus and its transactivation activity was diminished by silymarin and silibinin treatment in LNCaP cells (Zhu et al. 2001). Both compounds also inhibited androgen-regulated stimulation of PSA and human glandular kallikrein (hK2) secretion and expression of FKBP51, an immunophilin.

Recent studies have focused on the role of lipid metabolism in prostatic tumor progression. Studies have shown an effect of silibinin on aberrant lipid metabolism in prostate tumors (Deep et al. 2017; Nambiar et al. 2014; Ting et al. 2014). At physiological levels, silibinin interferes with lipid metabolism by reducing proliferative rates and the accumulation of lipid and cholesterol in prostate tumor cells (Nambiar et al. 2014). This effect was a result of decreased nuclear levels of sterol regulatory element binding protein 1 and 2 (SREBP1/2) and associated targets via SREBP1 phosphorylation as well as AMPK activation. Also, silibinin conferred an inhibitory effect on androgen-independent downstream targeting of SREBP1/2. Synthetic androgen R1881 was shown to induce lipid accumulation in LNCaP cells, but this induction was inhibited by silibinin (Nambiar et al. 2014). Additionally, aberrant metabolic tumor profiles were altered by silibinin in the TRAMP model (Raina et al. 2009). Hypoxic conditions promotes HIF-1α expression, acetyl-Co A carboxylase (ACC) and fatty acid synthase (FASN) activation, which leads to lipid accumulation and NOX activity as well as increased proliferation, and endothelial cells tube formation (Deep et al. 2017); these effects were reversed by silibinin treatment in in vitro and in vivo studies.

Limited clinical trials have evaluated the beneficial effects of silibinin in prostate cancer patients (Flaig et al. 2007a, 2010). The pharmacokinetics of oral silibinin was evaluated at varying dosages of its formulation, silybin-phytosome (Siliphos^R), in a phase I/II clinical trial in patients diagnosed with localized prostate cancer (Flaig et al. 2007a). In phase I trials, after Siliphos^R administration, patients exhibited interpatient viability in urine silibinin levels, gastrointestinal and minor hepatic toxicities shown at 15 g or 20 g, mild diarrhea, and one case of abnormal ALT and AST levels but this was normalized after 4 months (Flaig et al. 2007a).

In a phase II trial, over a 4-week period, prior to surgery, prostate cancer patients either received 13 g of silybin-phytosome for 14–31 days ($n = 6$) or served as untreated subjects ($n = 6$) (Flaig et al. 2010). This dose did achieve high plasma concentrations of silibinin but this was not maintained due to its short half-life, also very little was observed in prostatic tissue of patients. Although, disease stability was maintained in several patients, the serum prostate specific antigen (PSA) levels of patients did not achieve a partial or complete response to silibinin treatment.

6.5.2 *Silibinin-Based Combinatorial Treatments Against Prostate Cancer*

Silibinin has exhibited multiple antagonistic effects on prostate tumors while improving tumor cell sensitivity to chemotherapeutic agents associated with adverse side effects in patients. Prospective studies of clinical trials for FDA approved anti-androgen chemotherapeutic agents, abiraterone acetate and enzalutamide, showed castrant prostate cancer patients treated with these agents exhibited abnormal AST/ALT levels, cardiac events, hypertension and other adverse side effects (Iacovelli et al. 2018; Zhu et al. 2018). Co-administration of silibinin neo-adjuvant and/or adjuvant could aid in improved quality of life conditions during chemotherapy or harsh treatments. For instance, silibinin enhanced the sensitivity of DU145 prostate tumor cells to the cytotoxic activity of two clinical chemotherapeutic agents, cisplatin and carboplatin, which resulted in nearly a 50% induction in apoptotic death compared to silibinin alone (Dhanalakshmi et al. 2003). The cytotoxic effects of other anti-cancer agents were also improved by silibinin against prostate tumorigenesis (Flaig et al. 2007b; Tyagi et al. 2002). Silibinin induced G2-M arrest and enhanced DU145 cells sensitivity to doxorubicin via down-regulation of kinase activity (Cdc25C, Cdc2/p34, cyclin B1) in cell cycle mechanisms (Tyagi et al. 2002). A similar effect was shown in prostate cancer cell sensitivity to mitoxantrone in a report by Flaig and co-workers (2007), but this improvement in sensitivity only required a short incubation with silibinin in PC-3, LNCaP and DU145 cell lines (Flaig et al. 2007b). In a prostate cancer in vitro model, JAK-1 inhibitor- piceatannol combined with silibinin exerted G2/M cellular arrest, and induced pro-apoptotic signaling via suppressing phosho-Stat3 levels and triggering caspases-3/9-mediated cell death (Agarwal et al. 2007). Also, radiation therapy has shown to be more successful when used in combination with silibinin. In some cases, ionizing radiation (IR) resistance occurs in prostatic tumor cells, which limits IR cytotoxicity against tumor cells. In IR resistant prostate cancer cells, an induction was shown in angiogenic activity, mitogenic signaling and cellular invasion (Nambiar et al. 2015b), but these processes as well as DNA repair mechanisms were suppressed by silibinin by enhancing sensitivity to radiation (Nambiar et al. 2015a). Double stranded break repair mediators, EGFR and DNA-PK, were decreased by silibinin resulting in the prevention of DNA lesion repair and enhanced γ-H2AX (Ser139) foci repair. Furthermore, combination of radiation and silibinin treatment reduced tumor growth of DU145 xenografts in athymic nude mice (Nambiar et al. 2015a). This combination also suppressed tumor proliferation, and tube formation of endothelial cells (Nambiar et al. 2015b).

6.6 Lung Cancer

According to 2018 GLOBOCAN cancer estimates from over 185 countries, lung malignancy accounts for over 1.76 million deaths worldwide and one of highest incidence rates among women and men (Bray et al. 2018; Ferlay et al. 2019). In the U.S., metastatic lung cancer has a 4.7% 5-year survival rate and represents 57% of diagnoses for pulmonary malignancy for 2018 (2018 SEER Cancer Statistics). Moreover, lung cancer comprises over 25% of all cancer deaths in the U.S. Lung cancer has two major forms, non-small cell lung cancer (NSCLC) and small cell lung cancer (SCLC) (Gazdar et al. 2017; Herbst et al. 2008; Myers and Wallen 2019). Only 15% of lung cancers are classified as SCLC (Gazdar et al. 2017) while NSCLC (85%) is the most common lung cancer. Between the two major subtypes of lung cancer, SCLC has the lower 5-year survival rate (6%) (Society 2019). Approximately 81% of U.S. lung cancer mortalities are linked to tobacco product use (Society 2019). Specifically, most smokers tend to develop small cell and squamous cell lung tumors; whereas, lung adenocarcinoma tumors develop more frequently in non-smokers and this may be attributed to second-hand smoke and other factors (Herbst et al. 2008). Other high-risk factors associated with lung cancer development include second-hand smoke, hazardous metals (arsenic, cadmium, chromium), radiation, air pollution and occupational exposure (i.e., rubber manufacture, roofing, asbestos) (Society 2019).

Next-generation sequencing studies have identified multiple mutually exclusive molecular subtypes of lung cancer based on the accumulation of mutations, rearrangements and copy number variations (Devarakonda et al. 2017; Hirsch et al. 2017). Majority of lung adenocarcinomas are commonly characterized by mutations in receptor tyrosine kinase (RTK) signaling genes such as *EGFR*, *KRAS*, *BRAF*, *ERBB2*, and *MET* (Devarakonda et al. 2017; Mateen et al. 2013). Chromosomal rearrangements of *ALK*, *ROS1*, *RET* and *NTRK* are involved in the development of adenocarcinoma in the lung as well. SCLC and NSCLC tumors frequently show copy number alterations in chromosomes 3 and 14 as oncogenic drivers in tumorigenesis. Moreover, somatic mutations in tumor suppressors (*TP53*, *STK11*, *NF1*, *RB1*, *PTEN*, and *CDKN2A*) and oncogenes (*KRAS*, *EGFR*, *MET*, and *PIK3CA*) have been consistently reported in lung cancer (Devarakonda et al. 2017).

6.6.1 *Signaling Mechanisms in Lung Cancer Disrupted by Silibinin*

Extracellular matrix degradation is one of the primary cellular processes involved in the initiation of metastasis. Cellular motility and invasion of tumor cells is triggered by an imbalance between serine proteinase, metalloproteinases (MMPs), cathepsins, and plasminogen activator (PA) leading to extracellular matrix damage. Proteases such as MMP-2, and urokinase plasminogen activator (u-PA) are critical in wound healing, apoptosis, angiogenesis and other cancer-associated physiological processes, but endogenous tissue inhibitor of metalloproteinases (TIMPs) negatively regulate proteases. Transcriptional levels of proteases, MMP-2 and u-PA, and their potential to trigger ECM degradation were significantly reduced by silibinin in NSLC A549 cells via enhancing the levels of its natural inhibitor, TMIP-2 (Chu et al. 2004). Silibinin exerted a dose- and/or time-dependent suppression of the activation of Akt and ERK1/2, NF-κB and transcription factor AP-1 components and proto-oncogenes (c-Fos, c-Jun) and induction of cell invasion in A549 tumor cells (Chen et al. 2005). Enhancement of PI3K (LY294002) and MEK (U0126) inhibitors to impede cell invasion was observed on combination with silibinin in these cells (Chen et al. 2005). Silibinin (25–100 μM) induced cellular death via G1 cell cycle arrest in a time-dependent manner in both small cell lung (SHP-77) and non-small lung (A-549) carcinoma (Sharma et al. 2003). In comparison to another natural product, deguelin, silibinin (0.05, 0.1%) did not significantly inhibit the initiation of tobacco-specific benzo(*a*)pyrene (BP) lung carcinoma in A/J mice, but did effectively block the progression of benign tumors such as adenomas to malignancy (Mateen et al. 2013).

In both in vitro and urethane-induced lung cancer in vivo models, silibinin induced apoptosis, suppressed tumor proliferation, angiogenesis, tumor growth by inhibiting proliferative markers (PCNA, cyclin D1) and blocking the stimulation of VEGF by inducible nitric oxide synthase (iNOS) and COX-2 (Chittezhath et al. 2008; Singh et al. 2006a). Nitric oxide (NO) signaling positively stimulates angiogenesis in NSCLC tumors via synthesis of isoforms, eNOS, iNOS and nNOs. iNOS is highly expressed in lung cancer and its expression and activity directly correlates to high angiogenic and metastatic potential in tumors. Tumorigenesis in urethane-induced lung cancer was severely impaired in the iNOS knockout model evident by reduced tumor incidences and size; silibinin treatment did not further enhance this effect, however, considerable anti-tumor effects of silibinin were shown in urethane-WT mice associated with decreased proliferation (PCNA, Nestin), VEGFR protein, and nuclear levels of NF-κB p65 and STAT3 (Ramasamy et al. 2011). Furthermore, proliferation is tightly dependent on telomerase activity and in a recent study silibinin was shown to down-regulate a critical catalytic component of the human telomerase RNP, hTERT in A549 lung cancer cells (Amirsaadat et al. 2017).

Concomitant stimulation of NF-κB, STAT3/1, ERK1/2 and JNK1/2 signaling pathways by pro-inflammatory cytokines (IFN-γ, IL-1β and TNF-α) in A549 lung epithelial carcinoma cells was inhibited by silibinin as a result of it causing down-regulation of HIF-1α, iNOS and decreased phosphorylation of ERK1/2, c-Jun and c-Fos, major AP-1 transcription factor family members (Chittezhath et al. 2008). Similar effects for silibinin were also shown in the tumor microenvironment of tumor-derived mouse lung epithelial LM2 cells. Cytokine induction of ERK1/2, STAT3/1 and EGFR signaling and NF-κB interaction with DNA was inhibited by silibinin and its effects further reduced COX-2, iNOS and tumor cell migration via decrease MMP-2/9 levels (Tyagi et al. 2012). Pre-treatment with MEK, NF-κB, and EGFR inhibitors also showed comparable effects to silibinin. Furthermore, silibinin treatment of urethane-induced lung tumors resulted in low tumor incidence, size, blood vessel formation and expression levels of IL-13, TNF-α, HIF-1α and lung tumor macrophage population, but increased expression of protease inhibitors (TIMP-1/2) anti-angiogenic Angiopoietin-2 (Ang-2) and Ang-receptor tyrosine kinase (Tie-2) molecules (Tyagi et al. 2009).

In other NSCLC subtypes, silibinin targeted primary cell cycle and growth mechanisms to exert its anti-cancer activity. Both large cell carcinoma (H1299 and H460) and bronchioalveolar carcinoma (H322) cell cycle progression were halted at G1 phase by silibinin (50–75 μM) (Mateen et al. 2010). Silibinin mediated suppression of CDK2/4 activity and Rb phosphorylation lead to a subsequent reduction of G1 regulatory cyclins (CDKs 2, 4, 6, cyclins D1, D3, E) levels and release of E2F transcription factors required for G1 to S phase transition. In tumor metastasis, lysyl oxidase (LOX) overexpression in lung adenocarcinoma is linked to poor disease prognosis and strongly promotes cell invasion, migration and pre-metastatic niche development (Hou et al. 2018). Silibinin decreased LOX levels via inhibition of EGFR signaling and receptor-dependent metastasis of NCI-H1975 cells. Down-regulation of EMT markers by silibinin has been shown in EGFR-mutant, and gefitinib- and erlotinib unresponsive NSCLC tumors via suppressing STAT3 signaling and oncogenic microRNA (Cufi et al. 2013a, b; Cuyas et al. 2016).

6.6.2 *Silibinin-Based Combinatorial Treatments Against Lung Cancer*

Drug disease resistance is a major challenge for lung cancer treatment strategies (Corominas-Faja et al. 2013; Cufi et al. 2013a, b; Cuyas et al. 2016; Mateen et al. 2013; Sadava and Kane 2013). In an A549 xenograft model, silibinin treatment lead to decreased lung tumor cell proliferation, vascular network, and increased apoptosis; it also impeded chemoresistance to doxorubicin via inhibiting translocation of NF-κB signaling components, p65 and p50, and transcription of COX-2 caused by this chemotherapeutic agent in BALB/c nu/nu mice (Singh et al. 2004). In primary and acquired disease resistance in NSCLC cells, silibinin showed a time-dependent inhibition of EGFR activity, EGFR homo−/heterodimerization in H1975 and HCC827 lung cancer cells and significantly enhanced EGFR tyrosine kinase inhibitors, gefitinib and erlotinib, cytotoxicity in lung resistant cells harboring EGFR T790 M mutation as well as inhibited viability and growth of geftinib/erlotinib resistant lung cancer cell lines, and erlotinib-resistant xenograft tumors (Rho et al. 2010). This inhibitory effect was attributed to a suppression of pEGFR, pAKT, pERK in H1975, PC-9/GR, and PC-9ER cell lines. Silibinin treatment also overcame drug resistance disease to both etoposide and doxorubicin in a multidrug-resistant cell line, VPA17 SCLC, but not in NCI-H69 cells (Sadava and Kane 2013). The IC_{50} of etoposide and doxorubicin was significantly reduced and cytotoxicity enhanced by silibinin in VPA17 cells. Silibinin and etoposide or doxorubicin combination at a 1:1 ratio showed synergism in VPA17 cells (Sadava and Kane 2013).

A niche of reports have evaluated silibinin synergistic interaction with EGFR inhibitors to overcome drug resistance disease in lung cancer (Cufi et al. 2013a, b; Cuyas et al. 2016). Erlotinib-refractory lung cancer stem cells exhibited high levels of aldehyde dehydrogenase (ALDH) activity mediated by ALDH1/3 and percentage of $ALDH^{bright}$ population, but silibinin-meglumine suppressed spheroid and self-renewal potential in PC-9/erlotinib refractory cells by reversing their resistance to erlotinib (Corominas-Faja et al. 2013). This inhibitory effect was also showed for EMT-driven erlotinib resistant lung cancer (Cufi et al. 2013b). Silibinin reversed EMT and activated MET in erlotinib refractory and EGFR-mutant tumors (Cufi et al. 2013b). After silibinin-meglumine enhanced sensitivity to erlotinib in erlotinib-refractory cells (PC-9/Erl-R), mesenchymal-associated targets (SNAIL, ZEB1, N-cadherin), oncogenic miR-21 were reduced and tumor suppressor-related miR-200 family miR-200c was up-regulated in refractory cells compared to PC-9/Erl-R cells without silibinin in EGFR-T790 M mutant NSCLC xenografts in athymic nude murine model (Cufi et al. 2013b). The migratory pattern of these erlotinib refractory cells was impaired in vitro by silibinin treatment. Furthermore, silibinin-melglumine and gefitnib together impeded EMT progression (Vimentin, CDH2, TWIST-1, SNAIL2) tumor growth and regrowth in gefitnib unresponsive tumors in EGFR-mutant xenografts (Cufi et al. 2013a). Furthermore, co-treatment of erlotinib with silibinin reduced EMT markers and drivers, Vimentin, CDH2, TWIST, and SNAIL2 (Cufi et al. 2013b) and suppressed EMT-driven erlotinib resistance by reversing high *miR*-21/low *miR*-200c signature in vivo. In addition, silibinin also showed potent efficacy and overcame acquired resistance in crizotinib refractory lung cells by restoring its sensitivity to crizotinib via down-regulation of PD-L1 and EMT regulators (Cuyas et al. 2016).

Furthermore, silibinin inhibited HDAC activity via decreased expression of HDACs 1–3 and its combination with an HDAC inhibitor (Trichostatin A) promoted G2/M cell cycle arrest, increased p21 levels and reduced tumor growth (Mateen et al. 2012, 2013). Inhibition of PI3K and MAPK signaling via PI3K (LY294002) and MEK (U0126) inhibitors with silibinin decreased cellular invasion of lung tumor A549 cells via down-regulation of MMP-2, NF- κB and EKT1/2 signaling pathways (Mateen et al. 2012).

Silibinin and indole-3-carbinol (I3C) combination treatment strategies exhibited an inhibitory against pro-inflammatory, pro-carcinogenic, anti-proliferative proteins in the genetic signature of LPS-driven 4-(methyl-nitrosamino)-1-(3-pyridyl)-1-butanone (NNK)-induced lung tumorigenesis (Qian et al. 2015; Song et al. 2015). Compared to NNK and LPS treatment groups, ARNTL, Cyp1a1, NPAS2 were up-regulated whereas Spag11b was down-regulated by the combination treatment of silibinin and I3C (Qian et al. 2015). Liang et al. (2014) showed silibinin disruption of a NAD^+-dependent deacetylase and key regulator of cell survival, Silent information regulator 1 (SIRT1) signaling leads to its dose- and time-dependent reduction of cell viability, migration and increase of apoptosis ROS production (Liang et al. 2014). Moreover, down-regulation of SIRT1 signaling via its inhibitor, cambinol, further increased A549 lung adenocarcinoma cells sensitivity to silibinin. Thoracic irradiation (13 Gy) alone significantly reduced Lewis lung tumor derived nodules, but co-treatment with silibinin showed modest enhancement and minimized radiation-induced lung fibrosis, inflammatory cell infiltration and survival in C57BL/6 mice (Son et al. 2015). Some clinical trials have initiated studies on the efficacy of Indole-3-Carbinol/silibinin against smoking and Erlotinib (Tarceva) and Silybin-phytosome (Siliphos) against EGFR mutant lung cancer (NCT03687073, NCT02146118). However, additional clinical studies are required to fully understand silibinin synergistic effects on other cytotoxic agents including immune-, chemo- and radiation therapies.

6.7 Conclusion

Silibinin is a pleiotropic flavonoid that targets multiple signaling mechanisms that drive the initiation and progression of a diverse cluster of malignant diseases. As shown in the summation of pre-clinical and clinical evidence (Table 6.1), consistent findings illustrate silibinin implementation of anti-oncogenic changes in critical mechanisms in cellular development, processes and programmed death (cyclin/CDK interactions, caspases, LC3-II, LC3-I, SQSTM1), vasculature growth (angiogenesis), growth factor signaling (EGFR, TGF β, IGF-1, FGF2, VEGF), transcription factor activation (NF-κB, AP-1, Fos, Jun), EMT induction, kinase signaling cascade (PI3K, MAPK), maintenance of optimal free radical production, redox balance and infiltration of inflammatory mediators, that contribute to tumorigenesis. Therapeutic combinations with silibinin showed strong efficacy against the tumor phenotypic physiology such as enhanced proliferation, migration, invasion and tumorigenesis. Moreover, silibinin reprograms genetic machinery to exert its protective effect against different molecular subtypes of lung, prostate, bladder, colorectal and skin tumors as shown in Fig. 6.1. Collectively, the anti-inflammatory, anti-oxidant, and anti-oncogenic properties forms the basis of silibinin as an ideal chemopreventive agent to use in therapeutic strategies to counter mechanisms involved in cancer initiation, progression, and disease resistance.

Two of the major challenges faced by clinical management and treatment of cancer are cancer therapy-associated toxicities and refractory disease. As shown in this chapter, chemoprevention strategies utilizing nutraceutical silibinin dually target signaling that closely regulate tumor promoting mechanisms and reduce systemic toxicities produced by short- and long-term exposure to chemo-, immune- and radio-therapies. Pre-clinical and clinical data demonstrate silibinin is an excellent chemopreventive candidate for additional clinical studies on the basis of its enhancement of efficacy of cytotoxic agents, re-sensitization of resistant tumor cells to chemotherapeutic agents and protective effect against liver toxicity, a common adverse side effect of chemotherapy in cancer patients. A substantial volume of in vitro and in vivo studies have shown the wide-ranging anti-cancer effect of silibinin in various cancers, including colorectal, prostate, skin, bladder and lung, as well as on resistant tumors in response to Hedgehog inhibitors, EGFR tyrosine kinase inhibitors and several chemotherapeutic agents. Interestingly, silibinin anti-cancer activity were implicated to be p53-, NF-κB- and/or AR-dependent/

Table 6.1 Chemopreventive effects of silibinin in skin, bladder, prostate, colorectal and lung cancer (preclinical and clinical studies)

Agents	Model	Targets	Tumor phenotype	
Skin cancer				
Single treatment				
Silibinin	SKH-1 hairless mouse skin	↓ PCNA ↑ p53, CDKN1A/p21	↓ Proliferation ↑ Apoptosis	Dhanalakshmi et al. (2004b)
Silibinin	HaCaT cell line	↓ pERK1/2, Bclx(L) cytosol ↑ AP-1, Bclx(L) Mitochondria		Dhanalakshmi et al. (2004a)
Silibinin (post-UVB)		↑ pERK1/2, cleaved PARP, CASP-9, NF-κB, AP-1, pBcl-2, survivin		
Silibinin (post-UVB higher dose)		↓ AP-1, total PARP ↑ Cleaved PARP	↑ Apoptosis	
Silibinin (post-UVB), pan caspase inhibitor C1		↓ Cleaved PARP		
Silibinin (pre-/post UVB)	SKH-1 hairless mouse skin, xenograft in SKH-1 hairless mice	↓ PCNA, CDK2/4, cyclin A/D1/E, pAkt, survivin ↑ p53, cleaved CASP-3, pERK1/2, p38, pJNK1/2	↓ Proliferation, tumor growth, tumor multiplicity	Mallikarjuna et al. (2004)
Silibinin (pre-UVB)	A431 cell line	↓ Bcl-2 (mitochondrial/cytosol), Bax, Bak (cytosol), cyto c/Cytochrome c (mitochondrial), Bid (cell lysate) ↑ Cleaved CASP-3/7, pErk1/2, pJNK, p38	↑ Apoptosis	Mohan et al. (2004)
Silibinin (post-UVB)		↓ Cleaved CASP-3/7 ↑ Bcl-2, Bax, Bak, cyto c (mitochondrial)	↓ Apoptosis	

(continued)

Table 6.1 (continued)

Agents	Model	Targets	Tumor phenotype	
Silibinin	JB6 cell line	↓ p53 (Ser15), pAkt (Ser473), pERK1/2, Elk-1, pGSK-3α/β, pJNK1/2, cleaved CASP-3, DNA-PK, pATM (Ser1981), γH2A.X (Ser139)		Dhanalakshmi et al. (2005)
Silibinin (pre-UVB)		↑ p53 (Ser15), pAkt (Ser473), pERK1/2, Elk-1, pGSK-3, cleaved CASP-3, γH2A.X (Ser139), pATM (Ser1981), DNA-PK		
Silibinin (pre-UVB), MEK1/2 inhibitor PD98059		↓ pERK1/2 ↑ p53 (Ser15), cleaved CASP-3	↑ Apoptosis	
Silibinin, (pre-UVB), DNA-PK inhibitor LY294002		↓ pERK1/2, cleaved CASP-3, pAkt (Ser473), DNA-PK(180 kDa) ↑ p53 (Ser15)	↓ Apoptosis	
Silibinin, UVB, ATM/ATR inhibitor caffeine		↑ p53 (Ser15), DNA-PK(180 kDa)		
Silibinin (pre–/post-UVB)	SKH-1 hairless mouse skin	↓ pERK1/2, pJNK1/2, pAKT, p-p38/MAPK14, PCNA ↑ p53, p21, CDKN1B /Kip1/p27	↓ Proliferation, apoptosis	Gu et al. (2005a)
Silibinin (pre-UVB)	SKH-1 hairless mouse skin	↓ PCNA ↑ p53, p21	↓ Proliferation, apoptosis	Gu et al. (2005b)
Silibinin (post-UVB)	SKH-1 hairless mouse skin	↓ E2F2/3, total CDC25C, total CDC2/p34, cyclin A/B1/D1/E, CDK2/4, pERK1/2, pAkt, p-p38, PCNA, cleaved CASP-3, γH2A.X (Ser139)	↓ Proliferation	Gu et al. (2006)
		↑ E2F1, p53, p21, p27	↑ Apoptosis	
	Xenograft in SKH-1 hairless mice	↓ E2F1, PCNA ↑ p53, p21, p27, cleaved CASP-3, PARP	↓ Tumor growth, tumor multiplicity ↑ Apoptosis	

Silibinin (pre−/post-UVB)	JB6 cell line	↓ pERK1/2, pJNK1/2, p-p38, pAkt, NF-κB, AP-1		Singh et al. (2006b)
Silibinin (pre-EGF)		↓ pERK1/2, pJNK1/2, p-p38, pAkt, NF-κB, AP-1, p-c-Fos, c-Fos, p-c-Jun		
Silibinin (pre-UVA)	HaCaT cell line	↓ CHOP	↑ Apoptosis	Narayanapillai et al. (2012)
Silibinin (pre-UVB)	JB6 cell line	↓ Cleaved PARP, CASP-3	↓ Apoptosis	Roy et al. (2012)
	SKH1 hairless mouse skin	↑ p53 (nuclear), GADD45α		
siGAAD45α, Silibinin (pre-UVB)		↑ p53		
Silibinin (post-UVB)	Kunming mouse skin	↓ LC3-II/LC3-I, p53 (epidermal) ↑ p53 (dermis)	↓ Autophagy, migration, chemotaxis of neutrophils, mast cells	Wang et al. (2013)
Silibinin (pre-treatment)	DMBA + TPA-induced skin cancer in Swiss Albino mice	↓ TNF-α, IL-6, IL-1β, iNOS, COX-2, VEGF	↓ Tumor incidence, multiplicity	Khan et al. (2014)
Silibinin, Exogenous recombinant IL-12	JB6 cell line, SKH-1 hairless mice	↓ IL-12 ↑ Cleaved CASP-3, PARP	↑ Apoptosis	Narayanapillai et al. (2014)
Silibinin	DMBA/TPA-induced SCC cancer in			Tilley et al. (2016)
Silibinin	DMBA/TPA induced SCC model in LACA mice	↓ Taurine, glucose, lactate ↑ Guanine, LPO	↑ Apoptosis	Sati et al. (2016)
Silibinin (pre−/post-UVB)	Wildtype ($p53^{+/+}$) SKH-1 hairless mice	↓ NF-κB p50, COX-2, iNOS, TNF-α, IL-6, IL-12	↓ SSC lesions, tumor incidence, multiplicity	Rigby et al. (2017)
	Heterozygous ($p53^{+/-}$) SKH-1 hairless mice	↑ GADD45α, XPB, XPC		
	p53 knockout ($p53^{-/-}$) mice on SKH-1 hairless	↓ XPG ↑ GADD45α, XPB, XPC		
Silibinin, Hedgehog inhibitor Sant1	ASZ001-Sant1 resistant cell line	↓ pAKT (Ser 473), pERK1/2 (Thr202/Tyr 204), cyclin D1, Gli ↑ CASP-3, cleaved PARP, SUFU		Dheeraj et al. (2017)

(continued)

Table 6.1 (continued)

Agents	Model	Targets	Tumor phenotype	
Combination treatment				
Silibinin, Silymarin (pre-UVB)	C3H/HeN mice	↓ IL-10 ↑ IL-12	↓ Local immunosuppression	Meeran et al. (2006)
Silymarin, anti-IL-12 monoclonal (pre-UVB, pre-DNFB)			↓ Contact hypersensitivity response, ear thickness	
Silymarin, rat IgG1 (pre-UVB, pre-DNFB)			↑ Contact hypersensitivity response	
Silibinin	IL-12 wildtype C3H/HeN mice		↓ Contact hypersensitivity response, ear thickness	
Recombinant IL-12			↑ Contact hypersensitivity response, ear thickness	
Silymarin, Recombinant IL-12 (pre-UVB, pre-DNFB)	IL-12$^{-/-}$ C3H/HeN mice		↑ Contact hypersensitivity response, thickness	
IL-12 (pre-UVB, pre-DNFB)			↑ Contact hypersensitivity response, ear thickness	
Bladder cancer				
Single treatment				
Silymarin	OH-BBN induced bladder cancer in ICR mice	↓ Cyclin D1	↓ Proliferation, preneoplastric lesion, tumor incidence	Vinh et al. (2002)
Silibinin, Silymarin	OHBBN induced bladder cancer in ICR mice	↓ Cyclin D1, pERK1/2, PCNA, survivin, NF-κB p65 (Ser276 and Ser53)	↓ Proliferation, lesions	Tyagi et al. (2007)
		↑ Cleaved CASP-3, PARP	↑ Apoptosis	
Silibinin	RT4 xenograft in athymic nude mice	↓ Survivin, PCNA, CD31	↓ Proliferation, tumor microvasculature, tumor growth	Singh et al. (2008)
		↑ p53, CASP-3	↑ Apoptosis	
Silibinin, p53 siRNA		↓ Survivin ↑ Cleaved CASP-3		

Silibinin	5637 cell line, xenograft in athymic BALB/c nu/nu mice	↓ Survivin, cyto c, Omi/HtrA2, AIF	↓ Tumor growth, incidence superficial, invasive bladder lesion incidence	Zeng et al. (2011)
		↑ Cleaved CASP-3/9, PARP	Apoptosis	
Silibinin	T24-L cell line, xenograft in athymic BALB/c nu/nu mice	↓ Vimentin, MMP-2, pGSK-3β, CTNNB1/β-catenin, ZEB1, CD44	↓ Migration, invasion, lung metastatic lesion incidence, spheriod colony formation, lung/bone metastases	Wu et al. (2013)
		↑ Cytokeratins 18/19	↑ Apoptosis, animal survival	
Silibinin, NF-κB inhibitor PDTC	Cisplatin-resistant T24, J82 cell lines	↓ NF-κB, CDH 2/N-cadherin Vimentin, MMP-2/9, ABCB1	↓ Proliferation, migration, invasion	Sun et al. (2017)
Silibinin	UM-UC-3, T24 cell lines	↓ KRAS, H3K4me3, AcH3, HOTAIR, ZFAS1, EGFR, PI3K p85/p110, pAKT	↓ Proliferation, migration, invasion	Imai-Sumida et al. (2017)
		↑ SOS1, RAC1/2/3, PAK1, DDR1	↑ Apoptosis	
Silibinin	T24, RT4 cell lines	↓ FRAP/mTOR, pAKT2, FGFR-3, DNMT1, miRs-100/203	↓ Proliferation, colony formation	DE Oliveira et al. (2017)
		↑ miR-203	↑ Apoptosis	
Silibinin, TGF β1	T24, 253 J cell lines	↓ TGF β1, COX-2	↓ Cell migration, invasion	Li et al. (2018)
Combination treatment				
Silibinin, photodynamic therapy	MB49, T24 cell lines		↓ Viability, migration ↑ Apoptosis	Gandara et al. (2014)
Silibinin, radiation	MB49, MB49-I cell lines, C57BL/6 J mice	↓ NF-κB, survivin, pAkt	↓ Viability, colony formation, tumor growth	Prack Mc Cormick et al. (2018)
		↑ CASP-3, cleaved PARP	↑ Apoptosis	
Colorectal cancer				
Single treatment				
IdB 1016	Colorectal cancer patients at stages Dukes A, B, C, or D with liver metastates		↑ Concentration in colorectal mucosa, liver tissue (variable)	Hoh et al. (2006)

(continued)

Table 6.1 (continued)

Agents	Model	Targets	Tumor phenotype	
Silibinin (pre−/post-AOM)	AOM-induced colorectal cancer in Fisher 344 rats	↓ PCNA, cyclin D1, iNOS, COX-2	↓ Proliferation, aberrant crypt foci formation	Velmurugan et al. (2008)
		↑ Cleaved PARP, MCP-1/5, IL-4, TIMP-1	↑ Apoptosis	
Silibinin	DMH-induced colon cancer in albino Wistar rats	↓ TBARS, LOOH, CD, CTNNB1 ↑ SOD, CAT, GPX, UDPGT, GST, DTD	↓ Proliferation, preneoplastic lesions, aberrant crypt foci formation, tumor incidence	Sangeetha et al. (2009, 2010, 2012)
Silibinin	APC $^{min/+}$ mice	↓ PCNA, cyclin D1, CTNNB1, COX-2, PGE-2, nestin, HIF-1α, VEGF, eNOS Fas ligand, TNF-α, VCAM-1, eotoxin-2, VEGF, M-CSF, IL-1α, IL-1β, leptin, IFN-γ, P-selectin, leptin receptor	↓ Proliferation, angiogenesis, polyp incidence, tumor growth	Rajamanickam et al. (2010)
			↑ Apoptosis	
Silibinin	AOM-induced colorectal cancer in A/J mice	↓ PCNA, cyclin D1, iNOS, COX-2, p21, VEGF, pAkt, IGFBP-3, IGF-1Rβ, pGSK-3β, CTNNB1	↓ Proliferation, angiogenesis	Ravichandran et al. (2010)
		↑ Cleaved CASP-3, PARP		
Silibinin	SW480 xenograft in athymic (nu/nu) mice	↓ PCNA, CD31, cyclin D1, CTNNB1, p-GSK3β, c-Myc, survivin, VEGF, iNOS	↓ Proliferation, tumor growth	Velmurugan et al. (2010)
			↑ Apoptosis	
Silibinin, Exogenous IL-6, JNK inhibitor SP600125 / MMP-2 inhibitor	LoVo cell line	↓ MMP-2, AP-1	↓ Proliferation, invasion	Lin et al. (2012)
Silibinin	AOM-induced colon cancer in Wistar rats	↓ Bcl-2	↓ Aberrant crypt foci formation	Kauntz et al. (2012a)
		↑ Cleaved CASP-3, Bax, IL-1β, TNF-α, MMP-7	↑ Apoptosis	

Silibinin Silibinin + TRAIL	SW480, TRAIL-resistant SW620 metastatic cell lines	↓ Mcl-1, XIAP	↑ Apoptosis	Kauntz et al. (2012b)
		↑ DR4, DR5, cleaved CASP-3/8/9		
Silibinin	Primary colorectal cancer stem cells, xenograft in SCID mice	↓ $CD133^{+}$, pAKT (Ser473)/ mTOR, pJNK, p-p38, GSK-3β, RSK, pPP2Ac	↓ Cell growth, sphere formation, tumor formation rate, tumor growth	Wang et al. (2012)
Silibinin, C6-ceramide, LY294002, or rapamycin			↓ Tumor incidence	
Silibinin	SW480, LoVo, HT-29 cell lines, SW480 xenograft in athymic (nu/nu) nude male	↓ CYCS, SQSTM1, BECN1, EGF, AKT1, EGFR, MAPK1/3	↓ Colony formation	Raina et al. (2013)
		↑ HMOX1, GPX, CAT, LC3-II/ LC3-I, pMAP2K1/2, pELK1/2, mTOR, pPRKAA2	↑ Apoptosis, autophagy	
Silibinin	HT-29 cell line	↑ NAG-1, EGR-1, Cleavage PARP	↑ Apoptosis	Woo et al. (2014)
Silibinin	DMH-induced colon cancer in albino Wistar rats	↑ CDX2, GCC	↓ Adenocarcinoma incidence, mast cell infiltration	Sangeetha and Nalini (2015)
Silibinin, IL-4, IL-6	SW480, HT-29, LoVo cell lines	↓ IL-4, IL-6, CD44, CDv3–6, $CD44^{+}$ $EpCAM^{high}$, pSTAT3, NANOG, SOX-2, CD133, OCT-4, MSI-1, CDX2	↓ Colonosphere formation, colonsphere growth	Kumar et al. (2014)
			↑ Apoptosis	
Combination treatment				
Siliphos, PolyE	CT-26 cell line, CT-26 xenograft in BaLB/c mice		↓ Proliferation, tumor growth, liver nodule incidence	Yan et al. (2012)
			↑ Apoptosis	
Silibinin, Metformin	COLO205 cell line	↓ pAKT	↑ Apoptosis	Tsai et al. (2015)
		↑ AMPK, PTEN		
Silibinin, 1,25-dihydroxyvitamin D (1,25D)	HT-29 cell line	↓ TNF-α, Snail1/2	↓ Proliferation, migration	Bhatia and Falzon (2015)
		↑ VDR		

(continued)

Table 6.1 (continued)

Agents	Model	Targets	Tumor phenotype	
Silibinin, oxovanadium (IV) complexes	HT-29 cell line	↓ NF-κB, p70-S6K, p4EB-P1, pAKT, total AKT	↓ Proliferation	Leon et al. (2015)
		↑ CASP-3	↑ Apoptosis	
Silibinin, Kinase inhibitor Regoranfenib	SW48, SW48-CR, SW480, HCT15 cell lines	↓ pAKT, total AKT, p70-S6K, p4EB-P1	↓ Colony formation	Belli et al. (2017)
	Metastatic Colorectal cancer patients	↑ cleaved PARP, CASP-3, pro-CASP-9	↑ Apoptosis, overall survival	
Silibinin, 5FU	$CD44^+$ HCT116 cell line	↓ CD44v6, Nanog, CTNNB1, CDKN2A/p16INK4		Patel et al. (2018)
		↑ E-cadherin		
Prostate cancer				
Single treatment				
Silymarin	LNCaP cell line	↓ PSA, FKBP51	↓ hK2 secretion	Zhu et al. (2001)
Silibinin	$ARCaP_m$, DU145, 22Rv1 cell lines	↓ Cdk2, Skp-2	↓ Proliferation	Roy et al. (2007)
		↑ p21/p27	↑ Apoptosis	
Silibinin	TRAMP mice	↓ IGF, cyclin A, B1/E, CDK2/4/6	↓ PCNA, tumor growth, adeno-carcinoma incidence	Raina et al. (2007)
		↑ IGFBP-3, p21, p27	↑ PIN incidence	
$Siliphos^R$	Localized prostate cancer patients		↓ Inter/intra-patient viability in urine silibinin levels ↑ Plasma concentration (transient) disease stability	Flaig et al. (2007a)
Silibinin	LNCaP, PC-3, DU145 cell lines	↓ Vimentin, MMP-2	↓ Viability, proliferation, motility, migration, invasion	Wu et al. (2009)
$Siliphos^R$	Localized prostate cancer patients		↑ Plasma concentration (transient)	Flaig et al. (2010)

Silibinin	PC-3, PC-3MM2 C4-2B cell lines	↓ Slug, Snail, p-Akt (Ser473), CTNNB1, p-Src(tyr419), Hakai ↑ E-cadherin	↓ Migration, invasion	Deep et al. (2011)
Silybin A, Silybin B, Isosilybin A and Isosilybin B	HUVEC cell line, DU145 xenograft in athymic (nu/nu) nude mice	↓ PCNA, CD31, nestin, VEGF, VEGFR1/2, pAkt, HIF-1α	↓ Proliferation, microvasculation in mouse dorsal aortas, proliferation, capillary-like tube formation, invasion	Deep et al. (2012)
Silibinin	PC-3 cell line, Cancer associated fibroblasts	↓ pFAKT(Tyr-925), integrins α5/αV/β1/β3), pSrc, Cdc42, Rac, ARP2, cortactin, MMP-9	↓ Proliferation, motility, invasion	Deep et al. (2014)
			↑ Apoptosis	
Silibinin	HepG2, PC-3 cell lines	↓ sPLA2 of groups IB/III/V, hGIIA, NF-κB p65 (Ser536)		Hagelgans et al. (2014).
Silibinin, R1881	PWR-1E, LNCaP, DU145 cell lines	↓ SREBP1/2, FASN, AR ↑ AMPK		Nambiar et al. (2014)
Silibinin	Human prostate stromal cells (PrSCs) in control medium from PC-3 cells	↓ α-SMA, TGFβ2, IL-6, vimentin, FAP		Ting et al. (2015)
Silibinin	PC-3 cell line	↓ Pro-CASP-3, cleaved PARP ↑ LC3-II	↑ Autophagy	Kim et al. (2015)
Silibinin	PC-3 cell line	↑ NOX-4, cleaved PARP	↑ Apoptosis	Kim et al. (2016)
Silibinin, Curcumin, Resveratrol, Melatonin	LNCaP, PC-3 cell lines		↓ Viability	Rodriguez-Garcia et al. 2017)
5-O-Alkyl-2,3-dehydrosilybins	LNCaP, DU14, 5PC-3 cell lines		↓ Proliferation	Vue et al. (2017)
Silibinin	LNCaP, 22Rv1 cell lines	↓ HIF-1α, ACC, FASN, NOX	↓ Proliferation, colony formation, angiogenesis, endothelial cells tube formation	Deep et al. (2017)
	22Rv1 xenograft in athymic (nu/nu) nude mice	↓ HIF-1α, ACC, FASN	↓ Tumor growth, proliferation, angiogenesis	

(continued)

Table 6.1 (continued)

Agents	Model	Targets	Tumor phenotype	
Combination treatment				
Silibinin, Doxorubicin	DU145 cell line	↓ CDC25C, p34, cyclin B1	↑ Apoptosis	Tyagi et al. (2002)
Silibinin	DU145 cell line	↓ p34, cyclin B1, CDC25C	↓ Proliferation	Dhanalakshmi et al. (2003)
		↑ Cleaved PARP, CASP-3/7/9	↑ Apoptosis	
Silibinin, Cisplatin		↓ p34, cyclin B1, CDC25C ↑ Cleaved PARP, CASP-3/7/9		
Silibinin, Carboplatin		↓ p34, cyclin B1, CDC25C ↑ Cleaved PARP, CASP-3/7/9		
Silibinin, JAK-1 inhibitor piceatannol	DU145 cell line	↓ pStat3	↑ Apoptosis	Agarwal et al. (2007)
		↑ Cleaved CASP-3/9		
Silibinin, Mitoxantrone	PC-3, LNCaP, DU145 cell lines		↓ Viability ↑ Apoptosis	Flaig et al. (2007b)
Silibinin, Radiation	DU145, PC-3 cell lines, DU145 xenograft in athymic (nu/nu) nude mice	↓ Bcl-2, cyclin B1 Cdc2, Cdc25C, pATM, pChk1/2, pEGFR, pERK1/2	↓ Proliferation, colony formation, animal survival, tumor growth	Nambiar et al. (2015a)
		↑ Cleaved CASP-3	↑ Apoptosis	
Silibinin, Radiation	DU145 cell line, xenograft in athymic (nu/nu) male nude mice	↓ VEGF, iNOS, eNOS, MMP-2, u-PA, Vimentin, CDH2, pAKT, pERK1/2, PCNA	↓ Proliferation, migration invasion	Nambiar et al. (2015b)
		↑ E-cadherin		
Lung cancer				
Single treatment				
Silibinin	SHP-77, A549 cell lines		↓ Proliferation ↑ Apoptosis	Sharma et al. (2003)
Silibinin	A549 cell line	↓ MMP-2, u-PA	↓ Motility, invasion, adhesion	Chu et al. (2004)
		↑ TMIP-2		

Silibinin	Urethane-induced lung cancer in A/J mice	↓ PCNA, cyclin D1, VEGF, iNOS, COX-2	↓ Proliferation, angiogenesis, tumor growth, tumor incidence ↑ Apoptosis	Singh et al. (2006a)
Silibinin, IFNγ IL-1β, TNF-α	A549 cell line	↓ PCNA, Nestin, VEGFR, NF-κB p65, pSTAT1 (tyr-701), pSTAT3 (tyr-705), HIF-1α, iNOS, pERK1/2, c-Jun, c-Fos	↓ Proliferation, angiogenesis, tumor growth	Chittezhath et al. (2008)
			↑ Apoptosis	
Silibinin	Urethane-induced lung cancer in A/J mice	↓ IL-13, TNF-α, HIF-1α, NF-κB p65 (Ser276), pSTAT3 (Ser727), nestin	↓ Proliferation, angiogenesis macrophage infiltration, tumor growth, tumor incidence	Tyagi et al. (2009)
		↑ TIMP-1/2, Ang-2, Tie-2		
Silibinin	H1299, H460, H322 cell lines	↓ CDK2/4 6, cyclinD1/D3/E, p18/INK4C, p21, p27, pRb	↓ Proliferation	Mateen et al. (2010)
			↑ Apoptosis	
Silibinin	Urethane-induced lung cancer in B6/129-Nos2tm1Lau (iNOS$^{-/-}$) mice	↓ iNOS, VEGFR-2, pSTAT3 (Ser727), NF-κB p65 (Ser276), PCNA, nestin	↓ Proliferation, angiogenesis, tumor multiplicity	Ramasamy et al. (2011)
Silibinin, TNF-α, IFN-γ	LM2 cell line	↓ pSTAT3/1, pErk1/2, NF-kB, COX2, iNOS, MMP-2/9	↓ Viability, proliferation, migration	Tyagi et al. (2012)
Silibinin, EGFR inhibitor WZ4002, EGFR siRNA	NCI-H1975, HCC827 cell lines, NCI-H1975 xenograft in BALB/c mice	↓ pEGFR, pAKT (Ser473), pERK1/2, p-p38, LOX	↓ Migration, tumor nodule incidence	Hou et al. (2018)
			↑ Animal survival	
Combination treatment				
Silibinin, HDAC inhibitor Trichostatin A, DNMT inhibitor 5′-Aza-deoxycytidine	H1299 cell line	↓ HDACs 1–3, Mcl-1 L, Bcl x(L), Bcl-2, XIAP, Zeb1, cyclin B1, PCNA, p-histone H3	↓ Proliferation, migration, invasion	Mateen et al. (2012)
		↑ Cleaved CASP-3, PARP, CDKN1A/p21, AcH3, AcH4, E-cadherin		

(continued)

Table 6.1 (continued)

Agents	Model	Targets	Tumor phenotype	
Silibinin, PI3K (LY294002) and MEK (U0126) inhibitors	A549 cell line	↓ pAkt, pERK1/2, NF-κB, AP-1, c-Jun, c-Fos, MMP-9, u-PA	↓ Invasion	Chen et al. (2005)
Silibinin, Doxorubicin	Doxorubicin-resistant A549 cell line, A549 xenograft in BALB/c nu/nu mice	↓ NF-κB p65/p50, COX-2, PCNA, CD31	↓ Proliferation, angiogenesis, tumor growth	Singh et al. (2004)
			↑ Apoptosis	
Silibinin, Gefitinib, Erlotinib	H1975, HCC827, PC-9/GR, PC-9ER cell lines	↓ pEGFR (pErbB2/3), pAkt, pErk	↓ Viability, colony formation tumor growth	Rho et al. (2010)
			↑ Apoptosis	
Silibinin, Etoposide, Doxorubicin	NCI-H69, VPA17 cell lines	↓ CASP3 activity	↓ Viability	Sadava and Kane (2013)
		↑ Survivin		
Silibinin-meglumine, Erlotinib	PC-9/Erl-R cells	↓ ALDH1/3	↓ Spheroid formation, spheroid number	Corominas-Faja et al. (2013)
Silibinin-meglumine, gefitinib	PC-9, EGFR-mutant xenografts in NOD/ SCID mice	↓ Vimentin, CDH2, TWIST-1, SNAIL2	↓ Migration, tumor growth, tumor regrowth	Cufi et al. (2013a)
Silibinin-meglumine, erlotinib	PC-9, EGFR-mutant, PC-9/Erl-R xenografts in athymic nude mice	↓ SNAIL1, ZEB1, CDH2, miR-21	↓ Migration, tumor growth	Cufi et al. (2013b)
		↑ miR-200c		
Silibinin, Indole-3-carbinol (I3C)	A549 cell line, A549 xenograft in athymic nude mice	↓ SIRT1	↓ Viability, adhesion, migration, tumor growth, lung metastatic, colony formation	Liang et al. (2014)
		↑ p53, acetylated p53, Bax, cyto c (cytosol), CASP-3, GSH	↑ Apoptosis	

Silibinin, Indole-3-carbinol (I3C)	NNK-induced lung tumorigenesis in A/J mice	↓ ARNTL, Cyp1a1, NPAS2 ↑ Spag11b		Qian et al. (2015)
Silibinin, Radiation	Lewis lung cancer xenograft in C57BL/6 mice		↓ Tumor nodules, fibrosis, neutrophil/lymphocyte/macrophage cell infiltration	Son et al. (2015)

ABCB1 ATP binding cassette subfamily B member 1, *AcH3* acetylated histone H3, *AIF* allograft inflammatory factor 1, *ALDH* aldehyde dehydrogenase, *AKT* serine/threonine kinase, *AMPK* AMP-activated protein kinase, *Ang-2* angiopoietin 2, *AP-1* activator protein 1, *ATM* serine/threonine kinase, *BAX* BCL2 associated X, apoptosis regulator, *BCL-2* BCL2 apoptosis regulator, *Bclx(L)* BCL2 like 1, *BID* BH3 interacting domain death agonist, *CASP* caspase, *CAT* catalase, *CCM* control conditioned media, *CD* conjugated dienes, *CD31* platelet and endothelial cell adhesion molecule 1, *CD44* CD44 molecule (Indian blood group), *CD133* Prominin 1, *CDC2/p34* cyclin dependent kinase 1, *CDC25C* cell division cycle 25C, *CDH2* N-cadherin, *CDK* cyclin dependent kinase, *CDKN* cyclin dependent kinase inhibitor, *CDX2* caudal type homeobox 2 , *c-FOS* Fos proto-oncogene/AP-1 transcription factor subunit, *CHOP* DNA damage inducible transcript 3, *c-JUN* Jun proto-oncogene/AP-1 transcription factor subunit, *COX-2* prostaglandin-endoperoxide synthase 2, *CSF* colony stimulating factor, *Cyto c* Cytochrome, *DDR* discoidin domain receptor tyrosine kinase 1, *DNA-PK* DNA-dependent protein kinase, *DNMT1* DNA methyltransferase, *DR* HLA class II histocompatibility antigen, DRB beta, *DTD* DT-diaphorase, *E2F* E2F transcription factor, *EGFR* epidermal growth factor receptor, *EGR* early growth response, *ELK* ELK1 ETS transcription factor, *ERK1/2* mitogen-activated protein kinase 3/1, *FAP* fibroblast activation protein alpha, *FASN* fatty acid synthase, *FGFR* fibroblast growth factor receptor, *GADD45α* growth arrest and DNA damage inducible alpha, *GCC* guanylyl cyclase C, *GPX* glutathione peroxidase 1, *GSH* glutathione, *GSK-3β* glycogen synthase kinase 3 beta, *GST* glutathione S-transferase, *H3K4me3* Tri-methylation of histone H3 lysine 4, *HDAC* histone deacetylase, *HIF* hypoxia inducible factor 1, *HOTAIR* HOX transcript antisense RNA, *IFN* interferon, *IGF* insulin like growth factor, *IGFBP* insulin like growth factor binding protein, *IL* interleukin, *iNOS* inducible nitric oxide synthase, *JNK1/2* mitogen-activated protein kinase 8/9, *KRAS* KRAS proto-oncogene, *LC3* microtubule associated protein 1 light chain 3 alpha, *LOOH* lipid hydroperoxide, *LOX* lysyl oxidase, *LPO* lipid peroxidation, *MCL-1/MCL-1 L* MCL1 apoptosis regulator, *MCP-1* C-C motif chemokine ligand 2, *MCP-5* C-C motif chemokine ligand 12, *MMP* matrix metallopeptidase, *MSI-1* RNA-binding protein Musashi homolog 1, *mTOR/FRAP* mechanistic target of rapamycin kinase, *NAG1* non-steroidal anti-inflammatory drug-activated gene-1, *NF-κB* nuclear factor kappa B, *NOX* NADPH oxidase 1, *OCT*, POU class 2 homeobox 1, *p38* mitogen-activated protein kinase 14, *p53* tumor protein P53, *PAK* P21 (RAC1) activated kinase, *PARP* poly(ADP-ribose) polymerase, *PCNA* proliferating cell nuclear antigen, *PGE-2* prostaglandin E2, *PP2AC* protein phosphatase 2 catalytic subunit alpha, *PSA* prostate specific antigen, *PTEN* phosphatase and tensin homolog, *RAC1* Rac family small GTPase 1, *RB* retinoblastoma protein, *RG* complement C4A (Rodgers Blood Group), *RSK* ribosomal protein S6 kinase A1, *SIRT* Sirtuin 1, *α-SMA* actin alpha 2 smooth muscle, *SNAIL* Snail Family Transcriptional Repressor, *SOD1* superoxide dismutase 1, *SOS1* SOS Ras/Rac guanine nucleotide exchange factor 1, *SOX* SRY-Box, *SPAG11B* sperm associated antigen 11B, *STAT* signal transducer and activator of transcription, *SUFU* SUFU negative regulator of hedgehog signaling, *TBARS* thiobarbituric acid reactive substances, *TGFβ1* transforming growth factor beta 1, *Tie-2* TEK receptor tyrosine kinase, *TIMP* tissue inhibitor of metalloproteinases, *TNFα* tumor necrosis factor alpha, *TWIST-1* twist family BHLH transcription factor 1, *UDPGT* UDP-glucuronosyltransferase, *u-PA* plasminogen activator, Urokinase, *VCAM* vascular cell adhesion molecule 1, *VDR* vitamin D receptor, *VEGF* vascular endothelial growth factor, *VEGFR* vascular endothelial growth factor receptor, *XIAP* X-linked inhibitor of apoptosis, *XPB* ERCC excision repair 3, TFIIH core complex helicase subunit, *XPC* XPC complex subunit, DNA damage recognition and repair factor, *XPG* ERCC excision repair 5, endonuclease, *γH2A.X* H2A histone family member X, *ZEB1* zinc finger E-box binding homeobox 1, *ZFAS1* ZNFX1 antisense RNA 1

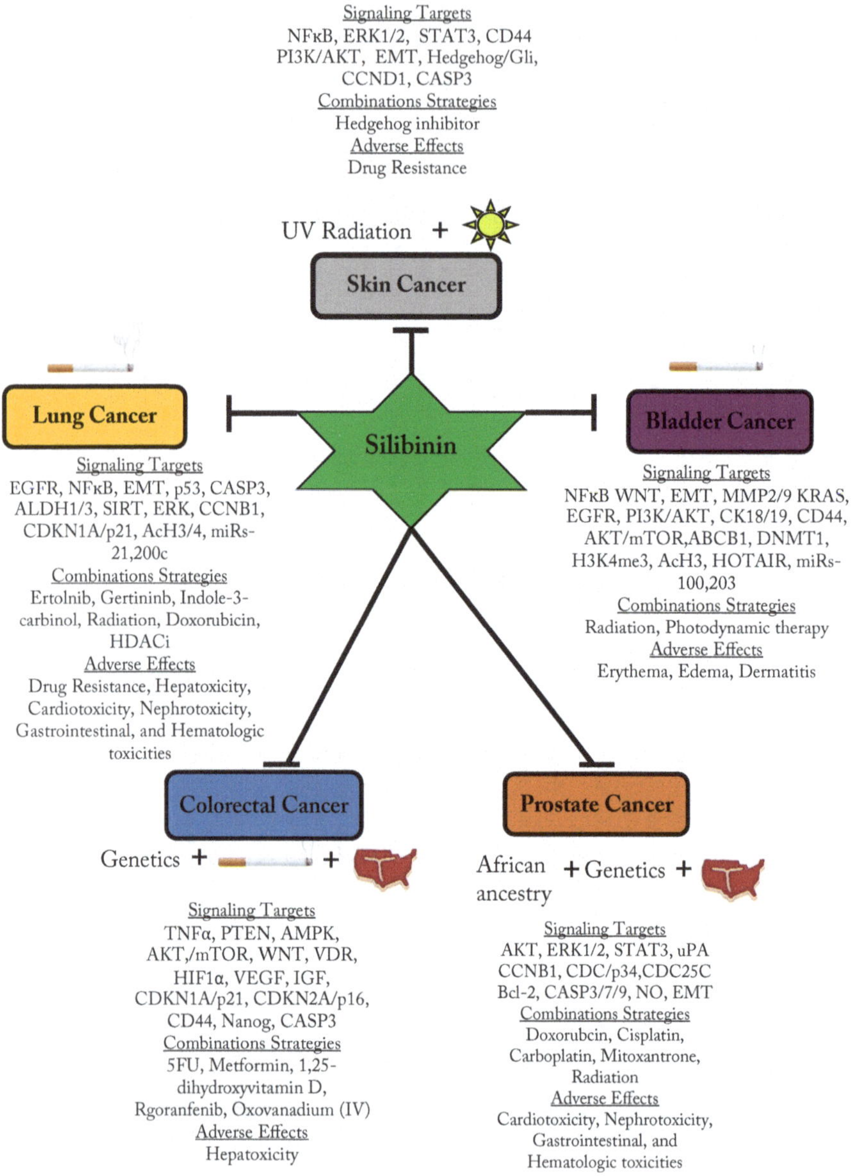

Fig. 6.1 Silibinin suppression of multiple-signaling mechanisms and adverse effects in combination treatment approaches against various cancers. Epidemiological evidence has identified major risk factors in the development of skin, lung, prostate and colorectal cancers. These risk factors can trigger the dysregulation of pro-oncogenic signaling pathways such as PI3K/AKT, NF-κB, MAPKs and KRAS in cancer initiation. Silibinin intervention in pre-clinical and clinical studies exert its anti-neoplastic effects by antagonizing multiple signaling pathways these malignancies. Silibinin as a nutraceutical has also shown efficacy in combination therapy strategies against chemotherapy resistant disease and associated adverse side effects

independent in bladder, colon and prostate tumors. In totality, use of silibinin as an adjuvant therapy in combination with leading cancer therapeutic agents could serve as a strong chemopreventive/intervention strategy for overall improvement in patient survival and treatment of acquired disease resistance in cancer.

Conflict of Interest Rajesh Agarwal is one of the founders and shareholders of a biotech company ProTechSure Scientific, Inc. that licensed Silibinin from UCD, and developed and marketed (OTC) its skin formulation as Difinsa53.

Grant Support Supported by NCI R01 grants CA140368 and CA195708 (to RA), R01 grant CA201112 (to KR), and R01 CA195708S (to DR).

References

Abenavoli L, Izzo AA, Milic N, Cicala C, Santini A, Capasso R (2018) Milk thistle (*Silybum marianum*): a concise overview on its chemistry, pharmacological, and nutraceutical uses in liver diseases. Phytother Res 32:2202–2213. https://doi.org/10.1002/ptr.6171

Agarwal C, Tyagi A, Kaur M, Agarwal R (2007) Silibinin inhibits constitutive activation of Stat3, and causes caspase activation and apoptotic death of human prostate carcinoma DU145 cells. Carcinogenesis 28:1463–1470. https://doi.org/10.1093/carcin/bgm042

Agarwal C, Wadhwa R, Deep G, Biedermann D, Gazak R, Kren V, Agarwal R (2013) Anti-cancer efficacy of silybin derivatives – a structure-activity relationship. PLoS One 8:e60074. https://doi.org/10.1371/journal.pone.0060074

Amirsaadat S, Pilehvar-Soltanahmadi Y, Zarghami F, Alipour S, Ebrahimnezhad Z, Zarghami N (2017) Silibinin-loaded magnetic nanoparticles inhibit hTERT gene expression and proliferation of lung cancer cells. Artif Cells Nanomed Biotechnol 45:1649–1656. https://doi.org/10.1080/21691401.2016.1276922

Arnold M, Sierra MS, Laversanne M, Soerjomataram I, Jemal A, Bray F (2017) Global patterns and trends in colorectal cancer incidence and mortality. Gut 66:683–691. https://doi.org/10.1136/gutjnl-2015-310912

Arora K, Barbieri CE (2018) Molecular subtypes of prostate cancer. Curr Oncol Rep 20:58. https://doi.org/10.1007/s11912-018-0707-9

Athanassiadou AM, Lazaris AC, Patsouris E, Tsipis A, Chelidonis G, Aroni K (2013) Significance of cyclooxygenase 2, EZH-2 polycomb group and p53 expression in actinic keratosis and squamous cell carcinomas of the skin. Am J Dermatopathol 35:425–431. https://doi.org/10.1097/DAD.0b013e318271292a

Belli V et al (2017) Regorafenib in combination with silybin as a novel potential strategy for the treatment of metastatic colorectal cancer. Oncotarget 8:68305–68316. https://doi.org/10.18632/oncotarget.20054

Bhatia V, Falzon M (2015) Restoration of the anti-proliferative and anti-migratory effects of 1,25-dihydroxyvitamin D by silibinin in vitamin D-resistant colon cancer cells. Cancer Lett 362:199–207. https://doi.org/10.1016/j.canlet.2015.03.042

Bijak M (2017) Silybin, a major bioactive component of milk thistle (*Silybum marianum* L. Gaernt.)-chemistry, bioavailability, and metabolism. Molecules 22. https://doi.org/10.3390/molecules22111942

Bray C, Bell LN, Liang H, Collins D, Yale SH (2017) Colorectal cancer screening. WMJ 116:27–33

Bray F, Ferlay J, Soerjomataram I, Siegel RL, Torre LA, Jemal A (2018) Global cancer statistics 2018: GLOBOCAN estimates of incidence and mortality worldwide for 36 cancers in 185 countries. CA Cancer J Clin 68:394–424. https://doi.org/10.3322/caac.21492
Chen PN, Hsieh YS, Chiou HL, Chu SC (2005) Silibinin inhibits cell invasion through inactivation of both PI3K-Akt and MAPK signaling pathways. Chem Biol Interact 156:141–150. https://doi.org/10.1016/j.cbi.2005.08.005
Chittezhath M, Deep G, Singh RP, Agarwal C, Agarwal R (2008) Silibinin inhibits cytokine-induced signaling cascades and down-regulates inducible nitric oxide synthase in human lung carcinoma A549 cells. Mol Cancer Ther 7:1817–1826. https://doi.org/10.1158/1535-7163.MCT-08-0256
Chu SC, Chiou HL, Chen PN, Yang SF, Hsieh YS (2004) Silibinin inhibits the invasion of human lung cancer cells via decreased productions of urokinase-plasminogen activator and matrix metalloproteinase-2. Mol Carcinog 40:143–149. https://doi.org/10.1002/mc.20018
Corominas-Faja B et al (2013) Stem cell-like ALDH(bright) cellular states in EGFR-mutant non-small cell lung cancer: a novel mechanism of acquired resistance to erlotinib targetable with the natural polyphenol silibinin. Cell Cycle 12:3390–3404. https://doi.org/10.4161/cc.26417
Cufi S et al (2013a) Silibinin meglumine, a water-soluble form of milk thistle silymarin, is an orally active anti-cancer agent that impedes the epithelial-to-mesenchymal transition (EMT) in EGFR-mutant non-small-cell lung carcinoma cells. Food Chem Toxicol 60:360–368. https://doi.org/10.1016/j.fct.2013.07.063
Cufi S et al (2013b) Silibinin suppresses EMT-driven erlotinib resistance by reversing the high miR-21/low miR-200c signature in vivo. Sci Rep 3:2459. https://doi.org/10.1038/srep02459
Cuyas E, Perez-Sanchez A, Micol V, Menendez JA, Bosch-Barrera J (2016) STAT3-targeted treatment with silibinin overcomes the acquired resistance to crizotinib in ALK-rearranged lung cancer. Cell Cycle 15:3413–3418. https://doi.org/10.1080/15384101.2016.1245249
Deep G, Agarwal R (2010) Antimetastatic efficacy of silibinin: molecular mechanisms and therapeutic potential against cancer. Cancer Metastasis Rev 29:447–463. https://doi.org/10.1007/s10555-010-9237-0
Deep G, Oberlies NH, Kroll DJ, Agarwal R (2007) Isosilybin B and isosilybin A inhibit growth, induce G1 arrest and cause apoptosis in human prostate cancer LNCaP and 22Rv1 cells. Carcinogenesis 28:1533–1542. https://doi.org/10.1093/carcin/bgm069
Deep G, Gangar SC, Agarwal C, Agarwal R (2011) Role of E-cadherin in antimigratory and antiinvasive efficacy of silibinin in prostate cancer cells. Cancer Prev Res (Phila) 4:1222–1232. https://doi.org/10.1158/1940-6207.CAPR-10-0370
Deep G et al (2012) Angiopreventive efficacy of pure flavonolignans from milk thistle extract against prostate cancer: targeting VEGF-VEGFR signaling. PLoS One 7:e34630. https://doi.org/10.1371/journal.pone.0034630
Deep G, Kumar R, Jain AK, Agarwal C, Agarwal R (2014) Silibinin inhibits fibronectin induced motility, invasiveness and survival in human prostate carcinoma PC3 cells via targeting integrin signaling. Mutat Res 768:35–46. https://doi.org/10.1016/j.mrfmmm.2014.05.002
Deep G et al (2017) Silibinin inhibits hypoxia-induced HIF-1alpha-mediated signaling, angiogenesis and lipogenesis in prostate cancer cells: In vitro evidence and in vivo functional imaging and metabolomics. Mol Carcinog 56:833–848. https://doi.org/10.1002/mc.22537
DeGeorge KC, Holt HR, Hodges SC (2017) Bladder cancer: diagnosis and treatment. Am Fam Physician 96:507–514
Derry MM, Raina K, Agarwal C, Agarwal R (2013) Identifying molecular targets of lifestyle modifications in colon cancer prevention. Front Oncol 3:119. https://doi.org/10.3389/fonc.2013.00119
Devarakonda S, Masood A, Govindan R (2017) Next-generation sequencing of lung cancers: lessons learned and future directions. Hematol Oncol Clin North Am 31:1–12. https://doi.org/10.1016/j.hoc.2016.08.008

DE Oliveira DT, Savio AL, Marcondes JP, Barros TM, Barbosa LC, Salvadori DM, GN DAS (2017) Cytotoxic and toxicogenomic effects of silibinin in bladder cancer cells with different TP53 status. J Biosci 42:91–101

Dhanalakshmi S, Agarwal P, Glode LM, Agarwal R (2003) Silibinin sensitizes human prostate carcinoma DU145 cells to cisplatin- and carboplatin-induced growth inhibition and apoptotic death. Int J Cancer 106:699–705. https://doi.org/10.1002/ijc.11299

Dhanalakshmi S, Mallikarjuna GU, Singh RP, Agarwal R (2004a) Dual efficacy of silibinin in protecting or enhancing ultraviolet B radiation-caused apoptosis in HaCaT human immortalized keratinocytes. Carcinogenesis 25:99–106. https://doi.org/10.1093/carcin/bgg188

Dhanalakshmi S, Mallikarjuna GU, Singh RP, Agarwal R (2004b) Silibinin prevents ultraviolet radiation-caused skin damages in SKH-1 hairless mice via a decrease in thymine dimer positive cells and an up-regulation of p53-p21/Cip1 in epidermis. Carcinogenesis 25:1459–1465. https://doi.org/10.1093/carcin/bgh152

Dhanalakshmi S, Agarwal C, Singh RP, Agarwal R (2005) Silibinin up-regulates DNA-protein kinase-dependent p53 activation to enhance UVB-induced apoptosis in mouse epithelial JB6 cells. J Biol Chem 280:20375–20383. https://doi.org/10.1074/jbc.M414640200

Dheeraj A, Rigby CM, O'Bryant CL, Agarwal C, Singh RP, Deep G, Agarwal R (2017) Silibinin treatment inhibits the growth of hedgehog inhibitor-resistant basal cell carcinoma cells via targeting EGFR-MAPK-Akt and hedgehog signaling. Photochem Photobiol 93:999–1007. https://doi.org/10.1111/php.12727

Drysdale E, Peng Y, Nguyen P, Baetz T, Hanna TP (2019) A population-based study of the treatment effect of first-line ipilimumab for metastatic or unresectable melanoma. Melanoma Res 29(6):635–642. https://doi.org/10.1097/CMR.0000000000000582

Ferlay J et al (2019) Estimating the global cancer incidence and mortality in 2018: GLOBOCAN sources and methods. Int J Cancer 144:1941–1953. https://doi.org/10.1002/ijc.31937

Flaig TW et al (2007a) A phase I and pharmacokinetic study of silybin-phytosome in prostate cancer patients. Investig New Drugs 25:139–146. https://doi.org/10.1007/s10637-006-9019-2

Flaig TW, Su LJ, Harrison G, Agarwal R, Glode LM (2007b) Silibinin synergizes with mitoxantrone to inhibit cell growth and induce apoptosis in human prostate cancer cells. Int J Cancer 120:2028–2033. https://doi.org/10.1002/ijc.22465

Flaig TW et al (2010) A study of high-dose oral silybin-phytosome followed by prostatectomy in patients with localized prostate cancer. Prostate 70:848–855. https://doi.org/10.1002/pros.21118

Flannery K, Cao X, He J, Zhong Y, Shah AY, Kamat AM (2018) Survival rates and health care costs for patients with advanced bladder cancer treated and untreated with chemotherapy. Clin Genitourin Cancer 16:e909–e917. https://doi.org/10.1016/j.clgc.2018.03.002

Gandara L et al (2014) The natural flavonoid silybin improves the response to photodynamic therapy of bladder cancer cells. J Photochem Photobiol B 133:55–64. https://doi.org/10.1016/j.jphotobiol.2014.03.006

Gazdar AF, Bunn PA, Minna JD (2017) Small-cell lung cancer: what we know, what we need to know and the path forward. Nat Rev Cancer 17:725–737. https://doi.org/10.1038/nrc.2017.87

Greenlee H, Abascal K, Yarnell E, Ladas E (2007) Clinical applications of *Silybum marianum* in oncology. Integr Cancer Ther 6:158–165. https://doi.org/10.1177/1534735407301727

Grignon DJ (2009) The current classification of urothelial neoplasms. Mod Pathol 22(Suppl 2): S60–S69. https://doi.org/10.1038/modpathol.2008.235

Gu M, Dhanalakshmi S, Mohan S, Singh RP, Agarwal R (2005a) Silibinin inhibits ultraviolet B radiation-induced mitogenic and survival signaling, and associated biological responses in SKH-1 mouse skin. Carcinogenesis 26:1404–1413. https://doi.org/10.1093/carcin/bgi096

Gu M, Dhanalakshmi S, Singh RP, Agarwal R (2005b) Dietary feeding of silibinin prevents early biomarkers of UVB radiation-induced carcinogenesis in SKH-1 hairless mouse epidermis. Cancer Epidemiol Biomark Prev 14:1344–1349. https://doi.org/10.1158/1055-9965.EPI-04-0664

Gu M, Singh RP, Dhanalakshmi S, Mohan S, Agarwal R (2006) Differential effect of silibinin on E2F transcription factors and associated biological events in chronically UVB-exposed skin versus tumors in SKH-1 hairless mice. Mol Cancer Ther 5:2121–2129. https://doi.org/10.1158/1535-7163.MCT-06-0052

Hagelgans A, Nacke B, Zamaraeva M, Siegert G, Menschikowski M (2014) Silibinin down-regulates expression of secreted phospholipase A2 enzymes in cancer cells. Anticancer Res 34:1723–1729

Herbst RS, Heymach JV, Lippman SM (2008) Lung cancer. N Engl J Med 359:1367–1380. https://doi.org/10.1056/NEJMra0802714

Higgins S, Nazemi A, Chow M, Wysong A (2018) Review of nonmelanoma skin cancer in African Americans, Hispanics, and Asians. Dermatol Surg 44:903–910. https://doi.org/10.1097/DSS.0000000000001547

Hirsch FR, Scagliotti GV, Mulshine JL, Kwon R, Curran WJ Jr, Wu YL, Paz-Ares L (2017) Lung cancer: current therapies and new targeted treatments. Lancet 389:299–311. https://doi.org/10.1016/S0140-6736(16)30958-8

Hodi FS et al (2010) Improved survival with ipilimumab in patients with metastatic melanoma. N Engl J Med 363:711–723. https://doi.org/10.1056/NEJMoa1003466

Hoh C et al (2006) Pilot study of oral silibinin, a putative chemopreventive agent, in colorectal cancer patients: silibinin levels in plasma, colorectum, and liver and their pharmacodynamic consequences. Clin Cancer Res 12:2944–2950. https://doi.org/10.1158/1078-0432.CCR-05-2724

Hou X et al (2018) Silibinin inhibits NSCLC metastasis by targeting the EGFR/LOX pathway. Front Pharmacol 9:21. https://doi.org/10.3389/fphar.2018.00021

Hwang SJE, Fernandez-Penas P (2018) Adverse reactions to biologics: melanoma (Ipilimumab, Nivolumab, Pembrolizumab). Curr Probl Dermatol 53:82–92. https://doi.org/10.1159/000478081

Iacovelli R et al (2018) The cardiovascular toxicity of abiraterone and enzalutamide in prostate cancer. Clin Genitourin Cancer 16:e645–e653. https://doi.org/10.1016/j.clgc.2017.12.007

Imai-Sumida M et al (2017) Silibinin suppresses bladder cancer through down-regulation of actin cytoskeleton and PI3K/Akt signaling pathways. Oncotarget 8:92032–92042. https://doi.org/10.18632/oncotarget.20734

Javed S, Kohli K, Ali M (2011) Reassessing bioavailability of silymarin. Altern Med Rev 16:239–249

Jeter JM et al (2019) Chemoprevention agents for melanoma: a path forward into phase 3 clinical trials. Cancer 125:18–44. https://doi.org/10.1002/cncr.31719

Jung HJ et al (2009) Silibinin inhibits expression of HIF-1alpha through suppression of protein translation in prostate cancer cells. Biochem Biophys Res Commun 390:71–76. https://doi.org/10.1016/j.bbrc.2009.09.068

Kaseb H, Aeddula NR (2019) Cancer, bladder. In: StatPearls [Internet]. StatPearls Publishing, Treasure Island (FL). https://www.ncbi.nlm.nih.gov/books/NBK536923/

Kauntz H, Bousserouel S, Gosse F, Marescaux J, Raul F (2012a) Silibinin, a natural flavonoid, modulates the early expression of chemoprevention biomarkers in a preclinical model of colon carcinogenesis. Int J Oncol 41(3):849–854. https://doi.org/10.3892/ijo.2012.1526

Kauntz H, Bousserouel S, Gosse F, Raul F (2012b) The flavonolignan silibinin potentiates TRAIL-induced apoptosis in human colon adenocarcinoma and in derived TRAIL-resistant metastatic cells. Apoptosis : Int J Program Cell Death 17(8):797–809. https://doi.org/10.1007/s10495-012-0731-4

Khan AQ et al (2014) Silibinin inhibits tumor promotional triggers and tumorigenesis against chemically induced two-stage skin carcinogenesis in Swiss albino mice: possible role of oxidative stress and inflammation. Nutr Cancer 66:249–258. https://doi.org/10.1080/01635581.2014.863365

Kim SH, Kim KY, Yu SN, Park SK, Choi HD, Ji JH, Ahn SC (2015) Autophagy inhibition enhances silibinin-induced apoptosis by regulating reactive oxygen species production in

human prostate cancer PC-3 cells. Biochem Biophys Res Commun 468(1–2):151–156. https://doi.org/10.1016/j.bbrc.2015.10.143
Kim SH, Kim KY, Yu SN, Seo YK, Chun SS, Yu HS, Ahn SC (2016) Silibinin induces mitochondrial NOX4-mediated endoplasmic reticulum stress response and its subsequent apoptosis. BMC cancer 16:452. https://doi.org/10.1186/s12885-016-2516-6
Klee NS, McCarthy CG, Martinez-Quinones P, Webb RC (2017) Out of the frying pan and into the fire: damage-associated molecular patterns and cardiovascular toxicity following cancer therapy. Ther Adv Cardiovasc Dis 11:297–317. https://doi.org/10.1177/1753944717729141
Kumar S, Raina K, Agarwal C, Agarwal R (2014) Silibinin strongly inhibits the growth kinetics of colon cancer stem cell-enriched spheroids by modulating interleukin 4/6-mediated survival signals. Oncotarget 5:4972–4989. https://doi.org/10.18632/oncotarget.2068
Kumar R, Deep G, Agarwal R (2015) An overview of ultraviolet B radiation-induced skin cancer chemoprevention by silibinin. Curr Pharmacol Rep 1:206–215. https://doi.org/10.1007/s40495-015-0027-9
Leon IE et al (2015) Oxidovanadium(IV) complexes with chrysin and silibinin: anticancer activity and mechanisms of action in a human colon adenocarcinoma model. J Biol Inorg Chem 20:1175–1191. https://doi.org/10.1007/s00775-015-1298-7
Li F et al (2018) Silibinin attenuates TGFbeta1induced migration and invasion via EMT suppression and is associated with COX2 downregulation in bladder transitional cell carcinoma. Oncol Rep 40:3543–3550. https://doi.org/10.3892/or.2018.6728
Liang Z et al (2014) Inhibition of SIRT1 signaling sensitizes the antitumor activity of silybin against human lung adenocarcinoma cells in vitro and in vivo. Mol Cancer Ther 13:1860–1872. https://doi.org/10.1158/1535-7163.MCT-13-0942
Lin CM, Chen YH, Ma HP, Wang BW, Chiu JH, Chua SK, Ong JR, Shyu KG (2012) Silibinin inhibits the invasion of IL-6-stimulated colon cancer cells via selective JNK/AP-1/MMP-2 modulation in vitro. J Agric Food Chem 60(51):12451–12457. https://doi.org/10.1021/jf300964f
Longo TA, Gopalakrishna A, Tsivian M, Van Noord M, Rasch CR, Inman BA, Geijsen ED (2016) A systematic review of regional hyperthermia therapy in bladder cancer. Int J Hyperth 32:381–389. https://doi.org/10.3109/02656736.2016.1157903
Mackiewicz J, Mackiewicz A (2018) BRAF and MEK inhibitors in the era of immunotherapy in melanoma patients. Contemp Oncol (Pozn) 22:68–72. https://doi.org/10.5114/wo.2018.73890
Mallikarjuna G, Dhanalakshmi S, Singh RP, Agarwal C, Agarwal R (2004) Silibinin protects against photocarcinogenesis via modulation of cell cycle regulators, mitogen-activated protein kinases, and Akt signaling. Cancer Res 64:6349–6356. https://doi.org/10.1158/0008-5472.CAN-04-1632
Manivannan E et al (2017) Design and discovery of silybin analogues as antiproliferative compounds using a ring disjunctive – based, natural product lead optimization approach. Eur J Med Chem 133:365–378. https://doi.org/10.1016/j.ejmech.2017.03.033
Mariotto AB, Yabroff KR, Shao Y, Feuer EJ, Brown ML (2011) Projections of the cost of cancer care in the United States: 2010-2020. J Natl Cancer Inst 103:117–128. https://doi.org/10.1093/jnci/djq495
Marmol I, Sanchez-de-Diego C, Pradilla Dieste A, Cerrada E, Rodriguez Yoldi MJ (2017) Colorectal carcinoma: a general overview and future perspectives in colorectal cancer. Int J Mol Sci 18. https://doi.org/10.3390/ijms18010197
Martinez Rodriguez RH, Buisan Rueda O, Ibarz L (2017) Bladder cancer: present and future. Med Clin 149:449–455. https://doi.org/10.1016/j.medcli.2017.06.009
Mateen S, Tyagi A, Agarwal C, Singh RP, Agarwal R (2010) Silibinin inhibits human nonsmall cell lung cancer cell growth through cell-cycle arrest by modulating expression and function of key cell-cycle regulators. Mol Carcinog 49:247–258. https://doi.org/10.1002/mc.20595
Mateen S, Raina K, Jain AK, Agarwal C, Chan D, Agarwal R (2012) Epigenetic modifications and p21-cyclin B1 nexus in anticancer effect of histone deacetylase inhibitors in combination with

silibinin on non-small cell lung cancer cells. Epigenetics 7:1161–1172. https://doi.org/10.4161/epi.22070

Mateen S, Raina K, Agarwal R (2013) Chemopreventive and anti-cancer efficacy of silibinin against growth and progression of lung cancer. Nutr Cancer 65(Suppl 1):3–11. https://doi.org/10.1080/01635581.2013.785004

Meeran SM, Katiyar S, Elmets CA, Katiyar SK (2006) Silymarin inhibits UV radiation-induced immunosuppression through augmentation of interleukin-12 in mice. Mol Cancer Ther 5:1660–1668. https://doi.org/10.1158/1535-7163.MCT-06-0095

Mengs U, Pohl RT, Mitchell T (2012) Legalon(R) SIL: the antidote of choice in patients with acute hepatotoxicity from amatoxin poisoning. Curr Pharm Biotechnol 13:1964–1970

Miller KD et al (2016) Cancer treatment and survivorship statistics, 2016. CA Cancer J Clin 66:271–289. https://doi.org/10.3322/caac.21349

Mohan S, Dhanalakshmi S, Mallikarjuna GU, Singh RP, Agarwal R (2004) Silibinin modulates UVB-induced apoptosis via mitochondrial proteins, caspases activation, and mitogen-activated protein kinase signaling in human epidermoid carcinoma A431 cells. Biochem Biophys Res Commun 320:183–189. https://doi.org/10.1016/j.bbrc.2004.05.153

Myers DJ, Wallen JM (2019) Cancer, lung adenocarcinoma. StatPearls, Treasure Island, FL

Nafees S, Mehdi SH, Zafaryab M, Zeya B, Sarwar T, Rizvi MA (2018) Synergistic Interaction of rutin and silibinin on human colon cancer cell line. Arch Med Res 49:226–234. https://doi.org/10.1016/j.arcmed.2018.09.008

Nambiar DK, Deep G, Singh RP, Agarwal C, Agarwal R (2014) Silibinin inhibits aberrant lipid metabolism, proliferation and emergence of androgen-independence in prostate cancer cells via primarily targeting the sterol response element binding protein 1. Oncotarget 5:10017–10033. https://doi.org/10.18632/oncotarget.2488

Nambiar DK, Rajamani P, Deep G, Jain AK, Agarwal R, Singh RP (2015a) Silibinin preferentially radiosensitizes prostate cancer by inhibiting DNA repair signaling. Mol Cancer Ther 14:2722–2734. https://doi.org/10.1158/1535-7163.MCT-15-0348

Nambiar DK, Rajamani P, Singh RP (2015b) Silibinin attenuates ionizing radiation-induced pro-angiogenic response and EMT in prostate cancer cells. Biochem Biophys Res Commun 456:262–268. https://doi.org/10.1016/j.bbrc.2014.11.069

Narayanapillai S, Agarwal C, Tilley C, Agarwal R (2012) Silibinin is a potent sensitizer of UVA radiation-induced oxidative stress and apoptosis in human keratinocyte HaCaT cells. Photochem Photobiol 88(5):1135–1140. https://doi.org/10.1111/j.1751-1097.2011.01050.x

Narayanapillai S, Agarwal C, Deep G, Agarwal R (2014) Silibinin inhibits ultraviolet B radiation-induced DNA-damage and apoptosis by enhancing interleukin-12 expression in JB6 cells and SKH-1 hairless mouse skin. Mol Carcinog 53:471–479. https://doi.org/10.1002/mc.22000

Patel S et al (2018) Silibinin, a natural blend in polytherapy formulation for targeting Cd44v6 expressing colon cancer stem cells. Sci Rep 8:16985. https://doi.org/10.1038/s41598-018-35069-0

Polachi N et al (2016) Modulatory effects of silibinin in various cell signaling pathways against liver disorders and cancer – a comprehensive review. Eur J Med Chem 123:577–595. https://doi.org/10.1016/j.ejmech.2016.07.070

Post-White J, Ladas EJ, Kelly KM (2007) Advances in the use of milk thistle (*Silybum marianum*). Integr Cancer Ther 6:104–109. https://doi.org/10.1177/1534735407301632

Prack Mc Cormick B, Langle Y, Belgorosky D, Vanzulli S, Balarino N, Sandes E, Eijan AM (2018) Flavonoid silybin improves the response to radiotherapy in invasive bladder cancer. J Cell Biochem 119:5402–5412. https://doi.org/10.1002/jcb.26693

Qian X, Khammanivong A, Song JM, Teferi F, Upadhyaya P, Dickerson E, Kassie F (2015) RNA-sequencing studies identify genes differentially regulated during inflammation-driven lung tumorigenesis and targeted by chemopreventive agents. Inflamm Res 64:343–361. https://doi.org/10.1007/s00011-015-0815-z

Raffa D, Maggio B, Raimondi MV, Plescia F, Daidone G (2017) Recent discoveries of anticancer flavonoids. Eur J Med Chem 142:213–228. https://doi.org/10.1016/j.ejmech.2017.07.034

Raina K et al (2007) Dietary feeding of silibinin inhibits prostate tumor growth and progression in transgenic adenocarcinoma of the mouse prostate model. Cancer Res 67:11083–11091. https://doi.org/10.1158/0008-5472.CAN-07-2222

Raina K, Serkova NJ, Agarwal R (2009) Silibinin feeding alters the metabolic profile in TRAMP prostatic tumors: 1H-NMRS-based metabolomics study. Cancer Res 69:3731–3735. https://doi.org/10.1158/0008-5472.CAN-09-0096

Raina K, Agarwal C, Wadhwa R, Serkova NJ, Agarwal R (2013) Energy deprivation by silibinin in colorectal cancer cells: a double-edged sword targeting both apoptotic and autophagic machineries. Autophagy 9(5):697–713. https://doi.org/10.4161/auto.23960

Raina K, Kumar S, Dhar D, Agarwal R (2016) Silibinin and colorectal cancer chemoprevention: a comprehensive review on mechanisms and efficacy. J Biomed Res 30:452–465. https://doi.org/10.7555/JBR.30.20150111

Rajamanickam S, Velmurugan B, Kaur M, Singh RP, Agarwal R (2010) Chemoprevention of intestinal tumorigenesis in APCmin/+ mice by silibinin. Cancer Res 70:2368–2378. https://doi.org/10.1158/0008-5472.CAN-09-3249

Rajput M, Kujur PK, Mishra A, Singh RP (2018) Flavonoids inhibit chronically exposed arsenic-induced proliferation and malignant transformation of HaCaT cells. Photodermatol Photoimmunol Photomed 34:91–101. https://doi.org/10.1111/phpp.12357

Ramasamy K, Agarwal R (2008) Multitargeted therapy of cancer by silymarin. Cancer Lett 269:352–362. https://doi.org/10.1016/j.canlet.2008.03.053

Ramasamy K et al (2011) Silibinin prevents lung tumorigenesis in wild-type but not in iNOS−/− mice: potential of real-time micro-CT in lung cancer chemoprevention studies. Clin Cancer Res 17:753–761. https://doi.org/10.1158/1078-0432.CCR-10-2290

Randhawa M, Archer C, Gaughran G, Miller A, Morey A, Dua D, Yip D (2019) Combined immune therapy grade IV dermatitis in metastatic melanoma. Asia Pac J Clin Oncol 15:262–265. https://doi.org/10.1111/ajco.13136

Ravichandran K, Velmurugan B, Gu M, Singh RP, Agarwal R (2010) Inhibitory effect of silibinin against azoxymethane-induced colon tumorigenesis in A/J mice. Clin Cancer Res 16:4595–4606. https://doi.org/10.1158/1078-0432.CCR-10-1213

Redondo-Blanco S, Fernandez J, Gutierrez-Del-Rio I, Villar CJ, Lombo F (2017) New insights toward colorectal cancer chemotherapy using natural bioactive compounds. Front Pharmacol 8:109. https://doi.org/10.3389/fphar.2017.00109

Reed D, Raina K, Agarwal R (2018) Nutraceuticals in prostate cancer therapeutic strategies and their neo-adjuvant use in diverse populations. NPJ Precis Oncol 2:15. https://doi.org/10.1038/s41698-018-0058-x

Rho JK et al (2010) Combined treatment with silibinin and epidermal growth factor receptor tyrosine kinase inhibitors overcomes drug resistance caused by T790M mutation. Mol Cancer Ther 9:3233–3243. https://doi.org/10.1158/1535-7163.MCT-10-0625

Rigby CM et al (2017) Role of p53 in silibinin-mediated inhibition of ultraviolet B radiation-induced DNA damage, inflammation and skin carcinogenesis. Carcinogenesis 38:40–50. https://doi.org/10.1093/carcin/bgw106

Rodriguez-Garcia A et al (2017) Thioredoxin 1 modulates apoptosis induced by bioactive compounds in prostate cancer cells. Redox Biol 12:634–647. https://doi.org/10.1016/j.redox.2017.03.025

Roy S, Deep G, Agarwal C, Agarwal R (2012) Silibinin prevents ultraviolet B radiation-induced epidermal damages in JB6 cells and mouse skin in a p53-GADD45alpha-dependent manner. Carcinogenesis 33(3):629–636. https://doi.org/10.1093/carcin/bgr299

Roy S, Kaur M, Agarwal C, Tecklenburg M, Sclafani RA, Agarwal R (2007) p21 and p27 induction by silibinin is essential for its cell cycle arrest effect in prostate carcinoma cells. Mol Cancer Ther 6:2696–2707. https://doi.org/10.1158/1535-7163.MCT-07-0104

Sadava D, Kane SE (2013) Silibinin reverses drug resistance in human small-cell lung carcinoma cells. Cancer Lett 339:102–106. https://doi.org/10.1016/j.canlet.2013.07.017

Salehi B et al (2018) Phytotherapeutics in cancer invasion and metastasis. Phytother Res 32:1425–1449. https://doi.org/10.1002/ptr.6087

Saller R, Brignoli R, Melzer J, Meier R (2008) An updated systematic review with meta-analysis for the clinical evidence of silymarin. Forsch Komplementmed 15:9–20. https://doi.org/10.1159/000113648

Sangeetha N, Felix AJ, Nalini N (2009) Silibinin modulates biotransforming microbial enzymes and prevents 1,2-dimethylhydrazine-induced preneoplastic changes in experimental colon cancer. Eur J Cancer Prev 18:385–394. https://doi.org/10.1097/CEJ.0b013e32832d1b4f

Sangeetha N, Aranganathan S, Panneerselvam J, Shanthi P, Rama G, Nalini N (2010) Oral supplementation of silibinin prevents colon carcinogenesis in a long term preclinical model. Eur J Pharmacol 643:93–100. https://doi.org/10.1016/j.ejphar.2010.05.060

Sangeetha N, Viswanathan P, Balasubramanian T, Nalini N (2012) Colon cancer chemopreventive efficacy of silibinin through perturbation of xenobiotic metabolizing enzymes in experimental rats. Eur J Pharmacol 674:430–438. https://doi.org/10.1016/j.ejphar.2011.11.008

Sangeetha N, Nalini N (2015) Silibinin modulates caudal-type homeobox transcription factor (CDX2), an intestine specific tumor suppressor to abrogate colon cancer in experimental rats. Hum Exp Toxicol 34(1):56–64. https://doi.org/10.1177/0960327114530741

Sati J, Mohanty BP, Garg ML, Koul A (2016) Pro-oxidant role of silibinin in DMBA/TPA induced skin cancer: 1H NMR metabolomic and biochemical study. PLoS One 11:e0158955. https://doi.org/10.1371/journal.pone.0158955

Shapiro CL (2018) Cancer survivorship. N Engl J Med 379:2438–2450. https://doi.org/10.1056/NEJMra1712502

Sharma G, Singh RP, Chan DC, Agarwal R (2003) Silibinin induces growth inhibition and apoptotic cell death in human lung carcinoma cells. Anticancer Res 23:2649–2655

Siegel AB et al (2014) A phase I dose-finding study of silybin phosphatidylcholine (milk thistle) in patients with advanced hepatocellular carcinoma. Integr Cancer Ther 13:46–53. https://doi.org/10.1177/1534735413490798

Singh RP et al (2004) Oral silibinin inhibits lung tumor growth in athymic nude mice and forms a novel chemocombination with doxorubicin targeting nuclear factor kappaB-mediated inducible chemoresistance. Clin Cancer Res 10:8641–8647. https://doi.org/10.1158/1078-0432.CCR-04-1435

Singh RP, Deep G, Chittezhath M, Kaur M, Dwyer-Nield LD, Malkinson AM, Agarwal R (2006a) Effect of silibinin on the growth and progression of primary lung tumors in mice. J Natl Cancer Inst 98:846–855. https://doi.org/10.1093/jnci/djj231

Singh RP, Dhanalakshmi S, Mohan S, Agarwal C, Agarwal R (2006b) Silibinin inhibits UVB- and epidermal growth factor-induced mitogenic and cell survival signaling involving activator protein-1 and nuclear factor-kappaB in mouse epidermal JB6 cells. Mol Cancer Ther 5:1145–1153. https://doi.org/10.1158/1535-7163.MCT-05-0478

Singh RP, Tyagi A, Sharma G, Mohan S, Agarwal R (2008) Oral silibinin inhibits in vivo human bladder tumor xenograft growth involving down-regulation of survivin. Clin Cancer Res 14:300–308. https://doi.org/10.1158/1078-0432.CCR-07-1565

Society AC (2016) Cancer Treatment and survivorship facts and figures 2016–2017. Altanta, GA

Society AC (2019) Cancer facts and figures 2019. Atlanta, GA

Son Y et al (2015) The ameliorative effect of silibinin against radiation-induced lung injury: protection of normal tissue without decreasing therapeutic efficacy in lung cancer. BMC Pulm Med 15:68. https://doi.org/10.1186/s12890-015-0055-6

Song JM et al (2015) Combinations of indole-3-carbinol and silibinin suppress inflammation-driven mouse lung tumorigenesis by modulating critical cell cycle regulators. Carcinogenesis 36:666–675. https://doi.org/10.1093/carcin/bgv054

Sun Y, Guan Z, Zhao W, Jiang Y, Li Q, Cheng Y, Xu Y (2017) Silibinin suppresses bladder cancer cell malignancy and chemoresistance in an NF-kappaB signal-dependent and signal-independent manner. Int J Oncol 51:1219–1226. https://doi.org/10.3892/ijo.2017.4089

Tilley C, Deep G, Agarwal R (2015) Chemopreventive opportunities to control basal cell carcinoma: current perspectives. Mol Carcinog 54:688–697. https://doi.org/10.1002/mc.22348

Tilley C et al (2016) Silibinin and its 2,3-dehydro-derivative inhibit basal cell carcinoma growth via suppression of mitogenic signaling and transcription factors activation. Mol Carcinog 55:3–14. https://doi.org/10.1002/mc.22253

Ting H, Deep G, Agarwal R (2013) Molecular mechanisms of silibinin-mediated cancer chemoprevention with major emphasis on prostate cancer. AAPS J 15:707–716. https://doi.org/10.1208/s12248-013-9486-2

Ting H, Deep G, Agarwal C, Agarwal R (2014) The strategies to control prostate cancer by chemoprevention approaches. Mutat Res 760:1–15. https://doi.org/10.1016/j.mrfmmm.2013.12.003

Ting HJ, Deep G, Jain AK, Cimic A, Sirintrapun J, Romero LM, Cramer SD, Agarwal C, Agarwal R (2015) Silibinin prevents prostate cancer cell-mediated differentiation of naive fibroblasts into cancer-associated fibroblast phenotype by targeting TGF beta2. Mol Carcinog 54(9):730–741. https://doi.org/10.1002/mc.22135

Tsai CC, Chuang TW, Chen LJ, Niu HS, Chung KM, Cheng JT, Lin KC (2015) Increase in apoptosis by combination of metformin with silibinin in human colorectal cancer cells. World J Gastroenterol 21:4169–4177. https://doi.org/10.3748/wjg.v21.i14.4169

Tyagi AK, Singh RP, Agarwal C, Chan DC, Agarwal R (2002) Silibinin strongly synergizes human prostate carcinoma DU145 cells to doxorubicin-induced growth Inhibition, G2-M arrest and apoptosis. Clin Cancer Res 8:3512–3519

Tyagi A et al (2007) Chemopreventive effects of silymarin and silibinin on N-butyl-N-(4-hydroxybutyl) nitrosamine induced urinary bladder carcinogenesis in male ICR mice. Mol Cancer Ther 6:3248–3255. https://doi.org/10.1158/1535-7163.MCT-07-2006

Tyagi A et al (2009) Growth inhibition and regression of lung tumors by silibinin: modulation of angiogenesis by macrophage-associated cytokines and nuclear factor-kappaB and signal transducers and activators of transcription 3. Cancer Prev Res (Phila) 2:74–83. https://doi.org/10.1158/1940-6207.CAPR-08-0095

Tyagi A, Agarwal C, Dwyer-Nield LD, Singh RP, Malkinson AM, Agarwal R (2012) Silibinin modulates TNF-alpha and IFN-gamma mediated signaling to regulate COX2 and iNOS expression in tumorigenic mouse lung epithelial LM2 cells. Mol Carcinog 51:832–842. https://doi.org/10.1002/mc.20851

Velmurugan B, Singh RP, Tyagi A, Agarwal R (2008) Inhibition of azoxymethane-induced colonic aberrant crypt foci formation by silibinin in male Fisher 344 rats. Cancer Prev Res (Phila) 1:376–384. https://doi.org/10.1158/1940-6207.CAPR-08-0059

Velmurugan B, Gangar SC, Kaur M, Tyagi A, Deep G, Agarwal R (2010) Silibinin exerts sustained growth suppressive effect against human colon carcinoma SW480 xenograft by targeting multiple signaling molecules. Pharm Res 27:2085–2097. https://doi.org/10.1007/s11095-010-0207-6

Vietor NO, George BJ (2012) Oxaliplatin-induced hepatocellular injury and ototoxicity: a review of the literature and report of unusual side effects of a commonly used chemotherapeutic agent. J Oncol Pharm Pract 18:355–359. https://doi.org/10.1177/1078155212437901

Vinh PQ et al (2002) Chemopreventive effects of a flavonoid antioxidant silymarin on N-butyl-N-(4-hydroxybutyl)nitrosamine-induced urinary bladder carcinogenesis in male ICR mice. Jpn J Cancer Res 93:42–49

Vue B et al (2017) 5- or/and 20-O-alkyl-2,3-dehydrosilybins: synthesis and biological profiles on prostate cancer cell models. Bioorg Med Chem 25:4845–4854. https://doi.org/10.1016/j.bmc.2017.07.035

Wang JY, Chang CC, Chiang CC, Chen WM, Hung SC (2012) Silibinin suppresses the maintenance of colorectal cancer stem-like cells by inhibiting PP2A/AKT/mTOR pathways. J Cell Biochem 113:1733–1743. https://doi.org/10.1002/jcb.24043

Wang Q et al (2013) p53-mediated autophagy adjustment is involved in the protection of silibinin against murine dermal inflammation and epidermal apoptosis induced by UVB irradiation. J Asian Nat Prod Res 15:117–129. https://doi.org/10.1080/10286020.2012.739616

Woo SM et al (2014) Silibinin induces apoptosis of HT29 colon carcinoma cells through early growth response-1 (EGR-1)-mediated non-steroidal anti-inflammatory drug-activated gene-1 (NAG-1) up-regulation. Chem Biol Interact 211:36–43. https://doi.org/10.1016/j.cbi.2014.01.004

Wu KJ, Zeng J, Zhu GD, Zhang LL, Zhang D, Li L, Fan JH, Wang XY, He DL (2009) Silibinin inhibits prostate cancer invasion, motility and migration by suppressing vimentin and MMP-2 expression. Acta Pharmacol Sin 30(8):1162–1168. https://doi.org/10.1038/aps.2009.94

Wu K et al (2013) Silibinin inhibits beta-catenin/ZEB1 signaling and suppresses bladder cancer metastasis via dual-blocking epithelial-mesenchymal transition and stemness. Cell Signal 25:2625–2633. https://doi.org/10.1016/j.cellsig.2013.08.028

Yan X et al (2012) Perioperative polyphenon E- and siliphos-inhibited colorectal tumor growth and metastases without impairment of gastric or abdominal wound healing in mouse models. Surg Endosc 26:1856–1864. https://doi.org/10.1007/s00464-011-2114-2

Zeng J et al (2011) Chemopreventive and chemotherapeutic effects of intravesical silibinin against bladder cancer by acting on mitochondria. Mol Cancer Ther 10:104–116. https://doi.org/10.1158/1535-7163.MCT-10-0577

Zhang QY, Wang FX, Jia KK, Kong LD (2018) Natural product interventions for chemotherapy and radiotherapy-induced side effects. Front Pharmacol 9:1253. https://doi.org/10.3389/fphar.2018.01253

Zhao J, Agarwal R (1999) Tissue distribution of silibinin, the major active constituent of silymarin, in mice and its association with enhancement of phase II enzymes: implications in cancer chemoprevention. Carcinogenesis 20:2101–2108

Zheng R et al (2018) Chemopreventive effects of silibinin on colitis-associated tumorigenesis by inhibiting IL-6/STAT3 signaling pathway. Mediat Inflamm 2018:1562010. https://doi.org/10.1155/2018/1562010

Zhu W, Zhang JS, Young CY (2001) Silymarin inhibits function of the androgen receptor by reducing nuclear localization of the receptor in the human prostate cancer cell line LNCaP. Carcinogenesis 22:1399–1403

Zhu J, Liao R, Su C, Liang D, Wu J, Qiu K, Li J (2018) Toxicity profile characteristics of novel androgen-deprivation therapy agents in patients with prostate cancer: a meta-analysis. Expert Rev Anticancer Ther 18:193–198. https://doi.org/10.1080/14737140.2018.1419871

Chapter 7
Adjuvant Value of Turmeric Extract (Containing Curcumin) in Colorectal Cancer Management

Clara Bik-San Lau and Grace Gar-Lee Yue

Abstract Turmeric, the rhizome of *Curcuma longa*, is a commonly used medicinal and culinary herb in Asian countries. One of its well-known components, curcumin, is becoming a rising star of dietary supplements in recent years due to its multi-targeted pharmacological benefits for health, including anticancer and antioxidant effects. However, poor oral absorption in intestine impedes the widespread clinical applications of curcumin. There have been prodigious efforts to develop new formulations of curcumin over the last decade. In fact, bioavailability of curcumin could be simply enhanced when it is used as a whole in turmeric extract, which has been hypothesized and proven in our cell-based and animal models, as well as in the recent clinical trials by other researchers. The mysteries of these interesting findings will be summarized in this chapter. Meanwhile, investigations on the pharmacological efficacies of curcumin or turmeric, especially on colorectal cancer, emerge from the concept of chemopreventive medicinal food and the advancement of oral bioavailability. Recent discoveries of the beneficial effects of curcumin or turmeric extract shown in preclinical studies (animal models and omics analysis) and clinical trials of colorectal cancer will be reviewed in this chapter. The potential adjuvant role of turmeric in colorectal cancer therapy will be explicitly explored and discussed.

7.1 Introduction

Turmeric, which is the dried rhizome of the plant *Curcuma longa* Linn., is a commonly used medicinal and culinary herb in India and China for centuries. *Curcuma longa* is a perennial plant of the ginger (Zingiberaceae) family with pulpy, orange tuberous rhizomes, which is widely cultivated in tropical and

C. B.-S. Lau (✉) · G. G.-L. Yue
Institute of Chinese Medicine and State Key Laboratory of Research on Bioactivities and Clinical Applications of Medicinal Plants, The Chinese University of Hong Kong, Shatin, New Territories, Hong Kong
e-mail: claralau@cuhk.edu.hk

J. M. Pezzuto, O. Vang (eds.), *Natural Products for Cancer Chemoprevention*,
https://doi.org/10.1007/978-3-030-39855-2_7

subtropical regions of India, China, Southeast Asia, and Latin America. In the last decade, this plant or its major constituent, curcumin, is commonly found in dietary supplement and cosmetics in Asian countries as well as in western countries (Aggarwal et al. 2007; Kunnumakkara et al. 2017b).

In Ayurvedic medicine, turmeric is used as a stimulant, tonic, stomachic and depurative, and can also be used in combinations for sprains and bruises (Government of India Ministry of Health and Family Welfare 2001). In traditional Chinese medicines, turmeric (Jianghuang) is for stabbing pain in the chest and hypochondrium, chest disorder and heart pain, dysmenorrhea, amenorrhea, abdominal masses, and relieving pain (Chinese Pharmacopoeia Commission 2015). Ancient Chinese and Ayurvedic medicine literatures have described the usefulness of turmeric in the treatment of a variety of ailments such as anorexia, sore throat, joint pain, wound dressing, hepatic and biliary disorders (Lodha and Bagga 2000).

The major chemical principles of turmeric are curcuminoids, which impart characteristic yellow color to it (Aggarwal et al. 2007). The curcuminoids (3–6%) and essential oil (3–5%) can be separated from turmeric by ethanol extraction (Gopalan et al. 2000). Curcumin (diferuloylmethane) is a low molecular weight polyphenol, first chemically characterized in 1910 (Milobedzka et al. 1910), which is generally regarded as the most active constituent of and comprises 2–8% of turmeric (Tayyem et al. 2006). Numerous in vitro and in vivo studies have reported the bioactivities of curcumin, which include anti-inflammatory, antioxidant, anti-atherosclerotic, anticancer, antidepressant, anti-aging, antidiabetic, etc. (Aggarwal et al. 2003, 2007; Kunnumakkara et al. 2017b). Nevertheless, curcumin-free turmeric (Aggarwal et al. 2013b) as well as other components in turmeric, such as turmerones (Aratanechemuge et al. 2002; Sandur et al. 2007; Yue et al. 2010a; Park et al. 2012), elemene (Li et al. 2012; Zhao et al. 2012), furanodiene (Xiao et al. 2007) and germacrone (Liu et al. 2013) have also been suggested to possess anti-inflammatory and anti-tumor activities. In addition, other studies proposed that degradation products/metabolic by-products of curcumin could also play roles in the polypharmacology of curcumin (Shen and Ji 2009; Schneider et al. 2015; Cavaleri 2018).

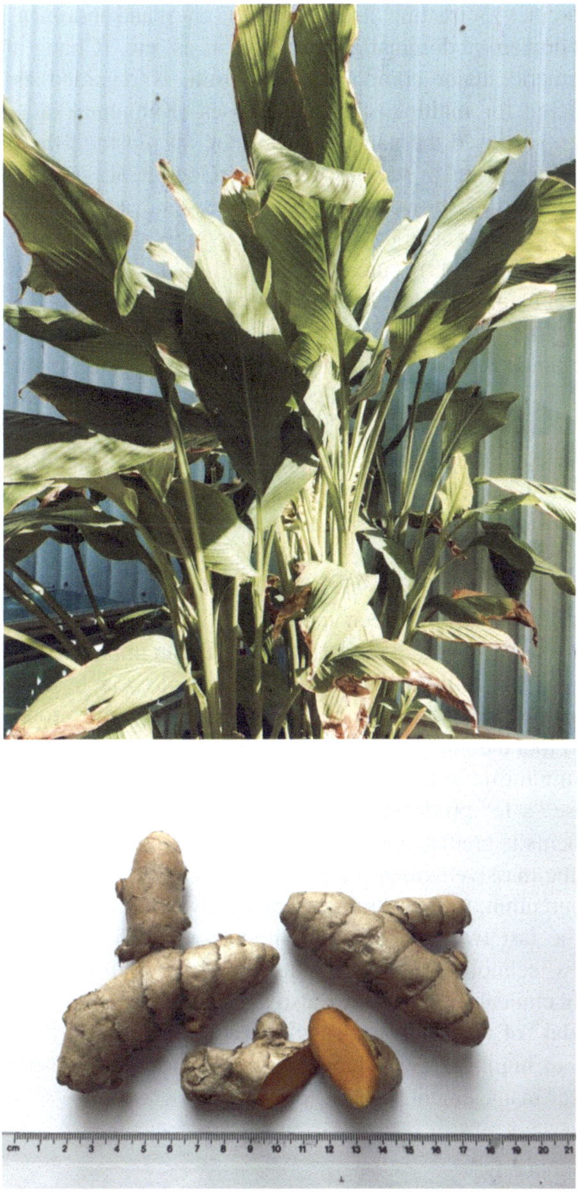

Upper: The growing *Curcuma longa* plant. Lower: Rhizome of the plant (*Photos taken by Clara B.S. Lau*)

Traditionally, turmeric was used for imparting color and flavor to food, religious ceremonies in India or as Indian medicines for biliary disorders, anorexia, coryza, cough, menstrual difficulties, etc. (Ammon and Wahl 1991; Gupta et al. 2013c), or as Chinese medicines for treating distention of the chest and abdomen, obstruction or lump in the abdomen, abdominal pain due to stasis, etc. (Chang and But 1987). Nowadays, turmeric major component, curcumin, is regarded as an important botanical medicine for multiple chronic diseases (Kunnumakkara et al. 2017b). Goel et al. even proposed the name "Curecumin" to illustrate the potential therapeutic roles for curcumin in various diseases (Goel et al. 2008). In fact, as the previous clinical studies showed good tolerability and accepted safety profile at single dose of 12 g (Lao et al. 2006) and following ingestion of 8 g/day over a 4 week period (Dhillon et al. 2008), curcumin as well as its parental turmeric extract, become common natural product health supplements.

Such a rising star in health supplements is increasing its popularity worldwide. Curcumin-containing/turmeric-based products, such as capsules, tablets, beverages, soaps, ointments, cream and cosmetics are commercially available in countries including the United States, India, China, Japan, Korea, Thailand, South Africa, Nepal, and Pakistan (Gupta et al. 2012, 2013a). In the United States, turmeric [including essential oils, oleoresins (solvent-free), and natural extractives (including distillates)] are listed as substances "Generally Recognized As Safe" (GRAS) for their intended use by the US Food and Drug Administration (U.S. FDA 2018). Whereas a turmeric extract BCM-95® (consists of no less than 85% curcuminoids and 5–7% volatile oils) has also been approved by FDA as GRAS (U.S. FDA 2017). According to a market research report, the global curcumin market size was estimated at over USD 44 million in 2016 (Grand View Research 2019). The demand for curcumin/turmeric-based herbal and Ayurvedic skin care products is growing and expected to fuel the market in the coming years. Advantages for these over-the-counter curcumin/turmeric-based products have been taken since the regulations applied on these "safe" products are limited. Hence, the market potential for such health supplements is predicted to be enormous.

In view of the massive evidence on the multi-targeted pharmacological benefits possessed by curcumin, to focus, most of the reviews on pharmacological activities published in the last two decades are summarized in this chapter. Besides, the advances in new technologies for surmounting technical hurdles (poor bioavailability) of curcumin clinical application are also discussed. Furthermore, we revealed the "hidden potential" of turmeric on managing varied health disorders. The intent of this chapter is to highlight the adjuvant value of turmeric extract, particularly in colorectal cancer management.

7.2 Curcumin: Overview of Biological Activities Published and the Proposed Mechanisms

Curcumin has been shown to interact with many signaling molecules, such as protein kinases (phosphorylase kinase, PKC), inflammatory molecules (COX-2), cell survival proteins, transcription factors (NF-κB, STAT), p-glycoprotein, multidrug resistance proteins, carrier proteins, and metal ions (Goel et al. 2008). The interaction of curcumin with protein-based macromolecules, e.g., human serum albumin (Pulla Reddy et al. 1999) and bovine serum albumin (Barik et al. 2003), was also suggested to play important role in its biological activities. On account of its β-diketone moiety, curcumin undergoes keto–enol tautomerization that has been reported as a favorable state for direct binding so as to exert multiple functions, such as antioxidant, anti-inflammatory, anticancer, etc., in prevention and treatment of diseases (Gupta et al. 2011; Priyadarsini 2013; Kunnumakkara et al. 2017a; Hewlings and Kalman 2017; Patel et al. 2019). On the other hand, some researchers argued that the exposed thiol groups of cysteine residues of proteins can react covalently with the 2 α,β-unsaturated ketones chemical groups, so that curcumin can exhibit multi-targeted biological activities (e.g., generate ROS, inactivate p53, etc.) in cells (Burgos-Morón et al. 2010).

Nevertheless, over the years, curcumin has been shown to exhibit advantageous anti-inflammatory and anti-oxidation properties, emerging as alternative treatments for gastric ailments, arthritis, Alzheimer's, viral/bacterial infections, as well as cancer. Among the wide-ranged pharmacological activities of curcumin, overview in particular on the anti-inflammatory, anticancer, antioxidant, cardioprotection, immunomodulatory, and neuroprotection activities are summarized in Table 7.1.

Despite all of these reports, recent reviews suggested that curcumin can be regarded as one of the pan assay interference compounds (PAINS) (Baell 2016), and an invalid metabolic panaceas (IMPs) (Bisson et al. 2016). Furthermore, Nelson et al. summarized the crucial medicinal chemistry of curcumin and raise sharp criticism on the stability, reactivity, bioavailability of curcumin (Nelson et al. 2017). In contrast, Bahadori and Demiray refuted this review and cited another list of references to demonstrate the beneficial side of curcumin and its potential role of being an adjunctive treatment agent for multiple diseases (Bahadori and Demiray 2017). Hence, the therapeutic potential of curcumin remains controversial.

7.3 Poor Oral Bioavailability of Curcumin: Advances in New Technologies for Surmounting Technical Hurdles

Even with noteworthy advancements in exploring the therapeutic potential of curcumin in various health disorders over the last two decades, the widespread clinical application of curcumin is still being impeded by its poor bioavailability. Low solubility in aqueous media, low oral absorption in intestine, high rate of metabolism, rapid systemic elimination and clearance of metabolic products, and low concentration of curcumin at the target sites could be the reasons behind (Anand et al. 2007; Kurien and Scofield 2009). The recognized poor absorption of curcumin was observed in early animal studies, in which most of the orally administered curcumin was excreted in the urine and faeces (Wahlström and Blennow 1978), and

Table 7.1 Multidimensional biological activities of curcumin reported in recent years

Biological activities	References
Anti-inflammatory	Basnet and Skalko-Basnet (2011)
	He et al. (2015)
	Panahi et al. (2015)
	Sahebkar et al. (2016)
	Hussain et al. (2017)
	Abdollahi et al. (2018)
	Cavaleri (2018)
Antioxidant	Anderson and Maes (2014)
	Kukongviriyapan et al. (2016)
	Xu et al. (2017)
Anticancer	Gupta et al. (2013b)
	Rahmani et al. (2014)
	Chen et al. (2015)
	Bimonte et al. (2016)
	Deng et al. (2016)
	Jordan et al. (2016)
	Kasi et al. (2016)
	Klinger and Mittal (2016)
	Momtazi et al. (2016)
	Pavan et al. (2016)
	Zheng et al. (2016)
	Allegra et al. (2017)
	Mahran et al. (2017)
	Crooker et al. (2018)
	Nabavi et al. (2018)
	Nagaraju et al. (2019)
	Subramani et al. (2017)
	Tajbakhsh et al. (2018)
	Farhood et al. (2019)
	Hesari et al. (2019)
	Naeini et al. (2019)
	Song et al. (2019)
	Sun et al. (2019)
Cardiovascular protection	Kapakos et al. (2012)
	Khurana et al. (2013)
	Sahebkar (2014)
	Pagliaro et al. (2015)
	Qin et al. (2017)
	Shehzad et al. (2017)
	Allawadhi et al. (2018)
	Kim and Clifton (2018)
Hepatoprotective	Hu et al. (2017)
	Zabihi et al. (2017)

(continued)

Table 7.1 (continued)

Biological activities	References
Immuno-regulatory	Sahebkar et al. (2016)
	Ghandadi and Sahebkar (2017)
	Abdollahi et al. (2018)
	Kinger et al. (2018)
Neuroprotective	Potter (2013)
	Brondino et al. (2014)
	Chen et al. (2018)
	Dhir (2018)
	Maiti and Dunbar (2018)
	Rakotoarisoa and Angelova (2018)
	Seo et al. (2018)
	Sun et al. (2018)
	Farkhondeh et al. (2019)
	Zhu et al. (2019)
Inflammatory bowel disease/colitis	Simadibrata et al. (2017)
	Grammatikopoulou et al. (2018)
	Mazieiro et al. (2018)

only minute amount of curcumin could be detected in blood (Ravindranath and Chandrasekhara 1980, 1981). While in the succeeding clinical studies, oral administration of curcumin in healthy subjects or cancer patients resulted in detectable plasma levels (Cheng et al. 2001; Sharma et al. 2001, 2004), although the detectable amounts of curcumin varied a great deal among studies (Garcea et al. 2004; Dhillon et al. 2008; Vareed et al. 2008). In contrast, some studies suggested that curcumin distribution in the gastrointestinal lumen is independent of its systemic concentration so that it could exert certain biological activities in intestinal mucosa regardless of its plasma concentration (Patel and Majumdar 2009). Another clinical study also demonstrated that both normal and malignant colorectal tissues were found to have taken up curcumin in colorectal cancer patient after ingesting curcumin (Garcea et al. 2005). Researchers from the University of Texas MD Anderson Cancer Centre have extensively reviewed the problems and improving progression for the bioavailability of curcumin in the last two decades (Anand et al. 2007; Goel et al. 2008; Prasad et al. 2014a).

There have been incredible efforts to develop new formulations of curcumin with enhanced bioavailability over the years by research groups worldwide. Attempts have been made through liposomal and other forms of microencapsulation, nanoparticles (Nair et al. 2019), localized or targeted delivery, use of adjuvants and structural analogues (Prasad et al. 2014b; Toden and Goel 2017; Mahran et al. 2017; Carolina Alves et al. 2019). In the meantime, strategies to increase the bioavailability of curcumin, including enhanced absorption by improved permeability, longer circulation, and resistance to metabolic processes, etc., have also been demonstrated in many studies. Here, those reviews summarized the aforementioned advancements are listed in Table 7.2.

Apart from the in vitro, in vivo and in silico studies regarding the improvement of curcumin solubility/absorption/bioavailability, there are various approaches to demonstrate how to increase the bioavailability and/or efficacies of curcumin in human participants (Hsu et al. 2007; Gupta et al. 2013b; Panahi et al. 2014). In the last decade, several clinical studies of curcumin products with improved bioavailability over conventional (unformulated) curcumin were reported and summarized in a review, in which the author pointed out that 3 out of 11 curcumin formulations exhibited over 100-fold higher bioavailability relative to reference unformulated curcumin (Jamwal 2018). Furthermore, the latest studies showed that the liposomal curcumin could be tolerated in patients with locally advanced or metastatic cancer (Greil et al. 2018) and the turmeric extract Curcumin C3® With BioPerine® could elicit antioxidant and epigenetic effects in healthy human volunteers (Cheng et al. 2019). Besides, a curcumin gum formulation was recently shown to be critical in improving curcumin release and absorption by enhancing mucosal contact, which may in turn help in the prevention of oral cavity head and neck squamous cell carcinoma (Boven et al. 2018).

In fact, bioavailability of curcumin could be simply enhanced when it is used as a whole in turmeric extract, which has been hypothesized and proven in cell-based and animal models in our previous studies. In our in vitro Caco-2 cell monolayer study, we showed that the presence of turmerones would affect the absorption of curcumin (Yue et al. 2012). Hence, we hypothesized the potential use of whole turmeric extract (including curcumin and turmerones), rather than curcumin alone, for treating diseases (Yue et al. 2016a). Later in our in vivo pharmacokinetic study, the plasma curcumin level of turmeric extract-fed mice was found to be higher than that of curcumin-fed mice (Yue et al. 2016b). These findings were consistent with another in vivo study, in which turmeric-containing diet was found to be more bioavailable when compared to curcumin-containing diet (Martin et al. 2012). The enhanced absorption and oral bioavailability of curcumin have also been shown in a clinical trial using a product containing unknown ratio of curcumin and non-curcuminoid components of turmeric (Antony et al. 2008). Another study strongly suggested that curcumin may be consumed as turmeric (a commercially available turmeric extract Biocurcumax® in lipophilic vehicles) instead of plain curcumin for maximum beneficial effects (Shishu and Maheshwari 2010). Our hypothesis on the use of whole turmeric extract was further verified in a recent clinical study in healthy human adult male subjects in India (Gopi et al. 2017). The researchers demonstrated that curcumin in a natural turmeric matrix exhibited greater bioavailability than the two comparator products (curcumin with volatile oil and curcumin with phospholipids and cellulose).

In view of the enhanced bioavailability of curcumin when it is present in turmeric extract relative to the compound alone, which was proven in studies by our research group or other laboratories mentioned above, the superior efficacies of crude turmeric extract to curcumin alone were then postulated. Attempts have been made by our group to confirm the stronger anti-proliferative and anti-angiogenic activities of

Table 7.2 Reviews on new technologies for enhancing the bioavailability of curcumin and new delivery systems for curcumin

Formulations	Effects/Improvement	References
Liposomal encapsulation	Curcumin based polymeric materials for biomedical applications	Mahmood et al. (2015)
	Liposomal curcumin and its application in cancer	Feng et al. (2017)
	Novel formulated forms of curcumin in the treatment of breast cancer	Tajbakhsh et al. (2018)
Nanoparticles	Delivery of anti-inflammatory nutraceuticals by nanoparticles	Nair et al. (2010)
	Plasma proteins interaction with curcumin nanoparticles	Yallapu et al. (2013)
	Transformation of curcumin from food additive to multifunctional medicine	Ahmad et al. (2014)
	Nanotechnology-applied curcumin for different diseases therapy	Ghalandarlaki et al. (2014)
	Curcumin nanoformulations	Naksuriya et al. (2014)
	Nano-curcumin formulations	Rahimi et al. (2016)
	Anticancerous potential of polyphenol-loaded polymeric nanotherapeutics	Ernest et al. (2018)
	Nanocarriers for encapsulation of curcumin	Rafiee et al. (2019)
	Amphiphilic nanocarrier systems for curcumin delivery	Rakotoarisoa and Angelova (2018)
	Augmentation of therapeutic potential of curcumin using nanotechnology	Sivasami and Hemalatha (2018)
	Nanoparticles for brain diseases	Del Prado-Audelo et al. (2019)
	Curcumin nanofibers for the purpose of wound healing	Fereydouni et al. (2019)
	Curcumin nanoparticles containing poloxamer or soluplus tailored by high pressure homogenization	Homayouni et al. (2019)
	Enhancing curcumin oral bioavailability through nanoformulations	Ipar et al. (2019)
	Curcumin nanoformulations for colorectal cancer	Wong et al. (2019)
	Curcumin-loaded nanopreparations: Improving bioavailability	Zhang et al. (2019)
Encapsulation of drugs into particles	Encapsulation of non-curcuminoid components in diverse drug delivery systems such as co-crystals, solid lipid nanoparticles, liposomes, microspheres, polar-non-polar sandwich (PNS) technology	Nair et al. (2019)

(continued)

Table 7.2 (continued)

Formulations	Effects/Improvement	References
	Curcumin-encapsulated and curcumin-primed exosomes	Oskouie et al. (2019)
	Chitosan-based delivery systems for curcumin	Saheb et al. (2019)
Analog	Implication of isoflavone, curcumin, and their synthetic analogs	Sarkar et al. (2010)
	Bioactivities of EF24	He et al. (2018)
	Biological and pharmacological effects of hexahydrocurcumin, a metabolite of curcumin	Huang et al. (2018)
Different routes of drug delivery rather than oral administration	Advanced drug delivery systems of curcumin for cancer chemoprevention	Bansal et al. (2011)
	Challenges of curcumin bioavailability: Novel aerosol remedies	Subramani and Narala (2013)
	Currently available lipid-based delivery systems	Mouhid et al. (2017)
	Nose-to-brain drug delivery	Agrawal et al. (2018)
Adjuvants/Natural product bioenhancers	Piperine, a major component of black pepper, known as inhibitor of hepatic and intestinal glucuronidation and is also shown to increase the bioavailability of curcumin	Prasad et al. (2014b)
	Piperine is the major active component of black pepper and when combined in a complex with curcumin, has been shown to increase bioavailability by 2000%	Hewlings and Kalman (2017)
	Review of strategies to enhance bioavailability and efficacy of curcumin	Mahran et al. (2017)
	Curcumin, a natural polyphenol for targeting molecular pathways	Maiti and Dunbar (2018)

curcumin in turmeric ethanolic extract than that of curcumin alone in colon cancer cells and endothelial cells, respectively (Yue et al. 2010b). Meanwhile, we also reported the immunomodulatory activities of turmeric polysaccharides (Yue et al. 2010a), as well as the anti-angiogenic activities of aromatic-turmerone (Yue et al. 2015). As summarized by Aggarwal et al. curcumin-free turmeric components (turmerones, elemene, sesquiterpenes, etc.) in fact possess various biological activities, such as anti-inflammatory, anticancer, and antidiabetic activities (Aggarwal et al. 2013b). Researchers from the same group further illustrated that curcumin-free turmeric exhibited greater anticancer potential in tumor-bearing mice than in cancer cells, against human colorectal cancer models, suggesting that turmeric might contain additional bioactive compounds other than curcumin (Prasad et al. 2017).

Taken together, the major reasons contributing to the better efficacies of turmeric appear to be due to its multi-targeted activities exerted by its multi-components, which might be with higher absorption, lower metabolism and systemic elimination than that of curcumin. We strongly believed that turmeric extract may represent a more viable therapeutic option.

In fact, a number of studies have tried to address the pharmacological activities of turmeric extracts over the years. Turmeric-containing diet was found to have greater effect on pro-inflammatory genes when compared to curcumin-containing diet in rats (Martin et al. 2012); while in an animal model, turmeric extract could protect against chronic CCl_4-induced liver damage by enhancing anti-oxidation (Lee et al. 2016). Turmeric extract was shown to act as anti-inflammatory as well as antioxidant agent in a dementia rat model (Yuliani et al. 2018) and it also demonstrated a protective effect against ethanol-induced liver injury by suppressing hepatic oxidation and inflammation (Uchio et al. 2017). On the other hand, turmeric/curcumin have long been suggested to maintain gastrointestinal health (Ammon and Wahl 1991; Aggarwal et al. 2007). Hence, the pharmacological activities in preclinical models and the health benefits, particularly in colorectal cancer management, are reviewed in the following section.

7.4 Curcumin/Turmeric and Colon Health: Current Evidence of Beneficial Effects

Colorectal cancer (CRC) represents the third most frequently diagnosed cancer and the second high cancer mortality worldwide in both sexes (Ferlay et al. 2018). The main modality of treatment with high cure rate in CRC is surgical (including surgery, radiofrequency ablation, cryosurgery), while chemotherapy, radiation therapy, targeted therapy and immunotherapy are also the common treatment options (PDQ Adult Treatment Editorial Board 2019). Most patients with metastasis disease are not curable and will require systemic therapy. First- and second-line therapies usually consist of a fluoropyrimidine combination (FOLFOX/CAPOX or FOLFIRI/CAPIRI) plus a biologic targeting angiogenesis (e.g., bevacizumab) (Loree and Kopetz 2017).

Approximately 20% of CRC patients present with relapse metastatic disease, and 25–30% of patients with stage II/III disease will have a recurrence within 5 years after curative intent surgery (Shah et al. 2016; Taieb et al. 2019). Diet and lifestyle modifications for patients are highly recommended in order to alleviate the impact from CRC on the quality of life (Gescher et al. 2001; Chan and Giovannucci 2010; Mehra et al. 2017; Rossi et al. 2018).

Investigations on the pharmacological efficacies of curcumin or turmeric, particularly on colorectal cancer, emerge from the concept of chemopreventive medicinal food. Turmeric has been used for adding color and taste to food (such as curry) in the Indian subcontinent (Aggarwal et al. 2007). The low rate of colorectal cancer in the Asian countries using turmeric in diet was supported by epidemiological data (Chauhan 2002; Sinha et al. 2003). Turmeric has also been recorded for hundreds of years in India for biliary and hepatic disorders (Ammon and Wahl 1991). In modern pharmacological studies, since the early 1990s, the chemopreventive effects of turmeric (which was added in diet or administered as aqueous extract), curcumin-free aqueous turmeric extract, or curcumin, against chemically-induced stomach and skin tumors were reported (Azuine and Bhide 1992; Azuine et al. 1992). The chemoprevention of colon carcinogenesis by dietary curcumin was also demonstrated (Rao et al. 1993, 1995; Huang et al. 1994; Kawamori et al. 1999). Reddy and Rao suggested that curcumin and certain phytosterols were effective naturally occurring COX-2 inhibitors for the prevention against colon carcinogenesis with minimal gastrointestinal toxicity (Reddy and Rao 2002). In fact, many studies reported the in vitro and in vivo activities of curcumin in colorectal cancer over the years and most of these studies have been summarized in review articles (Gescher et al. 2001; Goel et al. 2008; Gupta et al. 2010; Park and Conteas 2010; Goel and Aggarwal 2010; Shehzad et al. 2010; Ramasamy et al. 2015; Vallianou et al. 2015; Simental-Mendía et al. 2017; Imran et al. 2018; Jalili-Nik et al. 2018; Wong et al. 2019). Among these reports, only a few focused on the anti-metastatic activities of curcumin in colorectal cancer (Narayan 2004; Bandyopadhyay 2014; Tong et al. 2016).

On the other hand, research on the efficacy of turmeric extracts or non-cucurminoids components in colon cancer preclinical models has also drawn the attention of some researchers although these extracts might not be the first priority of study subjects. Turmeric extract was shown to protect the small intestine of rats from methotrexate-induced damage (Moghadam et al. 2013) and reduce inappropriate epithelial cell transport (SLC22A4, 503F) and increase anti-inflammatory cytokine gene promoter activity (IL-10, 1082A) in an inflammatory bowel disease cell culture model (McCann et al. 2014). Curcumin combined with turmerones abolished tumor formation in a model of dimethylhydradine-initiated and DSS-promoted mouse colon carcinogenesis and the authors suggested that this combination may become a powerful method for prevention of inflammation-associated colon carcinogenesis (Murakami et al. 2013). Besides, a diterpenoid from turmeric was found to inhibit proliferation and induce apoptosis in human colon adenocarcinoma cells acting via inhibiting MAPK signaling pathway (Shen et al. 2014). Another interesting study showed that a semi-bionic extract of turmeric was produced by mixing turmeric with artificial gastric juice or artificial intestinal juice and this extract was orally administered to rats with dextran sulfate sodium-induced acute enteritis. Results demonstrated that the semi-bionic turmeric extract exhibited potent protective effects on DSS-induced acute enteritis in rats through its anti-inflammatory and antioxidant activities (Wang et al. 2016).

Curcumin also appears to have beneficial therapeutic effects on inflammatory bowel disease (IBD), which is characterized by chronic inflammation of the colon and is a frequent complication of and risk factor for colorectal cancer. Numerous reports are found on the effectiveness of curcumin in IBD management and they were summarized in several review articles in the last decade (Hanai and Sugimoto 2009; White and Judkins 2011; Taylor and Leonard 2011; Baliga et al. 2012; Aggarwal et al. 2013a; Shehzad et al. 2013; Gupta et al. 2014; He et al. 2015;

Fadus et al. 2017; Simadibrata et al. 2017; Mazieiro et al. 2018; Quezada and Cross 2019). In contrast, the reports on turmeric extract in colitis studies were relatively fewer than those on curcumin. Rare studies demonstrated that a *Curcuma longa* extract has a myorelaxant effect on mouse ileum and colon, independent of the anti-inflammatory effect in the colitis model (Aldini et al. 2012), while curcumin and combined with turmerones abolished dextran sulfate sodium (DSS)-induced colon carcinogenesis (Murakami et al. 2013). Another study showed that turmeric powder treatment reduced oxidative stress associated with IBD in acetic acid-induced IBD rats (Bastaki et al. 2016).

In fact, our research group has also made attempts to illustrate the potential anti-tumor activities of turmeric extract in colon cancer mouse models. As mentioned earlier, we have proven in pharmacokinetic studies that curcumin present in turmeric extract could be better absorbed than curcumin alone in mice (Yue et al. 2016b). Hence, we hypothesized that turmeric extract could exert superior anti-tumor effects in tumor-bearing mice which was also demonstrated in our subsequent study (Yue et al. 2016a) (Fig. 7.1). Our hypotheses were further verified by a recent study, in which the anticancer activities of individual curcuminoids were found to be inferior to those of total extract of *Curcuma longa* (Kukula-Koch et al. 2018). Nevertheless, the adjuvant anti-tumor activities of turmeric extract with bevacizumab were first demonstrated in our study. The highlights of the findings were that the turmeric extract plus bevacizumab exerted comparable anti-tumor activities as the first line chemotherapeutics, 5-fluorouracil, leucovorin and oxaliplatin (FOLFOX), but without haematological side effects (Yue et al. 2016b). In view of the high incidence of

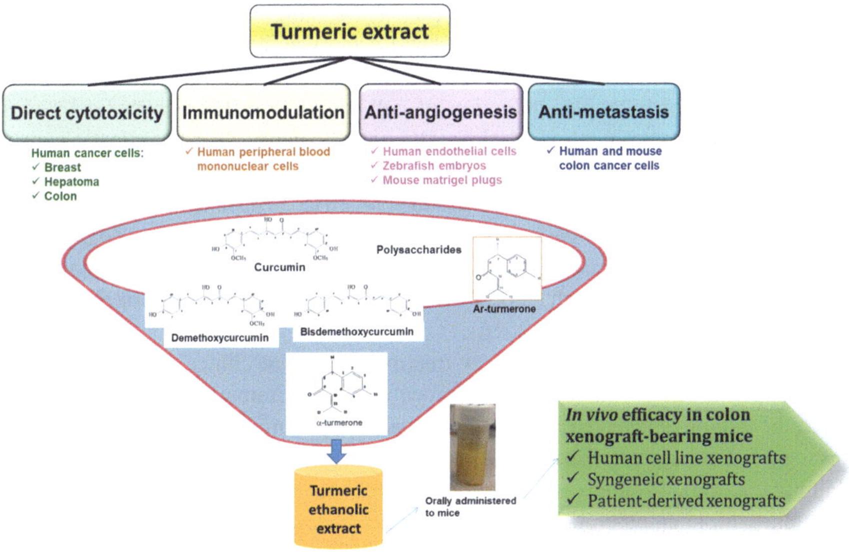

Fig. 7.1 Beneficial effects of turmeric extract (containing curcumin and other bioactive components) shown in our preclinical studies

metastasis in CRC, we further evaluated the anti-metastatic efficacies of turmeric extract using a syngeneic orthotopic colon tumor mouse model, in which the role of turmeric extract in regulating tumor microenvironment was revealed for the first time (Li et al. 2018). These promising findings in colon tumor-bearing mice further assert the importance of using the crude extract of turmeric for relatively better efficacy and bioavailability compared with curcumin alone. Such a holistic approach of research on turmeric was coincidently proposed by Nelson et al. who suggested that the PD/PK complexity and the broad traditional foundation of turmeric should be taken into account (Nelson et al. 2017).

7.5 Clinical and Translational Challenges for the Use of Curcumin/Turmeric

7.5.1 Combination of Curcumin with Chemotherapeutics in CRC

There is abundant evidence to support curcumin as an anticancer agent, which can regulate tumor growth via modulation of multiple cell signaling pathways (Kunnumakkara et al. 2017a), and at the same time help to overcome some of the drug-resistance and improve the efficacy of chemotherapeutic drugs when they were used in combination. Goel and Aggarwal listed the in vitro or in vivo chemosensitizing effects of curcumin in varied types of tumors including prostate, ovarian, gastric, liver, cervical, breast, pancreatic, lung, colon cancer as well as myeloma and erythroleukemic cells (Goel and Aggarwal 2010). In recent years, new data showed the enhancement of the combined use of curcumin and chemo- or targeted-drugs. For example, reduction of cell viability in lung cancer cells was augmented by curcumin plus erlotinib (Yamauchi et al. 2014); while curcumin combined with mitomycin C, suppression of ABCG2 expression in stem cell-like breast cancer cells could be improved (Zhou et al. 2015). The anti-tumor activities of cisplatin in bladder cancer cells (Park et al. 2016) and NSCLC cells (Zhang et al. 2018), or docetaxel in breast cancer cells (Sahu et al. 2016), could all be enhanced by curcumin. Curcumin also enhanced the effects of 5-fluorouracil and oxaliplatin in gastric cancer cells (Zhou et al. 2016).

In particular, for colorectal cancer treatment, the pre-clinical effectiveness of curcumin with and without chemotherapeutics was summarized in a review, in which the authors suggested that the combined use of curcumin with chemotherapy was regarded as a superior strategy for treatment of gastrointestinal cancer (Patel and Majumdar 2009). Whereas the recent preclinical studies on the combined use of curcumin with chemotherapeutics in colorectal cancer are listed in Table 7.3.

On the other hand, the VEGF-targeting drug, bevacizumab/ Avastin®, which is usually administered in combination with FOLFOX (5-fluorouracil, leucovorin, and oxaliplatin) for the second-line treatment of colorectal cancer (Cohen et al. 2007),

Table 7.3 Preclinical studies on the combined use of curcumin with chemotherapeutics in colorectal cancer

Combinations	Major results	References
Dasatinib	Dasatinib and curcumin eliminates chemo-resistant colon cancer cells	Nautiyal et al. (2011)
Doxorubicin	Favored the antineoplastic C26 murine colon carcinoma microenvironment	Sesarman et al. (2019)
5-Fluorouracil	Curcumin synergizes with 5-fluorouracil by impairing AMPK/ULK1-dependent autophagy	Zhang et al. (2017)
5-Fluorouracil and oxaliplatin	Enhanced growth inhibition of colon cancer cells by modulating EGFR and IGF-1R	Patel et al. (2008)
	Enhanced anti-proliferative and pro-apoptotic effects in a proportion of patient-derived explants	James et al. (2015)
FOLFOX	Curcumin targets FOLFOX-surviving colon cancer cells via inhibition of EGFRs and IGF-1R	Patel et al. (2010)
Irinotecan	Enhances the effects of irinotecan on colorectal cancer cells through the generation of reactive oxygen species	Huang et al. (2017)
	Attenuates resistance to irinotecan via induction of apoptosis of cancer stem cells in chemoresistant colon cancer cells	Su et al. (2018)
Oxaliplatin	Enhances inhibitory effects on cell growth, apoptosis, and angiogenesis in colorectal cancer.	Li et al. (2007)
	Ameliorates oxaliplatin induced chemoresistance in HCT116 colorectal cancer	Howells et al. (2011)
	Effectively suppress colorectal carcinoma in vivo	Guo et al. (2015)
	Oxaliplatin-acquired resistance reversion in colorectal cancer cell lines	Ruiz de Porras et al. (2016)
Platinum (II)-based anticancer drugs	Enhanced chemosensitivity of downregulation of nuclear endonuclease G and NF-κB	Wang et al. (2014)

has been tested in combination with curcumin in hepatocellular carcinoma cells. The synergistic effect of this combination was observed (Gao et al. 2015). Meanwhile our in vivo study using human colonic tumor-bearing mice model compared the efficacies and side effects of three combinations: turmeric extract, curcumin or FOLFOX with bevacizumab. Our data showed that the antitumor efficacy of turmeric extract plus bevacizumab was comparable to that of FOLFOX plus bevacizumab. Besides, the counts of neutrophils, eosinophils, RBC and platelets were decreased in FOLFOX-treated mice. However, such decreases were not found in turmeric extract- or curcumin-treated mice. Hence, the treatments of turmeric extract with bevacizumab in colonic tumor-bearing mice was effective and safe (Yue et al. 2016b). Coincidentally, a phase I dose escalation clinical study using combined curcumin with FOLFOX revealed curcumin to be a safe and tolerable adjunct to FOLFOX chemotherapy in patients with colorectal liver metastases (James et al. 2015). In addition, curcumin was shown to be a chemoprotector (Goel and Aggarwal 2010) and it could ameliorate chemotherapeutics-induced toxicity in cell-based or animal models (Kumar et al. 2017; Liu et al. 2018; Zangui et al. 2019). Taking together, beneficial interaction between turmeric (with absorbable curcumin) and bevacizumab (and/or other chemotherapeutics) in treating colorectal cancer is certainly worth further investigation in clinical trials and its application potentials will be infinite.

7.5.2 *Clinical Trials with Curcumin/Turmeric Products*

In the last two decades, more than 65 human clinical trials of curcumin have been completed (Aggarwal et al. 2013b; Schaffer et al. 2015). The majority of these studies were attempts to improve the bioavailability of curcumin, while the others aimed to assess the effects of curcumin in patients with various pathological disorders (Doello et al. 2018; Salehi et al. 2019). Here, special emphasis was given to curcumin efficacy, including improved tumor markers and symptomatic relief in cancer patients of colorectal cancer. A list of published trials on colorectal cancer patients is given in Table 7.4. Meanwhile, there are currently 13 clinical trials evaluating the effects of curcumin and/or other agents on colon disorders registered on ClinicalTrials.gov and they are shown in Table 7.5, which suggests great research interest worldwide.

7.6 Roles of Curcumin/Turmeric on Microbiota?

Recent perspectives on the carcinogenesis and progression of colorectal cancer (CRC) focused on diet and its impact on the composition and function of gut microbiota (Feng et al. 2015; Xu and Knight 2015; García-Castillo et al. 2016; Yang and Yu 2018). The growing interest in gut microorganisms and their influence on cancer development and treatment appear among scientists and clinicians all over the world. The gut microbiota such as anaerobic bacteria have been implicated in cellular dysplasia and carcinogenesis of CRC (Jahani-Sherafat et al. 2018). The recent research findings on the correlation between gut microbiota and CRC as well as the potential roles of modulating gut microbiota to become a viable adjunct to conventional anticancer therapies have been summarized in the latest review articles (Jahani-Sherafat et al. 2018; Park et al. 2018; Yang and Yu 2018; Helmink et al. 2019). Studies also suggested that gut microbes exert distinct impact on DNA damage and non-coding RNA expression in colon epithelial cells (Allen and Sears 2019). The microbiota also modulate the immune response by priming for the release of pro-inflammatory factors (Perez-Chanona and Trinchieri 2016).

Despite the multi-targeted pharmacological activities, curcumin is well-known for its poor absorption in gut, and a high concentration in the intestinal tract is expected. In view of the potential modulation on intestinal microorganisms by curcumin, research on the analysis of metabolic profile of curcumin in human intestinal flora has commenced since 2015 (Lou et al. 2015). Meanwhile, McFadden

Table 7.4 Clinical studies on the effect of curcumin in colorectal cancer patients

Study type	Intervention period, follow up study, population and treatment dose	Major outcomes	References
Phase I trial, dose-escalation pilot study	15 advanced colorectal cancer patients; 29 days; capsules (18 mg curcumin +2 mg desmethoxycurcumin) suspended in 200 mg essential oil derived from *Curcuma* spp.; oral administration 440–2200 mg/day (corresponding to 36–180 mg of curcumin)	Decreased lymphocytic GST activity (59%) at dose of 440 mg/day; leucocytic M1G levels were unaffected by any treatment; detectable levels of curcumin and its metabolites in feces [DNA adduct (M1G) formed by malondialdehyde]	Sharma et al. (2001)
Phase I clinical trial	15 patients with advanced colorectal cancer; 450 mg-3600 mg/day curcumin	A daily dose of 3.6 g curcumin engendered 62% and 57% decreases in inducible PGE(2) production in blood samples taken 1 h after dose on days 1 and 29, respectively	Sharma et al. (2004)
Prospective study	12 patients with colorectal cancer; 3600, 1800, or 450 mg/day curcumin	↓ M1G with 3.6 g curcumin Decreased M1G level; COX-2 levels were not affected; detected metabolites of curcumin in healthy and malignant colorectal tissue samples and trace levels in peripheral blood	Garcea et al. (2005)
Pilot study	5 familial adenomatous polyposis patients prior colectomy; tablets Oxy-CU containing curcumin (480 mg) and quercetin (20 mg); orally 3 times/day for 3–9 months	Decreased polyps' number (by 60.4%) and size (by 50.9%) after 6 month therapy	Cruz-Correa et al. (2006)
Double-blind placebo-controlled, randomized study	126 patients with colorectal cancer; 360 mg curcumin, thrice/day during the period ahead of surgery, between 10 and 30 days	↑ Body weight, ↓ serum TNF-α levels, ↑ Apoptotic tumor cells, enhanced expression of p53 molecule in tumor tissue, and modulated tumor cell apoptotic pathway	He et al. (2011)
Non-randomized, open labeled trial, phase IIa	44 patients (smokers); capsules in 2 doses: 2 and 4 g/day curcumin; oral administration for 30 days	Aberrant crypt foci were significantly reduced by higher curcumin dose	Carroll et al. (2011)

Table 7.5 Clinical trials evaluating the effects of curcumin on colon disorders registered on ClinicalTrials.gov (as of 28 March 2019)

NCT number	Study start	Study title	Recruitment status	Locations
NCT03061591	2017	Turmeric supplementation on polyp number and size in patients with familial adenomatous polyposis.	Not yet recruiting	Tel-Aviv Sourasky Medical Center, Israel
NCT02724202	2016	Curcumin in combination with 5FU for colon cancer	Unknown	Baylor Research Institute, USA
NCT02439385	2015	First line Avastin/FOLFIRI in combination with curcumin-containing supplement in colorectal cancer patients with unresectable metastasis	Active, not recruiting	Gachon University Gil Medical Center, USA
NCT01948661	2013	Anthocyanin extract and phospholipid curcumin in colorectal adenoma (MIRACOL)	Active, not recruiting	Ente Ospedaliero Ospedali Galliera, Italy
NCT01859858	2013	Effect of curcumin on dose limiting toxicity and pharmacokinetics of irinotecan in patients with solid tumors	Active, not recruiting	IU Simon Cancer Center Indianapolis, University of North Carolina at Chapel Hill Lineberger Comprehensive cancer Center, USA
NCT01490996	2012	Combining curcumin with FOLFOX chemotherapy in patients with inoperable colorectal cancer	Active, not recruiting	University of Leicester, UK
NCT01294072	2011	Study investigating the ability of plant exosomes to deliver curcumin to normal and colon cancer tissue	Active, not recruiting	James Graham Brown Cancer Center, USA
NCT01333917	2010	Curcumin biomarkers	Completed	University of North Carolina, Chapel Hill, USA
NCT00973869	2009	Curcumin in preventing colorectal cancer in patients undergoing colorectal endoscopy or colorectal surgery	Unknown	University of Leicester, UK
NCT00927485	2009	Use of curcumin for treatment of intestinal adenomas in familial adenomatous polyposis (FAP)	Completed	University of Puerto Rico, Puerto Rico
NCT00745134	2008	Radiation therapy and capecitabine with or without curcumin before surgery in treating patients with rectal cancer	Active, not recruiting	M.D. Anderson Cancer Center, USA
NCT00295035	2006	Phase III trial of gemcitabine, curcumin and celebrex in patients with metastatic colon cancer	Unknown	Tel-Aviv Sourasky Medical Center, Israel
NCT00027495	2001	Curcumin for the prevention of colon cancer	Completed	University of Michigan Rogel Cancer Center, USA

et al. hypothesized that curcumin would affect primarily colon epithelial cells and the gut microbiota. They suggested that the beneficial effect of curcumin on preventing progression of chronic colitis to colitis-associated colorectal cancer was associated with the maintenance of a more diverse colonic microbial ecology (McFadden et al. 2015). Afterwards, researchers have made attempts to investigate how curcumin regulates gut microbiota (Shen et al. 2017; An et al. 2017; Burapan et al. 2017). A review article highlighted the interaction between curcumin and gut microbiota and thoroughly summarized the animal studies and clinical trials of curcumin on microbiota (Zam 2018), while updates on the biotransformation of curcumin by digestive microbiota were summarized in other articles (Shen and Ji 2018; Lopresti 2018).

In summary, curcumin/turmeric might provide benefit by acting on gut microbiota. More clinical and preclinical studies are warranted to provide a basis for microbiota-based therapeutic applications of turmeric or other ideal curcumin formulations, which may result in reducing the risk of CRC.

7.7 Conclusion

Over the last two decades, remarkable advances in our understanding of a well-known spice, turmeric, and its renowned component, curcumin, for the multi-disciplinary pharmacological activities, which have led us to the realization of the great potential of these botanical products/dietary interventions for improving human health. Here, we summarized the research findings and the relevant reviews that will help better understand how curcumin/turmeric exerts the bioactivities, in particular in colorectal cancer management and how different approaches aimed to enhance the bioavailability of curcumin.

In our previous studies, we hypothesized that whole turmeric extract (including curcumin and turmerones), rather than curcumin alone, would exert better anti-tumor activities. We have successfully proven this hypothesis in various cell-based and animal models, while the novel efficacies of turmeric extract on managing colon cancer metastasis are further illustrated in syngeneic orthotopic colon tumor mice models (with tumor microenvironment concerned) and patient-derived xenograft mice models recently in our laboratory (Fig. 7.1). Together with current evidence which suggests that curcumin functions as an effective agent for restoring healthy gut homeostasis and microbial–host relationships, we suggest detailed investigation is necessary to define the full potential of the adjuvant role of turmeric extract (containing curcumin and other bioactive components) in CRC treatment and prevention. We strongly believe that all these findings would justify further clinical studies on whole turmeric extract in colorectal cancer patients.

In conclusion, with the current status and future prospective of the use of turmeric (with absorbable curcumin) being summarized and discussed in this chapter, the potential role of turmeric to become an adjuvant therapeutic agent in the management of colorectal cancer are affirmed, which may shed light on the widen clinical use of turmeric in the future.

References

Abdollahi E, Momtazi AA, Johnston TP, Sahebkar A (2018) Therapeutic effects of curcumin in inflammatory and immune-mediated diseases: a nature-made jack-of-all-trades? J Cell Physiol 233:830–848

Aggarwal BB, Kumar A, Bharti AC (2003) Anticancer potential of curcumin: preclinical and clinical studies. Anticancer Res 23:363–398

Aggarwal BB, Sundaram C, Malani N et al (2007) Curcumin: the Indian solid gold. Adv Exp Med Biol 595:1–75

Aggarwal BB, Gupta SC, Sung B (2013a) Curcumin: an orally bioavailable blocker of TNF and other pro-inflammatory biomarkers. Br J Pharmacol 169:1672–1692

Aggarwal BB, Yuan W, Li S et al (2013b) Curcumin-free turmeric exhibits anti-inflammatory and anticancer activities: identification of novel components of turmeric. Mol Nutr Food Res 57:1529–1542

Agrawal M, Saraf S, Antimisiaris SG et al (2018) Nose-to-brain drug delivery: an update on clinical challenges and progress towards approval of anti-Alzheimer drugs. J Control Release 281:139–177

Ahmad MZ, Akhter S, Mohsin N et al (2014) Transformation of curcumin from food additive to multifunctional medicine: nanotechnology bridging the gap. Curr Drug Discov Technol 11:197–213

Aldini R, Budriesi R, Roda G et al (2012) *Curcuma longa* extract exerts a myorelaxant effect on the ileum and colon in a mouse experimental colitis model, independent of the anti-inflammatory effect. PLoS One 7:e44650

Allawadhi P, Khurana A, Sayed N et al (2018) Isoproterenol-induced cardiac ischemia and fibrosis: plant-based approaches for intervention. Phytother Res 32:1908–1932

Allegra A, Innao V, Russo S et al (2017) Anticancer activity of curcumin and its analogues: preclinical and clinical studies. Cancer Investig 35:1–22

Allen J, Sears CL (2019) Impact of the gut microbiome on the genome and epigenome of colon epithelial cells: contributions to colorectal cancer development. Genome Med 11:11

Ammon HP, Wahl MA (1991) Pharmacology of *Curcuma longa*. Planta Med 57:1–7

An C, Sun Z, Shen L et al (2017) Biotransformation of food spice curcumin by gut bacterium Bacillus megaterium DCMB-002 and its pharmacological implications. Food Nutr Res 61(1):1412814

Anand P, Kunnumakkara AB, Newman RA et al (2007) Bioavailability of curcumin: problems and promises. Mol Pharm 4:807–818

Anderson G, Maes M (2014) Oxidative/nitrosative stress and immuno-inflammatory pathways in depression: treatment implications. Curr Pharm Des 20:3812–3847

Antony B, Merina B, Iyer VS et al (2008) A pilot cross-over study to evaluate human oral bioavailability of BCM-95CG (Biocurcumax), a novel bioenhanced preparation of curcumin. Indian J Pharm Sci 70:445–449

Aratanechemuge Y, Komiya T, Moteki H et al (2002) Selective induction of apoptosis by ar-turmerone isolated from turmeric (*Curcuma longa* L) in two human leukemia cell lines, but not in human stomach cancer cell line. Int J Mol Med 9:481–484

Azuine MA, Bhide SV (1992) Chemopreventive effect of turmeric against stomach and skin tumors induced by chemical carcinogens in Swiss mice. Nutr Cancer 17:77–83

Azuine MA, Kayal JJ, Bhide SV (1992) Protective role of aqueous turmeric extract against mutagenicity of direct-acting carcinogens as well as benzo [alpha] pyrene-induced genotoxicity and carcinogenicity. J Cancer Res Clin Oncol 118:447–452

Baell JB (2016) Feeling nature's PAINS: natural products, natural product drugs, and pan assay interference compounds (PAINS). J Nat Prod 79:616–628

Bahadori F, Demiray M (2017) A realistic view on "the essential medicinal chemistry of curcumin". ACS Med Chem Lett 8:893–896

Baliga MS, Joseph N, Venkataranganna MV et al (2012) Curcumin, an active component of turmeric in the prevention and treatment of ulcerative colitis: preclinical and clinical observations. Food Funct 3:1109–1117
Bandyopadhyay D (2014) Farmer to pharmacist: curcumin as an anti-invasive and antimetastatic agent for the treatment of cancer. Front Chem 2:113
Bansal SS, Goel M, Aqil F et al (2011) Advanced drug delivery systems of curcumin for cancer chemoprevention. Cancer Prev Res (Phila) 4:1158–1171
Barik A, Priyadarsini KI, Mohan H (2003) Photophysical studies on binding of curcumin to bovine serum albumins. Photochem Photobiol 77:597–603
Basnet P, Skalko-Basnet N (2011) Curcumin: an anti-inflammatory molecule from a curry spice on the path to cancer treatment. Molecules 16:4567–4598
Bastaki SMA, Al Ahmed MM, Al Zaabi A et al (2016) Effect of turmeric on colon histology, body weight, ulcer, IL-23, MPO and glutathione in acetic-acid-induced inflammatory bowel disease in rats. BMC Complement Altern Med 16:72
Bimonte S, Barbieri A, Leongito M et al (2016) Curcumin anticancer studies in pancreatic cancer. Nutrients 8(7):433
Bisson J, McAlpine JB, Friesen JB et al (2016) Can invalid bioactives undermine natural product-based drug discovery? J Med Chem 59:1671–1690
Boven L, Holmes SP, Latimer B et al (2018) Curcumin gum formulation for prevention of oral cavity head and neck squamous cell carcinoma. Laryngoscope 129(7):1597–1603
Brondino N, Re S, Boldrini A et al (2014) Curcumin as a therapeutic agent in dementia: a mini systematic review of human studies. ScientificWorldJournal 2014:174282
Burapan S, Kim M, Han J (2017) Curcuminoid demethylation as an alternative metabolism by human intestinal microbiota. J Agric Food Chem 65:3305–3310
Burgos-Morón E, Calderón-Montaño JM, Salvador J et al (2010) The dark side of curcumin. Int J Cancer 126:1771–1775
Carolina Alves R, Perosa Fernandes R, Fonseca-Santos B et al (2019) A critical review of the properties and analytical methods for the determination of curcumin in biological and pharmaceutical matrices. Crit Rev Anal Chem 49(2):138–149
Carroll RE, Benya RV, Turgeon DK et al (2011) Phase IIa clinical trial of curcumin for the prevention of colorectal neoplasia. Cancer Prev Res (Phila) 4:354–364
Cavaleri F (2018) Presenting a new standard drug model for turmeric and its prized extract, curcumin. Int J Inflamm 2018:5023429
Chan AT, Giovannucci EL (2010) Primary prevention of colorectal cancer. Gastroenterology 138:2029–2043.e10
Chang HM, But PPH (1987) Pharmacology and applications of Chinese materia medica. World Scientific Publishing, Singapore, pp 936–939
Chauhan DP (2002) Chemotherapeutic potential of curcumin for colorectal cancer. Curr Pharm Des 8:1695–1706
Chen J, Xu T, Chen C (2015) The critical roles of miR-21 in anticancer effects of curcumin. Ann Transl Med 3:330
Chen M, Du ZY, Zheng X et al (2018) Use of curcumin in diagnosis, prevention, and treatment of Alzheimer's disease. Neural Regen Res 13:742–752
Cheng AL, Hsu CH, Lin JK et al (2001) Phase I clinical trial of curcumin, a chemopreventive agent, in patients with high-risk or pre-malignant lesions. Anticancer Res 21:2895–2900
Cheng D, Li W, Wang L et al (2019) Pharmacokinetics, pharmacodynamics, and PKPD modeling of curcumin in regulating antioxidant and epigenetic gene expression in healthy human volunteers. Mol Pharm 16(5):1881–1889
Chinese Pharmacopoeia Commission (2015) Chinese Pharmacopoeia, Beijing
Cohen MH, Gootenberg J, Keegan P et al (2007) FDA drug approval summary: bevacizumab plus FOLFOX4 as second-line treatment of colorectal cancer. Oncologist 12:356–361
Crooker K, Aliani R, Ananth M et al (2018) A review of promising natural chemopreventive agents for head and neck cancer. Cancer Prev Res 11:441–450

Cruz-Correa M, Shoskes DA, Sanchez P et al (2006) Combination treatment with curcumin and quercetin of adenomas in familial adenomatous polyposis. Clin Gastroenterol Hepatol 4:1035–1038
Del Prado-Audelo ML, Caballero-Florán IH, Meza-Toledo JA et al (2019) Formulations of curcumin nanoparticles for brain diseases. Biomolecules 9(2):56
Deng Y, Verron E, Rohanizadeh R (2016) Molecular mechanisms of anti-metastatic activity of curcumin. Anticancer Res 36:5639–5647
Dhillon N, Aggarwal BB, Newman RA et al (2008) Phase II trial of curcumin in patients with advanced pancreatic cancer. Clin Cancer Res 14:4491–4499
Dhir A (2018) Curcumin in epilepsy disorders. Phytother Res 32:1865–1875
Doello K, Ortiz R, Alvarez PJ et al (2018) Latest in vitro and in vivo assay, clinical trials and patents in cancer treatment using curcumin: a literature review. Nutr Cancer 70:569–578
Ernest U, Chen HY, Xu MJ et al (2018) Anticancerous potential of polyphenol-loaded polymeric nanotherapeutics. Molecules 23(11):2787
Fadus MC, Lau C, Bikhchandani J et al (2017) Curcumin: an age-old anti-inflammatory and anti-neoplastic agent. J Tradit Complement Med 7:339–346
Farhood B, Mortezaee K, Goradel NH et al (2019) Curcumin as an anti-inflammatory agent: Implications to radiotherapy and chemotherapy. J Cell Physiol 234:5728–5740
Farkhondeh T, Samarghandian S, Pourbagher-Shahri AM et al (2019) The impact of curcumin and its modified formulations on Alzheimer's disease. J Cell Physiol 234(10):16953–16965
Feng Q, Liang S, Jia H et al (2015) Gut microbiome development along the colorectal adenoma-carcinoma sequence. Nat Commun 6:6528
Feng T, Wei Y, Lee RJ et al (2017) Liposomal curcumin and its application in cancer. Int J Nanomedicine 12:6027–6044
Fereydouni N, Darroudi M, Movaffagh J et al (2019) Curcumin nanofibers for the purpose of wound healing. J Cell Physiol 234:5537–5554
Ferlay J, Ervik M, Lam F et al. (2018) Global cancer observatory. Cancer Today. https://gco.iarc.fr/today. Accessed 1 Mar 2019
Gao JZ, Du JL, Wang YL et al (2015) Synergistic effects of curcumin and bevacizumab on cell signaling pathways in hepatocellular carcinoma. Oncol Lett 9:295–299
Garcea G, Jones DJ, Singh R et al (2004) Detection of curcumin and its metabolites in hepatic tissue and portal blood of patients following oral administration. Br J Cancer 90:1011–1015
Garcea G, Berry DP, Jones DJ et al (2005) Consumption of the putative chemopreventive agent curcumin by cancer patients: assessment of curcumin levels in the colorectum and their pharmacodynamic consequences. Cancer Epidemiol Biomark Prev 14:120–125
García-Castillo V, Sanhueza E, McNerney E et al (2016) Microbiota dysbiosis: a new piece in the understanding of the carcinogenesis puzzle. J Med Microbiol 65:1347–1362
Gescher AJ, Sharma RA, Steward WP (2001) Cancer chemoprevention by dietary constituents: a tale of failure and promise. Lancet Oncol 2:371–379
Ghalandarlaki N, Alizadeh AM, Ashkani-Esfahani S (2014) Nanotechnology-applied curcumin for different diseases therapy. Biomed Res Int 2014:394264
Ghandadi M, Sahebkar A (2017) Curcumin: an effective inhibitor of interleukin-6. Curr Pharm Des 23:921–931
Goel A, Aggarwal BB (2010) Curcumin, the golden spice from Indian saffron, is a chemosensitizer and radiosensitizer for tumors and chemoprotector and radioprotector for normal organs. Nutr Cancer 62:919–930
Goel A, Kunnumakkara AB, Aggarwal BB (2008) Curcumin as "Curecumin": from kitchen to clinic. Biochem Pharmacol 75:787–809
Gopalan B, Goto M, Kodama A et al (2000) Supercritical carbon dioxide extraction of turmeric (*Curcuma longa*). J Agric Food Chem 48:2189–2192
Gopi S, Jacob J, Varma K et al (2017) Comparative oral absorption of curcumin in a natural turmeric matrix with two other curcumin formulations: an open-label parallel-arm study. Phytother Res 31:1883–1891

Government of India Ministry of Health and Family Welfare, Department of Ayush India Government (2001) The Ayurvedic Pharmacopoeia of India
Grammatikopoulou MG, Gkiouras K, Theodoridis X et al (2018) Oral adjuvant curcumin therapy for attaining clinical remission in ulcerative colitis: a systematic review and meta-analysis of randomized controlled trials. Nutrients 10(11):1737
Grand View Research (2019) Curcumin market size, share and trends analysis report, and segment forecasts 2018–2025. https://www.grandviewresearch.com/industry-analysis/turmeric-extract-curcumin-market. Accessed 27 Mar 2019
Greil R, Greil-Ressler S, Weiss L et al (2018) A phase 1 dose-escalation study on the safety, tolerability and activity of liposomal curcumin (Lipocurc™) in patients with locally advanced or metastatic cancer. Cancer Chemother Pharmacol 82:695–706
Guo LD, Shen YQ, Zhao XH et al (2015) Curcumin combined with oxaliplatin effectively suppress colorectal carcinoma in vivo through inducing apoptosis. Phytother Res 29:357–365
Gupta SC, Kim JH, Prasad S et al (2010) Regulation of survival, proliferation, invasion, angiogenesis, and metastasis of tumor cells through modulation of inflammatory pathways by nutraceuticals. Cancer Metastasis Rev 29:405–434
Gupta SC, Prasad S, Kim JH et al (2011) Multitargeting by curcumin as revealed by molecular interaction studies. Nat Prod Rep 28:1937–1955
Gupta SC, Patchva S, Koh W et al (2012) Discovery of curcumin, a component of golden spice, and its miraculous biological activities. Clin Exp Pharmacol Physiol 39:283–299
Gupta SC, Kismali G, Aggarwal BB (2013a) Curcumin, a component of turmeric: from farm to pharmacy. Biofactors 39:2–13
Gupta SC, Patchva S, Aggarwal BB (2013b) Therapeutic roles of curcumin: lessons learned from clinical trials. AAPS J 15:195–218
Gupta SC, Sung B, Kim JH et al (2013c) Multitargeting by turmeric, the golden spice: from kitchen to clinic. Mol Nutr Food Res 57:1510–1528
Gupta SC, Tyagi AK, Deshmukh-Taskar P et al (2014) Downregulation of tumor necrosis factor and other proinflammatory biomarkers by polyphenols. Arch Biochem Biophys 559:91–99
Hanai H, Sugimoto K (2009) Curcumin has bright prospects for the treatment of inflammatory bowel disease. Curr Pharm Des 15:2087–2094
He ZY, Shi CB, Wen H et al (2011) Upregulation of p53 expression in patients with colorectal cancer by administration of curcumin. Cancer Investig 29:208–213
He Y, Yue Y, Zheng X et al (2015) Curcumin, inflammation, and chronic diseases: how are they linked? Molecules 20:9183–9213
He Y, Li W, Hu G et al (2018) Bioactivities of EF24, a novel curcumin analog: a review. Front Oncol 8:614
Helmink BA, Khan MAW, Hermann A et al (2019) The microbiome, cancer, and cancer therapy. Nat Med 25:377–388
Hesari A, Azizian M, Sheikhi A et al (2019) Chemopreventive and therapeutic potential of curcumin in esophageal cancer: current and future status. Int J Cancer 144:1215–1226
Hewlings S, Kalman D (2017) Curcumin: a review of its' effects on human health. Foods 6(10):92
Homayouni A, Amini M, Sohrabi M et al (2019) Curcumin nanoparticles containing poloxamer or soluplus tailored by high pressure homogenization using antisolvent crystallization. Int J Pharm 562:124–134
Howells LM, Sale S, Sriramareddy SN et al (2011) Curcumin ameliorates oxaliplatin-induced chemoresistance in HCT116 colorectal cancer cells in vitro and in vivo. Int J Cancer 129:476–486
Hsu C, Cheng A, Aggarwal B et al (2007) Clinical studies with curcumin. In: Aggarwal BB, Surh Y-J, Shishodia S (eds) Molecular targets and therapeutic uses of curcumin in health and disease, vol 595. Springer, New York, pp 471–480
Hu R, Carey E, Lindor K et al (2017) Curcumin in hepatobiliary disease: pharmacotherapeutic properties and emerging potential clinical applications. Ann Hepatol 16:835–841

Huang MT, Lou YR, Ma W et al (1994) Inhibitory effects of dietary curcumin on forestomach, duodenal, and colon carcinogenesis in mice. Cancer Res 54:5841–5847
Huang YF, Zhu DJ, Chen XW et al (2017) Curcumin enhances the effects of irinotecan on colorectal cancer cells through the generation of reactive oxygen species and activation of the endoplasmic reticulum stress pathway. Oncotarget 8:40264–40275
Huang Y, Cao S, Zhang Q et al (2018) Biological and pharmacological effects of hexahydrocurcumin, a metabolite of curcumin. Arch Biochem Biophys 646:31–37
Hussain Z, Thu HE, Amjad MW et al (2017) Exploring recent developments to improve antioxidant, anti-inflammatory and antimicrobial efficacy of curcumin: a review of new trends and future perspectives. Mater Sci Eng C Mater Biol Appl 77:1316–1326
Imran M, Ullah A, Saeed F et al (2018) Cucurmin, anticancer, and antitumor perspectives: a comprehensive review. Crit Rev Food Sci Nutr 58:1271–1293
Ipar VS, Dsouza A, Devarajan PV (2019) Enhancing curcumin oral bioavailability through nanoformulations. Eur J Drug Metab Pharmacokinet 44(4):459–480. https://doi.org/10.1007/s13318-019-00545-z
Jahani-Sherafat S, Alebouyeh M, Moghim S et al (2018) Role of gut microbiota in the pathogenesis of colorectal cancer; a review article. Gastroenterol Hepatol Bed Bench 11:101–109
Jalili-Nik M, Soltani A, Moussavi S et al (2018) Current status and future prospective of Curcumin as a potential therapeutic agent in the treatment of colorectal cancer. J Cell Physiol 233:6337–6345
James MI, Iwuji C, Irving G et al (2015) Curcumin inhibits cancer stem cell phenotypes in ex vivo models of colorectal liver metastases, and is clinically safe and tolerable in combination with FOLFOX chemotherapy. Cancer Lett 364:135–141
Jamwal R (2018) Bioavailable curcumin formulations: a review of pharmacokinetic studies in healthy volunteers. J Integr Med 16:367–374
Jordan B, Mock C, Thilagavathi R et al (2016) Molecular mechanisms of curcumin and its semisynthetic analogues in prostate cancer prevention and treatment. Life Sci 152:135–144
Kapakos G, Youreva V, Srivastava AK (2012) Cardiovascular protection by curcumin: molecular aspects. Indian J Biochem Biophys 49:306–315
Kasi P, Tamilselvam R, Skalicka-Wozniak K et al (2016) Molecular targets of curcumin for cancer therapy: an updated review. Tumor Biol 37:13017–13,028
Kawamori T, Lubet R, Steele VE et al (1999) Chemopreventive effect of curcumin, a naturally occurring anti-inflammatory agent, during the promotion/progression stages of colon cancer. Cancer Res 59:597–601
Khurana S, Venkataraman K, Hollingsworth A et al (2013) Polyphenols: benefits to the cardiovascular system in health and in aging. Nutrients 5:3779–3827
Kim Y, Clifton P (2018) Curcumin, cardiometabolic health and dementia. Int J Environ Res Public Health 15. https://doi.org/10.3390/ijerph15102093
Kinger M, Kumar S, Kumar V (2018) Some important dietary polyphenolic compounds: an anti-inflammatory and immunoregulatory perspective. Mini-Rev Med Chem 18:1270–1282
Klinger N, Mittal S (2016) Therapeutic potential of curcumin for the treatment of brain tumors. Oxidative Med Cell Longev 2016:9324085
Kukongviriyapan U, Apaijit K, Kukongviriyapan V (2016) Oxidative stress and cardiovascular dysfunction associated with cadmium exposure: beneficial effects of curcumin and tetrahydrocurcumin. Tohoku J Exp Med 239:25–38
Kukula-Koch W, Grabarska A, Łuszczki J et al (2018) Superior anticancer activity is demonstrated by total extract of *Curcuma longa* L. as opposed to individual curcuminoids separated by centrifugal partition chromatography. Phytother Res 32:933–942
Kumar P, Barua CC, Sulakhiya K et al (2017) Curcumin ameliorates cisplatin-induced nephrotoxicity and potentiates its anticancer activity in SD rats: potential role of curcumin in breast cancer chemotherapy. Front Pharmacol 8:132
Kunnumakkara AB, Bordoloi D, Harsha C et al (2017a) Curcumin mediates anticancer effects by modulating multiple cell signaling pathways. Clin Sci (Lond) 131:1781–1799

Kunnumakkara AB, Bordoloi D, Padmavathi G et al (2017b) Curcumin, the golden nutraceutical: multitargeting for multiple chronic diseases. Br J Pharmacol 174:1325–1348
Kurien BT, Scofield RH (2009) Increasing aqueous solubility of curcumin for improving bioavailability. Trends Pharmacol Sci 30:334–335. author reply 335
Lao CD, Ruffin MT, Normolle D et al (2006) Dose escalation of a curcuminoid formulation. BMC Complement Altern Med 6:10
Lee H, Kim S, Lee G et al (2016) Turmeric extract and its active compound, curcumin, protect against chronic CCl4-induced liver damage by enhancing antioxidation. BMC Complement Altern Med 16:316
Li L, Ahmed B, Mehta K et al (2007) Liposomal curcumin with and without oxaliplatin: effects on cell growth, apoptosis, and angiogenesis in colorectal cancer. Mol Cancer Ther 6:1276–1282
Li G, Xie B, Li X et al (2012) Down-regulation of survivin and hypoxia-inducible factor-1 α by β-elemene enhances the radiosensitivity of lung adenocarcinoma xenograft. Cancer Biother Radiopharm 27:56–64
Li M, Yue GGL, Tsui SK, Fung KP, Lau CBS (2018) Turmeric extract, with absorbable curcumin, has potent anti-metastatic effect in vitro and in vivo. Phytomedicine 46:131–141
Liu Y, Wang W, Fang B et al (2013) Anti-tumor effect of germacrone on human hepatoma cell lines through inducing G2/M cell cycle arrest and promoting apoptosis. Eur J Pharmacol 698:95–102
Liu Z, Huang P, Law S et al (2018) Preventive effect of curcumin against chemotherapy-induced side-effects. Front Pharmacol 9:1374
Lodha R, Bagga A (2000) Traditional Indian systems of medicine. Ann Acad Med Singap 29:37–41
Lopresti AL (2018) The problem of curcumin and its bioavailability: could its gastrointestinal influence contribute to its overall health-enhancing effects? Adv Nutr 9:41–50
Loree J, Kopetz S (2017) Recent developments in the treatment of metastatic colorectal cancer. Ther Adv Med Oncol 9:551–564
Lou Y, Zheng J, Hu H et al (2015) Application of ultra-performance liquid chromatography coupled with quadrupole time-of-flight mass spectrometry to identify curcumin metabolites produced by human intestinal bacteria. J Chromatogr B Anal Technol Biomed Life Sci 985:38–47
Mahmood K, Zia KM, Zuber M et al (2015) Recent developments in curcumin and curcumin based polymeric materials for biomedical applications: a review. Int J Biol Macromol 81:877–890
Mahran R, Hagras M, Sun D et al (2017) Bringing curcumin to the clinic in cancer prevention: a review of strategies to enhance bioavailability and efficacy. AAPS J 19:54–81
Maiti P, Dunbar G (2018) Use of curcumin, a natural polyphenol for targeting molecular pathways in treating age-related neurodegenerative diseases. Int J Mol Sci 19. https://doi.org/10.3390/ijms19061637
Martin RC, Aiyer HS, Malik D, Li Y (2012) Effect on pro-inflammatory and antioxidant genes and bioavailable distribution of whole turmeric vs curcumin: similar root but different effects. Food Chem Toxicol 50:227–231
Mazieiro R, Frizon RR, Barbalho SM et al (2018) Is curcumin a possibility to treat inflammatory bowel diseases? J Med Food 21:1077–1085
McCann MJ, Johnston S, Reilly K et al (2014) The effect of turmeric (*Curcuma longa*) extract on the functionality of the solute carrier protein 22 A4 (SLC22A4) and interleukin-10 (IL-10) variants associated with inflammatory bowel disease. Nutrients 6:4178–4190
McFadden RM, Larmonier CB, Shehab KW et al (2015) The role of curcumin in modulating colonic microbiota during colitis and colon cancer prevention. Inflamm Bowel Dis 21:2483–2494
Mehra K, Berkowitz A, Sanft T (2017) Diet, physical activity, and body weight in cancer survivorship. Med Clin North Am 101:1151–1165
Milobedzka J, Kostanecki V, Lampe V (1910) Structure of curcumin. Ber Dtsch Chem Ges 43:2163–2170
Moghadam AR, Mohajeri D, Namvaran-Abbas-Abad A et al (2013) Protective effect of turmeric extract on ethotrexate-induced intestinal damage and oxidative stress. Chin J Nat Med 11:477–483

Momtazi A, Shahabipour F, Khatibi S et al (2016) Curcumin as a microRNA regulator in cancer: a review. Rev Physiol Biochem Pharmacol 171:1–38

Mouhid L, Corzo-Martínez M, Torres C et al (2017) Improving in vivo efficacy of bioactive molecules: an overview of potentially antitumor phytochemicals and currently available lipid-based delivery systems. J Oncol 2017:7351976

Murakami A, Furukawa I, Miyamoto S et al (2013) Curcumin combined with turmerones, essential oil components of turmeric, abolishes inflammation-associated mouse colon carcinogenesis. Biofactors 39:221–232

Nabavi S, Russo G, Tedesco I et al (2018) Curcumin and melanoma: from chemistry to medicine. Nutr Cancer 70:164–175

Naeini MB, Momtazi AA, Jaafari MR et al (2019) Antitumor effects of curcumin: a lipid perspective. J Cell Physiol. https://doi.org/10.1002/jcp.28262

Nagaraju GP, Benton L, Bethi SR et al (2019) Curcumin analogs: their roles in pancreatic cancer growth and metastasis. Int J Cancer 145(1):10–19

Nair HB, Sung B, Yadav VR et al (2010) Delivery of antiinflammatory nutraceuticals by nanoparticles for the prevention and treatment of cancer. Biochem Pharmacol 80:1833–1843

Nair A, Amalraj A, Jacob J et al (2019) Non-curcuminoids from turmeric and their potential in cancer therapy and anticancer drug delivery formulations. Biomolecules 9. https://doi.org/10.3390/biom9010013

Naksuriya O, Okonogi S, Schiffelers R et al (2014) Curcumin nanoformulations: a review of pharmaceutical properties and preclinical studies and clinical data related to cancer treatment. Biomaterials 35:3365–3383

Narayan S (2004) Curcumin, a multi-functional chemopreventive agent, blocks growth of colon cancer cells by targeting beta-catenin-mediated transactivation and cell-cell adhesion pathways. J Mol Histol 35:301–307

Nautiyal J, Kanwar SS, Yu Y et al (2011) Combination of dasatinib and curcumin eliminates chemo-resistant colon cancer cells. J Mol Signal 6:7

Nelson KM, Dahlin JL, Bisson J et al (2017) The essential medicinal chemistry of curcumin. J Med Chem 60:1620–1637

Oskouie MN, Aghili Moghaddam NS, Butler AE et al (2019) Therapeutic use of curcumin-encapsulated and curcumin-primed exosomes. J Cell Physiol 234:8182–8191

Pagliaro B, Santolamazza C, Simonelli F et al (2015) Phytochemical compounds and protection from cardiovascular diseases: a state of the art. Biomed Res Int 2015:918069

Panahi Y, Saadat A, Beiraghdar F et al (2014) Adjuvant therapy with bioavailability-boosted curcuminoids suppresses systemic inflammation and improves quality of life in patients with solid tumors: a randomized double-blind placebo-controlled trial. Phytother Res 28:1461–1467

Panahi Y, Hosseini MS, Khalili N et al (2015) Antioxidant and anti-inflammatory effects of curcuminoid-piperine combination in subjects with metabolic syndrome: a randomized controlled trial and an updated meta-analysis. Clin Nutr 34:1101–1108

Park J, Conteas CN (2010) Anti-carcinogenic properties of curcumin on colorectal cancer. World J Gastrointest Oncol 2:169–176

Park SY, Kim YH, Kim Y et al (2012) Aromatic-turmerone attenuates invasion and expression of MMP-9 and COX-2 through inhibition of NF-κB activation in TPA-induced breast cancer cells. J Cell Biochem 113:3653–3662

Park BH, Lim JE, Jeon HG et al (2016) Curcumin potentiates antitumor activity of cisplatin in bladder cancer cell lines via ROS-mediated activation of ERK1/2. Oncotarget 7:63870–63,886

Park CH, Eun CS, Han DS (2018) Intestinal microbiota, chronic inflammation, and colorectal cancer. Intest Res 16:338–345

Patel BB, Majumdar AP (2009) Synergistic role of curcumin with current therapeutics in colorectal cancer: minireview. Nutr Cancer 61:842–846

Patel BB, Sengupta R, Qazi S et al (2008) Curcumin enhances the effects of 5-fluorouracil and oxaliplatin in mediating growth inhibition of colon cancer cells by modulating EGFR and IGF-1R. Int J Cancer 122:267–273

Patel BB, Gupta D, Elliott AA et al (2010) Curcumin targets FOLFOX-surviving colon cancer cells via inhibition of EGFRs and IGF-1R. Anticancer Res 30:319–325

Patel SS, Acharya A, Ray RS et al (2019) Cellular and molecular mechanisms of curcumin in prevention and treatment of disease. Crit Rev Food Sci Nutr:1–53. https://doi.org/10.1080/10408398.2018.1552244

Pavan A, da Silva G, Jornada D et al (2016) Unraveling the anticancer effect of curcumin and resveratrol. Nutrients 8(11):628

PDQ Adult Treatment Editorial Board (2002–2019) Colon Cancer Treatment (PDQ®): Patient Version. PDQ cancer information summaries. National Cancer Institute (US), Bethesda (MD)

Perez-Chanona E, Trinchieri G (2016) The role of microbiota in cancer therapy. Curr Opin Immunol 39:75–81

Potter PE (2013) Curcumin: a natural substance with potential efficacy in Alzheimer's disease. J Exp Pharmacol 5:23–31

Prasad S, Gupta SC, Tyagi AK et al (2014a) Curcumin, a component of golden spice: from bedside to bench and back. Biotechnol Adv 32:1053–1064

Prasad S, Tyagi AK, Aggarwal BB (2014b) Recent developments in delivery, bioavailability, absorption and metabolism of curcumin: the golden pigment from golden spice. Cancer Res Treat 46:2–18

Prasad S, Tyagi AK, Siddik ZH et al (2017) Curcumin-free turmeric exhibits activity against human HCT-116 colon tumor xenograft: comparison with curcumin and whole turmeric. Front Pharmacol 8:871

Priyadarsini KI (2013) Chemical and structural features influencing the biological activity of curcumin. Curr Pharm Des 19:2093–2100

Pulla Reddy AC, Sudharshan E, Appu Rao AG et al (1999) Interaction of curcumin with human serum albumin – a spectroscopic study. Lipids 34:1025–1029

Qin S, Huang L, Gong J et al (2017) Efficacy and safety of turmeric and curcumin in lowering blood lipid levels in patients with cardiovascular risk factors: a meta-analysis of randomized controlled trials. Nutr J 16:68

Quezada SM, Cross RK (2019) Cannabis and turmeric as complementary treatments for IBD and other digestive diseases. Curr Gastroenterol Rep 21:2

Rafiee Z, Nejatian M, Daeihamed M et al (2019) Application of different nanocarriers for encapsulation of curcumin. Crit Rev Food Sci Nutr 59(21):3468–3497

Rahimi HR, Nedaeinia R, Sepehri Shamloo A et al (2016) Novel delivery system for natural products: nano-curcumin formulations. Avicenna J Phytomed 6:383–398

Rahmani A, Al Zohairy M, Aly S et al (2014) Curcumin: a potential candidate in prevention of cancer via modulation of molecular pathways. Biomed Res Int 2014:761608

Rakotoarisoa M, Angelova A (2018) Amphiphilic nanocarrier systems for curcumin delivery in neurodegenerative disorders. Medicines (Basel) 5. https://doi.org/10.3390/medicines5040126

Ramasamy TS, Ayob AZ, Myint HH et al (2015) Targeting colorectal cancer stem cells using curcumin and curcumin analogues: insights into the mechanism of the therapeutic efficacy. Cancer Cell Int 15:96

Rao CV, Simi B, Reddy BS (1993) Inhibition by dietary curcumin of azoxymethane-induced ornithine decarboxylase, tyrosine protein kinase, arachidonic acid metabolism and aberrant crypt foci formation in the rat colon. Carcinogenesis 14:2219–2225

Rao CV, Rivenson A, Simi B et al (1995) Chemoprevention of colon cancer by dietary curcumin. Ann N Y Acad Sci 768:201–204

Ravindranath V, Chandrasekhara N (1980) Absorption and tissue distribution of curcumin in rats. Toxicology 16:259–265

Ravindranath V, Chandrasekhara N (1981) In vitro studies on the intestinal absorption of curcumin in rats. Toxicology 20:251–257

Reddy BS, Rao CV (2002) Novel approaches for colon cancer prevention by cyclooxygenase-2 inhibitors. J Environ Pathol Toxicol Oncol 21:155–164

Rossi M, Mirbagheri SEYE, Keshavarzian A et al (2018) Nutraceuticals in colorectal cancer: a mechanistic approach. Eur J Pharmacol 833:396–402

Ruiz de Porras V, Bystrup S, Martínez-Cardús A et al (2016) Curcumin mediates oxaliplatin-acquired resistance reversion in colorectal cancer cell lines through modulation of CXC-Chemokine/NF-κB signalling pathway. Sci Rep 6:24675

Saheb M, Fereydouni N, Nemati S et al (2019) Chitosan-based delivery systems for curcumin: a review of pharmacodynamic and pharmacokinetic aspects. J Cell Physiol 234(8):12325–12340

Sahebkar A (2014) A systematic review and meta-analysis of randomized controlled trials investigating the effects of curcumin on blood lipid levels. Clin Nutr 33:406–414

Sahebkar A, Cicero AFG, Simental-Mendía LE et al (2016) Curcumin downregulates human tumor necrosis factor-α levels: a systematic review and meta-analysis ofrandomized controlled trials. Pharmacol Res 107:234–242

Sahu BP, Hazarika H, Bharadwaj R et al (2016) Curcumin-docetaxel co-loaded nanosuspension for enhanced anti-breast cancer activity. Expert Opin Drug Deliv 13:1065–1074

Salehi B, Stojanović-Radić Z, Matejić J et al (2019) The therapeutic potential of curcumin: a review of clinical trials. Eur J Med Chem 163:527–545

Sandur SK, Pandey MK, Sung B et al (2007) Curcumin, demethoxycurcumin, bisdemethoxycurcumin, tetrahydrocurcumin and turmerones differentially regulate anti-inflammatory and anti-proliferative responses through a ROS-independent mechanism. Carcinogenesis 28:1765–1773

Sarkar FH, Li Y, Wang Z et al (2010) Lesson learned from nature for the development of novel anticancer agents: implication of isoflavone, curcumin, and their synthetic analogs. Curr Pharm Des 16:1801–1812

Schaffer M, Schaffer PM, Bar-Sela G (2015) An update on Curcuma as a functional food in the control of cancer and inflammation. Curr Opin Clin Nutr Metab Care 18:605–611

Schneider C, Gordon ON, Edwards RL et al (2015) Degradation of curcumin: from mechanism to biological implications. J Agric Food Chem 63:7606–7614

Seo EJ, Fischer N, Efferth T (2018) Phytochemicals as inhibitors of NF-κB for treatment of Alzheimer's disease. Pharmacol Res 129:262–273

Sesarman A, Tefas L, Sylvester B et al (2019) Co-delivery of curcumin and doxorubicin in PEGylated liposomes favored the antineoplastic C26 murine colon carcinoma microenvironment. Drug Deliv Transl Res 9:260–272

Shah M, Renfro L, Allegra C et al (2016) Impact of patient factors on recurrence risk and time dependency of oxaliplatin benefit in patients with colon cancer: analysis from modern-era adjuvant studies in the adjuvant colon cancer end points (ACCENT) database. J Clin Oncol 34:843–853

Sharma RA, McLelland HR, Hill KA et al (2001) Pharmacodynamic and pharmacokinetic study of oral Curcuma extract in patients with colorectal cancer. Clin Cancer Res 7:1894–1900

Sharma RA, Euden SA, Platton SL et al (2004) Phase I clinical trial of oral curcumin: biomarkers of systemic activity and compliance. Clin Cancer Res 10:6847–6854

Shehzad A, Khan S, Shehzad O et al (2010) Curcumin therapeutic promises and bioavailability in colorectal cancer. Drugs Today (Barc) 46:523–532

Shehzad A, Rehman G, Lee YS (2013) Curcumin in inflammatory diseases. Biofactors 39:69–77

Shehzad A, Qureshi M, Anwar M et al (2017) Multifunctional curcumin mediate multitherapeutic effects. J Food Sci 82:2006–2015

Shen L, Ji HF (2009) Contribution of degradation products to the anticancer activity of curcumin. Clin Cancer Res 15:7108. author reply 7108–9

Shen L, Ji HF (2018) Bidirectional interactions between dietary curcumin and gut microbiota. Crit Rev Food Sci Nutr 59(18):2896–2902

Shen Y, Lu B, Zhang S et al (2014) Diterpenoid C of Radix Curcumae: an inhibitor of proliferation and inducer of apoptosis in human colon adenocarcinoma cells acting via inhibiting MAPK signaling pathway. Pharm Biol 52:1158–1165

Shen L, Liu L, Ji HF (2017) Regulative effects of curcumin spice administration on gut microbiota and its pharmacological implications. Food Nutr Res 61:1361780
Shishu, Maheshwari M (2010) Comparative bioavailability of curcumin, turmeric, and BiocurcumaxTM in traditional vehicles using non-everted rat intestinal sac model. J Funct Foods 2:60–65
Simadibrata M, Halimkesuma CC, Suwita BM (2017) Efficacy of curcumin as adjuvant therapy to induce or maintain remission in ulcerative colitis patients: an evidence-based clinical review. Acta Med Indones 49:363–368
Simental-Mendía LE, Caraglia M, Majeed M et al (2017) Impact of curcumin on the regulation of microRNAs in colorectal cancer. Expert Rev Gastroenterol Hepatol 11:99–101
Sinha R, Anderson DE, McDonald SS et al (2003) Cancer risk and diet in India. J Postgrad Med 49:222–228
Sivasami P, Hemalatha T (2018) Augmentation of therapeutic potential of curcumin using nanotechnology: current perspectives. Artif Cells Nanomed Biotechnol 46:1004–1015
Song X, Zhang M, Dai E et al (2019) Molecular targets of curcumin in breast cancer (Review). Mol Med Rep 19:23–29
Su P, Yang Y, Wang G et al (2018) Curcumin attenuates resistance to irinotecan via induction of apoptosis of cancer stem cells in chemoresistant colon cancer cells. Int J Oncol 53:1343–1353
Subramani PA, Narala VR (2013) Challenges of curcumin bioavailability: novel aerosol remedies. Nat Prod Commun 8:121–124
Subramani PA, Panati K, Narala VR (2017) Curcumin nanotechnologies and its anticancer activity. Nutr Cancer 69:381–393
Sun J, Chen F, Braun C et al (2018) Role of curcumin in the management of pathological pain. Phytomedicine 48:129–140
Sun Y, Liu L, Wang Y et al (2019) Curcumin inhibits the proliferation and invasion of MG-63 cells through inactivation of the p-JAK2/p-STAT3 pathway. Onco Targets Ther 12:2011–2021
Taieb J, André T, Auclin E (2019) Refining adjuvant therapy for non-metastatic colon cancer, new standards and perspectives. Cancer Treat Rev 75:1–11
Tajbakhsh A, Hasanzadeh M, Rezaee M et al (2018) Therapeutic potential of novel formulated forms of curcumin in the treatment of breast cancer by the targeting of cellular and physiological dysregulated pathways. J Cell Physiol 233:2183–2192
Taylor RA, Leonard MC (2011) Curcumin for inflammatory bowel disease: a review of human studies. Altern Med Rev 16:152–156
Tayyem RF, Heath DD, Al-Delaimy WK et al (2006) Curcumin content of turmeric and curry powders. Nutr Cancer 55:126–131
Toden S, Goel A (2017) The holy grail of curcumin and its efficacy in various diseases: is bioavailability truly a big concern? J Restor Med 6:27–36
Tong W, Wang Q, Sun D et al (2016) Curcumin suppresses colon cancer cell invasion via AMPK-induced inhibition of NF-κB, uPA activator and MMP9. Oncol Lett 12:4139–4146
U.S. Food and Drug Administration (2017) Generally recognized as safe (GRAS) notice no. 686. https://www.fda.gov/downloads/food/ingredientspackaginglabeling/gras/noticeinventory/ucm549247.pdf. Accessed 29 Mar 2019
U.S. Food and Drug Administration (2018) Code of Federal Regulations Title 21, PART 182 – Substances Generally Recognized as Safe, Sec. 182.10 Spices and other natural seasonings and flavorings. https://www.accessdata.fda.gov/scripts/cdrh/cfdocs/cfcfr/cfrsearch.cfm?fr=182.20. Accessed 29 Mar 2019
Uchio R, Higashi Y, Kohama Y et al (2017) A hot water extract of turmeric. J Nutr Sci 6:e3
Vallianou NG, Evangelopoulos A, Schizas N et al (2015) Potential anticancer properties and mechanisms of action of curcumin. Anticancer Res 35:645–651
Vareed SK, Kakarala M, Ruffin MT et al (2008) Pharmacokinetics of curcumin conjugate metabolites in healthy human subjects. Cancer Epidemiol Biomark Prev 17:1411–1417
Wahlström B, Blennow G (1978) A study on the fate of curcumin in the rat. Acta Pharmacol Toxicol (Copenh) 43:86–92

Wang YT, Liu HS, Su CL (2014) Curcumin-enhanced chemosensitivity of FDA-approved platinum (II)-based anticancer drugs involves downregulation of nuclear endonuclease G and NF-κB as well as induction of apoptosis and G2/M arrest. Int J Food Sci Nutr 65:368–374

Wang R, Wu G, Du L et al (2016) Semi-bionic extraction of compound turmeric protects against dextran sulfate sodium-induced acute enteritis in rats. J Ethnopharmacol 190:288–300

White B, Judkins DZ (2011) Clinical inquiry. Does turmeric relieve inflammatory conditions? J Fam Pract 60:155–156

Wong KE, Ngai SC, Chan KG et al (2019) Curcumin nanoformulations for colorectal cancer: a review. Front Pharmacol 10:152

Xiao Y, Yang FQ, Li SP et al (2007) Furanodiene induces G2/M cell cycle arrest and apoptosis through MAPK signaling and mitochondria-caspase pathway in human hepatocellular carcinoma cells. Cancer Biol Ther 6:1044–1050

Xu Z, Knight R (2015) Dietary effects on human gut microbiome diversity. Br J Nutr 113(Suppl): S1–S5

Xu DP, Li Y, Meng X et al (2017) Natural antioxidants in foods and medicinal plants: extraction, assessment and resources. Int J Mol Sci 18. https://doi.org/10.3390/ijms18010096

Yallapu M, Ebeling M, Jaggi M et al (2013) Plasma proteins interaction with curcumin nanoparticles: implications in cancer therapeutics. Curr Drug Metab 14:504–515

Yamauchi Y, Izumi Y, Yamamoto J et al (2014) Coadministration of erlotinib and curcumin augmentatively reduces cell viability in lung cancer cells. Phytother Res 28:728–735

Yang J, Yu J (2018) The association of diet, gut microbiota and colorectal cancer: what we eat may imply what we get. Protein Cell 9:474–487

Yue GGL, Chan BC et al (2010a) Immunostimulatory activities of polysaccharide extract isolated from *Curcuma longa*. Int J Biol Macromol 47:342–347

Yue GGL, Chan BC et al (2010b) Evaluation of in vitro anti-proliferative and immunomodulatory activities of compounds isolated from *Curcuma longa*. Food Chem Toxicol 48:2011–2020

Yue GGL, Cheng SW et al (2012) The role of turmerones on curcumin transportation and P-glycoprotein activities in intestinal Caco-2 cells. J Med Food 15:242–252

Yue GGL, Kwok H et al (2015) Novel anti-angiogenic effects of aromatic-turmerone, essential oil isolated from spice turmeric. J Funct Foods 15:243–253

Yue GGL, Jiang L et al (2016a) Turmeric ethanolic extract possesses stronger inhibitory activities on colon tumour growth than curcumin – the importance of turmerones. J Funct Foods 22:565–577

Yue GGL, Kwok HF et al (2016b) Combined therapy using bevacizumab and turmeric ethanolic extract (with absorbable curcumin) exhibited beneficial efficacy in colon cancer mice. Pharmacol Res 111:43–57

Yuliani S, Mustofa, Partadiredja G (2018) Turmeric (*Curcuma longa* L.) extract may prevent the deterioration of spatial memory and the deficit of estimated total number of hippocampal pyramidal cells of trimethyltin-exposed rats. Drug Chem Toxicol 41:62–71

Zabihi N, Pirro M, Johnston T et al (2017) Is there a role for curcumin supplementation in the treatment of non-alcoholic fatty liver disease? The data suggest yes. Curr Pharm Des 23:969–982

Zam W (2018) Gut microbiota as a prospective therapeutic target for curcumin: a review of mutual influence. J Nutr Metab 2018:1367984

Zangui M, Atkin SL, Majeed M et al (2019) Current evidence and future perspectives for curcumin and its analogues as promising adjuncts to oxaliplatin: state-of-the-art. Pharmacol Res 141:343–356

Zhang P, Lai ZL, Chen HF et al (2017) Curcumin synergizes with 5-fluorouracil by impairing AMPK/ULK1-dependent autophagy, AKT activity and enhancing apoptosis in colon cancer cells with tumor growth inhibition in xenograft mice. J Exp Clin Cancer Res 36:190

Zhang W, Shi H, Chen C et al (2018) Curcumin enhances cisplatin sensitivity of human NSCLC cell lines through influencing Cu-Sp1-CTR1 regulatory loop. Phytomedicine 48:51–61

Zhang Y, Rauf Khan A, Fu M et al (2019) Advances in curcumin-loaded nanopreparations: improving bioavailability and overcoming inherent drawbacks. J Drug Target 27(9):917–931
Zhao YS, Zhu TZ, Chen YW et al (2012) B-elemene inhibits Hsp90/Raf-1 molecular complex inducing apoptosis of glioblastoma cells. J Neuro-Oncol 107:307–314
Zheng J, Zhou Y, Li Y et al (2016) Spices for prevention and treatment of cancers. Nutrients 8:495
Zhou Q, Ye M, Lu Y et al (2015) Curcumin improves the tumoricidal effect of mitomycin C by suppressing ABCG2 expression in stem cell-like breast cancer cells. PLoS One 10:e0136694
Zhou X, Wang W, Li P et al (2016) Curcumin enhances the effects of 5-fluorouracil and oxaliplatin in inducing gastric cancer cell apoptosis both in vitro and in vivo. Oncol Res 23:29–34
Zhu LN, Mei X, Zhang ZG et al (2019) Curcumin intervention for cognitive function in different types of people: a systematic review and meta-analysis. Phytother Res 33:524–533

Chapter 8
Cancer Prevention by Tea Polyphenols

Chung S. Yang

Abstract The cancer preventive activities of tea (*Camellia Sinensis* Theaceae) have been investigated extensively in laboratory and human studies. Green tea polyphenols, mainly catechins, have shown inhibitory activities against tumorigenesis in different animal models, including those for cancers of the lung, oral cavity, esophagus, stomach, small intestine, colon, bladder, liver, pancreas, skin, prostate and mammary glands. Similar activities have also been reported in some human studies. This chapter reviews the nature of these inhibitory actions and discusses possible mechanisms involved. These inhibitory activities are attributed to catechins, especially the most abundant (−)-epigallocatechin-3-gallate (EGCG). The antioxidant or pro-oxidant activities of catechins and their binding to molecular targets would affect signal transduction and metabolic pathways that enhance apoptosis, suppress cell proliferation, and inhibit angiogenesis, resulting in the inhibition of carcinogenesis and cancer cell growth. Tea is considered a healthy beverage. However, the effect of tea consumption on the prevention of cancer in humans still needs to be further investigated. This chapter discusses some future directions in this area of research and concerns about possible toxicity, especially with high doses of tea polyphenols in tablet form.

Keywords Tea polyphenols · Cancer prevention · Laboratory and human studies · Mechanisms

Abbreviations

67LR	67 kDa Laminin receptor
ACF	Aberrant crypt foci
AKT	Protein kinase B
AOM	Azoxymethane

C. S. Yang (✉)
Department of Chemical Biology, Ernest Mario School of Pharmacy, Rutgers, The State University of New Jersey, Piscataway, NJ, USA
e-mail: csyang@pharmacy.rutgers.edu

J. M. Pezzuto, O. Vang (eds.), *Natural Products for Cancer Chemoprevention*,
https://doi.org/10.1007/978-3-030-39855-2_8

CVDs	Cardiovascular diseases
DNMT	DNA methyltransferase
EC	(−)-Epicatechin
ECG	(−)-Epicatechin-3-gallate
EGC	(−)-Epigallocatechin
EGCG	(−)-Epigallocatechin-3-gallate
EGFR	Epidermal growth factor receptor
GTE	Green tea extract
HAT	Acetyltransferase
HCC	Hepatocellular carcinoma
HFD	High-fat diet
HGFR or c-Met	Hepatocyte growth factor receptor
hTERT	Human telomerase reverse transcriptase
IGF1	Insulin-like growth factor 1
IGF1R	IGF1 receptor
IGFBP3	IGF binding protein 3
IHC	Immunohistochemistry
M4	5-(3′, 4′, 5′-trihydroxyphenyl)-γ-valerolactone
M6	5-(3′, 4′-dihydroxyphenyl)-γ-valerolactone
M6′	5-(3′, 5′-dihydroxyphenyl)-γ-valerolactone
MAPK	Mitogen-activated protein kinases
MMP	Matrix metalloproteinase
MRP2	Multidrug resistant protein 2
NNK	4-(methylnitrosamino)-1-(3-pyridyl)-1-butanone
Nrf2	Nuclear factor erythroid 2-related factor 2
OR	Odds ratio
PDE5	Phosphodiesterase 5
PI3K	Phosphotidylinositol 3-kinase
PIN	Prostate intraepithelial neoplasia
PPE	Polyphenon E
RCT	Randomized clinical trial
ROS	Reactive oxygen species
RTKs	Receptor tyrosine kinases
SFRP	Secreted frizzled-related protein
SPR	Surface plasmon resonance
STAT1	Signal transduction activator of transcription 1
TAM	Tumor-associated macrophages
TRAMP	Transgenic adenocarcinoma of the mouse prostate
VEGFA	Vascular endothelial growth factor A
VEGFR	Vascular endothelial growth factor receptor

8.1 Introduction

Tea, a popular beverage, is made of the leaves of the plant *Camellia sinensis*. The potential beneficial health effects of tea have been studied extensively in recent decades. These include the prevention of cancer, excessive body weight gain, diabetes, cardiovascular diseases (CVDs) and other diseases [reviewed in Yang et al. (2009), Yang and Hong (2013), Yang and Zhang (2019), Crespy and Williamson (2004)]. Among these diseases, cancer prevention by tea is the first to receive major attention for research, and the earlier work was reviewed in 1993 (Yang and Wang 1993). Since then, extensive investigations have been conducted in animal models, cell lines and humans. Most of the cancer beneficial effects are believed to be due to the polyphenols (mostly catechins) in green tea, and possible mechanisms of their actions have been repeatedly reviewed (Yang et al. 2009; Yang and Hong 2013; Yang and Zhang 2019; Yang and Wang 2016; Shirakami and Shimizu 2018; Negri et al. 2018; Khan and Mukhtar 2018). This chapter reviews and assesses the current information in the literature in order to present a clearer understanding of cancer prevention by tea polyphenols.

Cancer is one of the most common diseases and the leading cause of death in many countries. If tea could prevent or delay the development of cancer, the public health implications would be tremendous. Because of this, there is immense scientific and public interest on this topic. A literature search on PubMed in March 2019 using the key words "Tea and cancer" yielded 4910 publications (starting from 1962). Some publications are based on strong evidence, while others may not. Many of the results observed in vitro may have been inappropriately extrapolated to beneficial effects on human health and propagated in the news media or internet.

This chapter reviews many of the key studies on cancer prevention by tea, especially on studies in animal models that are relevant to human health. Because of the large number of publications in this area of research, information from recently published systematic reviews and meta-analyses are used to help assess the relative strengths of the existing data. Selected examples are used to illustrate the cancer prevention effects and possible mechanisms involved. The limitation in using information derived from laboratory studies for human cancer prevention, the possible toxicity of high doses of tea catechins, and suggestions for future research are discussed.

8.2 Tea Polyphenols: Biochemical Properties, Bioavailability and Biotransformation

The commonly consumed types of tea are green, black and oolong teas. Their polyphenol compositions depend on the method of manufacture as discussed below.

8.2.1 Polyphenols in Green, Black and Oolong Tea

Green tea, which accounts for 18% of tea produced globally, are popular in Asian countries such as China and Japan. In the manufacture of green tea, the tea leaves are heated or steamed to inactivate enzymes, rolled and then dried. This process helps to stabilize the tea constituents during storage. The characteristic polyphenolic compounds in green tea are known as catechins, which include: (−)-epigallocatechin-3-gallate (EGCG), (−)-epigallocatechin (EGC), (−)-epicatechin-3-gallate (ECG) and (−)-epicatechin (EC). The structures of these catechins are shown in Fig. 8.1. Tea leaves also contain lower quantities of other polyphenols such as quercetin, kaempferol, and myricetin as well as alkaloids, such as caffeine and theobromine. A typical brewed green tea beverage (e.g., 2.5 g tea leaves in 250 ml of hot water) contains 240–320 mg of catechins, of which 60–65% is EGCG, and 20–50 mg of caffeine (Balentine et al. 1997; Sang et al. 2011).

Black tea accounts for 80% of tea produced, generally in tropical areas such as India, Sri Lanka, Africa and Argentina. It is consumed worldwide, including Europe and America. In the tropical areas, the tea leaves contain a high level of catechins, which are bitter and stringent. In the manufacture of black tea, the tea leaves are withered, crushed and the catechins undergo enzyme-catalyzed oxidation in a

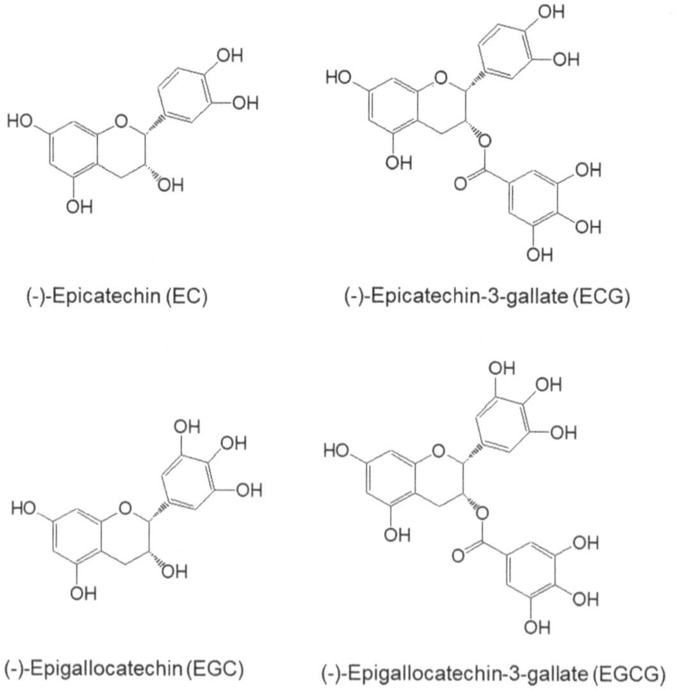

Fig. 8.1 Chemical structure of major green tea catechins. *EC* (−) epicatechin, *ECG* (−) epicatechin-gallate, *EGC* (−) epigallocatechin, *EGCG* (−)-epigallocatechin-3-gallate

process commonly known as "fermentation"; however, no microorganisms are involved. During this process, most of the catechins are oxidized, dimerized and polymerized to form dimers (theaflavins) and polymers (thearubigins) (Balentine et al. 1997; Sang et al. 2011). Therefore, the quantities of catechins are decreased. The "fermentation" process, converting catechins to dimers and polymers, makes black tea more palatable and flavorful. In brewed black tea, catechins, theaflavins, and thearubigins each account for 3–10%, 2–6%, and ≥20% of the dry weight, respectively.

Oolong tea is more popular in Taiwan, Fujian Province of China and Japan. Oolong tea is manufactured by crushing only the rims of the leaves and limiting fermentation to a short period of time to produce specific flavor and taste of the tea. In this process, some catechins are converted to derivatives and dimers. Dark tea, such as Pu-er tea, popular in some areas in southern China, is made by microbial fermentation of tea leaves and a large portion of catechins are converted to microbial metabolites. Yellow tea is made in certain areas in China by heating, rolling, keeping at room temperature and 70% humidity until the leaves turn yellow (in 6–8 h), and then are dried. Procedures for making different types of tea in laboratory scale and the compositions of these teas have recently been described (Wang et al. 2018).

8.2.2 Biochemical Properties of Tea Catechins

Tea catechins are strong antioxidants, which scavenge reactive oxygen species (ROS), and prevent their formation by chelating metal ions (Sang et al. 2011). Among tea catechins, the most abundant EGCG has the strongest antioxidant activity, and has been studied extensively. EGCG is also known to undergo superoxide-catalyzed autoxidation in vitro to produce ROS that can induce cell death (Hou et al. 2005). Nevertheless, such autoxidation of EGCG may not occur extensively in vivo under normal physiological conditions, because of the lower oxygen partial pressure (than in solution in vitro) and the presence of antioxidant enzymes in animal tissues (Hou et al. 2005). Therefore, results on EGCG obtained from cell culture studies need to be interpreted with caution. In vivo, EGCG and other catechins can serve as antioxidant in general; but at high concentrations, they may also cause the formation of ROS in mitochondria (Li et al. 2010; Tao et al. 2014). The ROS may activate nuclear factor erythroid 2-related factor 2 (Nrf2)-mediated antioxidant and other cytoprotective enzymes to protect against oxidative stress (Shen et al. 2005; Wang et al. 2015; James et al. 2015).

An important biochemical property of catechins is their strong binding to proteins, lipids and nucleic acids, through hydrogen-bonding and other interactions. Multiple hydrogen-bond formation provides high affinity binding of catechins to these biomolecules. As will be discussed subsequently, the binding of EGCG to many proteins has been proposed to be a key mechanism for its anti-cancer and other activities. The catechin dimers and polymers in black tea, with more phenolic groups, are expected to bind to biomolecules with even higher affinity than EGCG in vitro. Similar to catechins, these larger molecular weight molecules may inhibit digestive enzymes through binding and decrease the digestion and absorption of macronutrients in the digestive tract. However, their direct binding to macromolecules in internal organs depends on bioavailability and tissue distribution of the specific polyphenols.

8.2.3 Absorption and Biotransformation of Tea Polyphenols

The catechins are thought to enter cells mainly through passive diffusion, and the absorption rate is limited by the molecular mass, lipid solubility, as well as the number of hydrogen-bond donors and acceptors (Sang et al. 2011). However, the involvement of transporters, such as organic anion-transporting peptides 1A2 and 1B3, has also been suggested (Roth et al. 2011; Zhang et al. 2013). Some of the catechins are conjugated during absorption in the enterocytes. Multidrug resistant protein 2 (MRP2) has been suggested to limit the bioavailability of EGCG and ECG by actively exporting them from the enterocytes back into the intestinal lumen, either before or after conjugation (Sang et al. 2011). The catechins and their conjugated metabolites are absorbed into the portal circulation, enters the liver and are methylated and further conjugated (Sang et al. 2008). Catechins are methylated by catechol-*O*-methyltransferase, and conjugated by UDP-glucuronosyl transferases or sulfotransferases to form glucuronide or sulfate conjugates, respectively. The EGCG and its conjugates in the liver subsequently enter the blood and are transported to other organs or effluxed by MRP2 from the liver to the bile and then into the intestine (Sang et al. 2011; Liu et al. 2018). A large portion of EGCG in the ileum is reabsorbed and undergoes enterohepatic circulation, while the unabsorbed portion goes through the colon and are excreted in the feces as the major route of excretion. Depending on the animal species, a significant amount of EGCG (and ECG) is excreted in mouse urine, but not in the urine of humans or rats (Sang et al. 2011; Liu et al. 2018; Lee et al. 2002; Clifford et al. 2013). On the other hand, EGC (and EC) is more efficiently absorbed into the blood and excreted in the urine. Therefore, EGC can be used as an exposure marker for tea consumption in human studies (Sun et al. 2002). In addition, catechins can also be absorbed to a certain extent in the oral cavity and colon (Yang et al. 1999). Some dietary chemicals have been shown to affect the bioavailability of catechins through inhibiting their conjugations or efflux. For example, piperine, a compound found in black pepper, can inhibit gluconidation of EGCG and increase its bioavailability, when both compounds were co-administered orally to mice (Lambert et al. 2004).

In a previous study, the recovery in 24-h urine of gallocatechin conjugates (EGCG and ECG) after consumption of green tea was 11% of intake and that of non-gallocatechin conjugates (EGC and EC) was 28% (Stalmach et al. 2009). A similar tea preparation administered to individuals with ileostomy showed that the urinary excretion of gallocatechin conjugates was 8% of intake and that of non-gallocatechin conjugates was 27% (Stalmach et al. 2010). Because catechins need to be absorbed before urinary excretion, these results suggest that tea catechins are mostly absorbed in the small intestine and non-gallocatechins are more efficiently absorbed. It was estimated that 69% of catechin intake was recovered in the 0- to 24-h ileal fluid as mixtures of catechins and their metabolites (Stalmach et al. 2010), suggesting that this amount goes into the colon under normal physiological conditions.

Catechins are known to be degraded by microbes in the oral cavity and intestines (Yang et al. 1999; Meselhy et al. 1997; Li et al. 2000). The hydrolysis of the ester bonds of EGCG and ECG and the fission of the C-ring of catechins are carried out by microbial enzymes. Three metabolites, 5-(3′, 4′, 5′-trihydroxyphenyl)-γ-valerolactone (M4), 5-(3′, 4′-dihydroxyphenyl)-γ-valerolactone (M6) and 5-(3′, 5′--dihydroxyphenyl)-γ-valerolactone (M6′), have been identified in human and mouse plasma and urine samples (Sang et al. 2008; Li et al. 2000; Meng et al. 2002). These ring fission metabolites are further degraded to phenylvaleric acid, phenolic acid and smaller molecules, mostly in the colon and excreted as feces. These results strongly suggest that these microbial metabolites, together with intact catechins, are absorbed or reabsorbed in the small intestine, and are excreted in conjugated forms in the urine. Larger portions of these compounds are excreted as aglycones in the feces. A recent review article also indicated that a large portion of the ingested catechins passes through the intestine and undergoes ring fission degradation (Clifford et al. 2013). On the other hand, tea polyphenols can also modulate the composition of the gut microbiota, and this action has been proposed to mediate the health effects of tea (Chen et al. 2019; Henning et al. 2018).

8.3 Inhibition of Tumorigenesis in Animal Models

The research on tea and cancer prevention gained momentum in the early 1990s. Since then, tea and tea catechins have been shown to inhibit tumorigenesis in animal models for cancers of the oral cavity, esophagus, stomach, small intestine, colon, liver, pancreas, lung, bladder, prostate, mammary glands and skin (Yang et al. 2009; Yang and Wang 2016). Most of the studies were conducted with green tea extracts, tea catechin mixtures such as Polyphenon E (PPE, a standard tea catechin preparation containing 65% EGCG and other tea catechins) or pure EGCG, administered through drinking water or diet. Some examples of these studies are as follows.

8.3.1 Inhibition of Lung Tumorigenesis

The inhibition of lung tumorigenesis by tea extracts and catechins has been demonstrated in more than 20 studies using chemically induced and genetic rodent models (Yang et al. 2009, 2011). Administration of EGCG or EGC significantly decreased lung tumorigenesis in rats, mice or hamsters (Yang et al. 2009, 2011; Lu et al. 2006).

In A/J mice that had been treated with a single *i.p.* dose of 4-(methylnitrosamino)-1-(3-pyridyl)-1-butanone (NNK) 20 weeks earlier, oral administration of 0.5% PPE or 0.044% caffeine in the drinking water for 32 weeks significantly inhibited the progression of lung adenomas to adenocarcinomas (Lu et al. 2006). IHC analysis showed that PPE and caffeine treatment inhibited cell proliferation, enhanced apoptosis, and decreased levels of c-Jun and phospho-ERK1/2 in adenocarcinomas. In normal lung tissues, neither agent had a significant effect on cell proliferation or apoptosis, suggesting that the action is selective against tumor tissues. These and other studies demonstrate the broad inhibitory activity of tea catechins against lung carcinogenesis as well as the cancer preventive effects of caffeine. A recent study in the NNK-induced lung cancer model showed that 0.3% green tea extract (GTE) in drinking water decreased the tumor multiplicity and the percentage of PD-L1 positive cells, showing that EGCG acts as an alternative immune checkpoint inhibitor (Rawangkan et al. 2018).

In studies by Chung et al. in NNK-treated A/J mice (Xu et al. 1992), caffeine was effective in inhibiting lung tumorigenesis, but not as effective as the corresponding concentration of EGCG (in green tea). They also showed that the inhibitory effect of caffeine (680 ppm) was similar to that of 2% black tea (containing 680 ppm caffeine) against NNK-induced lung tumorigenesis in rats, suggesting that caffeine was responsible for the inhibitory effect (Chung et al. 1998). This conclusion is different from the experiments with A/J mice, which demonstrated the inhibition of lung tumorigenesis by decaffeinated green and black tea preparations (Wang et al. 1992). A possible interpretation of this difference is that the systemic bioavailability of catechins in mice are much higher than in rats, while the catechin dimers and polymers in black tea have little or no bioavailability in both species (Yang et al. 2008). That is, catechins from black tea are less bioavailable in the rat lung than the mouse lung; therefore, caffeine in rats is likely the major lung cancer preventive agent in black tea extracts.

A recent publication suggests that tea catechins may reduce the risk of lung cancer by trapping reactive aldehydes produced in tobacco smoke (Weng et al. 2018). This publication also reported that aldehydes from tobacco smoke is the predominant driving factor for lung carcinogenesis by causing aldehyde-induced γ-hydroxy-propano-deoxy-guanosine (γ-OH-PdG) and α-methyl-γ-OH-PdG formation and reducing the DNA repair capacity in the lung. PPE (0.1% in the diet) greatly reduced these effects of tobacco smoke (Weng et al. 2018).

8.3.2 Inhibition of Tumorigenesis in the Digestive Tract

The epithelial cells in the digestive tract have the opportunity of being directly exposed to orally ingested tea polyphenols. Thus, the action of tea polyphenols may not be limited by their systemic bioavailability. Inhibitory effects of tea catechins against tumorigenesis in chemically induced and genetic animal models in the oral cavity, esophagus, stomach, small intestine, and colon have been shown in more than 30 studies. For example, we showed that administration of EGCG at 0.02–0.32% in drinking water dose-dependently inhibited small intestinal tumorigenesis in *Apc*$^{Min/+}$ mice, while caffeine did not have an inhibitory effect (Ju et al. 2005). The inhibition was associated with increased levels of E-cadherin on the plasma membrane, as well as decreased levels of nuclear levels of β-catenin, c-Myc, phospho-AKT, and phospho-ERK1/2 in the tumors as determined by immunohistochemistry (IHC) (Ju et al. 2005). Administration of green tea extracts (0.6% in drinking fluid) also inhibited the formation of azoxymethane (AOM)-induced aberrant crypt foci (ACF) in CF-1 mice on a high-fat diet (Ju et al. 2003).

In male C57BL/KsJ-*db/db* mice, Shimizu et al. (2008a) demonstrated the inhibition of AOM-induced ACF formation by EGCG (0.01% and 0.1% in drinking water) was associated with suppression of insulin-like growth factor 1 (IGF1) signaling. The elevated levels of IGF1 receptor (IGF1R), phospho-IGF1R, phospho-GSK3β and β-catenin in the colonic mucosa were decreased by EGCG treatment; also decreased were the plasma levels of IGF1, insulin, triglyceride, cholesterol and leptin (Shimizu et al. 2008a).

In another set of experiments, treatment of rats with 0.24% of PPE in the diet for 8 weeks significantly decreased the total number of ACF in the colon of AOM-treated rats (Xiao et al. 2008). Treatment with 0.24% of PPE for 34 weeks significantly decreased the colon adenocarcinoma incidence (by 60%) and multiplicity (by 80%) (Hao et al. 2017). The inhibitory activity of PPE was associated with decreased levels of nuclear β-catenin and cyclin D1, enhanced cell apoptosis, and increased levels of retinoid X receptor-α, β and γ in adenocarcinoma and high-grade dysplasia (Xiao et al. 2008; Hao et al. 2017).

There have been suggestions that mixtures of catechins are more effective cancer preventive agents than pure EGCG due to synergistic actions. This hypothesis was tested in *Apc*$^{Min/+}$ mice by comparing the activities of PPE, EGCG and ECG administered in drinking fluid (Hao et al. 2007). The tumor multiplicity was decreased approximately 50% by both PPE (0.12%) and the corresponding amount of dietary EGCG (0.08%), and no difference was observed between PPE and EGCG. On the other hand, the inhibitory activity of ECG was not statistically significant. Examination of the tissues showed that PPE or EGCG treatment increased apoptosis, suppressed cell proliferation, and decreased the levels of phospho-AKT and nuclear β-catenin (Hao et al. 2007). Additional studies are required to further determine whether EGCG can interact with other catechins in PPE to generate synergistic actions to inhibit tumorigenesis in other models. In similar studies, we also found that the inhibitory activity of PPE was higher when administered in the diet than in the drinking water, both at 0.12% (Hao et al. 2007).

8.3.3 *Inhibition of Tumorigenesis in the Prostate and Liver*

In transgenic adenocarcinoma of the mouse prostate (TRAMP) mice, administration of a green tea polyphenol infusion (0.1% in drinking water) for 24 weeks markedly inhibited prostate cancer development and distant site metastases (Gupta et al. 2001;

Adhami et al. 2004). The inhibition was associated with decreased cell proliferation, increased apoptosis, decreased IGF1 level, and restored IGF binding protein 3 (IGFBP3) levels in both serum and the dorso-lateral prostate (Gupta et al. 2001; Adhami et al. 2004). This modulation of IGF1 and IGFBP3 levels was associated with reduced levels of phosphotidylinositol 3-kinase (PI3K) as well as phospho-AKT and phospho-ERK1/2. The green tea polyphenol treatment also significantly decreased levels of angiogenic and metastatic markers, such as vascular endothelial growth factor A (VEGFA), matrix metalloproteinase (MMP)2 and MMP9. These results suggest that the inhibition of the IGF1 signaling, VEGFA and MMPs contributes to the cancer preventive activity of green tea polyphenols.

On the prevention of liver carcinogenesis, there is a recent study on the inhibition of high-fat diet (HFD)-induced hepatocellular carcinoma (HCC) by Theaphenon E (a green tea catechin mixture similar to PPE) (Coia et al. 2018). In this study, mice were fed a HFD (60% of calories from fat) and had 42% incidence of HCC after 80 weeks. Interestingly, the formation of HCC was completely blocked by 2% Theaphenon E in the diet. The proposed mechanism is that catechins prevented lipid peroxidation-derived cyclic DNA-adduct (γ-OHPdG) formation. This aldehyde derived DNA-adduct is known to cause G to T and G to A mutations in many genes, including the tumor suppressor p53. The same group of investigators also showed that Theaphenon E (2% in the diet) inhibited HCC formation in nucleotide excision repair deficient (Xpa−/−) mice and diethylnitrosamine-treated mice, and the inhibition was associated with decreased γ-OHPdG formation in the liver (Yang and Malhi 2018). Considering the pandemic of obesity and fatty liver disease, the possible prevention of associated liver cancer by tea catechins in humans is an important topic for further research.

The above examples illustrate the broad cancer preventive activities of tea polyphenols in animal models and the nature of the data. Studies on other organ sites have been discussed in previous reviews (Negri et al. 2018; Khan and Mukhtar 2018; Yang et al. 2011). On the other hand, studies on some other organs, such as mammary glands (Yang et al. 2011), the cancer preventive activity of tea catechins is weak and inconsistent.

8.4 Effects of Tea or Catechin Consumption on Human Cancer Risk

In earlier human studies, tea consumption was suggested to increase the incidence of esophageal cancer (Yang and Wang 1993). Later, this cancer-promoting effect was attributed to the high temperature of the tea consumed. Since then, many epidemiological studies have been conducted concerning tea consumption and cancer risk in humans. Because of the various types and quantities of tea consumed and the different types of cancer studied in different populations, the results have not been consistent. Some of the studies, systematic reviews and meta-analyses are summarized as follows.

8.4.1 Observational Studies on Tea Consumption and Cancer Risk

In contrast to animal studies, in which the experimental conditions are well-defined, the human situation is more complex. Lifestyle factors, genetic differences and other interfering factors reduce the power of epidemiological studies. For example, the protective effect of green tea consumption against upper-gastrointestinal cancer became clear after adjusting for interfering factors (Yuan et al. 2011). Cigarette smoking appears to be a strong interfering factor. In a case-control study on the effect of green tea consumption on esophageal cancer in Shanghai by Gao et al. (1994), a protective effect was only observed in non-smokers, who were mostly women. A recent systematic review of cohort studies in Japan on green tea consumption and gastric cancer showed no overall preventive effect of green tea. However, a small consistent risk reduction was found in nonsmoking women, and the result became statistically significant after pooling data of six cohort studies (Sasazuki et al. 2012). The above results suggest the gastric cancer preventive effect of tea is only mild in humans.

Well-designed large cohort studies are instrumental in providing information on the effects of dietary habits on health. In the Ohsaki National health Insurance cohort Study, with 40,530 participants followed for 11 years (4209 deaths), tea consumption was shown to have no effect on cancer deaths (Kuriyama et al. 2006), even though tea consumption was dose-dependently associated with lower risk for deaths due to CVDs and deaths from all causes (Kuriyama et al. 2006). Similar negative results on cancer and protective effects on deaths due to CVDs and all causes combined by tea consumption were also observed in the combined cohort of the Shanghai women's and Shanghai men's studies, involving a total of 6571 deaths out of 136,432 individuals followed for 8.3–14.2 years (Zhao et al. 2017). On the other hand, in the Chinese Perspective Smoking Study involving 164,681 individuals followed for 11 years, tea drinking was associated with reduced risk of deaths due to cancer and CVDs, as well as deaths from all causes (Liu et al. 2016). These large long-term cohort studies suggest that tea drinking was more effective in reducing the deaths or preventing the development of CVDs than cancer.

The effects of tea consumption on **oral cancer** was analyzed recently in a dose-response meta-analysis of 12 case-control studies, showing a pooled odds ratio (OR) of 0.70 (90% C1 = 0.61–0.81, $p < 0.001$) (Zhou et al. 2018). Subgroup analysis also indicated an inverse association between tea intake and the risk for oral cancer, except in subgroup analysis of black tea and in American population. For tea consumption and lung cancer risk, a meta-analysis of 26 case-control studies and 12 cohort studies showed that tea consumption was significantly associated with overall decreased risk for lung cancer (RR, 0.78; CI, 0.70–0.87). Subgroup analyses showed that tea consumption was associated with reduced risk for lung cancer in women, but no significant associated was found in men or in cohort studies (Wang et al. 2014). However, results on the prevention of **liver cancer** have not been consistent among studies. For example, a protective effect of tea consumption was observed in a prospective cohort study in an European population (Bamia et al. 2015), but not in a Japanese cohort (Tamura et al. 2018). A meta-analysis of 9 prospective cohort studies in Asian populations in 2016 found a significant protective effect in females, but not in males (Huang et al. 2016). A meta-analysis including 4 case-control and 6 cohort studies in 2017 reported a lower liver cancer associated with green tea consumption, especially when consuming 4 cups/day or more (Ni et al. 2017). On the prevention of **biliary tract cancer**, a systematic review and dose-response meta-analysis of 8 observational studies found a dose-dependent protective effect of tea; the tea intake group, in comparison to the never intake group, had an OR of 0.66 (CI = 0.48–0.85), and the effect was stronger in women (Xiong et al. 2017). The effects of tea consumption on **colorectal cancer** have also been extensively studied. A dose-response meta-analysis of 29 publications on colorectal cancer did not find a clear protective effect of tea consumption; however, stratified analysis indicated that green tea consumption had a dose-response protective effect among females against rectal cancer (Chen et al. 2017).

On the prevention of **prostate cancer** by tea, although there are studies suggesting a preventive effect, a recent review article concluded that there is no general agreement among human studies on the prevention of prostate cancer by tea (Miyata et al. 2019). There is also no clear conclusion between tea consumption and **breast cancer** as reflected in three recent meta-analyses of observational studies: one showed a potential protective effect (Gianfredi et al. 2018), while the other two could not draw a conclusion on the beneficial effect (Najafi et al. 2018). However, more clear results have been reported in the prevention of **ovarian and endometrial cancers**. In systematic reviews and meta-analyses of observational studies, consumption of green tea, but not black tea, dose-dependently reduced the risk of ovarian (OR = 0.64, CI = 0.45–0.90) and endometrial cancer (OR = 0.78, CI = 0.66–0.92) (Zhang et al. 2018; Zhou et al. 2016).

8.4.2 Human Intervention Studies with Tea Polyphenols

Intervention trials are important in demonstrating a beneficial health effect of an agent. The results of human intervention studies with green tea polyphenols, mostly small randomized clinical trial (RCT), however, have been inconsistent. For example, an earlier RCT on **oral cancer** prevention in China, with a mixed tea product (3 g/day administered orally or topically) in patients with oral mucosa leukoplakia for 6 months, showed significant decrease in the number and total volume of proliferation index and silver-stained nucleoli organizer regions (Li et al. 1999). However, a later phase II RCT in the U.S. with GTE (500, 750 or 1000 mg/m^2, 2 times daily) for 12 weeks, to patients with oral pre-malignant lesions (n = 28), only showed possible beneficial effects nonsignificant in lessening oral pre-malignant lesions (Tsao et al. 2009).

In an RCT in Japan, subjects with a history of metachronous **colorectal adenoma**, supplementation with green tea extracts (1.5 g/day) for 1 year significantly decreased the recurrence of adenomas (Shimizu et al. 2008b). In a similar colorectal adenoma recurrence RCT in Korea, supplementation with GTE (0.9 g/day) for 1 year resulted in a recurrence rate of 23.6%, significantly lower than the 42.5% in the control group (n = 72 or 73 for each group) (Shin et al. 2018).

The most impressive intervention study with tea catechins was conducted in Italy on **prostate cancer**, in which 30 men with high-grade prostate intraepithelial neoplasia (PIN) were given 300 mg of green tea catechins, twice daily for 12 months (Bettuzzi et al. 2006). Only one subject developed prostate cancer, whereas 9 of the 30 subjects with high-grade PIN in the placebo group developed prostate cancer. The difference is highly statistically significant. However, a similar trial in Florida using PPE (containing 400 mg of EGCG) in 97 men with high-grade PIN and/or atypical small acinar proliferation (ASAP), supplementation for 6–12 months did not cause a reduction in the number of prostate cancer cases between the treatment and the placebo groups (Kumar et al. 2015). Kumar et al. (2018) recently reviewed several RCT on prostate cancer prevention and concluded that tea catechins can modulate several intermediate endpoint biomarkers and retard clinical progression of prostate cancer, without major side effects.

In a recent completed intervention trial on **breast cancer** prevention with GTE, the Minnesota Green Tea Trial with healthy postmenopausal women, 573 women received oral supplements of GTE twice a day (total of 1315 mg of catechins, including 843 mg of EGCG) for 1 year and 508 women received placebos. The intervention decreased the mammographic density of those who enrolled at the ages of 50–55 years but not in those enrolled at older ages (Samavat et al. 2017). It was also observed that 5.1% of the women in the GTE group had elevates serum alanine aminotransferase and aspartate aminotransferase activities, yielding an odds ratio of 7.0 (Yu et al. 2017). The elevation was reversible after the individual stopped the intake of GTE. The dose of 1315 mg of catechins per day was thought to be a safe dose in the design of this trial. The reason why approximately 5% of the women on GTE experience reversible liver toxicity is not clear.

Even with some of the above positive indications, the earlier optimistic expectation of cancer preventive activity by tea polyphenols, based on laboratory results, has not materialized in RCTs.

8.5 Possible Mechanisms of Cancer Prevention by Tea Catechins

The primary biological actions of catechins are due to their redox and physical binding activities, and this topic has been reviewed (Yang et al. 2009; Yang and Zhang 2019; Yang and Wang 2016). In the cancer prevention area, many mechanisms of action were derived from studies in cell lines. Using EGCG as an example, some of these actions are depicted in Fig. 8.2. These actions, other mechanisms and their relevance to cancer prevention are discussed below.

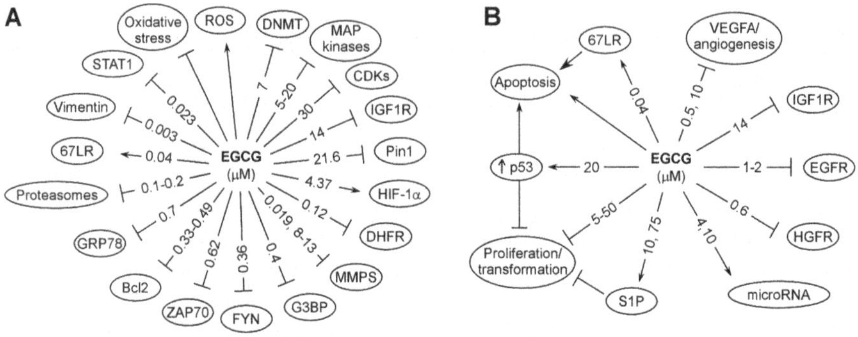

Fig. 8.2 Possible targets for the cancer preventive activity of EGCG (**a**) and subsequent cellular events (**b**). Some of these are through direct interactions, while others are affected indirectly (leftwards arrow, activation; turnstile symbol, inhibition). The reported effective concentrations, in IC50, Ki (inhibition constant) or Kd (dissociation constant) are shown in μM. All these are from studies in vitro. When two values are given, the first value is from cell-free systems and the second value is from studies in cell lines. *EGCG* (−)-epigallocatechin-3-gallate, *ROS* reactive oxygen species, *DNMT* DNA methyltransferase, *CDKs* cyclin-dependent kinases, *IGF1R* IGF1 receptor, *HIF-1α* hypoxia-inducible factor 1-alpha, *Pin1* peptidyl prolyl *cis/trans* isomerase, *DHFR* dihydrofolate reductase, *MMPS* matrix metalloproteinases, *G3BP* Ras-GTPase-activating protein SH3 domain-binding protein, *ZAP70* zeta-chain-associated protein kinase 70, *Bcl2* B-cell lymphoma 2, GRP78, glucose-regulated protein 78 kDa, *67LR* 67 kDa laminin receptor, *STAT1* signal transduction activator of transcription 1, *VEGFA* vascular endothelial growth factor A, *EGFR* epidermal growth factor, *HGFR* hepatocyte growth factor receptor, *SIP* sphingosine-1-phosphate receptor [from Yang and Hong (2013)]

8.5.1 Redox Activities and Carcinogen Detoxification

As discussed in earlier sections, catechins are well recognized as antioxidants, but they can also be pro-oxidants and generate ROS. ROS can alter the functions of cellular proteins, lipid and nucleic acids, and lead to different diseases (Dickinson and Chang 2011). Oxidative damage to DNA cause mutation and genomic instability, which are major contributing factors in the initiation, promotion and progression of carcinogenesis (Hussain et al. 2003). In animal models for carcinogenesis, ROS are induced by treatment with carcinogens, and EGCG could reduce the formation of 8-hydroxydeoxyguanosine (8-oxo-dG), a well-established marker for oxidative DNA damage that can mispair to induce mutations (Xu et al. 1992). As endogenously formed ROS are important in promoting carcinogenesis, tea catechins may have important roles in quenching these species at different stages of carcinogenesis. In human studies, administration of green tea to smokers for 4 weeks has been shown to significantly reduce the number of 8-oxo-dG-positive cells (Schwartz et al. 2005). Such antioxidant actions of tea catechins may reduce the risk of carcinogenesis.

Tea catechins can also be autoxidized to generate ROS in cell culture medium and cause cell death (Hou et al. 2005; Yang et al. 1998). After entering the cells, high concentrations of EGCG may also induce the production of ROS by a different mechanism, possibly involving the electron transport chain in the mitochondria (Tao et al. 2014). In our studies, oral administration of EGCG to mice bearing human lung cancer H1299 cell xenograft tumors inhibited tumor growth, enhanced tumor cell apoptosis, and produced ROS in the tumor cells (Li et al. 2010). The observed ROS accumulation in tumor cells is probably due to the lack of sufficient antioxidant enzymes in H1299 cells. It remains to be demonstrated whether the production of ROS is responsible for the induction of apoptosis in vivo. At modest doses (e.g., 0.5% EGCG in the diet), although increased levels of 8-oxo-dG and γ-H2AX (phosphorylated histone 2A variant X) were seen in xenograft tumors, 8-oxo-dG production and toxicity were not observed in the liver, kidney and other organs of the host mice (Li et al. 2010).

Cellular ROS may also activate the Nrf2-mediated signaling pathways to induce cytoprotective enzymes (Hayes and Dinkova-Kostova 2014). In human volunteers, supplementation with 800 mg PPE per day for 4 weeks increased glutathione *S*-transferase P activity in lymphocytes (Chow et al. 2007). In an intervention study in a high aflatoxin exposure area in China, supplementation with 500 or 1000 mg green tea polyphenols per day for 3 months increased the median urinary aflatoxin B1-mercapturic acid levels by more than ten-fold compared to baseline (Tang et al. 2008). This result is likely due to the induction of glutathione S-transferase by EGCG.

8.5.2 High Affinity Binding to Protein Targets

EGCG is known to bind to a variety of proteins with rather high affinities, through multiple hydrogen bonding to and hydrophobic interactions with proteins. In our previous work with molecular modeling, the inhibition of DNA methyltransferase (DNMT) 1 by EGCG was proposed to involve binding through 5 hydrogen bonds (Fang et al. 2003). Using an EGCG–Sepharose 4B column and 2D-gel electrophoresis, Dong et al. identified vimentin, IGF1R, FYN, glucose-regulated protein 78 kDa (GRP78), ZAP70 and Ras-GTPase-activating protein SH3 domain-binding protein 1 (G3BP1) (Shim et al. 2010) as high-affinity EGCG binding proteins [reviewed in Yang and Wang (2016)]. A subsequent X-ray crystallography study demonstrated the binding of EGCG to both the WW and PPIase domains of peptidyl prolyl cis/trans isomerase (Pin1) (Urusova et al. 2011). The direct binding of EGCG with Pin1 was confirmed and the binding inhibited Pin1 PPIase activity. This inhibition could have important biological consequences because Pin1 is required for full activation of AP-1, NFκB, β-catenin and other signaling pathways. Biochemical studies showed a dissociation constant of 21.6 μM for the binding of EGCG to Pin1. EGCG was shown to suppress the proliferation of cells expressing Pin1 and tumor growth in a xenograft mouse model Pin1 (Urusova et al. 2011).

Studies with surface plasmon resonance (SPR), molecular modeling and site directed mutagenesis found that EGCG (and ECG) could bind tightly to signal transduction activator of transcription 1 (STAT1) and block its phosphorylation by Janus kinase 2 (JAK2) in MDA-MB-231 breast cancer cells (Menegazzi et al. 2014).

Similar inhibitory mechanisms of EGCG may also occur in head and neck squamous carcinoma cells (Lin et al. 2012).

Although EGCG has been shown to bind many proteins with very low K_d valence, much higher EGCG concentrations are needed to inhibit the activities in cells. For example, vimentin bound to EGCG with a K_d of 3.3 nM, and studies in cultured cells showed that EGCG inhibited the phosphorylation of vimentin with $IC_{50} = 17$ μM. It is possible that EGCG binds nonspecifically to many macromolecules in the cells and therefore higher concentrations of EGCG needed to be added for sufficient amount of EGCG to reach the target molecule. The discovery of the aforementioned high-affinity EGCG-binding proteins is important; however, the direct involvement of these proteins in the action of EGCG in animal models and humans remains to be investigated. The binding of EGCG and other catechins to enzymes, receptors and transcription factors is likely the basis for the activities described in the following sections.

8.5.3 Inhibition of Enzyme Activities

EGCG and other catechins have been shown to bind and inhibit the activities of a variety of enzymes, such as different mitogen-activated protein (MAP) kinases, protein kinase B (AKT), chymotryptic activity of 20S proteasomes, MMP2, MMP9, DNMT1, dihydrofolate reductase, glucose-6-phosphate dehydrogenase, glyceraldehyde-3-phosphate dehydrogenase and carbonyl reductase [reviewed in Yang and Wang (2016)]. These results on enzyme inhibition are interesting. In many of the studies, however, the effective inhibitory concentration (or IC_{50}) was lower when lower concentrations of enzymes were used. This suggests nonspecific binding to the protein, and in order to inhibit these enzymes in vivo, the oral dose of catechins would be high. If some of these key enzymes in intermediate metabolism are inhibited in normal cells in vivo by tea consumption, the metabolic disturbance would be huge. Thus, these mechanisms may not be relevant for cancer prevention. For cancer therapy, the enzyme inhibition mechanism can only be relevant if catechins specifically target enzymes in cancer cells, but not normal cells.

8.5.4 Inhibition of Receptor Tyrosine Kinases and Other Receptors

Tea catechins have been shown to affect many receptor-mediated activities. Their inhibitory actions against receptor tyrosine kinases (RTKs) have been reviewed by Larsen et al. (2010) and Shimizu et al. (2011). All members of the RTK family, including epidermal growth factor receptor (EGFR), IGF1R, hepatocyte growth factor receptor (HGFR or c-Met) and vascular endothelial growth factor receptor

(VEGFR), consist of an extracellular ligand-binding domain, single membranes-spanning region and a cytoplasmic protein tyrosine kinase domain. All the receptors are known to involve cancer growth and progression. Many studies have demonstrated the inhibitory effects of EGCG on RTK signaling pathways (Liang et al. 1997; Adachi et al. 2007). Several mechanisms have been proposed for the inhibition of EGFR by EGCG: (a) interfering with the binding of EGF to EGFR and inhibiting EGFR tyrosine kinase activity, (b) altering lipid organization in the plasma membrane (lipid rafts) and inhibiting EGF binding to EGFR, and (c) inducing EGFR internalization without activation [reviewed in Yang and Wang (2016)].

8.5.5 *Effects on 67 kDa Laminin Receptor (67LR)*

The study on the activation of 67LR by EGCG is an impressive systematic study in different experimental systems. Binding of EGCG to the 67LR (with a K_d value of 0.04 μM) was first observed by Tachibana et al. using a SPR assay (Tachibana et al. 2004). Expression of the metastases-associated 67LR increased the responsiveness of MCF7 cells to low micromolar concentrations of EGCG (Tachibana et al. 2004). RNA interference (RNAi)-mediated silencing of 67LR abrogated EGCG-induced apoptosis in multiple myeloma (MM) cells (Umeda et al. 2008). Further studies in cultured macrophages showed that 67LR mediated anti-inflammation action of EGCG (Hong Byun et al. 2010). Anti-67LR antibody treatment or RNAi-mediated silencing of 67LR resulted in the abrogation of the inhibitory action of EGCG on lipopolysaccharide-induced activation of TLR4 and downstream signaling of inflammation. Subsequent work by Kumazoe et al. (2013) showed that the activation of 67LR by EGCG in primary MM cells and MM cell lines resulted in elevated levels of cGMP to initiate apoptosis. However, EGCG alone was not very effective in killing MM U266 cells (IC_{50} of 23.2 μM), because these cells overexpressed phosphodiesterase 5 (PDE5), which degrades cGMP. When a PDE5-selective inhibitor, vardenafil, was also added to cultured cells, it synergized with EGCG to reduce the IC_{50} of EGCG to 1.4 μM. This impressive synergism was also shown in a xenograft model, as well as in vitro in some breast, gastric, pancreatic and prostate cancer cell lines, which overexpresses both 67LR and PDE5 (Kumazoe et al. 2013). This line of studies may lead to advancements in cancer therapy. However, the involvement of 67LR in mediating the cancer prevention by EGCG still remains to be explored.

8.5.6 *Other Molecular Mechanisms*

Mixed or Unknown Mechanisms In some studies, signal pathways were modulated by catechins through direction or a combination of different mechanisms, for example, the Wnt signaling, which involves the nuclear translocation of β-catenin to transcriptionally activate effects on the genes such as c-Myc, cyclin D1 and COX-2. Studies in *Apc*$^{min/+}$ mice suggest that EGCG inhibits Wnt signaling. Treatment of HT29 human colon cancer cells with EGCG (20 μM) also decreased nuclear levels of β-catenin and the cellular levels of c-Myc and cyclin D1 (Hou et al. 2005). Subsequent studies also suggested that EGCG induced β-catenin *N*-terminal phosphorylation at the Ser33/37 residues and promoted its degradation (Oh et al. 2014; Singh and Katiyar 2013). EGCG was also shown to inhibit the Wnt signaling in hepatoblastoma cells, and this was found to be associated with the reexpression of the silenced tumor suppressor gene, secreted frizzled-related protein (SFRP)1, which is known to modulate Wnt signaling (Godeke et al. 2013). Another example is that many studies have demonstrated that EGCG treatment induces p53 expression and p53-dependent apoptosis: however, different mechanisms have been suggested in different cell line studies (Lee et al. 2011, 2010; Huang et al. 2009; Thakur et al. 2012). The involvement of p53 in the biological activity of EGCG requires additional studies in vitro and in vivo.

Epigenetic Mechanisms EGCG was reported to decrease the levels of 5-methylcytosine, DNMT activity, and expression levels of DNMT1, DNMT3a and DNMT3b in human epidermoid carcinoma A431 cells. It also decreased HDAC activity and affected levels of acetylated lysines on histones H3 and H4 (Nandakumar et al. 2011). Furthermore, EGCG inhibited acetyltransferase (HAT) enzymes (Choi et al. 2009) and inhibited the transcription of hTERT (human telomerase reverse transcriptase), the catalytic subunit of telomerase, through epigenetic mechanisms mediated at least partially through the inhibition of DNMT and HAT activities (Meeran et al. 2011).

Effect on microRNA MicroRNAs are small (about 22 bases) single-stranded, endogenous noncoding RNAs that negatively regulate the translation and/or stability of mRNAs (Bartel 2009). MicroRNA levels could be altered by EGCG to cause subtle changes in multiple molecular targets and pathways. It has been reported that EGCG upregulated miR-16 in HepG2 cells, and this led to the downregulation of Bcl2 and induction of apoptosis (Tsang and Kwok 2010). In our work in both human and mouse lung cancer cells in culture, we found that EGCG specifically upregulated the expression of mir-210, a major microRNA regulated by HIF-1α (Wang et al. 2011). The upregulation of mir-210 was found to be correlated with the transiently stabilized HIF-1α in lung cancer cell lines after EGCG treatment. We also demonstrated that EGCG could bind to the oxygen-dependent degradation (ODD) domain of the hypoxia-response element of HIF-1α promoter and prevented the hydroxylation-dependent ubiquitination and proteasome-mediated degradation of HIF-1α. The in vivo relevance of this observation, however, remains to be demonstrated. EGCG also upregulated miR-16 in breast cancer cell line 4T1 (Jang et al. 2013). The miR-16 could be transfected to tumor-associated macrophages (TAM) via exosomes and inhibited TAM infiltration and M2 microphage polarization. These actions were suggested to be responsible for the observed growth suppression of xenograft tumors from 4T1 cells in BALB/c mice treated with EGCG.

Binding to Lipids and Nucleic Acids The possibility that EGCG alters lipid organization in the plasma membrane (lipid rafts) and affect protein distribution and receptor functions has been proposed for the inhibition of the functions of EGFR, HGFR, and 67LR [reviewed in Yang and Wang (2016)]. Although interesting, it remains to be determined whether the effects occur in normal cells and cancer cells in vivo, and what concentrations of EGCG are required to exert an observable effect in vivo. Based on the physical binding of EGCG to nucleic acids, it has been suggested that DNA and RNA can also be targets of action of tea catechins (Kuzuhara et al. 2006). However, the relevance of this proposed binding depends on whether the catechins can bind selectively to specific nucleic acid in the genome of cancer or premalignant cells without affecting normal cells.

8.5.7 Indirect Physiological Effects

Tea catechins have been shown to reduce body weight gain and obesity (Yang and Hong 2013; Yang and Zhang 2019) and obesity enhances carcinogenesis at several organ sites (Khandekar et al. 2011). The possibility that green tea consumption decreases cancer risk through preventing obesity may occur in certain populations, and needs to be investigated. Consumption of tea polyphenols has been shown to affect gut microbiota in favor of the beneficial bacteria (Chen et al. 2019; Henning et al. 2018). Some of the anti-inflammatory activity of this microbiota may indirectly inhibit inflammation and carcinogenesis. Certain bacterial species (such as *Fusobacterium* nucleatum, colibactin *E. coli*, and enterotoxigenic *Bacteroides fragilis*) have been shown to promote or cause colon cancer (Tilg et al. 2018). It would be interesting to study the effect of TPP on the growth and activity of these bacteria.

There are also many recent studies on the effects of catechins, especially EGCG, on signal transduction pathways in different cancer cell lines [reviewed in Shirakami and Shimizu (2018), Negri et al. (2018), Khan and Mukhtar (2018)]. These actions are generally consistent to or in the same framework as the actions described above and are not described herein. Because of the broad cancer preventive activities of tea catechins in different animal models, multiple mechanisms are likely to be involved. Even in the same experimental system, a tea catechin, such as EGCG, may exhibit cancer inhibitory activities via more than one mechanism. It is interesting to consider the possibility that some of these actions may work additively or synergistically to exert the cancer preventive effects. Precise information about the mechanisms of cancer prevention by tea in humans is even more difficult to obtain. From the limited data that are available from human studies, actions of tea polyphenols in reducing oxidative stress, inhibiting inflammation and enhancing the metabolic elimination of carcinogens may be important.

8.6 Concluding Remarks

The above discussion on the cancer preventive activities of tea is based mostly on studies with green tea and green tea polyphenols. This will serve as a basis for understanding the cancer- preventive activities of other teas. For example, black teas are expected to have lower cancer-preventive activities because of the low or no systemic bioavailability of black tea polyphenols—theaflavins and thearubigins.

8.6.1 Issues in Extrapolating Studies In Vitro to Situations In Vivo

Many of the anti-cancer activities of tea polyphenols in the literature and most of the mechanistic information in the literature derived from studies in cell lines, mainly with EGCG. In relating observations in vitro to molecular events in vivo, an important issue is the concentrations used. In most animal cancer prevention studies, the EGCG levels in the blood and tissues were usually lower than 0.5 μM. How do we evaluate the relevance of an experiment using 10–100 μM EGCG in cell cultural studies? We previously compared the EGCG levels in blood and xenograft tumors of H1299 lung cancer cells and found that at conditions when tumor growth was inhibited ~50% (0.5% EGCG in the diet), the EGCG concentrations was 0.52 μM in blood and 0.18 μM in tumor tissues. These values were 2-orders of magnitude lower than the IC_{50} values of EGCG in the inhibition of H1299 cell growth in culture (Li et al. 2010). One possible reason for the observed discrepancy between the cell culture system and the xenograft model is the rather short-term exposure to EGCG in cell culture studies (24 or 48 h) compared to the long-term treatment in animal models. Prolonging the treatment period of cells in culture has been shown to reduce the effective concentration of EGCG (Shimizu et al. 2005). The environment for cells in culture is also very different from that in tumors. Therefore, we cannot rule out a mechanism just because the in vitro effective concentrations of EGCG are higher than we observed in vivo. However, it is reasonable to assume that activities effected by low concentrations of EGCG are likely to be more relevant than activities that are produced only at higher concentrations. Another concern is that events caused by ROS generated by EGCG extracellularly in cell culture studies may not occur in vivo (Hou et al. 2005). To avoid such a problem, we suggest the inclusion of SOD and catalase in the incubation mixture to prevent or minimize extracellular ROS generation.

8.6.2 Problems in Using Cancer Cell Lines for Cancer Prevention Research

A frequently asked question is whether all the actions of catechins observed in cancer cell lines are relevant for cancer prevention in vivo. Apparently, mechanisms suggested by cell line experiments and observed in cancer prevention studies in animal models are likely to be more relevant. These include the induction of apoptosis in different animal models, inhibition of the phosphorylation of c-Jun and ERK1/2 in lung tumorigenesis models, suppression of phospho-AKT and nuclear β-catenin levels in colon cancer models, inhibition of the IGF/IGF1R axis in colon and prostate cancer models, and suppression of VEGF-dependent angiogenesis in lung and prostate cancer models [reviewed in Yang and Wang (2016)]. It is still unclear whether these molecules are direct targets for EGCG or downstream events of the primary actions. A rationale for the use of cancer cell lines in cancer prevention research is that mechanisms observed in cancer cells may be applicable to inhibition of carcinogenesis, in particular cancer progression. However, the in vivo relevance of many of the reported mechanisms remain to be substantiated. In extrapolating results from laboratory studies to human cancer prevention, it is important to consider the relevance of the model system and the doses used in comparison to the doses of tea consumption by humans.

8.6.3 Possible Problems with Toxicity

Tea beverage is generally considered to be safe, even though some individuals may experience gastrointestinal irritation after drinking tea, established with an empty stomach. As was discussed in a previous section, in the Minnesota Green Tea Trial, daily consumption of 1315 mg of catechins (including 843 mg EGCG) by women caused elevated serum aminotransferase activities (indicative of liver toxicity) in 5.1% of the women. The dose was considered safe when we designed this trial based on information from human tea consumption. Even though the observed liver toxicity is reversible, this raises a concern for future chemoprevention trials with catechins. The liver toxicity of high doses of green tea extract-based weight-reduction supplements has been widely reported and the dose-dependent toxicity of catechins has been studied extensively in animal models [reviewed in Yang and Zhang (2019)]. Based on existing results, a tolerable upper intake level has been set at 300 mg of EGCG per day for humans by regulatory agents in some European countries, such as France and Italy (Yates et al. 2017; Dekant et al. 2017). This is for supplements in tablet forms. When the catechins are consumed in tea beverages throughout the day, the tolerable intake levels would be higher [reviewed in Yang and Zhang (2019)]. Clinical trials with PPE (2000 mg EGCG, twice daily for up to 6 months) have shown beneficial effects in patients with chronic lymphocytic leukemia (Shanafelt et al. 2013). There were side effects, which may be acceptable in short-term therapies for cancer patients, but are not acceptable for long-term use.

There are also many studies on the use of tea catechins and tea polyphenols in the form of nanoparticles to increase the efficiency of delivery in vitro and in vivo [reviewed in Khan and Mukhtar (2018)]. Indeed, the results are very impressive and may be useful in cancer therapy. However, if the nanoparticles do not specifically target cancer cells or specific organs, toxicity is still a concern. For cancer prevention, there will be more serious concerns on toxicity.

8.6.4 Future Studies

Even with the above reviewed laboratory and human studies, as well as the numerous mechanisms of action proposed for EGCG, the question whether tea consumption can prevent cancer in humans still remains unanswered. There seems to be enough evidence on cancer prevention from animal studies, but the classical approach of conducting human intervention trials has not provided clear answers. The current human trials have limitations in using high-risk populations with intervention for 1–3 years or even shorter. A long-term trial in a general population would be too expensive and too difficult to conduct. As described above, dose selection is also a major problem. In a double-blind trial, the tea polyphenols are usually delivered in tablet forms, and toxicity is a concern. Many investigators have conducted and advocated biomarker-based human cancer prevention trials. More efforts are needed to develop and use better biomarkers for tea exposure and effects that are relevant to cancer prevention.

In human cancer prevention, more specific questions should be asked about the protection against a specific type of cancer in a specified population, with environmental and genetic factors taken into consideration. Tea consumption apparently cannot "prevent all cancers" in different populations. As discussed in this chapter, the cancer preventive activity appeared stronger in women than men, but it is unclear whether this is mainly due to the more frequent use of tobacco in men or a gender difference. Well-conducted case-control studies with the dose of tea consumption in well-defined populations should be useful. More useful information on cancer prevention by tea will come from large, well-designed cohort studies. Laboratory scientists are in a good position to design and develop useful biomarkers for such studies.

Acknowledgements This work was supported by NIH grants CA120915, CA122474 and C141756. The author would like to thank Ms. Vi P. Dan for her assistance in preparing the manuscript.

References

Adachi S, Nagao T, Ingolfsson HI, Maxfield FR, Andersen OS, Kopelovich L, Weinstein IB (2007) The inhibitory effect of (−)-epigallocatechin gallate on activation of the epidermal growth factor receptor is associated with altered lipid order in ht29 colon cancer cells. Cancer Res 67:6493–6501

Adhami VM, Siddiqui IA, Ahmad N, Gupta S, Mukhtar H (2004) Oral consumption of green tea polyphenols inhibits insulin-like growth factor-i-induced signaling in an autochthonous mouse model of prostate cancer. Cancer Res 64:8715–8722

Balentine DA, Wiseman SA, Bouwens LC (1997) The chemistry of tea flavonoids. Crit Rev Food Sci Nutr 37:693–704

Bamia C, Lagiou P, Jenab M, Trichopoulou A, Fedirko V, Aleksandrova K, Pischon T, Overvad K, Olsen A, Tjonneland A, Boutron-Ruault MC, Fagherazzi G, Racine A, Kuhn T, Boeing H, Floegel A, Benetou V, Palli D, Grioni S, Panico S, Tumino R, Vineis P, Bueno-de-Mesquita HB, Dik VK, Bhoo-Pathy N, Uiterwaal CS, Weiderpass E, Lund E, Quiros JR, Zamora-Ros R, Molina-Montes E, Chirlaque MD, Ardanaz E, Dorronsoro M, Lindkvist B, Wallstrom P, Nilsson LM, Sund M, Khaw KT, Wareham N, Bradbury KE, Travis RC, Ferrari P, Duarte-Salles T, Stepien M, Gunter M, Murphy N, Riboli E, Trichopoulos D (2015) Coffee, tea and decaffeinated coffee in relation to hepatocellular carcinoma in a european population: multicentre, prospective cohort study. Int J Cancer 136:1899–1908

Bartel DP (2009) Micrornas: target recognition and regulatory functions. Cell 136:215–233

Bettuzzi S, Brausi M, Rizzi F, Castagnetti G, Peracchia G, Corti A (2006) Chemoprevention of human prostate cancer by oral administration of green tea catechins in volunteers with high-grade prostate intraepithelial neoplasia: a preliminary report from a one-year proof-of-principle study. Cancer Res 66:1234–1240

Chen YT, Wu Y, Du ML, Chu HY, Zhu LJ, Tong N, Zhang ZD, Wang ML, Gu DY, Chen JF (2017) An inverse association between tea consumption and colorectal cancer risk. Oncotarget 8:37367–37376

Chen T, Liu AB, Sun S, Ajami NJ, Ross MC, Wang H, Zhang L, Reuhl K, Kobayashi K, Onishi JC, Zhao L, Yang CS (2019) Green tea polyphenols modify the gut microbiome in db/db mice as co-abundance groups correlating with the blood glucose lowering effect. Mol Nutr Food Res 63: e1801064

Choi KC, Jung MG, Lee YH, Yoon JC, Kwon SH, Kang HB, Kim MJ, Cha JH, Kim YJ, Jun WJ, Lee JM, Yoon HG (2009) Epigallocatechin-3-gallate, a histone acetyltransferase inhibitor, inhibits ebv-induced b lymphocyte transformation via suppression of rela acetylation. Cancer Res 69:583–592

Chow HH, Hakim IA, Vining DR, Crowell JA, Tome ME, Ranger-Moore J, Cordova CA, Mikhael DM, Briehl MM, Alberts DS (2007) Modulation of human glutathione s-transferases by polyphenon e intervention. Cancer Epidemiol Biomark Prev 16:1662–1666

Chung FL, Wang M, Rivenson A, Iatropoulos MJ, Reinhardt JC, Pittman B, Ho CT, Amin SG (1998) Inhibition of lung carcinogenesis by black tea in fischer rats treated with a tobacco-specific carcinogen: caffeine as an important constituent. Cancer Res 58:4096–4101

Clifford MN, van der Hooft JJ, Crozier A (2013) Human studies on the absorption, distribution, metabolism, and excretion of tea polyphenols. Am J Clin Nutr 98:1619S–1630S

Coia H, Ma N, Hou Y, Dyba MD, Fu Y, Cruz MI, Benitez C, Graham GT, McCutcheon JN, Zheng YL, Sun B, Kallakury BV, Ma J, Fang HB, Berry DL, Muralidaran V, Chung FL (2018) Prevention of lipid peroxidation-derived cyclic DNA adduct and mutation in high-fat diet-induced hepatocarcinogenesis by theaphenon e. Cancer Prev Res (Phila) 11:665–676

Crespy V, Williamson G (2004) A review of the health effects of green tea catechins in in vivo animal models. J Nutr 134:3431S–3440S

Dekant W, Fujii K, Shibata E, Morita O, Shimotoyodome A (2017) Safety assessment of green tea based beverages and dried green tea extracts as nutritional supplements. Toxicol Lett 277:104–108

Dickinson BC, Chang CJ (2011) Chemistry and biology of reactive oxygen species in signaling or stress responses. Nat Chem Biol 7:504–511

Fang MZ, Wang Y, Ai N, Hou Z, Sun Y, Lu H, Welsh W, Yang CS (2003) Tea polyphenol (−)-epigallocatechin-3-gallate inhibits DNA methyltransferase and reactivates methylation-silenced genes in cancer cell lines. Cancer Res 63:7563–7570

Gao YT, McLaughlin JK, Blot WJ, Ji BT, Dai Q, Fraumeni JF Jr (1994) Reduced risk of esophageal cancer associated with green tea consumption. J Natl Cancer Inst 86:855–858

Gianfredi V, Nucci D, Abalsamo A, Acito M, Villarini M, Moretti M, Realdon S (2018) Green tea consumption and risk of breast cancer and recurrence-a systematic review and meta-analysis of observational studies. Nutrients 10. https://doi.org/10.3390/nu10121886

Godeke J, Maier S, Eichenmuller M, Muller-Hocker J, von Schweinitz D, Kappler R (2013) Epigallocatechin-3-gallate inhibits hepatoblastoma growth by reactivating the wnt inhibitor sfrp1. Nutr Cancer 65:1200–1207

Gupta S, Hastak K, Ahmad N, Lewin JS, Mukhtar H (2001) Inhibition of prostate carcinogenesis in tramp mice by oral infusion of green tea polyphenols. Proc Natl Acad Sci U S A 98:10350–10355

Hao X, Sun Y, Yang CS, Bose M, Lambert JD, Ju J, Lu G, Lee MJ, Park S, Husain A, Wang S (2007) Inhibition of intestinal tumorigenesis in apc(min/+) mice by green tea polyphenols (polyphenon e) and individual catechins. Nutr Cancer 59:62–69

Hao X, Xiao H, Ju J, Lee MJ, Lambert JD, Yang CS (2017) Green tea polyphenols inhibit colorectal tumorigenesis in azoxymethane-treated f344 rats. Nutr Cancer 69:623–631

Hayes JD, Dinkova-Kostova AT (2014) The nrf2 regulatory network provides an interface between redox and intermediary metabolism. Trends Biochem Sci 39:199–218

Henning SM, Yang J, Hsu M, Lee RP, Grojean EM, Ly A, Tseng CH, Heber D, Li Z (2018) Decaffeinated green and black tea polyphenols decrease weight gain and alter microbiome populations and function in diet-induced obese mice. Eur J Nutr 57(8):2759–2769

Hong Byun E, Fujimura Y, Yamada K, Tachibana H (2010) Tlr4 signaling inhibitory pathway induced by green tea polyphenol epigallocatechin-3-gallate through 67-kda laminin receptor. J Immunol 185:33–45

Hou Z, Sang S, You H, Lee MJ, Hong J, Chin KV, Yang CS (2005) Mechanism of action of (−)-epigallocatechin-3-gallate: auto-oxidation-dependent inactivation of epidermal growth factor receptor and direct effects on growth inhibition in human esophageal cancer kyse 150 cells. Cancer Res 65:8049–8056

Huang CH, Tsai SJ, Wang YJ, Pan MH, Kao JY, Way TD (2009) Egcg inhibits protein synthesis, lipogenesis, and cell cycle progression through activation of ampk in p53 positive and negative human hepatoma cells. Mol Nutr Food Res 53:1156–1165

Huang YQ, Lu X, Min H, Wu QQ, Shi XT, Bian KQ, Zou XP (2016) Green tea and liver cancer risk: a meta-analysis of prospective cohort studies in asian populations. Nutrition 32:3–8

Hussain SP, Hofseth LJ, Harris CC (2003) Radical causes of cancer. Nat Rev Cancer 3:276–285

James KD, Forester SC, Lambert JD (2015) Dietary pretreatment with green tea polyphenol, (−)-epigallocatechin-3-gallate reduces the bioavailability and hepatotoxicity of subsequent oral bolus doses of (−)-epigallocatechin-3-gallate. Food Chem Toxicol 76:103–108

Jang JY, Lee JK, Jeon YK, Kim CW (2013) Exosome derived from epigallocatechin gallate treated breast cancer cells suppresses tumor growth by inhibiting tumor-associated macrophage infiltration and m2 polarization. BMC Cancer 13:421

Ju J, Liu Y, Hong J, Huang MT, Conney AH, Yang CS (2003) Effects of green tea and high-fat diet on arachidonic acid metabolism and aberrant crypt foci formation in an azoxymethane-induced colon carcinogenesis mouse model. Nutr Cancer 46:172–178

Ju J, Hong J, Zhou JN, Pan Z, Bose M, Liao J, Yang GY, Liu YY, Hou Z, Lin Y, Ma J, Shih WJ, Carothers AM, Yang CS (2005) Inhibition of intestinal tumorigenesis in apcmin/+ mice by (−)-epigallocatechin-3-gallate, the major catechin in green tea. Cancer Res 65:10623–10631

Khan N, Mukhtar H (2018) Tea polyphenols in promotion of human health. Nutrients 11. https://doi.org/10.3390/nu11010039

Khandekar MJ, Cohen P, Spiegelman BM (2011) Molecular mechanisms of cancer development in obesity. Nat Rev Cancer 11:886–895

Kumar NB, Pow-Sang J, Egan KM, Spiess PE, Dickinson S, Salup R, Helal M, McLarty JW, Williams CR, Schreiber FMO, Parnes HL, Sebti S, Kazi A, Kang L, Quinn GP, Smith T, Yue B, Diaz K, Chornokur G, Crocker T, Schell MJ (2015) Randomized, placebo-controlled trial of green tea catechins for prostate cancer prevention. Cancer Prev Res (Phila) 8(10):879–887

Kumar NB, Dickinson SI, Schell MJ, Manley BJ, Poch MA, Pow-Sang J (2018) Green tea extract for prevention of prostate cancer progression in patients on active surveillance. Oncotarget 9:37798–37806

Kumazoe M, Sugihara K, Tsukamoto S, Huang Y, Tsurudome Y, Suzuki T, Suemasu Y, Ueda N, Yamashita S, Kim Y, Yamada K, Tachibana H (2013) 67-kda laminin receptor increases cgmp to induce cancer-selective apoptosis. J Clin Invest 123:787–799

Kuriyama S, Shimazu T, Ohmori K, Kikuchi N, Nakaya N, Nishino Y, Tsubono Y, Tsuji I (2006) Green tea consumption and mortality due to cardiovascular disease, cancer, and all causes in japan: the ohsaki study. JAMA 296:1255–1265

Kuzuhara T, Sei Y, Yamaguchi K, Suganuma M, Fujiki H (2006) DNA and rna as new binding targets of green tea catechins. J Biol Chem 281:17446–17456

Lambert JD, Hong J, Kim DH, Mishin VM, Yang CS (2004) Piperine enhances the bioavailability of the tea polyphenol (−)-epigallocatechin-3-gallate in mice. J Nutr 134:1948–1952

Larsen CA, Dashwood RH, Bisson WH (2010) Tea catechins as inhibitors of receptor tyrosine kinases: mechanistic insights and human relevance. Pharmacol Res 62:457–464

Lee MJ, Maliakal P, Chen L, Meng X, Bondoc FY, Prabhu S, Lambert G, Mohr S, Yang CS (2002) Pharmacokinetics of tea catechins after ingestion of green tea and (−)-epigallocatechin-3-gallate by humans: Formation of different metabolites and individual variability. Cancer Epidemiol Biomark Prev 11:1025–1032

Lee JH, Jeong YJ, Lee SW, Kim D, Oh SJ, Lim HS, Oh HK, Kim SH, Kim WJ, Jung JY (2010) Egcg induces apoptosis in human laryngeal epidermoid carcinoma hep2 cells via mitochondria with the release of apoptosis-inducing factor and endonuclease g. Cancer Lett 290:68–75

Lee MH, Han DW, Hyon SH, Park JC (2011) Apoptosis of human fibrosarcoma ht-1080 cells by epigallocatechin-3-o-gallate via induction of p53 and caspases as well as suppression of bcl-2 and phosphorylated nuclear factor-kappab. Apoptosis 16:75–85

Li N, Sun Z, Han C, Chen J (1999) The chemopreventive effects of tea on human oral precancerous mucosa lesions. Proc Soc Exp Biol Med 220:218–224

Li C, Lee MJ, Sheng S, Meng X, Prabhu S, Winnik B, Huang B, Chung JY, Yan S, Ho CT, Yang CS (2000) Structural identification of two metabolites of catechins and their kinetics in human urine and blood after tea ingestion. Chem Res Toxicol 13:177–184

Li GX, Chen YK, Hou Z, Xiao H, Jin H, Lu G, Lee MJ, Liu B, Guan F, Yang Z, Yu A, Yang CS (2010) Pro-oxidative activities and dose-response relationship of (−)-epigallocatechin-3-gallate in the inhibition of lung cancer cell growth: a comparative study in vivo and in vitro. Carcinogenesis 31:902–910

Liang YC, Lin-shiau SY, Chen CF, Lin JK (1997) Suppression of extracellular signals and cell proliferation through egf receptor binding by (−)-epigallocatechin gallate in human a431 epidermoid carcinoma cells. J Cell Biochem 67:55–65

Lin HY, Hou SC, Chen SC, Kao MC, Yu CC, Funayama S, Ho CT, Way TD (2012) (−)-epigallocatechin gallate induces fas/cd95-mediated apoptosis through inhibiting constitutive and il-6-induced jak/stat3 signaling in head and neck squamous cell carcinoma cells. J Agric Food Chem 60:2480–2489

Liu J, Liu S, Zhou H, Hanson T, Yang L, Chen Z, Zhou M (2016) Association of green tea consumption with mortality from all-cause, cardiovascular disease and cancer in a chinese cohort of 165,000 adult men. Eur J Epidemiol 31:853–865

Liu AB, Tao S, Lee MJ, Hu Q, Meng X, Lin Y, Yang CS (2018) Effects of gut microbiota and time of treatment on tissue levels of green tea polyphenols in mice. Biofactors. https://doi.org/10.1002/biof.1430

Lu G, Liao J, Yang G, Reuhl KR, Hao X, Yang CS (2006) Inhibition of adenoma progression to adenocarcinoma in a 4-(methylnitrosamino)-1-(3-pyridyl)-1-butanone-induced lung tumorigenesis model in a/j mice by tea polyphenols and caffeine. Cancer Res 66:11494–11501
Meeran SM, Patel SN, Chan TH, Tollefsbol TO (2011) A novel prodrug of epigallocatechin-3-gallate: differential epigenetic htert repression in human breast cancer cells. Cancer Prev Res 4:1243–1254
Menegazzi M, Mariotto S, Dal Bosco M, Darra E, Vaiana N, Shoji K, Safwat AA, Marechal JD, Perahia D, Suzuki H, Romeo S (2014) Direct interaction of natural and synthetic catechins with signal transducer activator of transcription 1 affects both its phosphorylation and activity. FEBS J 281:724–738
Meng X, Sang S, Zhu N, Lu H, Sheng S, Lee MJ, Ho CT, Yang CS (2002) Identification and characterization of methylated and ring-fission metabolites of tea catechins formed in humans, mice, and rats. Chem Res Toxicol 15:1042–1050
Meselhy MR, Nakamura N, Hattori M (1997) Biotransformation of (−)-epicatechin 3-o-gallate by human intestinal bacteria. Chem Pharm Bull (Tokyo) 45:888–893
Miyata Y, Shida Y, Hakariya T, Sakai H (2019) Anti-cancer effects of green tea polyphenols against prostate cancer. Molecules 24. https://doi.org/10.3390/molecules24010193
Najafi MN, Salehi M, Ghazanfarpour M, Hoseini ZS, Khadem-Rezaiyan M (2018) The association between green tea consumption and breast cancer risk: a systematic review and meta-analysis. Phytother Res 32:1855–1864
Nandakumar V, Vaid M, Katiyar SK (2011) (−)-epigallocatechin-3-gallate reactivates silenced tumor suppressor genes, cip1/p21 and p16ink4a, by reducing DNA methylation and increasing histones acetylation in human skin cancer cells. Carcinogenesis 32:537–544
Negri A, Naponelli V, Rizzi F, Bettuzzi S (2018) Molecular targets of epigallocatechin-gallate (egcg): a special focus on signal transduction and cancer. Nutrients 10. https://doi.org/10.3390/nu10121936
Ni CX, Gong H, Liu Y, Qi Y, Jiang CL, Zhang JP (2017) Green tea consumption and the risk of liver cancer: a meta-analysis. Nutr Cancer 69:211–220
Oh S, Gwak J, Park S, Yang CS (2014) Green tea polyphenol egcg suppresses wnt/beta-catenin signaling by promoting gsk-3beta- and pp2a-independent beta-catenin phosphorylation/degradation. Biofactors 40:586–595
Rawangkan A, Wongsirisin P, Namiki K, Iida K, Kobayashi Y, Shimizu Y, Fujiki H, Suganuma M (2018) Green tea catechin is an alternative immune checkpoint inhibitor that inhibits pd-l1 expression and lung tumor growth. Molecules 23. https://doi.org/10.3390/molecules23082071
Roth M, Timmermann BN, Hagenbuch B (2011) Interactions of green tea catechins with organic anion-transporting polypeptides. Drug Metab Dispos 39:920–926
Samavat H, Ursin G, Emory TH, Lee E, Wang R, Torkelson CJ, Dostal AM, Swenson K, Le CT, Yang CS, Yu MC, Yee D, Wu AH, Yuan JM, Kurzer MS (2017) A randomized controlled trial of green tea extract supplementation and mammographic density in postmenopausal women at increased risk of breast cancer. Cancer Prev Res (Phila) 10:710–718
Sang S, Lee MJ, Yang I, Buckley B, Yang CS (2008) Human urinary metabolite profile of tea polyphenols analyzed by liquid chromatography/electrospray ionization tandem mass spectrometry with data-dependent acquisition. Rapid Commun Mass Spectrom 22:1567–1578
Sang S, Lambert JD, Ho CT, Yang CS (2011) The chemistry and biotransformation of tea constituents. Pharmacol Res 64:87–99
Sasazuki S, Tamakoshi A, Matsuo K, Ito H, Wakai K, Nagata C, Mizoue T, Tanaka K, Tsuji I, Inoue M, Tsugane S (2012) Green tea consumption and gastric cancer risk: An evaluation based on a systematic review of epidemiologic evidence among the japanese population. Jpn J Clin Oncol 42:335–346
Schwartz JL, Baker V, Larios E, Chung FL (2005) Molecular and cellular effects of green tea on oral cells of smokers: a pilot study. Mol Nutr Food Res 49:43–51
Shanafelt TD, Call TG, Zent CS, Leis JF, LaPlant B, Bowen DA, Roos M, Laumann K, Ghosh AK, Lesnick C, Lee MJ, Yang CS, Jelinek DF, Erlichman C, Kay NE (2013) Phase 2 trial of daily, oral polyphenon e in patients with asymptomatic, rai stage 0 to ii chronic lymphocytic leukemia. Cancer 119:363–370

Shen G, Xu C, Hu R, Jain MR, Nair S, Lin W, Yang CS, Chan JY, Kong AN (2005) Comparison of (−)-epigallocatechin-3-gallate elicited liver and small intestine gene expression profiles between c57bl/6j mice and c57bl/6j/nrf2 (−/−) mice. Pharm Res 22:1805–1820
Shim JH, Su ZY, Chae JI, Kim DJ, Zhu F, Ma WY, Bode AM, Yang CS, Dong Z (2010) Epigallocatechin gallate suppresses lung cancer cell growth through ras-gtpase-activating protein sh3 domain-binding protein 1. Cancer Prev Res 3:670–679
Shimizu M, Deguchi A, Lim JT, Moriwaki H, Kopelovich L, Weinstein IB (2005) (−)-epigallocatechin gallate and polyphenon e inhibit growth and activation of the epidermal growth factor receptor and human epidermal growth factor receptor-2 signaling pathways in human colon cancer cells. Clin Cancer Res 11:2735–2746
Shimizu M, Shirakami Y, Sakai H, Adachi S, Hata K, Hirose Y, Tsurumi H, Tanaka T, Moriwaki H (2008a) (−)-epigallocatechin gallate suppresses azoxymethane-induced colonic premalignant lesions in male c57bl/ksj-db/db mice. Cancer Prev Res 1:298–304
Shimizu M, Fukutomi Y, Ninomiya M, Nagura K, Kato T, Araki H, Suganuma M, Fujiki H, Moriwaki H (2008b) Green tea extracts for the prevention of metachronous colorectal adenomas: A pilot study. Cancer Epidemiol Biomark Prev 17:3020–3025
Shimizu M, Adachi S, Masuda M, Kozawa O, Moriwaki H (2011) Cancer chemoprevention with green tea catechins by targeting receptor tyrosine kinases. Mol Nutr Food Res 55:832–843
Shin CM, Lee DH, Seo AY, Lee HJ, Kim SB, Son WC, Kim YK, Lee SJ, Park SH, Kim N, Park YS, Yoon H (2018) Green tea extracts for the prevention of metachronous colorectal polyps among patients who underwent endoscopic removal of colorectal adenomas: a randomized clinical trial. Clin Nutr 37:452–458
Shirakami Y, Shimizu M (2018) Possible mechanisms of green tea and its constituents against cancer. Molecules 23:2284
Singh T, Katiyar SK (2013) Green tea polyphenol, (−)-epigallocatechin-3-gallate, induces toxicity in human skin cancer cells by targeting beta-catenin signaling. Toxicol Appl Pharmacol 273:418–424
Stalmach A, Troufflard S, Serafini M, Crozier A (2009) Absorption, metabolism and excretion of choladi green tea flavan-3-ols by humans. Mol Nutr Food Res 53(Suppl 1):S44–S53
Stalmach A, Mullen W, Steiling H, Williamson G, Lean ME, Crozier A (2010) Absorption, metabolism, and excretion of green tea flavan-3-ols in humans with an ileostomy. Mol Nutr Food Res 54:323–334
Sun CL, Yuan JM, Lee MJ, Yang CS, Gao YT, Ross RK, Yu MC (2002) Urinary tea polyphenols in relation to gastric and esophageal cancers: a prospective study of men in shanghai, china. Carcinogenesis 23:1497–1503
Tachibana H, Koga K, Fujimura Y, Yamada K (2004) A receptor for green tea polyphenol egcg. Nat Struct Mol Biol 11:380–381
Tamura T, Wada K, Konishi K, Goto Y, Mizuta F, Koda S, Hori A, Tanabashi S, Matsushita S, Tokimitsu N, Nagata C (2018) Coffee, green tea, and caffeine intake and liver cancer risk: a prospective cohort study. Nutr Cancer 70(8):1210–1216
Tang L, Tang M, Xu L, Luo H, Huang T, Yu J, Zhang L, Gao W, Cox SB, Wang JS (2008) Modulation of aflatoxin biomarkers in human blood and urine by green tea polyphenols intervention. Carcinogenesis 29:411–417
Tao L, Forester SC, Lambert JD (2014) The role of the mitochondrial oxidative stress in the cytotoxic effects of the green tea catechin, (−)-epigallocatechin-3-gallate, in oral cells. Mol Nutr Food Res 58:665–676
Thakur VS, Gupta K, Gupta S (2012) Green tea polyphenols increase p53 transcriptional activity and acetylation by suppressing class i histone deacetylases. Int J Oncol 41:353–361
Tilg H, Adolph TE, Gerner RR, Moschen AR (2018) The intestinal microbiota in colorectal cancer. Cancer Cell 33:954–964
Tsang WP, Kwok TT (2010) Epigallocatechin gallate up-regulation of mir-16 and induction of apoptosis in human cancer cells. J Nutr Biochem 21:140–146

Tsao AS, Liu D, Martin J, Tang XM, Lee JJ, El-Naggar AK, Wistuba I, Culotta KS, Mao L, Gillenwater A, Sagesaka YM, Hong WK, Papadimitrakopoulou V (2009) Phase ii randomized, placebo-controlled trial of green tea extract in patients with high-risk oral premalignant lesions. Cancer Prev Res (Phila) 2:931–941

Umeda D, Yano S, Yamada K, Tachibana H (2008) Green tea polyphenol epigallocatechin-3-gallate signaling pathway through 67-kda laminin receptor. J Biol Chem 283:3050–3058

Urusova DV, Shim JH, Kim DJ, Jung SK, Zykova TA, Carper A, Bode AM, Dong Z (2011) Epigallocatechin-gallate suppresses tumorigenesis by directly targeting pin1. Cancer Prev Res 4:1366–1377

Wang ZY, Hong JY, Huang MT, Reuhl KR, Conney AH, Yang CS (1992) Inhibition of n-nitrosodiethylamine- and 4-(methylnitrosamino)-1-(3-pyridyl)-1-butanone-induced tumorigenesis in a/j mice by green tea and black tea. Cancer Res 52:1943–1947

Wang H, Bian S, Yang CS (2011) Green tea polyphenol egcg suppresses lung cancer cell growth through upregulating mir-210 expression caused by stabilizing hif-1alpha. Carcinogenesis 32:1881–1889

Wang L, Zhang X, Liu J, Shen L, Li Z (2014) Tea consumption and lung cancer risk: a meta-analysis of case-control and cohort studies. Nutrition 30:1122–1127

Wang D, Wang Y, Wan X, Yang CS, Zhang J (2015) Green tea polyphenol (−)-epigallocatechin-3-gallate triggered hepatotoxicity in mice: Responses of major antioxidant enzymes and the nrf2 rescue pathway. Toxicol Appl Pharmacol 283:65–74

Wang Y, Kan Z, Thompson HJ, Ling T, Ho CT, Li D, Wan X (2018) Impact of six typical processing methods on the chemical composition of tea leaves using a single camellia sinensis cultivar, longjing 43. J Agric Food Chem

Weng MW, Lee HW, Park SH, Hu Y, Wang HT, Chen LC, Rom WN, Huang WC, Lepor H, Wu XR, Yang CS, Tang MS (2018) Aldehydes are the predominant forces inducing DNA damage and inhibiting DNA repair in tobacco smoke carcinogenesis. Proc Natl Acad Sci U S A 115: E6152–E6161

Xiao H, Hao X, Simi B, Ju J, Jiang H, Reddy BS, Yang CS (2008) Green tea polyphenols inhibit colorectal aberrant crypt foci (acf) formation and prevent oncogenic changes in dysplastic acf in azoxymethane-treated f344 rats. Carcinogenesis 29:113–119

Xiong J, Lin J, Wang A, Wang Y, Zheng Y, Sang X, Xu Y, Lu X, Zhao H (2017) Tea consumption and the risk of biliary tract cancer: a systematic review and dose-response meta-analysis of observational studies. Oncotarget 8:39649–39657

Xu Y, Ho CT, Amin SG, Han C, Chung FL (1992) Inhibition of tobacco-specific nitrosamine-induced lung tumorigenesis in a/j mice by green tea and its major polyphenol as antioxidants. Cancer Res 52:3875–3879

Yang CS, Hong J (2013) Prevention of chronic diseases by tea: possible mechanisms and human relevance. Annu Rev Nutr 33:161–181

Yang JD, Malhi H (2018) Green tea consumption: a potential chemopreventive measure for hepatocellular carcinoma? Hepatology 67:10–12

Yang CS, Wang ZY (1993) Tea and cancer. J Natl Cancer Inst 85:1038–1049

Yang CS, Wang H (2016) Cancer preventive activities of tea catechins. Molecules 21:1679

Yang CS, Zhang J (2019) Studies on the prevention of cancer and cardiometabolic diseases by tea: issues on mechanisms, effective doses and toxicities. J Agric Food Chem 67(19):5446–5456

Yang GY, Liao J, Kim K, Yurkow EJ, Yang CS (1998) Inhibition of growth and induction of apoptosis in human cancer cell lines by tea polyphenols. Carcinogenesis 19:611–616

Yang CS, Lee MJ, Chen L (1999) Human salivary tea catechin levels and catechin esterase activities: implication in human cancer prevention studies. Cancer Epidemiol Biomark Prev 8:83–89

Yang CS, Sang S, Lambert JD, Lee MJ (2008) Bioavailability issues in studying the health effects of plant polyphenolic compounds. Mol Nutr Food Res 52(Suppl 1):S139–S151

Yang CS, Wang X, Lu G, Picinich SC (2009) Cancer prevention by tea: animal studies, molecular mechanisms and human relevance. Nat Rev Cancer 9:429–439

Yang CS, Wang H, Li GX, Yang Z, Guan F, Jin H (2011) Cancer prevention by tea: evidence from laboratory studies. Pharmacol Res 64:113–122

Yates AA, Erdman JW Jr, Shao A, Dolan LC, Griffiths JC (2017) Bioactive nutrients – time for tolerable upper intake levels to address safety. Regul Toxicol Pharmacol 84:94–101

Yu Z, Samavat H, Dostal AM, Wang R, Torkelson CJ, Yang CS, Butler LM, Kensler TW, Wu AH, Kurzer MS, Yuan JM (2017) Effect of green tea supplements on liver enzyme elevation: results from a randomized intervention study in the united states. Cancer Prev Res (Phila) 10:571–579

Yuan JM, Sun C, Butler LM (2011) Tea and cancer prevention: epidemiological studies. Pharmacol Res 64:123–135

Zhang Y, Hays A, Noblett A, Thapa M, Hua DH, Hagenbuch B (2013) Transport by oatp1b1 and oatp1b3 enhances the cytotoxicity of epigallocatechin 3-o-gallate and several quercetin derivatives. J Nat Prod 76:368–373

Zhang D, Kaushiva A, Xi Y, Wang T, Li N (2018) Non-herbal tea consumption and ovarian cancer risk: a systematic review and meta-analysis of observational epidemiologic studies with indirect comparison and dose-response analysis. Carcinogenesis 39:808–818

Zhao LG, Li HL, Sun JW, Yang Y, Ma X, Shu XO, Zheng W, Xiang YB (2017) Green tea consumption and cause-specific mortality: results from two prospective cohort studies in china. J Epidemiol 27:36–41

Zhou Q, Li H, Zhou JG, Ma Y, Wu T, Ma H (2016) Green tea, black tea consumption and risk of endometrial cancer: a systematic review and meta-analysis. Arch Gynecol Obstet 293:143–155

Zhou H, Wu W, Wang F, Qi H, Cheng Z (2018) Tea consumption is associated with decreased risk of oral cancer: a comprehensive and dose-response meta-analysis based on 14 case-control studies (moose compliant). Medicine (Baltimore) 97:e13611

Chapter 9
The Chemopreventive Power of Isothiocyanates

Sharadha Dayalan Naidu, Lidia Brodziak-Jarosz, Clarissa Gerhäuser, and Albena T. Dinkova-Kostova

Abstract Isothiocyanates are derived from their naturally-occurring glucosinolate precursors, which are abundant in cruciferous vegetables. Numerous scientific studies beginning more than half a century ago have documented the chemoprotective activities of these compounds. Isothiocyanates have numerous protein targets through which they exert protection in the context of various diseases such as cancer, neurodegeneration, inflammatory disease, metabolic disease and infection. The major mechanisms by which the isothiocyanates confer protection involve induction of stress response pathways that restore the cellular redox and protein homeostasis, and contribute to resolution of inflammation. However, high concentrations of isothiocyanates cause cell cycle arrest and selectively kill cancer cells by inducing

---

This chapter is dedicated to Paul Talalay MD (1923–2019) whose vision, scientific rigour, and insightful mentoring have inspired the work and influenced the lives of generations of scientists. He was a pioneer in cancer chemoprevention, famously saying of the early days of the field 'no room was small enough to accommodate the few who were interested'. His leadership in quantitative discovery science culminated in the isolation from broccoli of the isothiocyanate sulforaphane as inducer of cytoprotective enzymes, leading to the exponential growth of research on sulforaphane worldwide and its current development for disease prevention in humans. Although we have lost our hero, the treasure of his legacy will always be kept.

S. Dayalan Naidu
Department of Pharmacology and Molecular Sciences, Johns Hopkins University School of Medicine, Baltimore, MD, USA

L. Brodziak-Jarosz · C. Gerhäuser
Division of Epigenomics and Cancer Risk Factors, German Cancer Research Center, Heidelberg, Germany

A. T. Dinkova-Kostova (✉)
Department of Pharmacology and Molecular Sciences, Johns Hopkins University School of Medicine, Baltimore, MD, USA

Division of Cellular Medicine, School of Medicine, University of Dundee, Dundee, Scotland, UK

Department of Medicine, Johns Hopkins University School of Medicine, Baltimore, MD, USA
e-mail: adinkovakostova@dundee.ac.uk

J. M. Pezzuto, O. Vang (eds.), *Natural Products for Cancer Chemoprevention*,
https://doi.org/10.1007/978-3-030-39855-2_9

apoptosis, autophagy or necrosis. In this review, we present readers with a detailed overview of isothiocyanates functions and discuss their molecular targets and anti-neoplastic effects. Furthermore, we provide an up-to-date summary of the evidence on the chemoprotective activities of the most widely-studied isothiocyanates: sulforaphane, phenethyl isothiocyanate (PEITC) and benzyl isothiocyanate (BITC).

Keywords Isothiocyanates · Cancer · Chemoprevention · Sulforaphane · PEITC · BITC

9.1 Introduction

Isothiocyanates (ITCs) are biologically active molecules which are derived from glucosinolate phytochemical precursors. Glucosinolates are *S*-β-thioglucoside *N*-hydroxysulfates (Fig. 9.1) that are abundant in cruciferous (Brassicacea) plants. Chemically, there are three different types of glucosinolates, according to the origin of their side chain: (1) aromatic (from Phe or Tyr); (2) aliphatic (from Leu, Ile, Met, or Val); and (3) indole (from Trp) (Fahey et al. 2001; Halkier and Gershenzon 2006). The same plants which contain glucosinolates also have β-thioglucosidase enzymes, known as myrosinases (EC 3.2.3.1), which, however, are physically separated from their glucosinolate substrates. Enzyme and substrate only come in contact when the integrity of the plant tissue is compromised, such as during injury or chewing. The myrosinase reaction results in rapid hydrolysis of the glucosinolates to give rise to a variety of reactive compounds (Fig. 9.1). ITCs represent one of the major types of products of the myrosinase reaction and contribute to most of the biological effects that have been associated with glucosinolates. Around 120 natural ITCs have been identified so far (Verkerk et al. 2009; Herr and Buchler 2010).

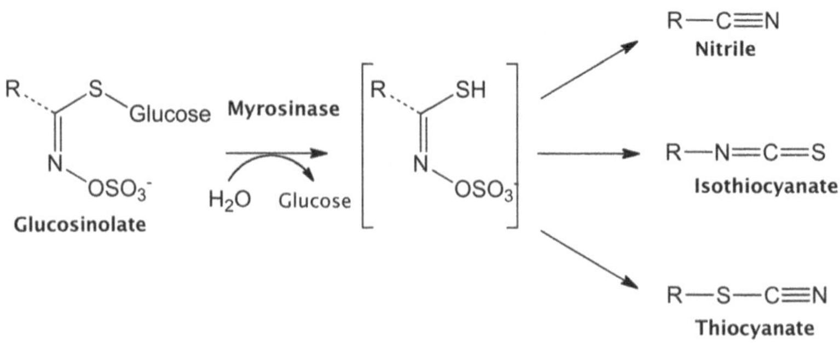

Fig. 9.1 The myrosinase reaction. Glucosinolates are hydrolyzed by β-thioglucosidases (myrosinases) to give unstable aglucones and liberate glucose. Depending on the reaction conditions, a variety of reactive products can be formed, the most common of which are nitriles, isothiocyanates and thiocyanates

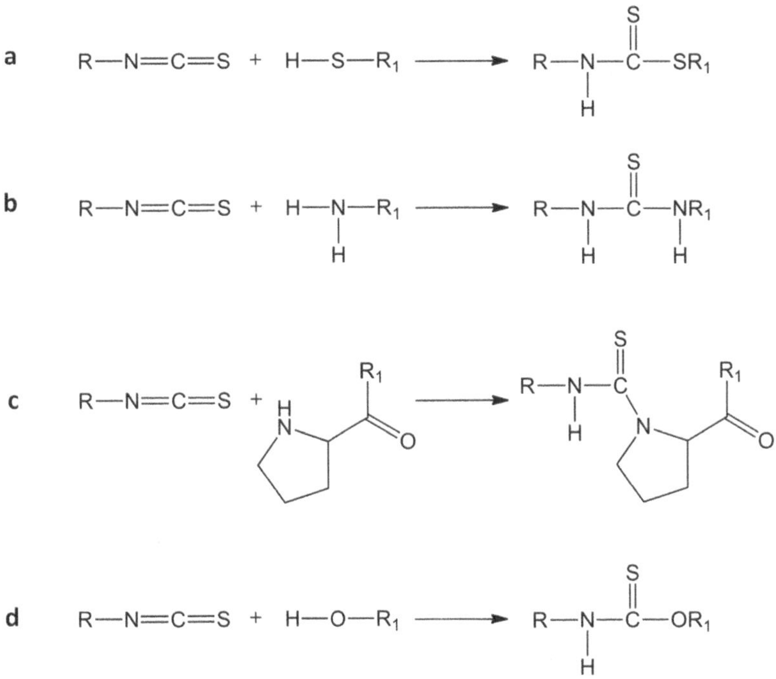

Fig. 9.2 Reactivity of isothiocyanates. The central carbon of the isothiocyante (—N=C=S) group is electrophilic and reacts readily with sulfur-, nitrogen-, and oxygen-centered nucleophiles. The most common reactions are: (**a**) conjugation with sulfhydryl groups, such as the sulfhydryl group of cysteine, (**b**) alkylation with α-amino groups in N-terminal residues and the ε-amino group of lysine, (**c**) reactions with the secondary amine in proline, and (**d**) reactions with hydroxyl group-containing residues, such as tyrosine

ITCs are characterized by high chemical reactivity due to the electrophilicity of the central carbon of the isothiocyanate (—N=C=S) group. The ITC group reacts readily with sulfur-, nitrogen-, and oxygen-centered nucleophiles (Fig. 9.2). Cysteine residues in proteins and glutathione (GSH) are the most common targets of ITCs, forming thiocarbamate products. The α-amino groups in N-terminal residues of proteins, the ε-amino groups of lysines, or even secondary amines, such as proline, can participate in alkylation reactions with ITCs, forming thiourea products. Finally, under certain although not physiological conditions, ITCs can also react with hydroxyl group-containing amino acid residues (e.g., tyrosine).

Natural ITCs or their synthetic analogs have been shown to prevent cancer development by limiting the exposure of cells to carcinogenic insults, thereby interfering with the initiation stage of carcinogenesis. The main mechanisms of early prevention include inhibition of intracellular activation of pro-carcinogens or acceleration of carcinogen detoxification. ITCs have been found to modulate transcript levels and inhibit phase I drug metabolizing enzymes, such as cytochrome P450 oxidases, involved in bioactivation of pro-carcinogens (Verkerk et al. 2009;

Herr and Buchler 2010). The potential and mechanisms of ITCs to induce cytoprotective enzymes are discussed in detail below, using sulforaphane as an example. Some of the mechanisms of cancer prevention by ITCs independent of their effects on carcinogen detoxification have been attributed at least in part to their cytotoxic properties. The current knowledge in this area will also be covered, emphasizing the molecular targets and signaling pathways contributing to ITCs toxicity towards cancer cells. In addition, ITCs have been reported to potently suppress the promotion and progression of carcinogenesis by affecting various signaling pathways related to inflammation (Heiss et al. 2001), angiogenesis (Xiao and Singh 2007; Bertl et al. 2006), autophagy (Powolny et al. 2011) metastasis formation (Wu et al. 2010), and dysregulation of gap junctional intercellular communications (Forster et al. 2014). Several reviews have discussed previously the various aspects of the mechanisms involved in the chemopreventive potential of ITCs (Antosiewicz et al. 2008; Cheung and Kong 2010; Fimognari et al. 2012; Jacob et al. 2011; Loo 2003; Prashar et al. 2012; Valgimigli and Iori 2009; Wu et al. 2009; Wu and Hua 2007; Zhang 2010; Zhang et al. 2005, 2006a).

9.2 The Diverse Family of Cytoprotective Proteins

A large family of proteins protects eukaryotic cells and organisms against the toxicities of electrophiles and oxidants which are the major causes of chronic degenerative diseases (Dinkova-Kostova and Talalay 2008, 2010). This family comprises enzymes that are involved in the metabolism and transport of a wide array of endo- and xenobiotics, as well as those that have direct and indirect antioxidant activities. Their functional diversity is truly extraordinary, and some examples are given in Table 9.1.

Notably, the distinction between *direct* and *indirect* antioxidant enzymes is not always straight-forward as many of these proteins perform both functions. For example, NQO1 is an *indirect* antioxidant enzyme because, by catalyzing the obligatory 2 electron-reduction of quinones, it prevents the formation of semiquinone radicals which, in the presence of oxygen, could lead to redox cycling, glutathione depletion, and oxidative stress (Dinkova-Kostova and Talalay 2010). NQO1 is also a *direct* antioxidant enzyme by virtue of its superoxide scavenging activity (Siegel et al. 2004). What is most important however is the fact that the inducibility and the enormous functional diversity of these cytoprotective enzymes underlie the capacity of the cell to mount a coordinate robust response to various conditions of stress, allowing adaptation and survival. It is thus not surprising that the genes coding for cytoprotective proteins share a common transcriptional regulation, with transcription factor Nrf2 (*N*F-E2 p45-*r*elated *F*actor *2*) being the master regulator of their expression (Motohashi and Yamamoto 2004). In addition to its direct influence on the transcription of cytoprotective genes, it is becoming increasingly clear that some of the protective effects of Nrf2 activation are mediated through cross-talks with other transcription factors, such as the aryl hydrocarbon receptor (AhR), nuclear factor κB (NF-κB), p53, and Notch1 (Wakabayashi et al. 2010).

Table 9.1 The diverse family of cytoprotective proteins

Protein function	Examples
Conjugation	Glutathione *S*-transferases (GSTs) UDP-glucuronosyltransferases (UGTs)
Export of xenobiotics and/or their metabolites	Solute carrier transporters ATP-binding cassette transporters
Synthesis, regeneration, utilization of glutathione	γ-Glutamate-cysteine ligase (γ-GCL) Glutathione reductase GSTs
Antioxidant enzymes	Heme oxygenase 1 (HO-1) NAD(P)H:Quinone oxidoreductase 1 (NQO1) GSTs
Synthesis of reducing equivalents	Glucose 6-phosphate dehydrogenase 6-Phosphogluconate dehydrogenase Malic enzyme 1 (ME1) Isocitrate dehydrogenase 1 (IDH1)
Anti-inflammatory enzymes	Leukotriene B_4 dehydrogenase
Prevention of damage by metal overload	Ferritin Metallothioneins
Repair and removal of misfolded or damaged proteins	Proteosomal subunits Proteins involved in autophagy

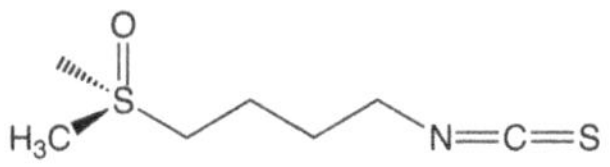

Fig. 9.3 Chemical structure of sulforaphane [1-isothiocyanato-(4*R*)-(methylsulfinyl)butane]

9.3 Sulforaphane

9.3.1 Induction of Endogenous Cytoprotective Enzymes In Vitro

Sulforaphane [1-isothiocyanato-(4*R*)-(methylsulfinyl)butane, Fig. 9.3] was isolated from extracts of broccoli (*Brassica oleracea*) as the principal inducer of the marker cytoprotective enzyme NQO1 using a highly quantitative bioassay in murine hepatoma Hepa1c1c7 cells (Zhang et al. 1992; Zhang and Tang 2007).

Over the years following this discovery, induction by sulforaphane of cytoprotective enzymes has been demonstrated in various cell culture and animal models by numerous independent research groups (Tables 9.2 and 9.3). In the Hepa1c1c7 cell line, sulforaphane treatment increased NQO1 and GST activities (Zhang et al. 1992; Gerhauser et al. 1997; Jiang et al. 2003; Matusheski et al. 2004; Anwar-Mohamed and El-Kadi 2009). Similar effects have been observed in rat bladder carcinoma NBT-II cells (Zhang et al. 2006b) and in murine NIH3T3 fibroblasts (Ernst et al. 2011). Exposure to sulforaphane in wild-type, but not

Table 9.2 Cytoprotective-inducing potential of sulforaphane in vitro

Organ	Cell line	Sulforaphane conc.	Treatment time	Cytoprotective enzymes induced	References
Liver	Hepa1c1c7	0.1–25 μM	24, 48 h	NQO1, GST	Zhang et al. (1992), Gerhauser et al. (1997), Jiang et al. (2003), Matusheski et al. (2004), Anwar-Mohamed and El-Kadi (2009)
	HepG2	5, 10, 12, 20, 25 μM	12, 24 h	NQO1, GST, UGT, HO-1, thioredoxin reductase 1, GSH	Jiang et al. (2003), Gan et al. (2010), Abdelhamid et al. (2010), Amara and El-Kadi (2011), Zhang et al. (2003), Bacon et al. (2003)
	Primary human hepatocytes	4–50 μM	48, 72 h	NQO1, GST	Gross-Steinmeyer et al. (2004), Maheo et al. (1997), Morel et al. (1997)
	Primary rat hepatocytes	10 μM	48, 72 h	GST	Maheo et al. (1997), Morel et al. (1997)
Breast	MCF7	25 μM	24 h	NQO1	Jiang et al. (2003)
	MCF10A	15 μM	24, 48 h	NQO1, AKRs, ALDH	Agyeman et al. (2012)
Prostate	LNCaP	0.1–25 μM	24, 48 h	NQO1, GST, HO-1	Jiang et al. (2003), Brooks and Paton (1999), Brooks et al. (2001), Clarke et al. (2011)
	LNCaPazaC	0.1–15 μM	48 h	NQO1, GST, γGCL	Brooks and Paton (1999)
	MDA PCa 2a	0.1–15 μM	48 h	NQO1, GST, γGCL	Brooks et al. (2001)
	MDA PCa 2b	0.1–15 μM	48 h	NQO1, GST, γGCL	Brooks et al. (2001)
	PC-3	0.1–15 μM	48 h	NQO1, GST, γGCL, HO-1	Brooks et al. (2001), Clarke et al. (2011)
	TSU-Pr1	0.1–15 μM	48 h	NQO1, GST, γGCL	Brooks et al. (2001)
	BPH1	15 μM	12 h	NQO1, HO-1	Clarke et al. (2011)
	PrEC	15 μM	12 h	NQO1, HO-1	Clarke et al. (2011)
Colon	HT-29	5–25 μM	2–24 h	NQO1, carbonyl reductase, γGCL, AKR1B1	Jiang et al. (2003), Ebert et al. (2010)
	Caco-2	1, 5, 10, 20, 50 μM	8, 24, 72 h	NQO1, GST, UGT, MRP2	Svehlikova et al. (2004), Jakubikova et al. (2005a), Traka et al. (2005)
Bladder	NBT-II	4, 8 μM	24 h	NQO1, GST	Zhang et al. (2006b)

Kidney	LLC-PK1	1, 3, 5 μM	24 h	NQO1, γGCL, GSH	Guerrero-Beltran et al. (2010)
Aorta	A10	0.5–5 μM	48 h	NQO1, GST, GSH, SOD, catalase, glutathione peroxidase, glutathione reductase	Zhu et al. (2008)
Spinal cord	Primary rat motor neurons	10 μM	48 h	NQO1, HO-1	Chang et al. (2010)
Brain	Primary murine cortical neurons	0.01–1 μM	24 h	NQO1, GST, glutathione reductase, thioredoxin reductase 1	Vauzour et al. (2010)
	Primary murine hippocampal neurons	0.5 μM	24 h	NQO1, HO-1, γGCL	Soane et al. (2010)
	Primary rat nigrostriatal cocultures	5 μM	48 h	NQO1	Siebert et al. (2009)
	Primary rat cortical astrocytes	5, 10 μM	24, 48 h	NQO1, HO-1, γGCL, thioredoxin reductase	Danilov et al. (2009), Bergstrom et al. (2011)
	SK-N-SH	0.5–5 μM	24 h	NQO1, GSH	Mas et al. (2012)
Retina	ARPE-19	0.625, 2.5 μM	24 h	NQO1, glucose-6-phosphate dehydrogenase, glutathione reductase	Gao et al. (2001)
Lung	Primary human bronchial epithelial cells	1 μM	24, 48 h	NQO1	Tan et al. (2010)
	HBEC	1 μM	24, 48 h	NQO1	Tan et al. (2010)
	BEAS-2B	5 μM	12, 24 h	NQO1, GST, HO-1, γGCL	Starrett and Blake (2011), Ritz et al. (2007)
Skin	Normal human keratinocytes	2.5, 5, 25 μM	24 h	NQO1, γGCL	Marrot et al. (2008)
	Normal human melanocytes	1, 5, 10 μM	24 h	NQO1, HO-1, γGCL	Marrot et al. (2008)
	HaCaT human keratinocytes	1–5 μM	24, 48 h	NQO1, GSH, HO-1, γGCL	Dinkova-Kostova et al. (2006), Wagner et al. (2010), Zhu and Bowden (2004)
	PE murine keratinocytes	0.2–5 μM	24, 48 h	NQO1, GSH	Dinkova-Kostova et al. (2006)

(continued)

Table 9.2 (continued)

Organ	Cell line	Sulforaphane conc.	Treatment time	Cytoprotective enzymes induced	References
Blood	CD34-derived human dendritic cells	2 μM	6, 24 h	NQO1, HO-1	Ade et al. (2009)
	THP-1 myeloid cells	2 μM	6, 24 h	NQO1, HO-1	Ade et al. (2009)
	Ramos 2G6 human B lymphocytes	5–20 μM	16 h	NQO1, GST	Wan and Diaz-Sanchez (2006)
	Human PBMC	5–20 μM	16 h	NQO1, GST	Wan and Diaz-Sanchez (2006)
Fibroblasts	Mouse embryonic fibroblast (MEFs)	3, 4, 5, 8 μM	24 h	NQO1, GST, γGCL, GSH	Zhang et al. (2006b), Nioi et al. (2003), Higgins and Hayes (2011)
	NIH3T3 fibroblasts	5, 10 μM	24 h	NQO1, γGCL, HO-1	Ernst et al. (2011)

Table 9.3 Cytoprotective-inducing potential of sulforaphane in vivo

Organ	Species	Sulforaphane dose and route of administration	Treatment duration	Cytoprotective enzymes induced	References
Liver	Mouse	15 μmol/day, *p.o.*	5 days	NQO1, GST	Zhang et al. (1992), Hu et al. (2006a)
		90 mg/kg, *p.o.*	Single dose	Phase 2 and 3 drug metabolizing enzymes, heat shock proteins, proteasomal subunits	
	Rat	40, 200, 500, or 1000 μmol/kg, *p.o.*	5 days	NQO1, GST	Matusheski and Jeffery (2001), Munday and Munday (2004)
Forestomach	Mouse	15 μmol/day, *p.o.*	5 days	NQO1, GST	Zhang et al. (1992)
Stomach	Mouse	15 μmol/day, *p.o.*	5 days	NQO1, GST	Zhang et al. (1992)
	Rat	40, 80, or 160 μmol/kg, *p.o.* As broccoli extract	14 days	NQO1, GST	Zhang et al. (2006b)
		40, 80, or 160 μmol/kg in diet as broccoli extract	14 days		
Small intestine	Mouse	15 μmol/day, *p.o.*	5 days	NQO1, GST	Zhang et al. (1992), McMahon et al. (2001), Thimmulappa et al. (2002)
		3 μmol/g of diet	14 days	NQO1, GST	
		9 μmol/day, *p.o.*	7 days	NQO1, GST, γGCL, UGT, epoxide hydrolase, glutathione peroxidase, glutathione reductase, ferritin, haptaglobin, NADPH regenerating enzymes (glucose 6-phosphate dehydrogenase, 6-phosphogluconate dehydrogenase, malic enzyme)	

(continued)

Table 9.3 (continued)

Organ	Species	Sulforaphane dose and route of administration	Treatment duration	Cytoprotective enzymes induced	References
Colon	Rat	40, 200, 500, or 1000 μmol/kg, *p.o.*	5 days	NQO1, GST	Matusheski and Jeffery (2001), Munday and Munday (2004)
Pancreas	Rat	40, 200, 500, or 1000 μmol/kg, *p.o.*	5 days	NQO1, GST	Matusheski and Jeffery (2001), Munday and Munday (2004)
Lung	Mouse	15 μmol/day, *p.o.*	5 days	NQO1, GST	Zhang et al. (1992)
Mammary gland	Mouse	3 mg/mouse, *p.o.*	4 days	NQO1, GST	Gerhauser et al. (1997)
	Rat	150 μmol, *p.o.*	Single dose	NQO1, HO-1	Cornblatt et al. (2007)
Retina	Mouse	0.5 mg/day, *i.p.*	3 days	Thioredoxin, thioredoxin reductase	Kong et al. (2007), Tanito et al. (2005)
Brain	Mouse	50 mg/kg, *i.p.*	16 h	NQO1, HO-1	Innamorato et al. (2008), Jazwa et al. (2011)
	Rat	5 mg/kg, *i.p.*	Single dose	NQO1, GST., SOD, catalase, HO-1	Zhao et al. (2007a), Hong et al. (2010), Ping et al. (2010), Chen et al. (2011)
Spinal cord	Rat	5 mg/kg, *i.p.*	Single dose	NQO1, HO-1, γGCL	Wang et al. (2012b)
Sciatic nerve	Mouse	0.5 or 1 mg/kg	14 days	NQO1, HO-1	Negi et al. (2011)
Skin	Mouse	1 μmol/day, topically	3 days	NQO1, K16, K17	Kerns et al. (2007), Talalay et al. (2007)

(continued)

Table 9.3 (continued)

Organ	Species	Sulforaphane dose and route of administration	Treatment duration	Cytoprotective enzymes induced	References
Bladder	Rat	40 μmol/kg, *p.o.*	5 days	NQO1, GST	Zhang et al. (2006b), Munday and Munday (2004), Munday et al. (2008)
		160 μmol/kg in diet as broccoli extract	6 and 12 weeks		
		40, 80, or 160 μmol/kg, *p.o.*, as broccoli extract	14 days		
		40, 80, or 160 μmol/kg in diet as broccoli extract	14 days		

Nrf2-knockout primary mouse embryonic fibroblasts (MEFs), caused an induction of 2- to 10-fold in the levels of mRNA for γ-glutamate-cysteine ligase (γ-GCL) catalytic (GCLC) and modifier (GCLM) subunits, GSTs and NQO1, and increased the levels of total GSH by 1.5- to 1.9-fold (Nioi et al. 2003; Higgins and Hayes 2011). In porcine renal epithelial cells (LLC-PK1), sulforaphane induced NQO1 and γGCL, increased the levels of GSH, and protected against cisplatin-mediated oxidative stress, mitochondrial membrane depolarization and cell death (Guerrero-Beltran et al. 2010). Furthermore, in isolated renal mitochondria from Wistar rats that had been treated with cisplatin, two intravenous injections of sulforaphane (the first one 24 h before and the second one 24 after cisplatin treatment) prevented the cisplatin-induced increase in reactive oxygen species and depletion of GSH, and restored the ATP content and oxygen consumption (Guerrero-Beltran et al. 2010). Similar protection was also observed in liver of cisplatin-treated animals (Gaona-Gaona et al. 2011). Exposure of rat aortic smooth muscle A10 cells to sulforaphane resulted in the induction of a number of cytoprotective enzymes in both whole-cell lysates as well as in mitochondrial fractions, including NQO1, superoxide dismutase (SOD), catalase, glutathione peroxidase, glutathione reductase, GST, increased the levels of GSH, and protected against the toxicities of oxidants and electrophiles, such as superoxide, H_2O_2, peroxynitrite, 4-hydroxy-2-nonenal, and acrolein (Zhu et al. 2008).

In motor neurons grown in organotypic cultures of rat spinal cord, sulforaphane induced NQO1 and heme oxygenase 1 (HO-1), and protected against glutamate-mediated excitotoxicity (Chang et al. 2010). Protection by sulforaphane against 5-*S*-cysteinyl-dopamine-induced neuronal injury was observed in cultures of primary murine cortical neurons and shown to correlate with increased expression and activity of the M-class (M1, M3 and M5) GSTs, glutathione reductase, thioredoxin reductase and NQO1 (Vauzour et al. 2010). In primary murine hippocampal neurons exposed to hemin or to the combination of oxygen and glucose deprivation, treatment with sulforaphane during the reoxygenation phase induced NQO1, HO-1 and GCLM, and protected against cell death (Soane et al. 2010). Dopaminergic neurons that were isolated from Sprague-Dawley rats and grown in organotypic nigrostriatal cocultures were protected against the toxicity of 6-hydroxydopamine by prior treatment with sulforaphane, and the observed protection was attributed to the increase in antioxidant capacity (Siebert et al. 2009). When primary cultures of rat cortical astrocytes were exposed to sulforaphane either 48 h prior to, or for 48 h after, a 4-h period of oxygen and glucose deprivation, both pre- and post-treatment was protective against oxidative stress (assessed by immunostaining for 8-hydroxy-2-deoxyguanosine) and cell death, with the concomitant induction of the levels of mRNA, protein, and enzyme activity of NQO1 (Danilov et al. 2009). In a similar cell culture system, sulforaphane exposure for 4 h induced the levels of mRNA for NQO1 and HO-1 (Bergstrom et al. 2011). Repeated sulforaphane administration resulted in an accumulation of mRNA and protein levels of NQO1 and was protective against oxidative damage. Similar effects of sulforaphane were also observed in human adult retinal pigment epithelial cells (ARPE-19), keratinocytes (HaCaT), and murine leukemia (L1210) cells (Gao et al. 2001).

In primary normal human bronchial epithelial cells as well as in the immortalized human bronchial epithelial cell line HBEC, sulforaphane caused a robust upregulation of NQO1 mRNA and protein levels (Tan et al. 2010). Induction of NQO1 by sulforaphane was also observed in primary cultures of human hepatocytes (Gross-Steinmeyer et al. 2004). In the Caco-2 human colon cancer cell line, NQO1, multidrug resistance-associated protein 2 (MRP2), GSTA1 and UDP-glucuronosyltransferase were elevated upon sulforaphane treatment (Svehlikova et al. 2004; Jakubikova et al. 2005a). In the human hepatoma cell line HepG2, sulforaphane treatment also increased the transcription of the endogenous NQO1 (Gan et al. 2010; Abdelhamid et al. 2010; Amara and El-Kadi 2011), thioredoxin reductase 1 (Zhang et al. 2003), and HO-1 (Gan et al. 2010). Moreover, in combination with selenium, sulforaphane treatment resulted in protection against paraquat-induced cell death (Zhang et al. 2003). In primary human and rat hepatocytes, sulforaphane induced the transcription of GSTA1/2 mRNA (Maheo et al. 1997; Morel et al. 1997). In HepG2 cells and in primary human hepatocytes, treatment with sulforaphane inhibited the formation of PhiP-DNA adducts; the protective effect correlated with transcriptional upregulation of UDP-glucuronosyltransferase and GSTA1 (Bacon et al. 2003). In the human dopaminergic neuroblastoma SK-N-SH cell line, sulforaphane induced NQO1 enzyme activity and increased the levels of glutathione (Mas et al. 2012). Induction of NQO1 was also observed in a number of human prostate cancer cell lines (Jiang et al. 2003; Brooks and Paton 1999; Brooks et al. 2001). The levels of GSH and GSH-related enzymes, such as GCLC and GSTs, were also upregulated (Brooks and Paton 1999). In the human BEAS-2B epithelial cell line, sulforaphane increased the expression of NQO1, HO-1, and GCLM (Starrett and Blake 2011). Sulforaphane also increased the levels of mRNA for HO-1 and NQO1 in normal (PrEC), benign hyperplastic (BPH1) and cancerous (LNCaP and PC3) human prostate epithelial cells (Clarke et al. 2011), and the mRNA for carbonyl reductase 3, a member of the short-chain dehydrogenase/reductase superfamily, in HT-29 colon cancer cells (Ebert et al. 2010). Upregulation of NQO1 was observed when cultured normal human keratinocytes and melanocytes were exposed to sulforaphane (Marrot et al. 2008). In murine and human (HaCaT) keratinocytes, the enzyme activity of NQO1, the GSH content (Zhu et al. 2004; Dinkova-Kostova et al. 2006) and the mRNA and protein levels for NQO1, HO-1 and γ-GCL (Wagner et al. 2010) were all upregulated by exposure to sulforaphane. NQO1 and HO-1 were also induced by sulforaphane in human CD34-derived dendritic cells isolated from umbilical cord blood, and in the THP-1 myeloid cell line (Ade et al. 2009). Sulforaphane treatment also caused increased gene expression of *NQO1*, *GSTM1* and *GSTP1* in cultured Ramos 2G6 human B lymphocytes and PBMCs isolated from blood (Wan and Diaz-Sanchez 2006), as well as in the airway epithelial cell line BEAS-2B (Ritz et al. 2007). In the estrogen receptor negative human breast epithelial MCF10A cell line, sulforaphane exposure led to a profound upregulation of the aldo-keto reductase family members AKR1B10, AKR1C1, AKR1C2 and AKR1C3, the aldehyde dehydrogenase 3 family member ALDH3A1, and of NQO1, as revealed by the use of both microarray and stable isotopic labeling with amino acids in culture (SILAC) approaches (Agyeman et al. 2012).

9.3.2 Activation of the Antioxidant/Electrophile Responsive Element in Reporter Systems

The upstream regulatory regions of the genes coding for cytoprotective proteins contain single or multiple copies of the antioxidant/electrophile response element (ARE/EpRE, consensus sequence: 5′-A/GTGAC/GNNNGCA/G-3′) (Rushmore and Pickett 1990; Friling et al. 1990; Hayes et al. 2010). Activation of gene expression through the ARE requires binding of transcription factor Nrf2 as a heterodimer with a small Maf protein (Motohashi and Yamamoto 2004). Thus, in addition to the effects on endogenous gene expression, ARE- and Nrf2-dependent induction by sulforaphane has been demonstrated in a number of reporter systems. In the human hepatoma cell line HepG2 stably transfected with the chloramphenicol acetyltransferase (CAT) reporter gene under the transcriptional control of the rat GSTYa promoter, treatment with sulforaphane caused a dose-dependent induction of the reporter gene (Fei et al. 1996). Similarly, a second reporter HepG2 cell line that was developed by a stable transfection with the gene encoding green fluorescent protein (GFP) under the transcriptional control of the thymidine kinase (TK) promoter adjacent to the ARE, also showed an increase in fluorescence upon sulforaphane treatment (Zhu and Fahl 2000). When HepG2 cells were transiently transfected with a CAT reporter under the control of the 5′-regulatory region of the rat NQO1 gene and then exposed to sulforaphane, enhanced CAT expression was also observed (Gerhauser et al. 1997). Sulforaphane caused induction of the

ARE-luciferase reporter in the stably transfected MCF7-derived AREc32 human breast cancer cell line, which contains a luciferase reporter construct controlled by eight copies of the ARE that is present in both rat *GSTA2* and mouse *gsta1 genes* (Wang et al. 2006, 2010; Dinkova-Kostova and Wang 2011). The pARE-TI-luciferase reporter in the stably transfected HepG2-ARE-C8 cell line was also induced by sulforaphane (Saw et al. 2011). Upregulation of the luciferase reporter was observed in the reporter cell line EpRE(mGST-Ya)-LUX, which is a Hepa1c1c7 cell line that contains the ARE from the promoter region of the murine *gstya* gene (Vermeulen et al. 2009). Sulforaphane was also shown to activate a reporter in which the Neh2 domain of Nrf2 that is responsible for binding to its negative regulator, Kelch-like ECH-associated protein 1 (Keap1) (Itoh et al. 1999), was fused to firefly luciferase (Neh2-luciferase) allowing the direct monitoring of the response to inducers based on the time course of reporter activation (Smirnova et al. 2011).

9.3.3 Cytoprotective Effects of Sulforaphane In Vivo

Induction of cytoprotective enzymes by sulforaphane also occurs in vivo (Table 9.3). Sulforaphane administered to mice daily, *p.o.*, at a dose of 15 μmol/day, for 5 days, resulted in induction of NQO1 and GST activities in liver, forestomach, glandular stomach, small intestine, and lung (Zhang et al. 1992). Induction of both NQO1 and GST occurred in mammary glands of mice that had been given 4 daily doses of 3 mg of sulforaphane per animal, *p.o.* (Gerhauser et al. 1997). In liver, colon, and pancreas of rats given either 200, 500, or 1000 μmol/kg (Matusheski and Jeffery 2001) or 40 μmol/kg of sulforaphane, *p.o.* for 5 days, NQO1 and GST activities were also upregulated (Munday and Munday 2004). Especially high was the magnitude of induction in bladder (Zhang et al. 2006b; Munday and Munday 2004; Munday et al. 2008). Feeding sulforaphane (3 μmol/g of diet) for 14 days induced the activities of NQO1 and GST in the small intestine in wild-type mice (McMahon et al. 2001). In contrast, an identical treatment had no effect in Nrf2-knockout animals (McMahon et al. 2001). Topical application of sulforaphane to the mouse skin induced the gene expression of keratins 16 (K16) and 17 (K17) in the basal layer of the epidermis (Kerns et al. 2007). K17 is homologous and functionally redundant with K14, and the sulforaphane-dependent induction of K17 was evaluated as a potential strategy for reducing skin blistering in K14-knockout mice, a model for the human skin blistering disease epidermolysis bullosa simplex (EBS). Systemic (*i.p.*) administration of 5 μmol of sulforaphane to a pregnant mouse every other day in the week before delivery followed by topical applications of 1 μmol of sulforaphane to the newborn pups on the day of birth, day 1 and day 3 after birth, restored the skin integrity in these animals (Kerns et al. 2007). A subsequent study revealed that the induction of K17 is independent of Nrf2 activity and parallels the decrease in glutathione levels that occur after topical administration of sulforaphane (Kerns et al. 2010).

A pharmacokinetics/pharmacodynamics preclinical study for breast cancer prevention by sulforaphane was conducted in Sprague-Dawley rats (Cornblatt et al. 2007). It was found that orally administered sulforaphane reaches the mammary gland and increases the levels of cytoprotective enzymes in this tissue. The levels of dithiocarbamates (sulforaphane and its glutathione-derived conjugates) peaked at 1 h after oral administration of 150 μmol sulforaphane, reaching concentrations of 60 μM and 18.8 pmol/mg tissue in plasma and mammary gland, respectively. After 1 h, the plasma concentration of dithiocarbamates declined rapidly and exhibited a minor second peak of 22 μM at 12 h. The mRNA levels for NQO1 in the mammary gland were significantly induced as early as 2 h after dosing, and maximally elevated at 12 h. The NQO1 enzymatic activity in the mammary gland was also increased, peaking at 24 h after dosing. A biphasic pattern of HO-1 transcript induction was observed, with an initial peak at 2 h followed by a second peak at 12 h, indicating a more complex mode of regulation.

Microarray analyses in cells and tissues isolated from mice, rats and humans have further confirmed and expanded the list of transcriptional targets of sulforaphane (Agyeman et al. 2012; Thimmulappa et al. 2002; Hu et al. 2004, 2006a; Traka et al. 2005, 2008). The most prominent changes are in genes encoding proteins that are involved in xenobiotic metabolism, glutathione homeostasis, carbohydrate metabolism, and NADH/NADPH regeneration, and are thus tightly linked to cellular defense mechanisms, inhibition of proliferation, and induction of differentiation. The multitude of effects of sulforaphane on such fundamental cellular processes has led to numerous investigations evaluating the ability of this isothiocyanate to protect against the development of chronic degenerative diseases. Indeed, protection by sulforaphane has been demonstrated in animal models of carcinogenesis (Zhang et al. 1994; Chung et al. 2000; Fahey et al. 2002; Conaway et al. 2005; Kuroiwa et al. 2006; Myzak et al. 2006; Hu et al. 2006b; Gills et al. 2006; Xu et al. 2006; Singh et al. 2009), cardiovascular disease (Piao et al. 2010), diabetes (Zheng et al. 2011; Negi et al. 2011), neurotoxicity (Innamorato et al. 2008; Toyama et al. 2011), neurodegeneration (Kong et al. 2007; Rojo et al. 2010; Innamorato et al. 2010; Jazwa et al. 2011), and neuronal tissue injury (Tanito et al. 2005; Zhao et al. 2005, 2007a, b; Dash et al. 2009; Hong et al. 2010; Ping et al. 2010; Chen et al. 2011; Mao et al. 2011; Wang et al. 2012a). Notably, all of these disease models have both oxidative stress and inflammatory components underlying their pathogenesis. The protective effects of sulforaphane in animal models are being reflected in multiple human studies, in which various broccoli preparations or dietary supplements have been used as delivery vehicles for sulforaphane. The published studies have been summarized in a recent review (Dinkova-Kostova et al. 2017), and there are 20 ongoing clinical trials. In addition, a stabilized version of suforaphane encapsulated in cyclodextrin (SFX-01) is currently in two clinical trials, in patients with subarachnoid haemorrhage (NCT02614742) and metastatic breast cancer (NCT02970682) (Cuadrado et al. 2019).

9.3.4 Long Lasting Indirect Antioxidant Properties Via Induction of Cytoprotective Enzymes

The ability to upregulate the expression of a plethora of cytoprotective genes and to inhibit pro-inflammatory responses makes sulforaphane a particularly efficient, albeit indirect antioxidant. The "ultimate antioxidants," namely, the cytoprotective enzymes, act catalytically, are not consumed in the course of their antioxidant functions, have relatively long (usually several days) half-lives, and catalyze a wide variety of chemical reactions, such that their concerted actions protect cells and organisms and allows their adaptation to conditions of stress. A study using human adult retinal pigment epithelial cells (ARPE-19) as a model demonstrated that induction of cytoprotective enzymes by sulforaphane is a powerful strategy for enhancing the cellular antioxidant defense (Gao et al. 2001). Furthermore, such intervention provides efficient protection against chemically-induced oxidative stress produced by oxidants of several different types, such as the redox cycling agent menadione, the water-soluble peroxide *tert*-butyl hydroperoxide, the genotoxic alkenal 4-hydroxynonenal, and the highly damaging product of the reaction of superoxide with nitric oxide, peroxynitrite. Unlike the short-lived effects of direct antioxidants, protection against menadione toxicity at the end of a 24-h treatment with sulforaphane is prolonged and maintained for several days. Importantly, the duration of sulforaphane-mediated resistance to menadione paralleled the time period of increased cytoprotective enzyme activities: NQO1, glucose-6-phosphate dehydrogenase, and glutathione reductase in cells treated with sulforaphane continued to rise for 48 h after removal of sulforaphane from the medium and remained high during the ensuing 48–72 h. The levels of GSH after 24-h exposure to sulforaphane were increased by 50%, remained at this level for another 24 h, and then declined to control cell levels in the subsequent 96 h. In primary cultures of rat cortical astrocytes, sulforaphane exposure for 4 h induced the levels of mRNA for NQO1 and HO-1 (Bergstrom et al. 2011). These levels remained high for 24 h, and the corresponding protein levels were increased for more than 48 h. The long-lasting effects of sulforaphane treatment on induction of NQO1 were also observed in several different human prostate cancer cell lines (Jiang et al. 2003; Brooks and Paton 1999; Brooks et al. 2001). Transcriptional induction by sulforaphane was transient: it was evident at 4 h after exposure, reached a peak at 8 h, and returned to basal levels by 12 h. However, the enzyme activity remained elevated for up to 5 days after treatment. The levels of glutathione and glutathione-related enzymes, such as GCLC and GSTs, were also upregulated (Brooks and Paton 1999). Thus, even a transient exposure to sulforaphane causes an elevation of endogenous antioxidant systems, which by virtue of their long half-lives ultimately result in long-lasting protection. Moreover, protection against oxidative stress is quantitatively related to the indirect antioxidant action of sulforaphane, which is the result from induction of cytoprotective enzymes.

Table 9.4 Structure, chemical names and dietary sources of selected isothiocyanates (Cheung and Kong 2010; Prashar et al. 2012)

Structure	Chemical name/ Glucosinolate precursor	Origin
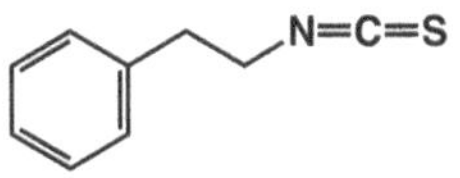	2-Phenethyl-ITC (PEITC) 2-Isothiocyanatoethyl benzene/Gluconasturtiin	Watercress, radishes, turnips
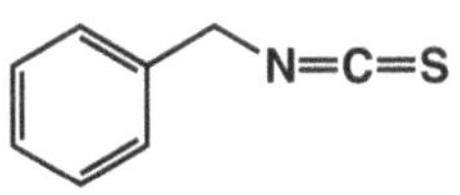	Benzyl-ITC (BITC) Isothiocyanatomethyl benzene/Glucotropaeolin	Lepidium cress, cabbage, papaya
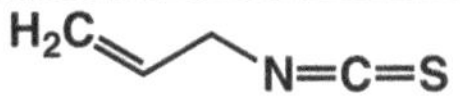	Allyl ITC (AITC) 3-Isothiocyanatoprop-1-ene/Sinigrin	Mustards, horseradish, wasabi, cabbage, brussels sprouts, kale, cauliflower

9.4 Phenethyl Isothiocyanate, Benzyl Isothiocyanate, Allyl Isothiocyanate

Phenethyl isothiocyanate (PEITC), benzyl isothiocyanate (BITC) and allyl isothiocyanate (AITC) occurring commonly in the human diet (Table 9.4) have been widely investigated with respect to their cancer chemopreventive properties.

AITC, also known as mustard oil, is responsible for the pungent taste of several cruciferous vegetables. This is due to its effects on the transient receptor potential A1 channel in sensory neurons and plays a role in plant defense against herbivores (Zhang 2010). Moreover AITC, as well as sulforaphane, PEITC and BITC, manifest antimicrobial activity against a wide spectrum of pathogens (Zhang 2010; Fahey et al. 2002; Navarro et al. 2011; Haristoy et al. 2005; Johansson et al. 2008; Yanaka et al. 2009). Many studies have presented AITC, sulforaphane, PEITC and BITC as promising cancer preventive phytochemicals, with anti-cancer activity in both cancer cells and animal models (Zhang 2010; Navarro et al. 2011). Many examples of comparison studies performed with use of aliphatic AITC and sulforaphane and aromatic PEITC and BITC have enabled to draw conclusions about their structure-activity relationships amongst compounds belonging to the ITC family (Prashar et al. 2012). Other ITCs, like sulforaphane, are able to induce cytoprotective enzymes responsible for detoxification and augmentation of anti-oxidant defense, as outlined above. The potency of ITCs to induce apoptosis or inhibit cell cycle progression of cancer cells is determined by their ability to affect various molecular targets involved in regulating these processes (Fig. 9.4). Furthermore, these ITCs are also able to modulate these processes through their interaction with unique molecular targets dictated by their structure.

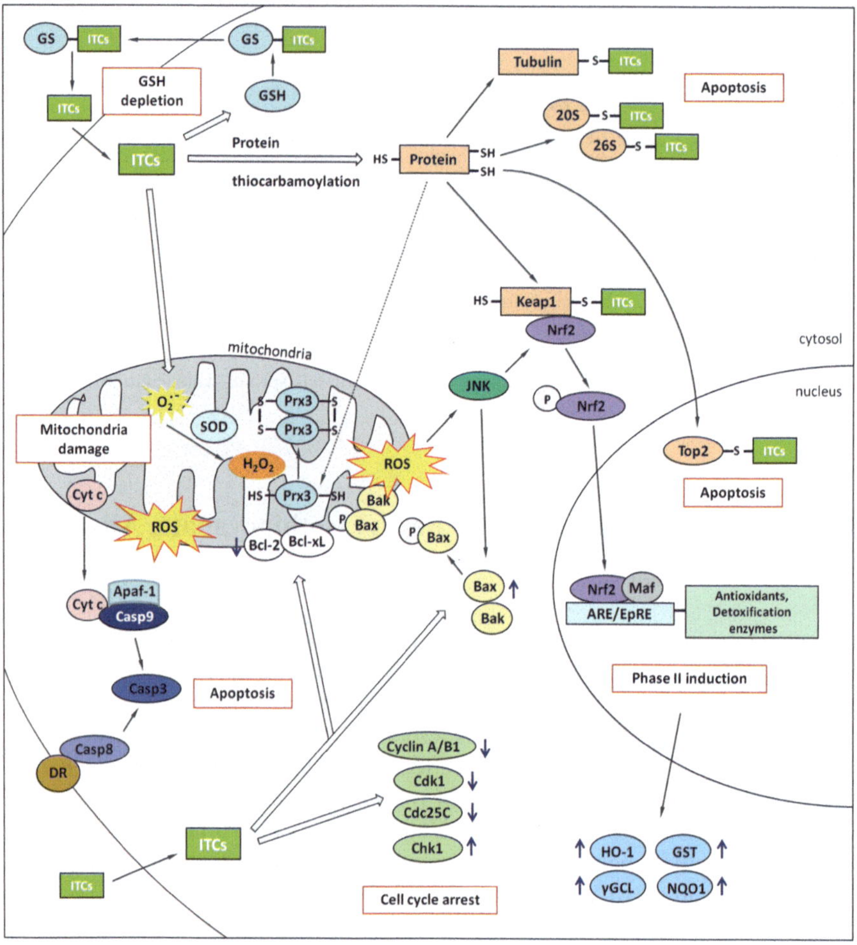

Fig. 9.4 Schematic representation of the signaling pathways contributing to ITC-induced cytotoxicity and indirect antioxidant effects (details are described in the text). *ITCs* isothiocyanates, *GSH* glutathione, *Top2* DNA topisomerase II, *Keap1* Kelch-like ECH-associated protein 1, *Nrf2* NF-E2 p45-related factor 2, *Maf* small musculoaponeurotic fibrosarcoma, *ARE/EpRE* antioxidant/electrophile response element, *γGCL* γ-glutamate-cysteine ligase, *GST* glutathione *S*-transferase, *HO-1* heme oxygenase 1, *NQO1* NAD(P)H:quinone oxidoreductase 1, *Bcl-2* B-cell lymphoma 2, *Bcl-xL* B-cell lymphoma-extra large, *Bak* Bcl-2 homologous antagonist killer, *Bax* Bcl-2–associated X protein, *SOD* superoxide dismutase, *Prx3* peroxiredoxin 3, *ROS* reactive oxygen species, *Cyt c* cytochrome c, *Apaf-1* apoptotic protease activating factor 1, *Casp3,8,9* caspase-3,-8,-9, *DR* death receptor, *JNK* c-Jun N-terminal kinase, *Cdk1* cyclin-dependent kinase 1, *Cdc25C* cell division cycle 25 homolog C, *Chk1* checkpoint kinase 1

9.4.1 Cellular Accumulation of ITCs and Depletion of Glutathione (GSH)

ITCs upon crossing the cell membrane accumulate in the cytosol as dithiocarbamates due to their rapid reaction with molecules containing thiol (-SH) group(s), or other nucleophilic moieties. As shown in Fig. 9.4, the main targets of ITCs for thiocarbamoylation are GSH and various cellular proteins. Intracellular conditions, such as high concentration of GSH (1–10 mM) and abundance of GSTs catalyzing the conjugation of GSH to the carbon of the –N=C=S moiety contribute to a rapid and highly efficient accumulation of ITCs. The intracellular concentration of ITCs can exceed the extracellular one over 100–200-fold within 1 to 3 h of exposure (Zhang 2000, 2001). Total intracellular BITC and PEITC accumulation levels were 1.04 and 0.66 mM, respectively, when UM-UC-3 cells were exposed to each ITC at 7.5 μM for 1 h (Tang and Zhang 2005). Then, as a means of detoxification, ITC-glutathione (ITC-SG) conjugates are transported out of the cell. Since the reaction between GSH and ITCs is reversible, the breakage of ITC-SG conjugates extracellularly promotes accumulation of ITCs and depletion of intracellular GSH exploited by the detoxification of ITCs re-entering cells. Measurements of GSH level in Jurkat T lymphoma cells upon 20 and 60 min of stimulation with 15 μM sulforaphane or PEITC showed a prominent reduction of GSH levels of around 60 and 30% of the control, respectively (Brown et al. 2008). Depletion of GSH, widely recognized as the main cellular redox buffer, can disrupt redox homeostasis and induce signaling pathways aimed at restoring the redox balance. Nevertheless, the cell survival/cell death fate is context dependent, and is contingent on drug concentration, duration of treatment, cell type (origin, normal vs. cancer cells) (Fig. 9.4) (Nakamura and Miyoshi 2010).

9.4.2 Apoptosis Induction by ITCs

One mechanism by which ITCs are able to wield their anti-cancer prowess is through the activation of apoptotic pathways. ITCs have been shown to suppress proliferation of different types of cancer cells (see Tables 9.5 and 9.6 for overview). Induction of apoptosis and cell cycle arrest by ITCs has been attributed to their pro-oxidative activity mediated via triggering mitochondrial signaling, as well as their electrophilic nature which causes the thiocarbamoylation of proteins of which the proper functioning is necessary for viability (Fig. 9.4). Multiple reports in the existing literature have shown that ITCs are potent inducers of apoptosis in a time- and dose-dependent manner. Interestingly, differences in molecular targets, mechanisms, and potency of apoptosis induction by ITCs have been identified. This underlines the importance of the side chain, unique to different compounds bearing an isothiocyanate moiety. Exemplary, the effectiveness of six different ITCs in dissipation of the mitochondrial membrane potential and apoptosis induction in leukemia cells (HL60) followed the

Table 9.5 Cytotoxicity attributed to pro-oxidative activities of ITCs

Organ	Cell line	ITCs concentration	Treatment time	Effect	References
Bladder	UM-UC-3	7.5, 15, 30 μM BITC, PEITC	3, 24 h	Procaspase-9 cleavage	Tang and Zhang (2005)
				PARP cleavage	
		7.5, 15, 30 μM BITC, PEITC, AITC, sulforaphane		Loss of MTMP	
				Cytochrome c release	
		7.5, 15, 30 μM BITC, PEITC		Damage of plasma membrane	
				Bak translocation to the mitochondria	
	Mitochondria from UM-UC-3	7.5, 15, 30 μM BITC, PEITC	30 min	Disturb association of Bcl-xL with both Bak and Bax	Tang and Zhang (2005)
		15, 50, 100 μM BITC, PEITC, AITC, sulforaphane		Loss of MTMP	
Bone	U2OS	5–15 μM BITC, PEITC	6–48 h	↓ Viable cells	Wu et al. (2011)
		5 μM BITC, 5 and 7.5 μM PEITC	48 h	G_2/M-phase cell cycle arrest	
		7.5 μM BITC, 10 μM PEITC	12, 18, 24 h	Apoptosis induction (sub-G_1 fraction)	
			24, 48 h	Chromatin condensation	
				DNA damage	
			0.5, 1, 2 h	↑ ROS	
			2, 4, 6 h	↑ NO	
				↑ Catalase level	
		7.5 μM BITC	6 h	↓ MnSOD level	
		7.5 μM BITC 10 μM PEITC	12, 24, 48 h	Loss of MTMP	
			12, 18, 24 h	↑ Cytochrome c, caspase-9, −3, AIF, cleaved PARP proteins	
			24 h	Cytochrome c and AIF translocation	

Brain	GBM8401	0.5–20 μM AITC	24 h	↓ Viable cells $IC_{50} = 9.25 \pm 0.69$ μM	Chen et al. (2010)
		10 μM AITC	24 h	G_2/M-phase cell cycle arrest	
				Apoptosis induction (sub-G_1 fraction)	
				Chromatin condensation	
			6, 12, 24 h	↓ Cdk1 activity	
			6, 12, 24, 48 h	↓ CDK1, cyclin B, cyclin A protein levels	
				↑ Cytochrome c, Apaf-1, pro-caspase-9, AIF, Endo G proteins in cytosolic fraction	
			24 h	↑ Caspase-3, −9 activity	
reast	MDA-MB-231, MCF-7	2.5–20 μM BITC, PEITC, sulforaphane	24 h	↓ Viable cells	Xiao et al. (2006)
		0.5, 1, 2.5 μM BITC	3, 6, 12, 24 h	G_2/M-phase cell cycle arrest	
				Apoptosis induction (sub-G_1 fraction)	
		2.5 or 10 μM BITC	1, 3, 6, 12 h	↓ Level of cyclin B1, Cdk1, Cdc25C	
		1, 2.5 μM BITC	24 h	Apoptosis induction (cells with condensed chromatin)	
		1, 2.5, 5, 10 μM BITC	24 h	Apoptosis induction (DNA fragmentation)	
		2.5 or 10 μM BITC	2–24 h	↑ Bax, Bak ↓ Bcl-2, Bcl-xL	
		2.5 or 5, 10 μM BITC	1, 2, 4, 6 h	Loss of MTMP	
		2.5 μM BITC	1, 3, 6, 12, 24 h	Cytochrome c release	
			6 h	Autophagososmes	
			1, 2, 4 h	↑ ROS	
			1, 3, 6, 12, 24 h	Procaspase-3, -9, -8 cleavage	

(continued)

Table 9.5 (continued)

Organ	Cell line	ITCs concentration	Treatment time	Effect	References
Breast	MDA-MB-231, MCF-7	2.5 μM BITC	2 h	↑ ROS	Xiao et al. (2008)
			24 h	Apoptosis induction (DNA fragmentation),	
				Procaspase-3 cleavage Caspase-3 activation	
			16, 24 h	Cytochrome c release	
			24 h	↓ Viable cells	
			6 h	Loss of MTMP	
			8, 16 h	Bax activation	
				PARP cleavage	
		5 μM BITC	1, 3, 6 h	↓ Complex III activity	
		2.5, 5 μM BITC	2, 4, 8, 16 h	↑ JNK, p38 MAPK activity	
	MCF7	5 μM BITC	24 h	↑Apoptosis induction	Sehrawat and Singh (2016)
		1–5 μM BITC	12	↓ Viable cells	
		5 μM BITC	6 h	↑ ROS	
	MDA-MB-361	5 μM BITC	24 h	↑ Apoptosis induction	
		5 μM BITC	6 h	↑ ROS	
Leukemia	Jurkat T lymphoma cells	2.5–60 μM PEITC	5–120 min	↑ Oxidation of mitochondrial Prx3	Brown et al. (2008)
		10–60 μM PEITC, Sulforaphane	1 h	↓ TrxR activity	
		10–60 μM PEITC, Sulforaphane	1 h	↓ GR activity	
		15 μM PEITC, Sulforaphane	20, 60 min	↓ GSH level	
		15 μM PEITC, BITC, AITC, Sulforaphane	24 h	↓ Viable cells	

	HL60, HL60/ADR, HL60/VCR[a]	0.5–25 μM AITC, BITC, PEITC, Sulforaphane, ERN, IBN	72 h	↓ Viable cells	Jakubikova et al. (2005b)
		5–20 μM AITC, BITC, PEITC, Sulforaphane, ERN, IBN	6, 24 h	G_2/M-phase cell cycle arrest	
				Apoptosis induction (sub-G_1 fraction)	
				Apoptosis and necrosis induction	
				Loss of MTMP	
Liver	RL34[b]	20, 50 μM BITC	8, 24 h	↓ Viable cells	Nakamura et al. (2002)
		20 μM BITC	8 h	Nuclear fragmentation	
				↑ Caspase-3 activity	
		5, 50 μM BITC	0.5 h	Loss of MTMP	
		5–100 μM BITC		↑ ROS	
Larynx	Hep-2	2.5–10 μM PEITC	24, 48, 72 h	↓ Viable cells	Dai et al. (2016)
		5, 7.5, 10 μM PEITC	24 h	Apoptosis induction	
		5, 7.5, 10 μM PEITC	48 h	↓ Cell invasion	
		7.5, 10 μM PEITC	24 h	G_2/M-phase cell cycle arrest	
Lung	L9981	1–40 μM BITC or PEITC	48 h	↓ Viable cells $IC_{50} = 5.0 \pm 0.22$ μM $IC_{50} = 9.7 \pm 0.39$ μM	Wu et al. (2010)
		5 μM BITC, 10 μM PEITC	30 h	↓ Cell migration (reduced to 8.1 and 16.5% of control)	
			24 h	↓ Cell invasion (reduced to 2.7 and 7.3% of control)	
			4 h	↓ mRNA of pro-metastasis genes: MMP-2, twist ↑ mRNA of anti-metastasis genes: β-catenin	
		5–20 μM BITC or PEITC	24 h	↓ MMP-2 and twist protein level	
		5 μM BITC, 10 μM PEITC	4 h	↑ ROS	
		5 or 10 μM BITC or PEITC	3 and 6 h	↓ GSH	
		5–20 μM BITC or PEITC	24 h	↓ Akt phosphorylation (activity)	
			18 h	↓ NF-κB transcriptional activation	
	L9981	7.5 or 10 μM BITC 12.5 or 20 μM PEITC	24 h	Apoptosis induction	Yan et al. (2011)

(continued)

Table 9.5 (continued)

Organ	Cell line	ITCs concentration	Treatment time	Effect	References
		7.5 μM BITC, 12.5 μM PEITC	24 h	G_2/M-phase cell cycle arrest	
		7.5 or 10 μM BITC 12.5 or 20 μM PEITC	24 h	↑ Phosphorylated JNK, p44/42 MAPK, p38	
Marrow	DA1-3b[c]	5, 10 μM PEITC	24 h	↓ Viable cells	Trachootham et al. (2006)
Myeloma	MM.1S, OPM1	1.6–50 μM PEITC, Sulforaphane	24, 48 h	↓ Viable cells	Jakubikova et al. (2011)
		2.5, 5, 10, 20 μM PEITC, Sulforaphane	12, 24, 48 h	G_2/M-phase cell cycle arrest	
				Apoptosis induction (sub-G_1 fraction)	
			12 h	Changes in level of cell cycle-related proteins	
			24, 48 h	↓ Viable cells (among death cells: ~30% necrotic, ~70% apoptotic)	
			24 h	Procaspase-3 cleavage, PARP cleavage	
			2, 6, 12, 24 h	Transient ↑ of JNK, c-Jun, MEK1, p38, ERK1/2, Akt, GSK3α/β	
	Bone marrow CD138[+] tumor cells	1.6–50 μM PEITC, Sulforaphane	48 h	↓ Viable cells	Jakubikova et al. (2011)
Ovary	T72Ras[d]	5, 10 μM PEITC	1, 3, 5 h	↑ ROS, ↑ NO	Trachootham et al. (2006)
		1–20 μM PEITC	1–48 h	↓ Viable cells	
		0.3–10 μM PEITC	10 days	↓ Cell proliferation, $IC_{50} = 0.49 \pm 0.1$ μM	
		10 μM PEITC	2, 4, 6, 8 h	↑ Cardiolipin oxidation	
				Loss of MTMP	
		5 μM PEITC	1, 3 h	↓ GSH	
		5, 10 μM PEITC	5 h	↓ GPX activity	
		5 μM PEITC	0.5, 1 h	↑ JNK activity	
	SKOV3	10 μM PEITC	6 h	↑ ROS	Trachootham et al. (2006)
		0.3–10 μM PEITC	10 days	↓ Cell proliferation	
		10 μM PEITC	23 h	↓ Viable cells	
Ovary	A2008	10 μM PEITC	24 h	↓ Viable cells	Trachootham et al. (2006)
		0.3–30 μM PEITC	3 days	↓ Cell proliferation	

	HEY	0.3–30 μM PEITC	3 days	↓ Cell proliferation	Trachootham et al. (2006)
	PA-1 SKOV3	1–40 μM PEITC	24, 48 h	↓ Viable cells PA-1 – IC_{50} = 7 (24 h), 5.09 (48 h) μM SKOV3 – IC_{50} = 7.95 (24 h), 4.67 (48 h) μM	Hong et al. (2015)
		5 μM PEITC	12, 24 h	↑ ROS	
		5 μM PEITC	12, 24 h	↑ UPR	
		5 μM PEITC	24, 48 h	↑ Apoptosis	
Skin	A375	5 μM PEITC, BITC, sulforaphane	48 h	G_2/M-phase cell cycle arrest	Mantso et al. (2019)
Prostate	LNCaP, PC-3	5 μM PEITC	2, 4, 6 h	↑ ROS	Xiao et al. (2010)
		2.5 μM PEITC	4 h		
		5 μM PEITC	6 h		
		2.5, 5 μM PEITC	24 h	Inhibition of complex III activity	
		5 μM PEITC	6 h	↓ Oxidative phophorylation rate	
				↓ Glycolysis rate	
			45 min	↓ ATP	
			4 h	Loss of MTMP	
		2.5 μM PEITC	8 h	Bax activation	
		5 μM PEITC	24 h	Apoptotic DNA fragmentation	
				Caspase-3 activation	
			6, 9 h	Autophagy induction	

ITCs isothiocyanates, *AITC* allyl ITC, *BITC* benzyl ITC, *PEITC* phenylethyl ITC, *ERN* erucin, *IBN* iberin, *PARP* poly (ADP-ribose) polymerase, *MTMP* mitochondrial transmembrane potential

[a]Multidrug resistant cells derived from HL60

[b]Rat liver epithelial RL34 cells

[c]Bcr-Abl transformed murine myeloid progenitor cells

[d]Ras-transformed ovarian epithelial cells

Table 9.6 Cytotoxicity attributed to electrophilic activities of ITCs

Organ	Cell line	ITCs conc.	Treatment time	Effect	References
Breast	MCF10A-Ras	BITC, PEITC, Sulforaphane	4 days	↓ Viable cells $IC_{50} = 3.2 \pm 0.7$; 3.4 ± 0.5; 10 ± 1.3	Lin et al. (2011)
		10 μM PEITC	6 h	↑ DNA damage	
		0.1 mM BITC, 1 mM BITC	1 and 5 min, 30 min	In vitro covalent binding to DNA topoisomerase II	
Lung	A549	1–100 μM BITC, PEITC, Sulforaphane	24 h	↓ Viable cells $IC_{50} = 13.8$; 18.3; 43	Mi et al. (2008)
		10 μM BITC or PEITC, 30 μM SFN	4–24 h	G_2/M-phase cell cycle arrest	
			24 h	Accumulation of mitotic cells	
		10 or 20 μM BITC, PEITC, Sulforaphane	24, 48, 72 h	Apoptosis induction (sub-G_1 fraction)	
			4–24 h	Caspase-3 activity	
		20 μM ^{14}C-PEITC, ^{14}C-SFN;	1 h	α- and β-tubulin binding	
		30 μM BITC, PEITC, Sulforaphane (in vitro)	Not stated	Tubulin polymerization inhibition	
		5 μM BITC or PEITC	0.5 or 1 h	Microtubule network disruption	
		20 μM	1 h	Covalent binding to cysteine residues in tubulin	
Myeloma Ovary Lung Prostate Colon Breast	U266 RPMI-8226 HeLa A549 PC-3 HT-29 MCF-7	10, 20, 30 μM BITC or PEITC	2–24 h	Inhibition of proteosome (26S and 20S) activity by direct binding	Mi et al. (2011)
Myeloma	U266	10 or 20 μM BITC, PEITC, SFN	1 h	↓ GSH	Mi et al. (2011)
		10 μM BITC or PEITC	24 h	G_2/M-phase cell cycle arrest	
		10 or 20 μM BITC, PEITC, SFN	24 h	Apoptosis induction (sub-G_1 fraction)	

(continued)

Table 9.6 (continued)

Organ	Cell line	ITCs conc.	Treatment time	Effect	References
		5, 10, 15 μM BITC	24 h	Apoptosis induction (PARP cleavage)	
		2.5–40 μM BITC	24, 48 h	↓ viable cells	
		10–40 μM BITC, PEITC, SFN	4 h	α- and β-tubulin aggregation and depletion	
Ovary	HeLa	10 μM BITC	20 h	Apoptosis induction (sub-G_1 fraction)	Mi et al. (2009)
		10 μM BITC	20 h	G_2/M-phase cell cycle arrest	

order: BITC = PEITC > ERN (erucin) = IBN (iberin) > AITC > sulforaphane (Jakubikova et al. 2005b). A 24-h exposure of human breast cancer cells to as little as 2.5 μM PEITC and BITC resulted in about 70% and 30% decrease in cell viability, respectively for MDA-MB-231 and MCF-7 cell lines (Xiao et al. 2006). The increase in each of the compound's concentration to 20 μM caused severe elevation in the number of dead cells (above 90%) in the case of PEITC and complete cell death with BITC. Sulforaphane, also used in this study, showed a relatively lower potential in inducing cell death. On the basis of analysis of DNA fragmentation, chromatin condensation, and percentage of cells in the sub-G_1 fraction, apoptosis induction was identified as a mechanism responsible for reduction of the number of viable cells (Xiao et al. 2006). Treatment of the same cell lines with low concentrations of BITC over 2–24 h resulted in an increase in the levels of the pro-apoptotic proteins Bax and Bak and down-regulation of the anti-apoptotic proteins Bcl-2 and Bcl-xL (Xiao et al. 2006). Interestingly, RNA interference of Bax and Bak conferred significant protection against PEITC-induced apoptosis (Xiao et al. 2010). Bcl-2 family members are known to influence the integrity of the mitochondrial membrane: the anti-apoptotic proteins are normally located at the mitochondrial membrane to protect its stability; the pro-apoptotic proteins translocate from the cytosol to the mitochondrial membrane in order to destabilize it in response to apoptotic stimuli. The results from a study performed in human bladder cancer cells (UM-UC3) showed ITC-mediated phosphorylation of Bcl-2, mitochondrial translocation of Bak, and disruption of the association of Bcl-xL with both Bak and Bax in the mitochondrial membrane, indicating that ITC-induced mitochondrial damage results at least in part from modulation of selected Bcl-2 family members (Tang and Zhang 2005). This effect was further complemented in breast cancer cells through the presence of the loss of mitochondrial membrane potential, cytochrome c release and finally activation of caspase-9, -3 and -8. Pre-treatment of cells with specific inhibitors for caspase-9 or -8 was associated with decreased cleavage of pro-caspase-3 and decreased DNA fragmentation, pointing at the involvement of both, the mitochondrial pathway (mediated by caspase-9) and the death receptor pathway (mediated by caspase-8) in apoptosis induction (Xiao et al. 2006). The capacity of ITCs to induce apoptosis is also observed in various cell culture (Pappa et al. 2006, 2007a, b) as well as in vivo systems where researchers have linked this ability to the antineoplastic effects seen in their studies (Yeh et al. 2016a, b; Herz et al. 2014; Wang et al. 2014; Stan et al. 2014; Ni et al. 2013). For example, both BITC (Huang et al. 2018) and PEITC (Chou et al. 2018) have been found to inhibit the growth of xenograft tumors of glioblastoma multiforme in mice, in part, due to their capability to induce apoptosis in these cells through the down regulation of several anti-apoptotic proteins. In a highly metastatic human non-small cell lung cancer cell line L9981, BITC and PEITC have shown to potently induce apoptosis as well as cause the upregulation of the MAPK signaling pathway (a signaling pathway implicated in apoptosis induction), and that their effects were abrogated by the pretreatment with the anti-oxidant N-acetyl-cysteine (NAC) (Yan et al. 2011). Also, using the Affymetrix GeneChip microarray, treatment of these cells with 10 μM BITC for 24 h exhibited an upregulation of 77 and 52 genes involved in apoptosis and cell cycle progression respectively (Yan et al. 2011).

Another molecular mechanism by which these ITCs induce apoptosis could be through the modulation of the short form Recepteur d'Origine Nantais (sfRON), a receptor tyrosine kinase. Sehrawat and Singh reported that MCF7 cells overexpressing sfRON (MCF7/sfRON) treated with 5 μM BITC for 24 h had an approximately two-fold higher apoptotic-induction compared to the wild-type cells (Sehrawat and Singh 2016). MCF7/sfRON and MDA-MB-361/sfRON cells treated with 5 μM BITC for 6 h exhibited an increase in activated apoptotic proteins Bak and Bax compared to their respective wild-type counterparts (Sehrawat and Singh 2016). Also, it is interesting to note that MCF7/sfRON cells had increased basal ROS production and BITC-induced ROS production in these cells was significantly attenuated compared to their wild-type counterparts (Sehrawat and Singh 2016).

The combinatorial effects of ITCs in inducing cancer cell death has also been studied. It has been shown that in the non-small cell lung cancer cell line A549, the synergistic effects of AITC and sulforaphane led to a more extensive apoptosis induction compared to when the ITCs were singly administered (Rakariyatham et al. 2019). It will be interesting to evaluate the synergistic potential of ITCs for their antineoplastic potential in animal models.

Although there is a large body of evidence linking ITCs to apoptosis induction, it is noteworthy that there has been an instance where they have been implicated in the inhibition of apoptosis (Ho et al. 2012). In particular, in the left ventricle of the heart of a murine acquired immune deficiency syndrome (AIDS) model, Ho and colleagues found that sulforaphane, PEITC and BITC inhibit apoptosis by increasing the Bcl-2/Bax ratio when compared to the vehicle treated mice (Ho et al. 2012) and that mice treated with the ITCs survived at least 25 days longer than the control group.

9.4.3 The Role of ROS Induction in ITC-Mediated Cytotoxicity

Pro-oxidative properties of BITC, as potentially important for triggering apoptosis, were investigated by use of dihydroethidium (DHE) bromide (hydroethidine) and 2′,7′-dichlorodihydrofluorescein diacetate (H_2DCF-DA), fluorescent probes designed to indicate superoxide anion radicals and more general ROS levels, respectively (Table 9.5). MDA-MB-231 cells treated with 2.5 μM of BITC for 2 h were loaded with the dyes. Subsequent measurements of oxidized fluorescent products ethidium bromide and 2′,7′-dichlorofluorescein (DCF) fluorescence indicated increased signals for BITC-treated samples compared to a vehicle control. Moreover, apoptosis induction by BITC was significantly attenuated in the presence of combined superoxide dismutase and catalase mimetic EUK134, supporting the notion that ROS generation is critical for triggering the death pathway (Xiao et al. 2006). Further studies by the same authors demonstrated that increased ROS levels by BITC treatment were due to inhibition of Complex III of the mitochondrial respiratory chain (Xiao et al. 2008). BITC-induced ROS production and apoptosis were significantly inhibited by overexpression of the anti-oxidant enzymes catalase and Cu,Zn-superoxide dismutase and by pharmacological inhibition of the mitochondrial respiratory chain (Xiao et al. 2008). In accordance, the mitochondrial DNA-deficient Rho-0 variant of MDA-MB-231 cells was almost completely resistant to BITC-stimulated ROS generation and apoptosis induction (Xiao et al. 2008). Treatment with BITC caused activation of c-Jun N-terminal kinase (JNK) and the mitogen-activated protein kinase p38 (Xiao et al. 2008); the latter is s also observed upon treatment with PEITC (Dayalan Naidu et al. 2016). Pharmacological inhibition of both JNK and p38 ensured partial protection against BITC-induced apoptosis (Xiao et al. 2008). Concerning the cascade of events triggered by BITC, it can be concluded from this study that ROS production is up-stream of JNK and p38 activation, and such activation is up-stream of Bax conformational changes.

Hence, overexpression of catalase abolished activation of JNK and p38 in BITC treated cells, and BITC-mediated activation of Bax was suppressed by ectopic expression of a catalytically inactive mutant of JNKK2, which is a JNK specific kinase (Xiao et al. 2008). The importance of JNK, p38 and related signaling in mediating cytotoxic effects of sulforaphane and PEITC was examined in the MM.1S myeloma cell line (Jakubikova et al. 2011). Multiplex analysis of phosphorylation of diverse components of signaling cascades revealed transient changes in JNK, c-Jun, MEK1, p38, extracellular signal-regulated kinase (ERK)1/2, Akt, GSK3α/β and p53 activation in sulforaphane- and PEITC-treated cells, which may result from ITC-induced oxidative stress or potential targeting of phosphatases (Jakubikova et al. 2011). Studies done in human prostate cancer cells (LNCaP and PC-3) showed similarly that PEITC-induced cell death initiated by production of ROS (measured here by electron paramagnetic resonance spectroscopy: EPR) correlated with inhibition of Complex III activity, suppression of oxidative phosphorylation, and ATP depletion (Xiao et al. 2010). Pre-treatment of cells with 4 mM N-acetyl cysteine

(NAC) for 2 h, followed by further PEITC/NAC co-treatment, caused a decrease of ROS production and readouts for apoptotic markers (Xiao et al. 2010).

Nevertheless, a study by Mi et al. (2010) with use of [^{14}C]PEITC and [^{14}C] sulforaphane demonstrated that NAC pretreatment significantly reduced ITC cellular uptake by conjugating with ITCs extracellularly in the cell culture medium, suggesting that reduced uptake of ITCs, rather than the antioxidant activity of NAC itself, is responsible for the diminished downstream apoptotic effect (Mi et al. 2010). Therefore, other approaches, such as Rho-0 cells characterized by non-functional mitochondria or up-/down-regulation of antioxidant enzymes level would be more reliable to demonstrate the importance of ROS signaling induced by ITCs for downstream effects. Indeed, counterparts of LNCaP and PC-3 cells with overexpressed Mn-SOD or Cu,Zn-SOD, or unfunctional respiratory chain (Rho-0 cells), were more resistant to PEITC-mediated ROS generation and subsequent apoptosis induction (Xiao et al. 2010).

It is recognized now that the superoxide anion radical production by Complex III of the mitochondrial respiratory chain is directed towards both matrix and intermembrane space (Han et al. 2003). This would clarify why overexpression of SOD localized to the mitochondrial matrix (Mn-SOD) and SOD localized to the mitochondrial intermembrane space and cytosol (Cu,Zn-SOD) could decrease PEITC-mediated ROS generation (Xiao et al. 2010). On the other hand, there have been some studies reporting ITC-stimulated ROS-independent cell death (Wiczk et al. 2012; Hsu et al. 2013). Measuring [^{3}H]-leucine incorporation, Wiczk et al. observed that sulforaphane dose-dependently (10, 20 and 40 μM) reduced protein synthesis in PC-3 cells by 80, 50 and 20% when compared to the vehicle-treated cells (Wiczk et al. 2012). They further found that SFN-induced protein synthesis blockade occurred in a ROS-independent manner, and that cell death induced by SFN was due to the decrease in the levels of the short-lived protein survivin (Wiczk et al. 2012).

ROS accumulation activates the unfolded protein response (UPR), which causes ER stress, which if not alleviated, leads to activation of cell death pathways. In ovarian cancer cell lines SKOV3 and PA-1, exposure to 5 μM PEITC for 48 h caused cellular ROS accumulation, subsequent UPR activation and apoptotic cell death. These effects observed upon PEITC exposure were abrogated in the presence of the ROS scavenger NAC, signifying that PEITC-induced ROS is crucial for the UPR-induced apoptosis (Hong et al. 2015).

Studies by Brown et al. brought interesting insights into the exact topology of PEITC-mediated ROS generation (Brown et al. 2008). There exist several enzymes dedicated to remove intracellular hydrogen peroxide (H_2O_2), a product of superoxide dismutation by SOD. One type is represented by peroxiredoxins (Prxs) that in course of peroxide decomposition by specific cysteine residues generate a disulfide-linked intermolecular dimer. Hence, their oxidation can be analyzed by western blotting detection of a band shift from monomer (reduced Prx) to dimer (oxidized Prx). Interestingly, oxidation of mitochondrial peroxiredoxin 3 (Prx3) was detected as early as 5 min after exposure of Jurkat T lymphoma cells to PEITC. Time- (5–120 min with 15 μM) and dose- (2.5–60 μM for 60 min) dependent analyses revealed that such oxidation is specific to the mitochondrial isoform, with cytoplasmic Prx1 and Prx2 remaining in their reduced forms (Brown et al. 2008). Treatment of the cells with sulforaphane under similar conditions had no influence on Prx3 dimerization. Moreover, the ability to disturb mitochondrial redox homeostasis by selected ITCs was correlated to their pro-apoptotic activity (from the most to least potent: PEITC, BITC, phenylhexyl ITC, phenylbutyl ITC, phenylpropyl ITC, AITC, sulforaphane) (Brown et al. 2008). In addition to regulation of Prx oxidation, ITCs are able to modulate cellular redox conditions by affecting the activity of other antioxidant enzymes, including thioredoxin reductase (Brown et al. 2008, 2010; Heiss and Gerhauser 2005), glutathione peroxidase (Trachootham et al. 2006), and glutathione reductase (Brown et al. 2008).

9.4.4 ITC-Related Electrophilicity and Apoptosis Induction

Cysteine residues present in diverse classes of proteins often have regulatory roles. They can be subjected to modifications such as oxidation, nitrosylation or glutathionylation, and also have the ability to bind to metals contained within proteins. Such cysteine modifications on proteins may have different biological consequences. Not all cysteine residues are equally reactive. Cysteine reactivity to electrophiles greatly varies across different proteins and also within the same protein. The protonation state of the cysteine residue determines the extent of its reactivity and nucleophilicity that is indicated by its pKa value, which in turn is affected by the proximate amino acids. Free cysteine residues usually have a pKa value of 8.6 whereas a reactive cysteine has a pKa value in the neutral or even acidic range, and thus typically exists in a thiolate form (Roos et al. 2013).

Keap1, the main negative regulator of transcription factor Nrf2 (Itoh et al. 1999), is equipped with highly reactive cysteines that serve as sensors for electrophiles (Dinkova-Kostova et al. 2002; McMahon et al. 2010; Saito et al. 2016), including ITCs, leading to Nrf2 stabilization and enhanced Nrf2-target gene expression (Fig. 9.4). Cysteine 151 in Keap1, which is surrounded by a cluster of basic amino acids (H129, K131, R135, K150, and H154), is the primary sensor for sulforaphane and PEITC (Zhang and Hannink 2003; Dayalan Naidu et al. 2018). However, at high concentration of PEITC (7.5 μM for immortalized mouse embryonic fibroblast cells), Nrf2 stabilization proceeds in the absence of cysteine 151 (Zhang and Hannink 2003; Dayalan Naidu et al. 2018), indicating that other cysteines are also modified within Keap1 as well as other proteins. Thus, mass spectrometric analyses have demonstrated that PEITC directly interacts with two cysteines of purified Prx3 in vitro (Brown et al. 2008). Also, by use of high-resolution mass spectrometry, it has been shown in vitro that PEITC modifies the single cysteine in GSTA1 as well as cysteines 14, 47 and 169 in GSTP1 causing the irreversible inhibition of the catalytic activity of these enzymes. This observation suggests that PEITC is capable of suppressing its own metabolism in the cells through its sulfhydryl reactivity (Kumari et al. 2016). It has been speculated that the inhibition of Complex III by PEITC may be caused by covalent modification of critical sulfhydryl groups on subunit(s) of Complex III driven by the electrophilicity of the isothiocyanate moiety. In this regard, direct covalent modification of cellular proteins has been suggested to be an important early event in the induction of apoptosis by ITCs (Mi et al. 2007) (Table 9.6). So far, several specific protein targets have been identified (Mi et al. 2008, 2009, 2011; Lin et al. 2011). A study using two-dimensional gel electrophoresis of human lung cancer A549 cells treated with radiolabeled PEITC and sulforaphane revealed that tubulin may be an intracellular binding target for ITCs. The potency exerted by selected ITCs to cause mitotic arrest and apoptosis correlated positively with their ability to disrupt microtubule polymerization, with the established order of activity: BITC > PEITC > sulforaphane ($IC_{50} = 13.8 > 18.3 > 43$ μM) (Mi et al. 2008). Immunofluorescent microscopy showed disruption and degradation of the microtubule network in A549 cells treated with 5 μM of BITC or PEITC for 0.5 h and 1 h, respectively, while treatment with 10 μM sulforaphane over 4 h did not affect cells so potently. In contrast, exposure of cells to N-methyl phenethylamine, a structural analog of PEITC lacking the isothiocyanate functionality, did not interfere with tubulin polymerization, and consequently did not reduce cell viability (Mi et al. 2008). Additionally, tubulin precipitation was detected in BITC- and PEITC-treated cells, suggesting that this is a result of structural misfolding caused by ITCs. Further mass spectrometric data of tubulin purified from the insoluble fraction revealed that cysteine 347 of α-tubulin was covalently modified by BITC (Mi et al. 2008). The authors concluded that variation in ITCs activity to bind to tubulin and cause apoptosis results from the differences in their structure, which determines compound hydrophobicity, size, shape, and electrophilicity, all together influencing binding preferences (Mi et al. 2008). Exemplarily, the alkyl linkage joining the –N=C=S moiety to the aromatic ring is shorter in BITC then in PEITC. This might explain differences in covalent interaction between these ITCs and tubulin. Further studies by the same group demonstrated that ITCs can selectively induce degradation of both α- and β-tubulin in a variety of human cancer cell lines. Tubulin aggregation was found as the initial step in its proteasome-dependent degradation, which is triggered by ITC binding to tubulin and is independent from oxidative stress (Mi et al. 2009).

Other identified protein targets of ITCs are components of the 20S and 26S proteasomes. Their activities in cancer cells of different tissue origin were significantly inhibited by BITC or PEITC binding. This binding was unrelated to either ROS generation or ITC-induced protein degradation (Mi et al. 2011). Recent investigations have indicated that ITC-induced apoptosis of oncogene-transformed cells (MCF-10A-Ras) involved thiol modification of DNA topoisomerase II (Top2). siRNA-mediated knockdown of Top2α resulted in reduced sensitivity towards ITCs, showing that the Top2α protein level is important for mediating ITC-induced growth inhibition, DNA damage and apoptosis. In addition, proteomic analysis revealed that several cysteine residues on human Top2α were covalently modified by BITC, possibly contributing to formation of lethal Top2α-DNA covalent adducts (Top2α cleavage complex) (Lin et al. 2011).

MEK kinase 1 (MEKK1) is a MAP3K that regulates ERK and JNK MAPK pathways, pro-apoptotic and pro-survival pathways. Cross and colleagues found that oxidative stress induced by menadione exposure inhibits the function of MEKK1 *via* the glutathionylation of its cysteine residue 1238 which is found in the ATP-binding domain (Cross and Templeton 2004). In a following study by the same group, MEKK1 overexpressed in CV-1 cells showed that 1 h exposure to PEITC from 50 μM to 200 μM showed reduction it is catalytic activity when the kinases were purified from these cells an assayed in an in vitro kinase assay. Importantly, using purified recombinant full length MEKK1 and the mutant MEKK1 C1238V which retains its wild-type kinase function whilst resistant to oxidative stimuli, it was shown that PEITC dose dependently (6.5 μM to 200 μM) caused a loss of kinase activity in the wild-type MEKK1 and that the mutant MEKK1 C1238V retained its kinase activity, indicating that C1238 is modified by PEITC thereby inhibiting its kinase activity (Cross et al. 2007). However, it remains to be seen whether inhibition of MEKK1 by PEITC affects its pro-apoptotic or its pro-survival activity. The MEK1/MEKK1/FLT3 inhibitor E6201 dose-dependently induced apoptosis in acute myeloid leukemia cells, therefore, it is possible that chemical inhibition of MEKK1 through PEITC may allow it to exert it pro-apoptotic effects.

Under basal conditions, the apoptosis signal-regulating kinase 1 (ASK1), a mitogen-activated protein kinase kinase kinase (MAP3K), is negatively regulated by the redox-sensitive protein thioredoxin 1 (Txn1) through direct interaction (Bishopric and Webster 2002). ASK1, is an upstream regulator of the MAPK family members p38 and JNK and when activated, signals pro-apoptotic pathways mediated by these kinases (Liu et al. 2000). Mutagenesis studies using purified recombinant proteins reveal that the Txn1 binds to ASK1 through its cysteines C32 and C35, where the former residue exhibits a relatively higher binding affinity (Kylarova et al. 2016). Oxidation of Txn1 has been implicated in its dissociation from ASK1 and the subsequent activation of the kinase (Nadeau et al. 2007; Saitoh et al. 1998). It has been found that in the hepatocellular carcinoma cell line MHCC97H, a 24 h exposure to 20 and 30 μM PEITC caused the reduction in the levels of reduced Txn1 and increased the levels of oxidized Txn1 in a dose-dependent manner (Zhang et al. 2012). In CV-1 cells expressing full length ASK1, exposure to PEITC does not affect its kinase activity (Cross et al. 2007). Since oxidation status of Txn1 is perturbed by PEITC, possibly through its electrophilic nature, it is highly conceivable that apoptosis induced by this isothiocyanate is mediated via ASK1 activation through the release of Txn1 from the kinase.

9.4.5 Necrosis, Autophagy, and Cell Cycle Arrest Triggered by ITCs

The cellular processes other than apoptosis triggered by ITCs-initiated oxidative stress or protein thiocarbamoylation deserve some attention and include induction of necrosis, autophagy, and cell cycle arrest. Such events triggered by ITCs can represent the responses interrelated to or distinct from apoptosis induction (Xiao et al. 2006).

Effects of sulforaphane and PEITC on induction of apoptosis and necrosis in myeloma cells (MM.1S) were quantified by flow cytometry upon staining with annexinV-FITC and PI (propidium iodide). The percentage ratio of apoptotic to necrotic death was about 70% to 30%, respectively (Jakubikova et al. 2011), demonstrating a significant contribution of necrosis to the overall mechanisms responsible for a drop of cell survival. The study performed in leukemia cells (HL60) treated with different ITCs for 6 h revealed an over 50% contribution of necrotic cells to the total pool of dead cells. This phenomenon was especially visible when higher concentrations of ITCs were used (Jakubikova et al. 2005b). Consistently, apoptosis was induced when rat liver cells were treated with 20 μM BITC, but increasing its concentration to 50 μM caused necrosis (Nakamura et al. 2002).

ROS resulting from the disturbance of the mitochondrial electron transport chain or catalase degradation can induce autophagy (Azad et al. 2009). Autophagy, a self-digestion process that degrades intracellular structures in response to stress caused by nutrient starvation, mitochondrial toxins, hypoxia, or ROS, can be involved in both cell survival and cell death. Autophagic degradation of cellular material generates amino acids and fatty acids, which can be used for protein synthesis and ATP generation during stressful conditions such as starvation. Autophagy also removes protein aggregates (which can trigger apoptosis) and damaged mitochondria (as a source of apoptotic proteins and toxic ROS). However, prolonged autophagy can lead to cell death through excessive self-digestion or activation of apoptosis (Azad et al. 2009; Kondo et al. 2005).

Xiao et al. investigated the induction of autophagy as an additional mechanism downstream of ROS generation by PEITC (Xiao et al. 2010). PEITC-initiated autophagy was partially dependent on ROS production in prostate LNCaP and PC-3 cancer cells, since their Rho-0 counterparts were less affected when autophagy markers were analyzed. Xiao et al. suggested that autophagy may represent a clearing mechanism for mitochondria involved in ROS production. Nevertheless, a possible influence of autophagy on apoptosis induction in this study could not be excluded and remains to be elucidated (Xiao et al. 2010). In triple negative breast cancer cell lines, MDA-MB-231, MDA-MB-468 and BT549, by the use of fluorescence microscopy techniques, it was reported that sulforaphane induced autophagy by downregulating HDAC6-mediated PTEN activation (Yang et al. 2018), where the latter is an important driver of autophagy (Ueno et al. 2008). BITC induced autophagy in the human colorectal cancer cells HCT-116 where increases in the lipidated form of LC3B and p62 which are proteins required for the formation of autophagic vesicles were observed (Liu et al. 2017). A similar effect was observed with the use of sulforaphane in the U2OS osteosarcoma cells (Olagnier et al. 2017) and PEITC in a prostate cancer mouse model (Powolny et al. 2011).

A common phenomenon caused by ITCs in different cancer cell lines is the inhibition of cell cycle progression. Most reports describe ITC-induced cell cycle arrest at the G_2-M phase. Statistically significant enrichment of the G_2-M fraction of MDA-MB-231 cells treated with 2.5 μM BITC was evident as early as 3 h after treatment and this effect was sustained, correlating with increased growth inhibition (Xiao et al. 2006). Studies by Jakubikova and colleagues showed that AITC (10 μM,

24 h) was the most potent inducer of G_2-M arrest among the six tested ITCs where 52% of the HL60 cells accumulated at the G_2-M phase (Jakubikova et al. 2005b). PEITC- and sulforaphane-induced G_2-M cell cycle arrest was accompanied by phosphorylation of histone H3 at serine 10 (a mitotic marker) in human myeloma cell lines (Jakubikova et al. 2011). Immunobloting analysis revealed that BITC-mediated cell cycle arrest was associated with a decrease in levels of proteins involved in regulation of G_2-M transition, including cyclin B1, cyclin-dependent kinase 1 (Cdk1), and cell division cycle 25C (Cdc25C) (Fig. 9.4) (Xiao et al. 2006). Expression patterns of cell cycle-related proteins were studied also in myeloma cells (MM.1S) and revealed a decrease of cyclin B1, p-Cdc2 and Cdc25C (Jakubikova et al. 2011). Similarly, the BITC- and PEITC-induced G_2-M phase arrest of human osteosarcoma U2OS cells was due to a reduction in cyclin A and B1 levels, accompanied by an increase of Chk1 and p53 levels, events that lead to G_2-M arrest (Wu et al. 2011). Along these lines, it has been demonstrated that treatment of glioma cells with AITC markedly reduced Cdk1/cyclin B activity and protein levels (Chen et al. 2010). Interestingly, experiments using phase-specific synchronized cells demonstrated that G_2-M phase-arrested cells are more sensitive to undergo apoptotic stimulation by BITC than cells in other phases (Miyoshi et al. 2004). A recent study conducted by Mantso and colleagues found that using low concentrations of sulforaphane, BITC and PEITC (5 μM) in the human melanoma cell line A375 for 48 h with a replenishment of cell growth media with the compounds after 24 h of exposure showed that these cells, in agreement with other independent reports in the literature, were arrested at the G_2-M phase (Mantso et al. 2019). BITC caused the highest proportion of A375 cells to arrest at G_2-M followed by sulforaphane and PEITC (Mantso et al. 2019). In this study, all three ITCs induced p21, p27, cyclin D1, cyclin D3, CDK2 and p53 phosphoserine 15 and caused a reduction in the cyclin dependent kinases (CDK) 4 and 6, where the levels of all of these proteins when perturbed cause cell cycle arrest (Mantso et al. 2019).

9.4.6 ITC-Mediated Selective Killing of Transformed and Cancer Cells

It is of great importance to address the question of whether normal cells are sensitive to ITC-induced oxidative and/or electrophilic stress and the following signals leading to cell death. Studies performed by Xiao et al. indicated that normal mammary epithelial cell lines (MCF-10A or HMEC) were significantly more resistant to growth arrest and apoptosis induction by BITC compared to breast cancer cell lines (MDA-MB-231 and MCF-7) (Xiao et al. 2006, 2008). Similarly, investigations done in human prostate cancer cell lines (LNCaP and PC-3) and their representative normal prostate epithelial cells (PrEC) revealed that ROS generation by PEITC is more harmful to cancer cells than to normal cells (Xiao et al. 2010). These results suggest that ITCs may selectively target cancer cells but spare normal breast or prostate epithelium, which is a highly desirable property of potential anticancer agents (Xiao et al. 2006, 2010).

In ovarian cancer cell lines SKOV3 and PA-1, exposure to PEITC induced cell death, however, in the same study, this effect of PEITC was not observed in normal ovarian epithelial cells (Hong et al. 2015). Similarly, in human laryngeal carcinoma Hep-2 cells, exposure to a maximum of 10 μM PEITC exerted its anti-cancer properties by causing cell cycle arrest at G_2-M, inhibiting cell proliferation and inducing apoptosis, and these effects were not observed in the normal human bronchial epithelial cells 16HBE. This finding shows the sensitivity of the Hep-2 cells to PEITC compared to the normal cells (Dai et al. 2016). Furthermore, findings from this study provide a therapeutic strategy where a safe range (up to 10 μM in vitro) of administration of PEITC will confer minimal toxicity to normal cells and at the same time has the ability to exert its antineoplastic effects on cancer cells (Dai et al. 2016).

Trachootham et al. developed an interesting model, consisting of immortalized ovarian epithelial cells (T72) and their H-Ras^{V12} transformed counterparts (T72Ras), to test the concept that increased ROS generation associated with oncogenic transformation may serve as a biochemical basis to selectively kill cancer cells using agents that cause further oxidative stress (Trachootham et al. 2006). Indeed, oxidative stress facilitated by exposure to PEITC was significantly more pronounced in T72Ras cells comparing to parental T72 cells, corresponding with a lowered survival of transformed cells in response to treatment (10 days treatment: $IC_{50} = 0.49 \pm 0.1$ μM for T72Ras vs. $IC_{50} = 1.95 \pm 0.1$ μM for T72) (Trachootham et al. 2006). The selective killing of Ras-transformed cells by PEITC was attributed to ROS-mediated damage of mitochondria. PEITC was also proved to be effective in killing naturally occurring human ovarian cancer cells (SKOV3, A2008, HEY) and exhibited significant therapeutic activity in vivo by prolonging survival of mice bearing Ras-transformed ovarian cancer cells (Trachootham et al. 2006). Similar pro-survival effects combined with decreased tumor volume were achieved with sulforaphane and PEITC in a myeloma xenograft mouse model (Jakubikova et al. 2011). As important factor for therapeutic applications, and shown in later studies, ITCs concentrations required to produce statistically significant inhibition of cancer cell growth may be achievable in vivo.

9.5 Summary

Isothiocyanates are promising multitarget cancer preventive agents. They exert health promoting effects mainly through induction of cytoprotective enzymes or selective toxicity towards cancer cells, processes critical for decreasing the risk of cancer onset and retardation or inhibition of tumor growth, respectively. Various investigations performed in cultured cancer cells support the notion that pro-oxidative and electrophilic activities of ITCs serve as a main driving force of their anti-tumor properties. The electrophilic nature of ITCs determines their targeting to molecules containing nucleophilic moieties. Indeed, upon entering cells ITCs are metabolized by conjugation with the cysteine residue of GSH, and due to extracellular exclusion of such conjugates during the detoxification process, cause depletion of this main cellular redox buffer. This, together with direct reactivity with cysteine residues within their target proteins and oxidative stress mediated *via* the mitochondrial pathway, challenges the cellular anti-oxidant defense. Such conditions stimulate the response of redox-sensitive proteins. One of them is Keap1, which upon sensor cysteine modification by ITCs loses its ability to target Nrf2 for ubiquitination and proteasomal degradation, enabling Nrf2 to accumulate, translocate to the nucleus and act as a transcription factor for cytoprotective genes regulated via ARE/EpRE. Subsequent increase of cytoprotective enzymes determines the restoration of the GSH pool and re-balancing of the cellular redox homeostasis. Nevertheless, this pro-survival signaling can be confronted by cell death-promoting pathways that are turned on in response to ITC-mediated cellular stress. Thiocarbamoylation of proteins, such as tubulin, proteasome or topoisomerase II, has been demonstrated as an early and critical event for induction of apoptosis and cell cycle arrest by ITCs. Similar reactivity of ITCs toward Complex III of the mitochondrial respiratory chain has been suggested to trigger ROS production and further mitochondrial damage, contributing to caspase-executed apoptosis.

Undoubtedly, ITCs possess potential to exhibit various biological activities. This renders this family of compounds highly effective in providing protection against cancer in animal models, induced by a variety of chemical carcinogens. In addition to preventing chemically induced cancers, several ITC compounds have also been shown to inhibit growth of cancer cells in vivo. In translating the anti-cancer efficacy of ITCs into the clinic, combinatorial therapy has been suggested whereby chemopreventive compounds are given in association with drugs currently used in chemotherapy, to achieve synergistic interaction for anti-cancer activity and reduce harmful effects (Russo et al. 2010).

References

Abdelhamid G, Anwar-Mohamed A, Elmazar MM, El-Kadi AO (2010) Modulation of NAD(P)H: quinone oxidoreductase by vanadium in human hepatoma HepG2 cells. Toxicol in Vitro 24 (6):1554–1561

Ade N, Leon F, Pallardy M, Peiffer JL, Kerdine-Romer S, Tissier MH et al (2009) HMOX1 and NQO1 genes are upregulated in response to contact sensitizers in dendritic cells and THP-1 cell line: role of the Keap1/Nrf2 pathway. Toxicol Sci 107(2):451–460

Agyeman AS, Chaerkady R, Shaw PG, Davidson NE, Visvanathan K, Pandey A et al (2012) Transcriptomic and proteomic profiling of KEAP1 disrupted and sulforaphane-treated human breast epithelial cells reveals common expression profiles. Breast Cancer Res Treat 132 (1):175–187

Amara IE, El-Kadi AO (2011) Transcriptional modulation of the NAD(P)H:quinone oxidoreductase 1 by mercury in human hepatoma HepG2 cells. Free Radic Biol Med 51(9):1675–1685

Antosiewicz J, Ziolkowski W, Kar S, Powolny AA, Singh SV (2008) Role of reactive oxygen intermediates in cellular responses to dietary cancer chemopreventive agents. Planta Med 74 (13):1570–1579

Anwar-Mohamed A, El-Kadi AO (2009) Down-regulation of the detoxifying enzyme NAD(P)H: quinone oxidoreductase 1 by vanadium in Hepa 1c1c7 cells. Toxicol Appl Pharmacol 236 (3):261–269

Azad MB, Chen Y, Gibson SB (2009) Regulation of autophagy by reactive oxygen species (ROS): implications for cancer progression and treatment. Antioxid Redox Signal 11(4):777–790

Bacon JR, Williamson G, Garner RC, Lappin G, Langouet S, Bao Y (2003) Sulforaphane and quercetin modulate PhIP-DNA adduct formation in human HepG2 cells and hepatocytes. Carcinogenesis 24(12):1903–1911

Bergstrom P, Andersson HC, Gao Y, Karlsson JO, Nodin C, Anderson MF et al (2011) Repeated transient sulforaphane stimulation in astrocytes leads to prolonged Nrf2-mediated gene expression and protection from superoxide-induced damage. Neuropharmacology 60(2–3):343–353

Bertl E, Bartsch H, Gerhauser C (2006) Inhibition of angiogenesis and endothelial cell functions are novel sulforaphane-mediated mechanisms in chemoprevention. Mol Cancer Ther 5(3):575–585

Bishopric NH, Webster KA (2002) Preventing apoptosis with thioredoxin: ASK me how. Circ Res 90(12):1237–1239

Brooks JD, Paton V (1999) Potent induction of carcinogen defence enzymes with sulforaphane, a putative prostate cancer chemopreventive agent. Prostate Cancer Prostatic Dis 2(S3):S8

Brooks JD, Paton VG, Vidanes G (2001) Potent induction of phase 2 enzymes in human prostate cells by sulforaphane. Cancer Epidemiol Biomark Prev 10(9):949–954

Brown KK, Eriksson SE, Arner ES, Hampton MB (2008) Mitochondrial peroxiredoxin 3 is rapidly oxidized in cells treated with isothiocyanates. Free Radic Biol Med 45(4):494–502

Brown KK, Cox AG, Hampton MB (2010) Mitochondrial respiratory chain involvement in peroxiredoxin 3 oxidation by phenethyl isothiocyanate and auranofin. FEBS Lett 584 (6):1257–1262

Chang G, Guo Y, Jia Y, Duan W, Li B, Yu J et al (2010) Protective effect of combination of sulforaphane and riluzole on glutamate-mediated excitotoxicity. Biol Pharm Bull 33 (9):1477–1483

Chen NG, Chen KT, Lu CC, Lan YH, Lai CH, Chung YT et al (2010) Allyl isothiocyanate triggers G2/M phase arrest and apoptosis in human brain malignant glioma GBM 8401 cells through a mitochondria-dependent pathway. Oncol Rep 24(2):449–455

Chen G, Fang Q, Zhang J, Zhou D, Wang Z (2011) Role of the Nrf2-ARE pathway in early brain injury after experimental subarachnoid hemorrhage. J Neurosci Res 89(4):515–523

Cheung KL, Kong AN (2010) Molecular targets of dietary phenethyl isothiocyanate and sulforaphane for cancer chemoprevention. AAPS J 12(1):87–97

Chou YC, Chang MY, Lee HT, Shen CC, Harnod T, Liang YJ et al (2018) Phenethyl isothiocyanate inhibits in vivo growth of xenograft tumors of human glioblastoma cells. Molecules 23(9). https://doi.org/10.3390/molecules23092305

Chung FL, Conaway CC, Rao CV, Reddy BS (2000) Chemoprevention of colonic aberrant crypt foci in Fischer rats by sulforaphane and phenethyl isothiocyanate. Carcinogenesis 21 (12):2287–2291

Clarke JD, Hsu A, Yu Z, Dashwood RH, Ho E (2011) Differential effects of sulforaphane on histone deacetylases, cell cycle arrest and apoptosis in normal prostate cells versus hyperplastic and cancerous prostate cells. Mol Nutr Food Res 55(7):999–1009

Conaway CC, Wang CX, Pittman B, Yang YM, Schwartz JE, Tian D et al (2005) Phenethyl isothiocyanate and sulforaphane and their N-acetylcysteine conjugates inhibit malignant progression of lung adenomas induced by tobacco carcinogens in A/J mice. Cancer Res 65 (18):8548–8557

Cornblatt BS, Ye L, Dinkova-Kostova AT, Erb M, Fahey JW, Singh NK et al (2007) Preclinical and clinical evaluation of sulforaphane for chemoprevention in the breast. Carcinogenesis 28 (7):1485–1490

Cross JV, Templeton DJ (2004) Oxidative stress inhibits MEKK1 by site-specific glutathionylation in the ATP-binding domain. Biochem J 381(Pt 3):675–683

Cross JV, Foss FW, Rady JM, Macdonald TL, Templeton DJ (2007) The isothiocyanate class of bioactive nutrients covalently inhibit the MEKK1 protein kinase. BMC Cancer 7:183

Cuadrado A, Rojo AI, Wells G, Hayes JD, Cousin SP, Rumsey WL et al (2019) Therapeutic targeting of the NRF2 and KEAP1 partnership in chronic diseases. Nat Rev Drug Discov 18 (4):295–317

Dai MY, Wang Y, Chen C, Li F, Xiao BK, Chen SM et al (2016) Phenethyl isothiocyanate induces apoptosis and inhibits cell proliferation and invasion in Hep-2 laryngeal cancer cells. Oncol Rep 35(5):2657–2664

Danilov CA, Chandrasekaran K, Racz J, Soane L, Zielke C, Fiskum G (2009) Sulforaphane protects astrocytes against oxidative stress and delayed death caused by oxygen and glucose deprivation. Glia 57(6):645–656

Dash PK, Zhao J, Orsi SA, Zhang M, Moore AN (2009) Sulforaphane improves cognitive function administered following traumatic brain injury. Neurosci Lett 460(2):103–107

Dayalan Naidu S, Sutherland C, Zhang Y, Risco A, de la Vega L, Caunt CJ et al (2016) Heat shock factor 1 is a substrate for p38 mitogen-activated protein kinases. Mol Cell Biol 36 (18):2403–2417

Dayalan Naidu S, Suzuki T, Yamamoto M, Fahey JW, Dinkova-Kostova AT (2018) Phenethyl isothiocyanate, a dual activator of transcription factors NRF2 and HSF1. Mol Nutr Food Res 62 (18):e1700908

Dinkova-Kostova AT, Talalay P (2008) Direct and indirect antioxidant properties of inducers of cytoprotective proteins. Mol Nutr Food Res 52(Suppl 1):S128–S138

Dinkova-Kostova AT, Talalay P (2010) NAD(P)H:quinone acceptor oxidoreductase 1 (NQO1), a multifunctional antioxidant enzyme and exceptionally versatile cytoprotector. Arch Biochem Biophys 501(1):116–123

Dinkova-Kostova AT, Wang XJ (2011) Induction of the Keap1/Nrf2/ARE pathway by oxidizable diphenols. Chem Biol Interact 192(1–2):101–106

Dinkova-Kostova AT, Holtzclaw WD, Cole RN, Itoh K, Wakabayashi N, Katoh Y et al (2002) Direct evidence that sulfhydryl groups of Keap1 are the sensors regulating induction of phase 2 enzymes that protect against carcinogens and oxidants. Proc Natl Acad Sci U S A 99 (18):11908–11913

Dinkova-Kostova AT, Jenkins SN, Fahey JW, Ye L, Wehage SL, Liby KT et al (2006) Protection against UV-light-induced skin carcinogenesis in SKH-1 high-risk mice by sulforaphane-containing broccoli sprout extracts. Cancer Lett 240(2):243–252

Dinkova-Kostova AT, Fahey JW, Kostov RV, Kensler TW (2017) KEAP1 and done? Targeting the NRF2 pathway with sulforaphane. Trends Food Sci Technol 69(Pt B):257–269

Ebert B, Kisiela M, Malatkova P, El-Hawari Y, Maser E (2010) Regulation of human carbonyl reductase 3 (CBR3; SDR21C2) expression by Nrf2 in cultured cancer cells. Biochemistry 49 (39):8499–8511

Ernst IM, Schuemann C, Wagner AE, Rimbach G (2011) 3,3′-Diindolylmethane but not indole-3-carbinol activates Nrf2 and induces Nrf2 target gene expression in cultured murine fibroblasts. Free Radic Res 45(8):941–949

Fahey JW, Zalcmann AT, Talalay P (2001) The chemical diversity and distribution of glucosinolates and isothiocyanates among plants. Phytochemistry 56(1):5–51

Fahey JW, Haristoy X, Dolan PM, Kensler TW, Scholtus I, Stephenson KK et al (2002) Sulforaphane inhibits extracellular, intracellular, and antibiotic-resistant strains of Helicobacter pylori and prevents benzo[a]pyrene-induced stomach tumors. Proc Natl Acad Sci U S A 99 (11):7610–7615

Fei P, Matwyshyn GA, Rushmore TH, Kong AN (1996) Transcription regulation of rat glutathione S-transferase Ya subunit gene expression by chemopreventive agents. Pharm Res 13 (7):1043–1048

Fimognari C, Turrini E, Ferruzzi L, Lenzi M, Hrelia P (2012) Natural isothiocyanates: genotoxic potential versus chemoprevention. Mutat Res 750(2):107–131

Forster T, Rausch V, Zhang Y, Isayev O, Heilmann K, Schoensiegel F et al (2014) Sulforaphane counteracts aggressiveness of pancreatic cancer driven by dysregulated Cx43-mediated gap junctional intercellular communication. Oncotarget 5(6):1621–1634

Friling RS, Bensimon A, Tichauer Y, Daniel V (1990) Xenobiotic-inducible expression of murine glutathione S-transferase Ya subunit gene is controlled by an electrophile-responsive element. Proc Natl Acad Sci U S A 87(16):6258–6262

Gan N, Mi L, Sun X, Dai G, Chung FL, Song L (2010) Sulforaphane protects microcystin-LR-induced toxicity through activation of the Nrf2-mediated defensive response. Toxicol Appl Pharmacol 247(2):129–137

Gao X, Dinkova-Kostova AT, Talalay P (2001) Powerful and prolonged protection of human retinal pigment epithelial cells, keratinocytes, and mouse leukemia cells against oxidative damage: the indirect antioxidant effects of sulforaphane. Proc Natl Acad Sci U S A 98 (26):15221–15226

Gaona-Gaona L, Molina-Jijon E, Tapia E, Zazueta C, Hernandez-Pando R, Calderon-Oliver M et al (2011) Protective effect of sulforaphane pretreatment against cisplatin-induced liver and mitochondrial oxidant damage in rats. Toxicology 286(1–3):20–27

Gerhauser C, You M, Liu J, Moriarty RM, Hawthorne M, Mehta RG et al (1997) Cancer chemopreventive potential of sulforamate, a novel analogue of sulforaphane that induces phase 2 drug-metabolizing enzymes. Cancer Res 57(2):272–278

Gills JJ, Jeffery EH, Matusheski NV, Moon RC, Lantvit DD, Pezzuto JM (2006) Sulforaphane prevents mouse skin tumorigenesis during the stage of promotion. Cancer Lett 236(1):72–79

Gross-Steinmeyer K, Stapleton PL, Liu F, Tracy JH, Bammler TK, Quigley SD et al (2004) Phytochemical-induced changes in gene expression of carcinogen-metabolizing enzymes in cultured human primary hepatocytes. Xenobiotica 34(7):619–632

Guerrero-Beltran CE, Calderon-Oliver M, Martinez-Abundis E, Tapia E, Zarco-Marquez G, Zazueta C et al (2010) Protective effect of sulforaphane against cisplatin-induced mitochondrial alterations and impairment in the activity of NAD(P)H: quinone oxidoreductase 1 and gamma glutamyl cysteine ligase: studies in mitochondria isolated from rat kidney and in LLC-PK1 cells. Toxicol Lett 199(1):80–92

Halkier BA, Gershenzon J (2006) Biology and biochemistry of glucosinolates. Annu Rev Plant Biol 57:303–333

Han D, Canali R, Rettori D, Kaplowitz N (2003) Effect of glutathione depletion on sites and topology of superoxide and hydrogen peroxide production in mitochondria. Mol Pharmacol 64 (5):1136–1144

Haristoy X, Fahey JW, Scholtus I, Lozniewski A (2005) Evaluation of the antimicrobial effects of several isothiocyanates on Helicobacter pylori. Planta Med 71(4):326–330

Hayes JD, McMahon M, Chowdhry S, Dinkova-Kostova AT (2010) Cancer chemoprevention mechanisms mediated through the Keap1-Nrf2 pathway. Antioxid Redox Signal 13 (11):1713–1748

Heiss E, Gerhauser C (2005) Time-dependent modulation of thioredoxin reductase activity might contribute to sulforaphane-mediated inhibition of NF-kappaB binding to DNA. Antioxid Redox Signal 7(11–12):1601–1611

Heiss E, Herhaus C, Klimo K, Bartsch H, Gerhauser C (2001) Nuclear factor kappa B is a molecular target for sulforaphane-mediated anti-inflammatory mechanisms. J Biol Chem 276 (34):32008–32015

Herr I, Buchler MW (2010) Dietary constituents of broccoli and other cruciferous vegetables: implications for prevention and therapy of cancer. Cancer Treat Rev 36(5):377–383

Herz C, Hertrampf A, Zimmermann S, Stetter N, Wagner M, Kleinhans C et al (2014) The isothiocyanate erucin abrogates telomerase in hepatocellular carcinoma cells in vitro and in an orthotopic xenograft tumour model of HCC. J Cell Mol Med 18(12):2393–2403

Higgins LG, Hayes JD (2011) The cap'n'collar transcription factor Nrf2 mediates both intrinsic resistance to environmental stressors and an adaptive response elicited by chemopreventive agents that determines susceptibility to electrophilic xenobiotics. Chem Biol Interact 192 (1–2):37–45

Ho JN, Yoon HG, Park CS, Kim S, Jun W, Choue R et al (2012) Isothiocyanates ameliorate the symptom of heart dysfunction and mortality in a murine AIDS model by inhibiting apoptosis in the left ventricle. J Med Food 15(9):781–787

Hong Y, Yan W, Chen S, Sun CR, Zhang JM (2010) The role of Nrf2 signaling in the regulation of antioxidants and detoxifying enzymes after traumatic brain injury in rats and mice. Acta Pharmacol Sin 31(11):1421–1430

Hong YH, Uddin MH, Jo U, Kim B, Song J, Suh DH et al (2015) ROS accumulation by PEITC selectively kills ovarian cancer cells via UPR-mediated apoptosis. Front Oncol 5:167

Hsu YC, Chang SJ, Wang MY, Chen YL, Huang TY (2013) Growth inhibition and apoptosis of neuroblastoma cells through ROS-independent MEK/ERK activation by sulforaphane. Cell Biochem Biophys 66(3):765–774

Hu R, Hebbar V, Kim BR, Chen C, Winnik B, Buckley B et al (2004) In vivo pharmacokinetics and regulation of gene expression profiles by isothiocyanate sulforaphane in the rat. J Pharmacol Exp Ther 310(1):263–271

Hu R, Xu C, Shen G, Jain MR, Khor TO, Gopalkrishnan A et al (2006a) Gene expression profiles induced by cancer chemopreventive isothiocyanate sulforaphane in the liver of C57BL/6J mice and C57BL/6J/Nrf2 (−/−) mice. Cancer Lett 243(2):170–192

Hu R, Khor TO, Shen G, Jeong WS, Hebbar V, Chen C et al (2006b) Cancer chemoprevention of intestinal polyposis in ApcMin/+ mice by sulforaphane, a natural product derived from cruciferous vegetable. Carcinogenesis 27(10):2038–2046

Huang YP, Jiang YW, Chen HY, Hsiao YT, Peng SF, Chou YC et al (2018) Benzyl isothiocyanate induces apoptotic cell death through mitochondria-dependent pathway in gefitinib-resistant NCI-H460 human lung cancer cells in vitro. Anticancer Res 38(9):5165–5176

Innamorato NG, Rojo AI, Garcia-Yague AJ, Yamamoto M, de Ceballos ML, Cuadrado A (2008) The transcription factor Nrf2 is a therapeutic target against brain inflammation. J Immunol 181 (1):680–689

Innamorato NG, Jazwa A, Rojo AI, Garcia C, Fernandez-Ruiz J, Grochot-Przeczek A et al (2010) Different susceptibility to the Parkinson's toxin MPTP in mice lacking the redox master regulator Nrf2 or its target gene heme oxygenase-1. PLoS One 5(7):e11838

Itoh K, Wakabayashi N, Katoh Y, Ishii T, Igarashi K, Engel JD et al (1999) Keap1 represses nuclear activation of antioxidant responsive elements by Nrf2 through binding to the amino-terminal Neh2 domain. Genes Dev 13(1):76–86

Jacob C, Jamier V, Ba LA (2011) Redox active secondary metabolites. Curr Opin Chem Biol 15 (1):149–155

Jakubikova J, Sedlak J, Mithen R, Bao Y (2005a) Role of PI3K/Akt and MEK/ERK signaling pathways in sulforaphane- and erucin-induced phase II enzymes and MRP2 transcription, G2/M arrest and cell death in Caco-2 cells. Biochem Pharmacol 69(11):1543–1552

Jakubikova J, Bao Y, Sedlak J (2005b) Isothiocyanates induce cell cycle arrest, apoptosis and mitochondrial potential depolarization in HL-60 and multidrug-resistant cell lines. Anticancer Res 25(5):3375–3386

Jakubikova J, Cervi D, Ooi M, Kim K, Nahar S, Klippel S et al (2011) Anti-tumor activity and signaling events triggered by the isothiocyanates, sulforaphane and phenethyl isothiocyanate, in multiple myeloma. Haematologica 96(8):1170–1179

Jazwa A, Rojo AI, Innamorato NG, Hesse M, Fernandez-Ruiz J, Cuadrado A (2011) Pharmacological targeting of the transcription factor Nrf2 at the basal ganglia provides disease modifying therapy for experimental parkinsonism. Antioxid Redox Signal 14(12):2347–2360

Jiang ZQ, Chen C, Yang B, Hebbar V, Kong AN (2003) Differential responses from seven mammalian cell lines to the treatments of detoxifying enzyme inducers. Life Sci 72 (20):2243–2253

Johansson NL, Pavia CS, Chiao JW (2008) Growth inhibition of a spectrum of bacterial and fungal pathogens by sulforaphane, an isothiocyanate product found in broccoli and other cruciferous vegetables. Planta Med 74(7):747–750

Kerns ML, DePianto D, Dinkova-Kostova AT, Talalay P, Coulombe PA (2007) Reprogramming of keratin biosynthesis by sulforaphane restores skin integrity in epidermolysis bullosa simplex. Proc Natl Acad Sci U S A 104(36):14460–14465

Kerns M, DePianto D, Yamamoto M, Coulombe PA (2010) Differential modulation of keratin expression by sulforaphane occurs via Nrf2-dependent and -independent pathways in skin epithelia. Mol Biol Cell 21(23):4068–4075

Kondo Y, Kanzawa T, Sawaya R, Kondo S (2005) The role of autophagy in cancer development and response to therapy. Nat Rev Cancer 5(9):726–734

Kong L, Tanito M, Huang Z, Li F, Zhou X, Zaharia A et al (2007) Delay of photoreceptor degeneration in tubby mouse by sulforaphane. J Neurochem 101(4):1041–1052

Kumari V, Dyba MA, Holland RJ, Liang YH, Singh SV, Ji X (2016) Irreversible inhibition of glutathione S-transferase by phenethyl isothiocyanate (PEITC), a dietary cancer chemopreventive phytochemical. PLoS One 11(9):e0163821

Kuroiwa Y, Nishikawa A, Kitamura Y, Kanki K, Ishii Y, Umemura T et al (2006) Protective effects of benzyl isothiocyanate and sulforaphane but not resveratrol against initiation of pancreatic carcinogenesis in hamsters. Cancer Lett 241(2):275–280

Kylarova S, Kosek D, Petrvalska O, Psenakova K, Man P, Vecer J et al (2016) Cysteine residues mediate high-affinity binding of thioredoxin to ASK1. FEBS J 283(20):3821–3838

Lin RK, Zhou N, Lyu YL, Tsai YC, Lu CH, Kerrigan J et al (2011) Dietary isothiocyanate-induced apoptosis via thiol modification of DNA topoisomerase IIalpha. J Biol Chem 286 (38):33591–33600

Liu H, Nishitoh H, Ichijo H, Kyriakis JM (2000) Activation of apoptosis signal-regulating kinase 1 (ASK1) by tumor necrosis factor receptor-associated factor 2 requires prior dissociation of the ASK1 inhibitor thioredoxin. Mol Cell Biol 20(6):2198–2208

Liu X, Abe-Kanoh N, Liu Y, Zhu B, Munemasa S, Nakamura T et al (2017) Inhibition of phosphatidylinositide 3-kinase impairs the benzyl isothiocyanate-induced accumulation of autophagic molecules and Nrf2 in human colon cancer cells. Biosci Biotechnol Biochem 81 (11):2212–2215

Loo G (2003) Redox-sensitive mechanisms of phytochemical-mediated inhibition of cancer cell proliferation (review). J Nutr Biochem 14(2):64–73

Maheo K, Morel F, Langouet S, Kramer H, Le Ferrec E, Ketterer B et al (1997) Inhibition of cytochromes P-450 and induction of glutathione S-transferases by sulforaphane in primary human and rat hepatocytes. Cancer Res 57(17):3649–3652

Mantso T, Anestopoulos I, Lamprianidou E, Kotsianidis I, Pappa A, Panayiotidis MI (2019) Isothiocyanate-induced cell cycle arrest in a novel in vitro exposure protocol of human malignant melanoma (A375) cells. Anticancer Res 39(2):591–596

Mao L, Wang H, Wang X, Liao H, Zhao X (2011) Transcription factor Nrf2 protects the spinal cord from inflammation produced by spinal cord injury. J Surg Res 170(1):e105–e115

Marrot L, Jones C, Perez P, Meunier JR (2008) The significance of Nrf2 pathway in (photo)-oxidative stress response in melanocytes and keratinocytes of the human epidermis. Pigment Cell Melanoma Res 21(1):79–88

Mas S, Gasso P, Trias G, Bernardo M, Lafuente A (2012) Sulforaphane protects SK-N-SH cells against antipsychotic-induced oxidative stress. Fundam Clin Pharmacol 26(6):712–721

Matusheski NV, Jeffery EH (2001) Comparison of the bioactivity of two glucoraphanin hydrolysis products found in broccoli, sulforaphane and sulforaphane nitrile. J Agric Food Chem 49 (12):5743–5749

Matusheski NV, Juvik JA, Jeffery EH (2004) Heating decreases epithiospecifier protein activity and increases sulforaphane formation in broccoli. Phytochemistry 65(9):1273–1281

McMahon M, Itoh K, Yamamoto M, Chanas SA, Henderson CJ, McLellan LI et al (2001) The Cap'n'Collar basic leucine zipper transcription factor Nrf2 (NF-E2 p45-related factor 2) controls both constitutive and inducible expression of intestinal detoxification and glutathione biosynthetic enzymes. Cancer Res 61(8):3299–3307

McMahon M, Lamont DJ, Beattie KA, Hayes JD (2010) Keap1 perceives stress via three sensors for the endogenous signaling molecules nitric oxide, zinc, and alkenals. Proc Natl Acad Sci U S A 107(44):18838–18843

Mi L, Wang X, Govind S, Hood BL, Veenstra TD, Conrads TP et al (2007) The role of protein binding in induction of apoptosis by phenethyl isothiocyanate and sulforaphane in human non-small lung cancer cells. Cancer Res 67(13):6409–6416

Mi L, Xiao Z, Hood BL, Dakshanamurthy S, Wang X, Govind S et al (2008) Covalent binding to tubulin by isothiocyanates. A mechanism of cell growth arrest and apoptosis. J Biol Chem 283 (32):22136–22146

Mi L, Gan N, Cheema A, Dakshanamurthy S, Wang X, Yang DC et al (2009) Cancer preventive isothiocyanates induce selective degradation of cellular alpha- and beta-tubulins by proteasomes. J Biol Chem 284(25):17039–17051

Mi L, Sirajuddin P, Gan N, Wang X (2010) A cautionary note on using N-acetylcysteine as an antagonist to assess isothiocyanate-induced reactive oxygen species-mediated apoptosis. Anal Biochem 405(2):269–271

Mi L, Gan N, Chung FL (2011) Isothiocyanates inhibit proteasome activity and proliferation of multiple myeloma cells. Carcinogenesis 32(2):216–223

Miyoshi N, Uchida K, Osawa T, Nakamura Y (2004) A link between benzyl isothiocyanate-induced cell cycle arrest and apoptosis: involvement of mitogen-activated protein kinases in the Bcl-2 phosphorylation. Cancer Res 64(6):2134–2142

Morel F, Langouet S, Maheo K, Guillouzo A (1997) The use of primary hepatocyte cultures for the evaluation of chemoprotective agents. Cell Biol Toxicol 13(4–5):323–329

Motohashi H, Yamamoto M (2004) Nrf2-Keap1 defines a physiologically important stress response mechanism. Trends Mol Med 10(11):549–557

Munday R, Munday CM (2004) Induction of phase II detoxification enzymes in rats by plant-derived isothiocyanates: comparison of allyl isothiocyanate with sulforaphane and related compounds. J Agric Food Chem 52(7):1867–1871

Munday R, Mhawech-Fauceglia P, Munday CM, Paonessa JD, Tang L, Munday JS et al (2008) Inhibition of urinary bladder carcinogenesis by broccoli sprouts. Cancer Res 68(5):1593–1600

Myzak MC, Dashwood WM, Orner GA, Ho E, Dashwood RH (2006) Sulforaphane inhibits histone deacetylase in vivo and suppresses tumorigenesis in Apc-minus mice. FASEB J 20(3):506–508

Nadeau PJ, Charette SJ, Toledano MB, Landry J (2007) Disulfide Bond-mediated multimerization of Ask1 and its reduction by thioredoxin-1 regulate H(2)O(2)-induced c-Jun NH(2)-terminal kinase activation and apoptosis. Mol Biol Cell 18(10):3903–3913

Nakamura Y, Miyoshi N (2010) Electrophiles in foods: the current status of isothiocyanates and their chemical biology. Biosci Biotechnol Biochem 74(2):242–255

Nakamura Y, Kawakami M, Yoshihiro A, Miyoshi N, Ohigashi H, Kawai K et al (2002) Involvement of the mitochondrial death pathway in chemopreventive benzyl isothiocyanate-induced apoptosis. J Biol Chem 277(10):8492–8499

Navarro SL, Li F, Lampe JW (2011) Mechanisms of action of isothiocyanates in cancer chemoprevention: an update. Food Funct 2(10):579–587

Negi G, Kumar A, Sharma SS (2011) Nrf2 and NF-kappaB modulation by sulforaphane counteracts multiple manifestations of diabetic neuropathy in rats and high glucose-induced changes. Curr Neurovasc Res 8(4):294–304

Ni WY, Hsiao YP, Hsu SC, Hsueh SC, Chang CH, Ji BC et al (2013) Oral administration of benzyl-isothiocyanate inhibits in vivo growth of subcutaneous xenograft tumors of human malignant melanoma A375.S2 cells. In Vivo 27(5):623–626

Nioi P, McMahon M, Itoh K, Yamamoto M, Hayes JD (2003) Identification of a novel Nrf2-regulated antioxidant response element (ARE) in the mouse NAD(P)H:quinone oxidoreductase 1 gene: reassessment of the ARE consensus sequence. Biochem J 374(Pt 2):337–348

Olagnier D, Lababidi RR, Hadj SB, Sze A, Liu Y, Naidu SD et al (2017) Activation of Nrf2 signaling augments vesicular stomatitis virus oncolysis via autophagy-driven suppression of antiviral immunity. Mol Ther 25(8):1900–1916

Pappa G, Lichtenberg M, Iori R, Barillari J, Bartsch H, Gerhauser C (2006) Comparison of growth inhibition profiles and mechanisms of apoptosis induction in human colon cancer cell lines by isothiocyanates and indoles from Brassicaceae. Mutat Res 599(1–2):76–87

Pappa G, Bartsch H, Gerhauser C (2007a) Biphasic modulation of cell proliferation by sulforaphane at physiologically relevant exposure times in a human colon cancer cell line. Mol Nutr Food Res 51(8):977–984

Pappa G, Strathmann J, Lowinger M, Bartsch H, Gerhauser C (2007b) Quantitative combination effects between sulforaphane and 3,3′-diindolylmethane on proliferation of human colon cancer cells in vitro. Carcinogenesis 28(7):1471–1477

Piao CS, Gao S, Lee GH, Kim do S, Park BH, Chae SW et al (2010) Sulforaphane protects ischemic injury of hearts through antioxidant pathway and mitochondrial K(ATP) channels. Pharmacol Res 61(4):342–348

Ping Z, Liu W, Kang Z, Cai J, Wang Q, Cheng N et al (2010) Sulforaphane protects brains against hypoxic-ischemic injury through induction of Nrf2-dependent phase 2 enzyme. Brain Res 1343:178–185

Powolny AA, Bommareddy A, Hahm ER, Normolle DP, Beumer JH, Nelson JB et al (2011) Chemopreventative potential of the cruciferous vegetable constituent phenethyl isothiocyanate in a mouse model of prostate cancer. J Natl Cancer Inst 103(7):571–584

Prashar A, Siddiqui F, Singh AK (2012) Synthetic and green vegetable isothiocyanates target red blood leukemia cancers. Fitoterapia 83(2):255–265

Rakariyatham K, Yang X, Gao Z, Song M, Han Y, Chen X et al (2019) Synergistic chemopreventive effect of allyl isothiocyanate and sulforaphane on non-small cell lung carcinoma cells. Food Funct 10(2):893–902

Ritz SA, Wan J, Diaz-Sanchez D (2007) Sulforaphane-stimulated phase II enzyme induction inhibits cytokine production by airway epithelial cells stimulated with diesel extract. Am J Physiol Lung Cell Mol Physiol 292(1):L33–L39

Rojo AI, Innamorato NG, Martin-Moreno AM, De Ceballos ML, Yamamoto M, Cuadrado A (2010) Nrf2 regulates microglial dynamics and neuroinflammation in experimental Parkinson's disease. Glia 58(5):588–598

Roos G, Foloppe N, Messens J (2013) Understanding the pK(a) of redox cysteines: the key role of hydrogen bonding. Antioxid Redox Signal 18(1):94–127

Rushmore TH, Pickett CB (1990) Transcriptional regulation of the rat glutathione S-transferase Ya subunit gene. Characterization of a xenobiotic-responsive element controlling inducible expression by phenolic antioxidants. J Biol Chem 265(24):14648–14653

Russo M, Spagnuolo C, Tedesco I, Russo GL (2010) Phytochemicals in cancer prevention and therapy: truth or dare? Toxins 2(4):517–551

Saito R, Suzuki T, Hiramoto K, Asami S, Naganuma E, Suda H et al (2016) Characterizations of three major cysteine sensors of Keap1 in stress response. Mol Cell Biol 36(2):271–284

Saitoh M, Nishitoh H, Fujii M, Takeda K, Tobiume K, Sawada Y et al (1998) Mammalian thioredoxin is a direct inhibitor of apoptosis signal-regulating kinase (ASK) 1. EMBO J 17 (9):2596–2606

Saw CL, Cintron M, Wu TY, Guo Y, Huang Y, Jeong WS et al (2011) Pharmacodynamics of dietary phytochemical indoles I3C and DIM: Induction of Nrf2-mediated phase II drug metabolizing and antioxidant genes and synergism with isothiocyanates. Biopharm Drug Dispos 32 (5):289–300

Sehrawat A, Singh SV (2016) Short-form RON overexpression augments benzyl isothiocyanate-induced apoptosis in human breast cancer cells. Mol Carcinog 55(5):473–485

Siebert A, Desai V, Chandrasekaran K, Fiskum G, Jafri MS (2009) Nrf2 activators provide neuroprotection against 6-hydroxydopamine toxicity in rat organotypic nigrostriatal cocultures. J Neurosci Res 87(7):1659–1669

Siegel D, Gustafson DL, Dehn DL, Han JY, Boonchoong P, Berliner LJ et al (2004) NAD(P)H: quinone oxidoreductase 1: role as a superoxide scavenger. Mol Pharmacol 65(5):1238–1247

Singh SV, Warin R, Xiao D, Powolny AA, Stan SD, Arlotti JA et al (2009) Sulforaphane inhibits prostate carcinogenesis and pulmonary metastasis in TRAMP mice in association with increased cytotoxicity of natural killer cells. Cancer Res 69(5):2117–2125

Smirnova NA, Haskew-Layton RE, Basso M, Hushpulian DM, Payappilly JB, Speer RE et al (2011) Development of Neh2-luciferase reporter and its application for high throughput screening and real-time monitoring of Nrf2 activators. Chem Biol 18(6):752–765

Soane L, Li Dai W, Fiskum G, Bambrick LL (2010) Sulforaphane protects immature hippocampal neurons against death caused by exposure to hemin or to oxygen and glucose deprivation. J Neurosci Res 88(6):1355–1363

Stan SD, Singh SV, Whitcomb DC, Brand RE (2014) Phenethyl isothiocyanate inhibits proliferation and induces apoptosis in pancreatic cancer cells in vitro and in a MIAPaca2 xenograft animal model. Nutr Cancer 66(4):747–755

Starrett W, Blake DJ (2011) Sulforaphane inhibits de novo synthesis of IL-8 and MCP-1 in human epithelial cells generated by cigarette smoke extract. J Immunotoxicol 8(2):150–158

Svehlikova V, Wang S, Jakubikova J, Williamson G, Mithen R, Bao Y (2004) Interactions between sulforaphane and apigenin in the induction of UGT1A1 and GSTA1 in CaCo-2 cells. Carcinogenesis 25(9):1629–1637

Talalay P, Fahey JW, Healy ZR, Wehage SL, Benedict AL, Min C et al (2007) Sulforaphane mobilizes cellular defenses that protect skin against damage by UV radiation. Proc Natl Acad Sci U S A 104(44):17500–17505

Tan XL, Shi M, Tang H, Han W, Spivack SD (2010) Candidate dietary phytochemicals modulate expression of phase II enzymes GSTP1 and NQO1 in human lung cells. J Nutr 140 (8):1404–1410

Tang L, Zhang Y (2005) Mitochondria are the primary target in isothiocyanate-induced apoptosis in human bladder cancer cells. Mol Cancer Ther 4(8):1250–1259

Tanito M, Masutani H, Kim YC, Nishikawa M, Ohira A, Yodoi J (2005) Sulforaphane induces thioredoxin through the antioxidant-responsive element and attenuates retinal light damage in mice. Invest Ophthalmol Vis Sci 46(3):979–987

Thimmulappa RK, Mai KH, Srisuma S, Kensler TW, Yamamoto M, Biswal S (2002) Identification of Nrf2-regulated genes induced by the chemopreventive agent sulforaphane by oligonucleotide microarray. Cancer Res 62(18):5196–5203

Toyama T, Shinkai Y, Yasutake A, Uchida K, Yamamoto M, Kumagai Y (2011) Isothiocyanates reduce mercury accumulation via an Nrf2-dependent mechanism during exposure of mice to methylmercury. Environ Health Perspect 119(8):1117–1122

Trachootham D, Zhou Y, Zhang H, Demizu Y, Chen Z, Pelicano H et al (2006) Selective killing of oncogenically transformed cells through a ROS-mediated mechanism by beta-phenylethyl isothiocyanate. Cancer Cell 10(3):241–252

Traka M, Gasper AV, Smith JA, Hawkey CJ, Bao Y, Mithen RF (2005) Transcriptome analysis of human colon Caco-2 cells exposed to sulforaphane. J Nutr 135(8):1865–1872

Traka M, Gasper AV, Melchini A, Bacon JR, Needs PW, Frost V et al (2008) Broccoli consumption interacts with GSTM1 to perturb oncogenic signalling pathways in the prostate. PLoS One 3(7): e2568

Ueno T, Sato W, Horie Y, Komatsu M, Tanida I, Yoshida M et al (2008) Loss of Pten, a tumor suppressor, causes the strong inhibition of autophagy without affecting LC3 lipidation. Autophagy 4(5):692–700

Valgimigli L, Iori R (2009) Antioxidant and pro-oxidant capacities of ITCs. Environ Mol Mutagen 50(3):222–237

Vauzour D, Buonfiglio M, Corona G, Chirafisi J, Vafeiadou K, Angeloni C et al (2010) Sulforaphane protects cortical neurons against 5-S-cysteinyl-dopamine-induced toxicity through the activation of ERK1/2, Nrf-2 and the upregulation of detoxification enzymes. Mol Nutr Food Res 54(4):532–542

Verkerk R, Schreiner M, Krumbein A, Ciska E, Holst B, Rowland I et al (2009) Glucosinolates in Brassica vegetables: the influence of the food supply chain on intake, bioavailability and human health. Mol Nutr Food Res 53(Suppl 2):S219

Vermeulen M, Boerboom AM, Blankvoort BM, Aarts JM, Rietjens IM, van Bladeren PJ et al (2009) Potency of isothiocyanates to induce luciferase reporter gene expression via the electrophile-responsive element from murine glutathione S-transferase Ya. Toxicol in Vitro 23(4):617–621

Wagner AE, Ernst I, Iori R, Desel C, Rimbach G (2010) Sulforaphane but not ascorbigen, indole-3-carbinole and ascorbic acid activates the transcription factor Nrf2 and induces phase-2 and antioxidant enzymes in human keratinocytes in culture. Exp Dermatol 19(2):137–144

Wakabayashi N, Slocum SL, Skoko JJ, Shin S, Kensler TW (2010) When NRF2 talks, who's listening? Antioxid Redox Signal 13(11):1649–1663

Wan J, Diaz-Sanchez D (2006) Phase II enzymes induction blocks the enhanced IgE production in B cells by diesel exhaust particles. J Immunol 177(5):3477–3483

Wang XJ, Hayes JD, Wolf CR (2006) Generation of a stable antioxidant response element-driven reporter gene cell line and its use to show redox-dependent activation of nrf2 by cancer chemotherapeutic agents. Cancer Res 66(22):10983–10994

Wang XJ, Hayes JD, Higgins LG, Wolf CR, Dinkova-Kostova AT (2010) Activation of the NRF2 signaling pathway by copper-mediated redox cycling of para- and ortho-hydroquinones. Chem Biol 17(1):75–85

Wang X, de Rivero Vaccari JP, Wang H, Diaz P, German R, Marcillo AE et al (2012a) Activation of the nuclear factor E2-related factor 2/antioxidant response element pathway is neuroprotective after spinal cord injury. J Neurotrauma 29(5):936–945

Wang Y, Chen Y, Wang J, Chen J, Aggarwal BB, Pang X et al (2012b) Xanthohumol, a prenylated chalcone derived from hops, suppresses cancer cell invasion through inhibiting the expression of CXCR4 chemokine receptor. Curr Mol Med 12(2):153–162

Wang D, Upadhyaya B, Liu Y, Knudsen D, Dey M (2014) Phenethyl isothiocyanate upregulates death receptors 4 and 5 and inhibits proliferation in human cancer stem-like cells. BMC Cancer 14:591

Wiczk A, Hofman D, Konopa G, Herman-Antosiewicz A (2012) Sulforaphane, a cruciferous vegetable-derived isothiocyanate, inhibits protein synthesis in human prostate cancer cells. Biochim Biophys Acta 1823(8):1295–1305

Wu XJ, Hua X (2007) Targeting ROS: selective killing of cancer cells by a cruciferous vegetable derived pro-oxidant compound. Cancer Biol Ther 6(5):646–647

Wu X, Zhou QH, Xu K (2009) Are isothiocyanates potential anti-cancer drugs? Acta Pharmacol Sin 30(5):501–512

Wu X, Zhu Y, Yan H, Liu B, Li Y, Zhou Q et al (2010) Isothiocyanates induce oxidative stress and suppress the metastasis potential of human non-small cell lung cancer cells. BMC Cancer 10:269

Wu CL, Huang AC, Yang JS, Liao CL, Lu HF, Chou ST et al (2011) Benzyl isothiocyanate (BITC) and phenethyl isothiocyanate (PEITC)-mediated generation of reactive oxygen species causes cell cycle arrest and induces apoptosis via activation of caspase-3, mitochondria dysfunction and nitric oxide (NO) in human osteogenic sarcoma U-2 OS cells. J Orthop Res 29(8):1199–1209

Xiao D, Singh SV (2007) Phenethyl isothiocyanate inhibits angiogenesis in vitro and ex vivo. Cancer Res 67(5):2239–2246

Xiao D, Vogel V, Singh SV (2006) Benzyl isothiocyanate-induced apoptosis in human breast cancer cells is initiated by reactive oxygen species and regulated by Bax and Bak. Mol Cancer Ther 5(11):2931–2945

Xiao D, Powolny AA, Singh SV (2008) Benzyl isothiocyanate targets mitochondrial respiratory chain to trigger reactive oxygen species-dependent apoptosis in human breast cancer cells. J Biol Chem 283(44):30151–30163

Xiao D, Powolny AA, Moura MB, Kelley EE, Bommareddy A, Kim SH et al (2010) Phenethyl isothiocyanate inhibits oxidative phosphorylation to trigger reactive oxygen species-mediated death of human prostate cancer cells. J Biol Chem 285(34):26558–26569

Xu C, Huang MT, Shen G, Yuan X, Lin W, Khor TO et al (2006) Inhibition of 7,12-dimethylbenz (a)anthracene-induced skin tumorigenesis in C57BL/6 mice by sulforaphane is mediated by nuclear factor E2-related factor 2. Cancer Res 66(16):8293–8296

Yan H, Zhu Y, Liu B, Wu H, Li Y, Wu X et al (2011) Mitogen-activated protein kinase mediates the apoptosis of highly metastatic human non-small cell lung cancer cells induced by isothiocyanates. Br J Nutr 106(12):1779–1791

Yanaka A, Fahey JW, Fukumoto A, Nakayama M, Inoue S, Zhang S et al (2009) Dietary sulforaphane-rich broccoli sprouts reduce colonization and attenuate gastritis in Helicobacter pylori-infected mice and humans. Cancer Prev Res (Phila) 2(4):353–360

Yang F, Wang F, Liu Y, Wang S, Li X, Huang Y et al (2018) Sulforaphane induces autophagy by inhibition of HDAC6-mediated PTEN activation in triple negative breast cancer cells. Life Sci 213:149–157

Yeh YT, Hsu YN, Huang SY, Lin JS, Chen ZF, Chow NH et al (2016a) Benzyl isothiocyanate promotes apoptosis of oral cancer cells via an acute redox stress-mediated DNA damage response. Food Chem Toxicol 97:336–345

Yeh CC, Ko HH, Hsieh YP, Wu KJ, Kuo MY, Deng YT (2016b) Phenethyl isothiocyanate enhances TRAIL-induced apoptosis in oral cancer cells and xenografts. Clin Oral Investig 20 (9):2343–2352

Zhang Y (2000) Role of glutathione in the accumulation of anticarcinogenic isothiocyanates and their glutathione conjugates by murine hepatoma cells. Carcinogenesis 21(6):1175–1182

Zhang Y (2001) Molecular mechanism of rapid cellular accumulation of anticarcinogenic isothiocyanates. Carcinogenesis 22(3):425–431

Zhang Y (2010) Allyl isothiocyanate as a cancer chemopreventive phytochemical. Mol Nutr Food Res 54(1):127–135

Zhang DD, Hannink M (2003) Distinct cysteine residues in Keap1 are required for Keap1-dependent ubiquitination of Nrf2 and for stabilization of Nrf2 by chemopreventive agents and oxidative stress. Mol Cell Biol 23(22):8137–8151

Zhang Y, Tang L (2007) Discovery and development of sulforaphane as a cancer chemopreventive phytochemical. Acta Pharmacol Sin 28(9):1343–1354

Zhang Y, Talalay P, Cho CG, Posner GH (1992) A major inducer of anticarcinogenic protective enzymes from broccoli: isolation and elucidation of structure. Proc Natl Acad Sci U S A 89 (6):2399–2403

Zhang Y, Kensler TW, Cho CG, Posner GH, Talalay P (1994) Anticarcinogenic activities of sulforaphane and structurally related synthetic norbornyl isothiocyanates. Proc Natl Acad Sci U S A 91(8):3147–3150

Zhang J, Svehlikova V, Bao Y, Howie AF, Beckett GJ, Williamson G (2003) Synergy between sulforaphane and selenium in the induction of thioredoxin reductase 1 requires both transcriptional and translational modulation. Carcinogenesis 24(3):497–503

Zhang Y, Li J, Tang L (2005) Cancer-preventive isothiocyanates: dichotomous modulators of oxidative stress. Free Radic Biol Med 38(1):70–77

Zhang Y, Yao S, Li J (2006a) Vegetable-derived isothiocyanates: anti-proliferative activity and mechanism of action. Proc Nutr Soc 65(1):68–75

Zhang Y, Munday R, Jobson HE, Munday CM, Lister C, Wilson P et al (2006b) Induction of GST and NQO1 in cultured bladder cells and in the urinary bladders of rats by an extract of broccoli (Brassica oleracea italica) sprouts. J Agric Food Chem 54(25):9370–9376

Zhang T, Liu H, Zhu C, Briggs K, Kang Y, Fleming JA et al (2012) Silencing thioredoxin induces liver cancer cell senescence under hypoxia. Hepatol Res 42(7):706–713

Zhao J, Moore AN, Clifton GL, Dash PK (2005) Sulforaphane enhances aquaporin-4 expression and decreases cerebral edema following traumatic brain injury. J Neurosci Res 82(4):499–506

Zhao X, Sun G, Zhang J, Strong R, Dash PK, Kan YW et al (2007a) Transcription factor Nrf2 protects the brain from damage produced by intracerebral hemorrhage. Stroke 38 (12):3280–3286

Zhao J, Moore AN, Redell JB, Dash PK (2007b) Enhancing expression of Nrf2-driven genes protects the blood brain barrier after brain injury. J Neurosci 27(38):10240–10248

Zheng H, Whitman SA, Wu W, Wondrak GT, Wong PK, Fang D et al (2011) Therapeutic potential of Nrf2 activators in streptozotocin-induced diabetic nephropathy. Diabetes 60(11):3055–3066

Zhu M, Bowden GT (2004) Molecular mechanism(s) for UV-B irradiation-induced glutathione depletion in cultured human keratinocytes. Photochem Photobiol 80(2):191–196

Zhu M, Fahl WE (2000) Development of a green fluorescent protein microplate assay for the screening of chemopreventive agents. Anal Biochem 287(2):210–217

Zhu M, Zhang Y, Cooper S, Sikorski E, Rohwer J, Bowden GT (2004) Phase II enzyme inducer, sulforaphane, inhibits UVB-induced AP-1 activation in human keratinocytes by a novel mechanism. Mol Carcinog 41(3):179–186

Zhu H, Jia Z, Strobl JS, Ehrich M, Misra HP, Li Y (2008) Potent induction of total cellular and mitochondrial antioxidants and phase 2 enzymes by cruciferous sulforaphane in rat aortic smooth muscle cells: cytoprotection against oxidative and electrophilic stress. Cardiovasc Toxicol 8(3):115–125

Chapter 10
Xanthohumol and Structurally Related Prenylflavonoids for Cancer Chemoprevention and Control

Jan F. Stevens

Abstract Humans are almost exclusively exposed to the prenylated hop chalcone, xanthohumol, by consumption of beer and hop-derived dietary supplements. Its spontaneous isomerization into the flavanone, isoxanthohumol, in conjunction with gut microbial and hepatic metabolism, produces several xanthohumol-derived prenylated flavonoids that exert bioactivities relevant to cancer chemoprevention. The mechanisms by which these prenylflavonoids may act to counter tumorigenesis, as well as carcinogenesis and metastasis, include detoxifying carcinogens, reducing inflammation and inflammation-driven angiogenesis, and promoting apoptotic cell death. Following our discoveries that xanthohumol has the ability to inhibit cytochrome P450 enzymes that metabolically activate procarcinogens and induce the carcinogen-detoxifying quinone reductase, other researchers have investigated the effects of xanthohumol on the activity of these metabolic enzymes in various cancer cell lines using carcinogenic substrates as well as its effects on transcriptional activation of metabolic genes in animal models. Another group of metabolic enzymes, glutathione *S*-transferases, detoxify electrophilic carcinogens and appear to be transcriptionally induced by xanthohumol via activation of Nrf2. Various human malignancies have in common that they activate the pro-inflammatory NFκB pathway to induce the expression of inflammatory cytokines, growth factors, and anti-apoptotic genes. Many researchers, including our laboratory, have shown that xanthohumol and related flavonoids inhibit NFκB activation in various cancer cell lines. Furthermore, xanthohumol can inhibit tumor growth in vivo by inhibiting the pro-angiogenic NFκB and Akt pathways. Tumor cells differ from normal cells by their increased metabolic rate and demand for oxygen, which forces them to switch from oxidative phosphorylation to aerobic glycolysis to meet energy demands while coping with increased oxidative stress and apoptotic risk. Acting as mild mitochondrial uncouplers, prenylated flavonoids lower the mitochondrial inner membrane potential thereby promoting apoptosis, counteracting anti-apoptotic pathways in

J. F. Stevens (✉)
Department of Pharmaceutical Sciences, Oregon State University, Corvallis, OR, USA

The Linus Pauling Institute, Oregon State University, Corvallis, OR, USA
e-mail: fred.stevens@oregonstate.edu

J. M. Pezzuto, O. Vang (eds.), *Natural Products for Cancer Chemoprevention*,
https://doi.org/10.1007/978-3-030-39855-2_10

tumor cells, and decreasing the metastatic potential of cancer cells. While xanthohumol and other prenylated flavonoids have low potential for use as effective cancer therapeutics by themselves, they hold promise for combination therapy because tumor cells cannot develop resistance against the mitochondrial uncoupling effects of prenylated flavonoids.

Keywords Apoptosis · Cancer · Chemoprevention · Hops · *Humulus lupulus* · Metabolism · Mitochondria · 8-prenylnaringenin · Xanthohumol

10.1 Introduction

The hop flavonoid, xanthohumol, has received increasing attention in the last 20 years due to its multitude of health-related effects in cell culture and preclinical models of disease. A large proportion of the >400 publications on xanthohumol to date reported anti-oxidant, anti-inflammatory, anti-proliferative, anti-bacterial, anti-obesity, and anti-carcinogenic effects. Several excellent review articles on xanthohumol have appeared over the years (Bolton et al. 2019; Gerhauser 2005; Gerhauser et al. 2002; Gerhäuser and Frank 2005; Jiang et al. 2018; Stevens and Page 2004; Venturelli et al. 2016). This review focuses on the anticarcinogenic mechanisms of xanthohumol and its metabolites. Because the same mechanisms can underlie antiproliferative effects in multiple cell lines, this review is not organized by cancer type. It would also be difficult to discuss effects of xanthohumol on various cancers because there were no clinical data available on the anticancer effects of xanthohumol at the time of collecting articles for this review. This review cites 161 articles, of which 51 were published since 2015 (32%). Despite efforts to provide a comprehensive overview of the topic, the author cannot not claim that this review is exhaustive and apologizes for any relevant articles on xanthohumol that are not cited here.

10.2 Occurrence and Human Exposure

In the plant kingdom, three major biosynthetic pathways produce the vast majority of natural products: terpenoids, alkaloids, and polyphenols. Within the class of polyphenolic natural products, there are an estimated 10,000 molecular species that meet the definition of a flavonoid (Dixon and Pasinetti 2010). Flavonoids consist of two aromatic/phenyl rings, often substituted with hydroxyl or methoxy groups, connected to one another through a three-carbon bridge. They are further subdivided into chalcones, flavanones, flavones, flavonols, flavanols, and isoflavones based on variation in their carbon skeleton. One of the two aromatic rings of flavonoids originates from the shikimic acid pathway while the acetate pathway delivers the other ring by combining three acetate molecules. Prenylated flavonoids differ from other flavonoids by carrying a substituent on a carbon or oxygen atom that is provided by the mevalonate pathway. Most prenylated flavonoids carry a 5-carbon isopentenyl or 10-carbon geranyl substituent. Approximately 1000 natural products meet the characteristics of a prenylated flavonoid (Barron and Ibrahim 1996). A 2019 SciFinder substructure search for naturally occurring prenylated chalcones, flavanones, flavones, flavonols, and isoflavones returned 1157 compounds, indicating that only a few hundred additional prenylated flavonoids have been reported since Barron and Ibrahim's 1996 survey (Barron and Ibrahim 1996). Unlike non-prenylated flavonoids, prenylated flavonoids are sporadically distributed among the plant kingdom, with the Asteraceae, Fabaceae, Moraceae and Cannabinaceae being rich producers of prenylated flavonoids. Specialized secretory cell systems, such as glandular trichomes, secrete prenylated flavonoids into the extracellular space as part of resin, epicuticular wax, or latex, and in non-glycosylated form.

Prenylated flavonoids make up a small fraction of the total dietary intake of polyphenols in a habitual diet, quantitatively the most important food source being beer. The prenylated flavonoids in beer originate from its ingredient, hops (Fig. 10.1). Hops are the inflorescences of the female hops plant, *Humulus lupulus* (Cannabinaceae). Although *Humulus* is the sister genus of *Cannabis*, hemp and marijuana do not contain substantial amounts of prenylated flavonoids. Major brand beers contain up to about 0.5 mg total prenylated flavonoids per liter, while a bitter microbrew beer may contain up to 4 mg/L (Stevens et al. 1999b). The major prenylated flavonoid in beer is isoxanthohumol, which is formed by thermal isomerization of xanthohumol in the brew kettle (Stevens et al. 1999a). Habitual consumption of beer is unlikely to confer health benefit resulting from intake of prenylated flavonoids. The steady increase in the number of publications claiming health properties of hop-derived prenylated flavonoids has undoubtedly contributed to the market appearance of dietary supplements containing (milligram) doses of xanthohumol that would not be attainable through consumption of beer.

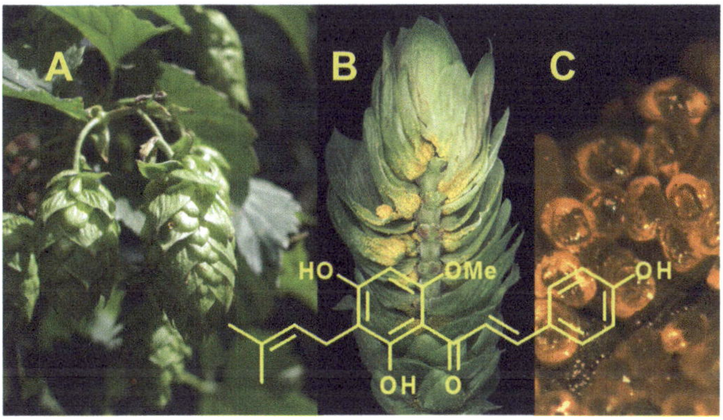

Fig. 10.1 Panel (**a**) and (**b**): Hops or hop cones are the inflorescences of the female hop plant (*Humulus lupulus*). Panel (**c**): Glandular trichomes covering the bracts of hops excrete a resin (lupulin) which consists of bitter acids, essential oils, and prenylated flavonoids. Xanthohumol makes up about 90% of the prenylflavonoid fraction

10.3 Hepatic and Gut Microbial Metabolism

Dietary polyphenols are generally characterized as xenobiotics with low bioavailability, usually defined as the fraction of the ingested xenobiotic that is absorbed and circulating in intact, non-metabolized form. Many researchers have attempted to link the low bioavailability, often translating into plasma levels in the low nanomolar range, to biological effects in the mammalian host, probably requiring tissue concentrations in the high nanomolar to low micromolar range. The large difference in concentration levels can be attributed to metabolism and accumulation of parent compounds and metabolites in tissues. In the case of dietary polyphenols, it is often not known whether or which metabolites contribute to their bioactivity. In such cases it is advisable to determine a total exposure profile and adjust the bioavailability accordingly. Using this broader definition of bioavailability, Legette et al. (2012) determined the absolute bioavailability of xanthohumol in Sprague-Dawley rats by comparing area under the curve (AUC) after administration of a single intravenous and oral dose of xanthohumol. The authors found that the oral bioavailability of the sum of xanthohumol and its metabolites, calculated as $F = (AUC_{p.o.}/AUC_{i.v.}) \times (Dose_{i.v.} \times Dose_{p.o.})$, ranged from 0.11 at a human equivalent oral dose of 180 mg to 0.33 at a human equivalent dose of 20 mg. The main compounds detected in the circulation were the *O*-glucuronides of xanthohumol, isoxanthohumol, and 8-prenylnaringenin (the *O*-demethylated metabolite of isoxanthohumol). The elimination half-life appeared to be dose-dependent and ranged from 18 to 30 h. The authors repeated the studies in humans taking single doses of 20, 60, and 180 mg by mouth (Legette et al. 2014). In humans, the main circulating flavonoids were the *O*-glucuronides of xanthohumol and isoxanthohumol, while the levels of 8-prenylnaringenin or its *O*-glucuronides were either very low or not detectable. The half-life of xanthohumol was about 20 h.

Exposure to hops and its products has been associated with estrogenic effects for over a century. Before mechanical harvesting, hops were harvested manually and women who hand-picked hop cones commonly experienced menstrual disturbances. Early experimental studies to verify the estrogenic activity of hops had variable outcomes: some researchers reported high estrogen activity of hops (Zenisek and Bednar 1960) while others could not substantiate these findings (Fenselau and Talalay 1973). The estrogenic activity of hops could not be attributed to xanthohumol (Verzele 1986). Milligan and coworkers identified 8-prenylnaringenin as the estrogenic principle of hops (Milligan et al. 1999, 2000, 2002). Our research group detected 8-prenylnaringin in beer at concentrations of up to 0.24 mg/L (Stevens et al. 1999b). While these concentrations are probably too low to exert estrogenic effects, isoxanthohumol can be converted metabolically into 8-prenylnaringenin by liver cytochrome P450s (Guo et al. 2006) and by gut microbiota (Bolca et al. 2007; Possemiers et al. 2005, 2006, 2008). Ex vivo incubation of human fecal samples with isoxanthohumol revealed that about 40% of the humans participating in the study possessed a gut microbiome capable of converting isoxanthomumol, the major beer prenylflavonoid [up to 4 mg/L (Stevens et al. 1999b)], into 8-prenylnaringenin

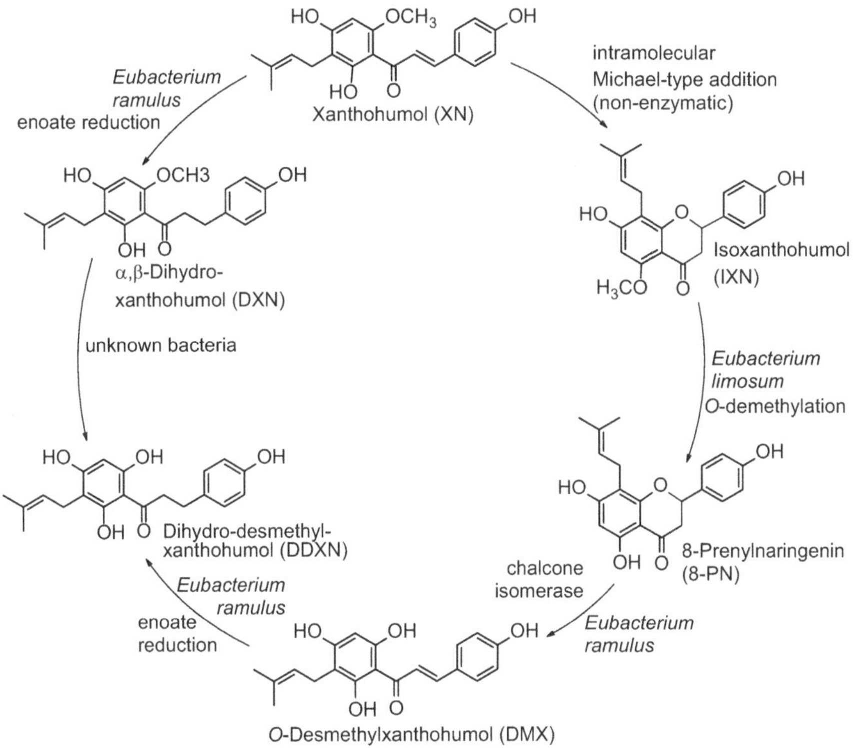

Fig. 10.2 Gut microbioal metabolism of xanthohumol. Adapted from Paraiso et al. (2018)

(Possemiers et al. 2006). Possemiers and coworkers reported that the human gut bacterium *Eubacterium limosum* is capable of *O*-demethylating isoxanthohumol into 8-prenylnaringenin (Possemiers et al. 2008).

Paraiso and coworkers (2018) were able to confirm that *E. limosum* converts isoxanthohumol into 8-prenylnaringenin, but they also found that 8-prenylnaringenin is a substrate for a reductase expressed by *E. ramulus* which produces *O*-desmethyl-α,β-dihydroxanthohumol (3′-prenylphloretin) from 8-prenylnaringenin (Fig. 10.2). In addition, they found that *E. limosum* converts xanthohumol directly into α,β-dihydroxanthohumol. The latter metabolite cannot form 8-prenylnaringenin metabolically and it appears to be devoid of estrogenic activity determined by estrogen receptor binding assays and by lack of ability to induce the expression of the progesterone receptor, a recognized biomarker of estrogen receptor-α activity, in MCF-7 breast cancer cells (Miranda et al. 2018). These new insights into the gut microbial metabolism of xanthohumol and isoxanthohumol are certainly relevant to the possible estrogenic effects of hops and hop-derived supplements and they highlight the importance of the gut microbiome in the metabolism of xenobiotics.

10.4 Multiple Links Between Oxidative Stress and Carcinogenesis

Oxidative stress, or the excessive production of reactive oxygen species (ROS), can result from a toxicological insult and from chronic inflammation. ROS cause oxidative damage to nuclear DNA, in which the oxidative conversion of guanine into 8-oxo-guanine is quantitively the most important. Because 8-oxo-guanine does not pair with cytosine but with adenine, the mismatch will lead to base-pair transversion in the following round of DNA synthesis, resulting in a point mutation and possibly in the initiation of carcinogenesis. It has been estimated that DNA in a cell is hit by an oxidative event 1.5×10^5 times per day, the majority of which are undone by excision of the oxidized nucleotide and repair (Boelsterli 2007). 8-Oxo-deoxyguanosine (8-hydroxy-deoxyguanosine) excreted in the urine is a popular biomarker of DNA damage. Oxidative DNA damage cannot be completely prevented but it can be reduced to a level at which mismatch repair can cope with it. Besides mismatch repair, the body has the ability to activate antioxidant mechanisms that eliminate ROS (Halliwell and Gutteridge 1999). Dietary polyphenols are unlikely to act as direct scavengers of ROS in vivo because their attainable cellular concentrations are in the low micromolar range and cannot compete with the two most important cellular antioxidants, glutathione (GSH) and ascorbic acid, whose cellular concentrations are in the low millimolar range (Halliwell and Gutteridge 1999; Traber and Stevens 2011). However, dietary polyphenols and dietary supplements containing polyphenols may exert an indirect antioxidant effect by reducing inflammation through interfering with prooxidant/proinflammatory pathways and by boosting the natural antioxidant systems in response to oxidative stress.

Ferk and coworkers (2016) studied the effects of oral administration of xanthohumol to humans on DNA stability. The study was a placebo-controlled cross-over design with a dose was 12 mg xanthohumol (in the form of a beverage) per day for 14 days. The authors evaluated single and double strand-break DNA damage in peripheral lymphocytes by the single cell gel electrophoresis assay. No changes in DNA damage were observed between the xanthohumol treatment and placebo groups. However, when they treated the nuclei with formamidopyrimidine glycolase in order to detect oxidized purines, they observed a 33% reduction of comet formation (a measure of DNA damage). When isolated lymphocytes were exposed to hydrogen peroxide (50 μM), DNA damage was smaller in the xanthohumol treatment groups. These findings are consistent with the lower urinary excretion of 8-oxo-deoxyguanosine of the volunteers in the xanthohumol treatment group. Taken together, these data suggest that low doses of xanthohumol protect against DNA damage (Ferk et al. 2016).

10.4.1 Prenylated Flavonoids Interfere with Xenobiotics-Induced Oxidative Stress and with Bioactivation of Procarcinogens

Many halogenated xenobiotics undergo reductive dehalogenation by cytochrome P450 enzymes which produce radical intermediates that react with molecular oxygen to form ROS. For example, carbon tetrachloride (CCl_4), widely used as an industrial solvent and a popular agent to induce ROS formation in rodent models of oxidative stress and liver injury, is converted by CYP2E1 into $CCl_3^{\bullet}$ which subsequently reacts with O_2 to form $CCl_3OO^{\bullet}$ (Boelsterli 2007). This peroxyl radical causes cellular damage by abstraction of allylic hydrogens from polyunsaturated fatty acids. The resulting lipid radicals react with O_2 to form lipid peroxyl radicals and lipid hydroperoxides with relatively short half-lives. The majority of lipid hydroperoxides are reductively converted into hydroxylipids by glutathione peroxidases, but a small fraction forms reactive aldehydes, notably 2-alkenals, which can covalently modify proteins and DNA (Halliwell and Gutteridge 1999).

Pinto and coworkers (2012) examined the effects of xanthohumol on the prevention of CCl_4-induced liver injury in Wistar rats. They found that oral pretreatment of the rats with xanthohumol at daily doses of 0.1–0.4 mg/kg body weight for 8 days offered significant protection against liver injury. They also found that xanthohumol-pretreated animals had lower production of thiobarbituric acid reactive substances, a general biomarker of reactive lipid peroxidation products, and higher levels of GSH compared to vehicle-pretreated rats. The authors attributed the protective effects to an antioxidant mechanism. The authors did not test the alternative hypothesis that xanthohumol directly inhibited or reduced the expression of the CYP enzymes responsible for the activation of CCl_4. Dorn and coworkers (2012) pretreated female BALB/c mice with xanthohumol at a daily dose of 1 mg/kg body weight for 2 days prior to induction of liver injury by CCl_4 injection and for 3 days post CCl_4 injection. Unlike the Pinto group, they found that xanthohumol pretreatment did not reduce the acute hepatoxic effects of CCl_4, measured by the release of transaminase enzymes from the liver. But they detected a profound inhibitory effect of xanthohumol pretreatment on the CCl_4-induced production of inflammatory cytokines and activation of NFκB. These xanthohumol-associated effects translated into a mitigated fibrogenic response following CCl_4 administration. The authors hypothesized that the effective low oral dose of xanthohumol is due to direct exposure of hepatic stellate cells (responsible for extracellular matrix deposition) to portal vein blood in which the concentration of xenobiotics is higher than in the general circulation. The authors attributed the protective effects of xanthohumol against liver inflammation and fibrosis to inhibition of the pro-inflammatory NFκB pathway. As liver inflammation and fibrosis can progress to liver cancer, the study shows potential of xanthohumol in the prevention or amelioration of liver cancer.

Other xenobiotics that can induce carcinogenesis in the liver and gastro-intestinal tract include polyaromatic hydrocarbons (PAHs), cooked food-derived heterocyclic amines and aflatoxins. These xenobiotics are considered pro-carcinogens because they require cytochrome P540-mediated bioactivation, notably by CYP1A1 and CYP1A2, into ultimate carcinogens. A prominent example of a bioactivation reaction is epoxidation, which gives the xenobiotic metabolites electrophilic properties and ability to covalently modify DNA and so initiate the carcinogenesis process. The 7-ethoxyresorufin-*O*-deethylase (EROD) activity of CYP1A1 is often used to monitor the cancer chemopreventive potential of test compounds. Henderson and coworkers (2000) tested the inhibitory effects of xanthohumol on cDNA-expressed human CYP1A1, CYP1B1, CYP1A2, CYP3A4, and CYP2E1 in vitro. They found that xanthohumol, at a concentration of 10 μM, almost completely inhibited the EROD activity of CYP1A1 and CYP1B1. Using acetanilide as a model substrate for the acetanilide 4-hydroxylase activity of CYP1A2, the authors found isoxanthohumol and 8-prenylnaringenin to be the most potent inhibitors of CYP1A2, inhibiting the enzyme by 90% at 10 μM and suppressing the bioactivation of the procarcinogen aflatoxin B1. The three tested prenylflavonoids appeared to be poor inhibitors of CYP2E1 (Henderson et al. 2000). Gerhauser and coworkers (2002) also observed xanthohumol's ability to inhibit CYP1A activity using 3-cyano-ethoxycoumarin as enzyme substrate. Miranda and coworkers studied the effects of xanthohumol, isoxanthohumol, and 8-prenylnaringenin on the CYP1A2-mediated bioactivation of the cooked meat mutagen, 2-amino-3-methylimidazo [4,5-*f*]quinoline (IQ). They found that cDNA-expressed human CYP1A2 activated IQ as measured by the covalent binding of IQ metabolites to calf thymus DNA. In this assay, the three tested prenylflavonoids inhibited the enzyme-induced covalent binding of IQ to DNA by 60–90% at the tested concentration of 10 μM (Miranda et al. 2000c). Plazar and coworkers reported that xanthohumol, at non-toxic concentrations in the range 0.01 to 10 μM, dose-dependently inhibited CYP1A activity using 7-ethoxycoumarin as the enzyme substrate, in rat microsomes but not in rat liver slices, even though xanthohumol completely prevented IQ- and PAH-induced DNA damage (Plazar et al. 2008). Ferk and coworkers (2010) observed that xanthohumol-treated rats challenged with IQ showed less DNA damage in both colon and liver tissue and they developed fewer (50%) and smaller (44%) glutathione *S*-transferase positive foci (GST-p+, a biochemical marker for preneoplastic lesions) in the liver. In a human ex vivo study, Pichler and coworkers (2017) investigated the effects of xanthohumol in volunteers consuming 12 mg/day via a beverage. When lymphocytes isolated from blood samples were exposed to IQ and the PAH benzo(*a*)pyrene, the authors detected lower levels of DNA damage in the volunteers taking xanthohumol which correlated with higher levels of glutathione *S*-transferase-α (α-GST) by ELISA and which provides a partial explanation for the protection against DNA damage. This study is one of the very few examples showing that xanthohumol exerts anticarcinogenic effects in humans (Pichler et al. 2017).

10.4.2 Prenylflavonoids as Inhibitors of the NFκB Signaling Pathway and Other Pro-inflammatory Pathways

The pro-inflammatory nuclear factor kappa B (NFκB) pathway fulfills a physiological role in the innate immune system to defend the host against infections. Under conditions of chronic inflammation in age-related pathologies, the NFκB pathway proceeds in a sustained fashion, thereby producing pro-inflammatory cytokines that promote the progression of cardiovascular and metabolic diseases. Stimulation of the transmembrane Toll-like receptor 4 (TLR4) by circulating microbial constituents, notably lipopolysaccharides released from the outer membrane of Gram-negative bacteria, initiates NFκB signaling and results in an inflammatory response. At the molecular level, activation of TLR4 by LPS induces heterodimerization of TLR4 with myeloid differentiation protein-2 (MD-2) in response to binding of the fatty acid residues of LPS to a hydrophobic cavity of MD-2. The TLR4-MD-2 heterodimerization leads to phosphorylation, ubiquitinylation, and degradation of the IκB, thereby releasing free NFκB for translocation to the nucleus to activate transcription. We (Colgate et al. 2007) and others (Cho et al. 2008; Dorn et al. 2010) established that xanthohumol and related prenylflavonoids inhibit the NFκB pathway as an anticarcinogenic mechanism. Harikumar and coworkers (2009) discovered that xanthohumol has the ability to modify cysteine residues in IκB kinase and in the p65 unit of NFκB, thereby inhibiting NFκB signaling and promoting apoptosis. Cho and coworkers (2008) found that xanthohumol reduces the expression of TLR4 and MD-2, resulting in suppression of NFκB activation in LPS-activated RAW264.7 mouse macrophages. We hypothesized that prenylated flavonoids would be more potent inhibitors of the NFκB pathway than non-prenylated counterparts due to their greater lipophilicity and binding of the prenyl groups to the hydrophobic cavity of MD-2 (Peluso et al. 2010). To test this hypothesis, we tested the anti-inflammatory effects of 16 prenylated flavonoids, found in hops (*Humulus lupulus*), in LPS-activated THP-1 monocytes using the release of the pro-inflammatory cytokine monocyte chemo-attractant protein-1 (MCP-1) and interleukin-6 (IL-6) as endpoints. In support of this hypothesis, we showed that prenylated chalcones inhibit cytokine release to a greater extent than their corresponding flavanone isomers at the tested concentration of 20 μM (Peluso et al. 2010). Geranylated flavonoids inhibited cytokine release to a greater extent than their corresponding dimethylallyl-substituted flavonoids, consistent with the hypothesis that hydrophobicity contributes to the inhibitory effect on cytokine release. To examine the relationship between binding of prenylated flavonoids to the hydrophobic MD-2 pocket and cytokine release, we conducted molecular docking studies in silico and found a statistically significant inverse correlation between MCP-1 release and flavonoid-MD-2 complementarity. Using a combination of experimental and theoretical modeling analysis, Fu and coworkers (2016) confirmed our work that xanthohumol has the ability to bind to the hydrophobic pocket of MD-2 and they established that xanthohumol forms hydrogen bonds with arginine-90 and tyrosine-102 of MD-2. Based on the xanthohumol pharmacophore,

Chen and coworkers (2017) synthesized a series of 39 bisaryl-1,4-dien-3-ones and tested an compared their binding to the MD-2 protein in a cell-free system and determined the inhibitory effect on cytokine production in primary mouse macrophases. Compared to xanthohumol (49% inhibition at 10 μM), two analogues in the series inhibited cytokine production by 52% and 61% and they offered significant protection in LPS-induced septic death in mice.

Downstream of NFκB (whose activation produces cytokines such as IL-6), the signal transducer and activator of transcription (Stat3) pathway is activated by cytokine (IL-6) receptor agonism which controls a wide spectrum of cellular processes, including cell proliferation, downregulation of the tumor suppressor gene p53, promoting cell survival by upregulating apoptosis inhibitors, induction of angiogenesis by activating vascular endothelial growth factor (VEGF) and hypoxia inducible factor 1α (HIF1α), and promotion of cell invasion by upregulating metalloproteinases 2 and 9 (MMP-2/9) (Niit et al. 2015). The Stat3 pathway is activated in the development of cholangiocarcinoma (CCA, biliary tract cancer), the second most prevalent hepatic cancer for which there is no effective therapy (Bridgewater et al. 2016). Infection with the liver fluke, *Opisthorchis viverrini*, can cause CCA through consumption of raw fish dishes (Alsaleh et al. 2019) which is common in northeast Thailand (Kaewpitoon et al. 2008; Sripa and Pairojkul 2008) and other parts of East Asia (Alsaleh et al. 2019). Dokduang and coworkers (2016) tested the hypothesis that xanthohumol can inhibit proliferation of CCA cells and whether it can do so by inhibiting Stat3 activation. In support of their hypothesis, they found that xanthohumol (20–50 μM) dose-dependently suppressed IL-6 stimulated growth of CCA cells in vitro. Xanthohumol's antiproliferative effect paralleled a reduction in Stat3 phosphorylation (activation) and induction of apoptosis. When BALB/c mice were subcutaneously inoculated with KKU-M241 CCA cells, treatment of the mice with xanthohumol, administered via the drinking water (50 μM, about 3.2 mg/kg body weight/day), caused a reduction of tumor volume by about half after 30 days of treatment compared to the no-treatment group. The xenograft experiment also showed that xanthohumol suppressed Akt activation and NFκB translocation to the nucleus, from which the authors concluded that xanthohumol suppresses Stat3 activation in CCA by inhibiting Akt-NFκB signaling (Dokduang et al. 2016). Jammongkan and coworkers (2018) studied CCA in Syrian gold hamsters infected with *Opisthorchis viverrini* cysts by intragastric intubation. Animals received various treatments: *N*-nitrosodimethylamine (NDMA, a carcinogen), praziquantel (anti-helmintic, single dose of 400 mg/kg 30 days after cyst infection), and xanthohumol (via the drinking water, 171 mg/kg body weight/day). The authors observed a reduction of periductal fibrosis in the animals treated with praziquantel and especially in the animals co-treated with praziquantel and xanthohumol. By immunostaining, they observed high levels of activated p38 MAPK in the nuclei of the hyperplastic bile duct cells from untreated animals and significantly lower levels in animals treated with praziquantel, xanthohumol, or the combination. They concluded that the combination therapy of praziquantel and xanthohumol has potential to prevent *Opisthorchis viverrini*-induced cholangiocarcinogenesis (Jamnongkan et al. 2018). Stat3 suppression was also implicated in the radio-sensitizing effect of xanthohumol on doxorubicin-resistant MCF-7 breast cancer cells (Kang et al. 2013).

The Notch signaling pathway, whose malfunction has been associated with tumorigenesis of several cancers including CCA (Maemura et al. 2014), provides a means for Notch receptor-bearing cells to receive signals from neighboring cells to differentiate, proliferate, or undergo apoptosis. The signal from one cell to another is transmitted through physical interaction between the Notch receptor and the membrane-bound Notch ligand embedded in the cell membrane of the signaling cell. The molecular biology has been summarized in (Hori et al. 2013). Walden and co-workers (2017) examined the antiproliferative and pro-apoptotic effects of xanthohumol (5–15 μM) on the CCA cell lines CCLP-1, SG-231, and CC-SW-1. They attributed the effects of xanthohumol to reduced Notch1 and Akt expression. In mice xenografted with CCLP-1 and SG-231 cells, xanthohumol treatment (i.p. injection of 0.125 mg every other day for 16 days) reduced CCA growth measured by tumor volume compared to the no-treatment group (Walden et al. 2017). Krajnović and coworkers (2016) observed a dose-dependent decrease of viability of two melanoma cell lines (B16 and A375) exposed to xanthohumol, isoxanthohumol, and 8-prenylnaringenin. Xanthohumol was most cytotoxic and 8-prenylnaringenin least with IC_{50} values in the range 9–48 μM. They examined the mechanistic actions of isoxanthohumol and contributed its antiproliferative effect to apoptosis, but no clear molecular pathway could be identified responsible for the observed effects. While the IC_{50} values indicate moderate cytotoxic potency, isoxanthohumol (20 mg/kg) was able to sensitize melanoma cells to treatment with subtoxic doses of paclitaxel in xenografted C57BL/6 mice (Krajnović et al. 2016). Suppression of Notch1 signaling was also implicated in the anti-proliferative activity of xanthohumol against the human pancreatic cancer cell lines, AsPC-1, PANC-1, L3.6pl, MiaPaCa-2, 512, and 651) (Kunnimalaiyaan et al. 2015) and against the breast cancer cell lines, MCF-7 and MDA-MB-231 (Sun et al. 2018).

The serine/threonine protein kinase Akt pathway can also be activated by IL-6, demonstrating its connectivity with the NFκB pathway. Akt is often overactive in human cancer. Activation of the PI3K/Akt pathway (phosphatidylinositol 3-kinase, PI3K, is upstream of Akt; it activates Akt by phosphorylation) is associated with resistance to apoptosis, cell survival and proliferation, and with metastasis. The endogenous antagonist of Akt is the tumor repressor PTEN, whose inactivation often occurs in metastatic prostate cancer. Akt can activate the mammalian target of rapamycin (mTOR) which functions as a kinase to regulate cell proliferation, cell survival and autophagy. Taken together, the PI3K/Akt/mTOR pathway is tumorigenic and cancer chemoprevention strategies are designed to inhibit the pathway. Guo and coworkers (2018) tested the hypothesis that xanthohumol induces apoptosis of human gastric cancer SGC-7901 cells, in vitro and in a BALB/c mouse xenograft model, by inhibiting the PI3K/Akt/mTOR pathway. By Western blot analysis, the authors found that xanthohumol treatment in the low micromolar range suppressed the phosphorylation (activation) of Akt and mTOR and that it promoted the phosphorylation (activation) of PTEN. Treatment of the xenografted mice with xanthohumol with low doses of 0.5 and 1 mg/kg body weight per day resulted in smaller tumors, lower levels of phosphorylated Akt and mTOR and higher numbers of apoptotic cells compared with the no-treatment tumors (Guo et al. 2018). Albini and co-workers (2006) identified inhibition of the NFκB and Akt pathways as a mechanism by which xanthohumol suppressed proliferation of Kaposi's sarcoma-derived KS-IMM cells in vitro and by which it inhibited in vivo angiogenesis in the matrigel sponge model. In this model, angiogenesis was induced by vascular endothelial growth factor (VEGF) and TNF-α and inhibited by direct injection of xanthohumol into the matrigel as well as by oral administration of xanthohumol to the mice via the drinking water. Angiogenesis was quantified by measuring hemoglobin content. Mice xenografted with KS-IMM cells had about 60% reduced tumor volume when treated with xanthohumol (20 μM in the drinking water, about 1.2 mg/kg body weight/day) for 23 days (Albini et al. 2006). The authors collaborated with synthetic chemists to prepare a series of 13 novel xanthohumol derivatives with *O*- and *C*-substitutions on the phenolic rings and tested their antiangiogenic activity in vitro. One of the derivatives, 2-fluroro-4-*O*-methylxanthohumol, exerted greater antiangiogenic activity than xanthohumol (Nuti et al. 2017). Isoxanthohumol (10 μM) inhibited angiogenesis in human umbilical endothelial (HUVEC) and human aortic smooth muscle cell (HASMC) culture, which the authors attributed to inhibition of the NFκB and Akt pathways (Negrão et al. 2013). Similarly, xanthohumol inhibited angiogenesis of HUVECs co-cultured with pancreatic BxPC-3 cancer cells in vitro as well as in BxPC-3 xenografted BALB/c nu-nu mice by suppressing NFκB activity (Saito et al. 2018). Shikata and coworkers identified valosin-containing protein (VCP, also known as p97) as a mediator in xanthohumol-inhibition of the NFκB pathway and a player in the anticarcinogenic activity of xanthohumol (Sasazawa et al. 2012; Shikata et al. 2017).

Cell invasion defines the ability of cells to migrate through the extracellular matrix to infiltrate neighboring tissues so to potentially form metastatic tumors. Overexpression of the Cysteine X Cysteine chemokine receptor 4 (CXCR4) is a characteristic of nearly every major malignancy (Sleightholm et al. 2017). CXCR4-expressing cancer cells can migrate to other tissues whose cells express CXCL12, a ligand with affinity for CXCR4. Wang and co-workers (2012) found that xanthohumol inhibits expression of CXCR4 in various cancer cell types, thereby suppressing cell invasion. Equally relevant to metastatic potential of cells in organ tissues is the ability of cells to maintain affinity for each other. The invasive potential of cells depends on the function of the E-cadherin/catenin complex as an invasion suppressor. The mechanism of this suppressor action can be explained by enhanced cell-cell adhesion in which E-cadherin plays the role of a transmembrane glycoprotein whose cytosolic domain binds to the cytoskeleton via catenin proteins. Upregulation of the E-cadherin/catenin complex can potentially be exploited therapeutically in gastro-intestinal and breast cancers. Vanhoecke and coworkers investigated the inhibitory effect of xanthohumol on the invasive potential of three breast cancer cell lines (MCF-7/6, MCF-7/AZ, and T47-D) in the chick heart invasion assay (Vanhoecke et al. 2005). They examined the cell-cell adhesion of the human MCF-7/6 cells which have a functionally defective E-cadherin/catenin complex. Xanthohumol was able to stimulate aggregation of MCF-7/6 cells in suspension by restoring the function of the complex. The stimulating effect could be inhibited by a monoclonal antibody against the extracellular domain of E-cadherin (Vanhoecke et al. 2005). These findings show the potential of xanthohumol as an inhibitor of metastasis. Other researchers have studied the anti-proliferative effects of xanthohumol on doxorubicin-resistant MCF-7/ADR cells and found a synergistic effect between xanthohumol and doxorubicin which appears to associate with downregulation of the cancer stem-like properties of the MCF-7/ADR cells (Liu et al. 2016). In MCF-7 breast cancer spheroids grown on lymphendothelial cells, xanthohumol inhibited expression of the adhesion molecule ICAM-1 and it prevented adherence of the MCF-7 cells to the lymphendothelial cells by inhibiting NFκB activity, which shows the antimetastatic potential of xanthohumol (Viola et al. 2013).

As an Akt/NFκB inhibitor, xanthohumol showed low micromolar cytotoxicity to acute (AML) and chronic myelogenous leukemia (AML) cell lines (Dell'Eva et al. 2007) as well as to Bcr/Abl-expressing, imatinib-resistant K562 leukemia cells (Monteghirfo et al. 2008). The Bcr/Abl oncogene appears to be essential for the pathogenesis of CML while the tyrosine kinase activity of ABL is essential for Bcr/Abl-mediated transformation, which makes the ABL kinase an attractive target for therapy. Imatinib mesylate (Gleevec), developed to inhibit ABL kinase, has been used with therapeutic success in CML (Deininger et al. 2005) despite the emergence of drug resistance (Quintas-Cardama et al. 2007). When the imatinib-resistant K562 cells were cultured for 48 h in the presence of a non-lethal concentration of xanthohumol in an attempt to develop resistance to xanthohumol, the cells remained susceptible to apoptosis induced by xanthohumol at a concentration of 5 μM, which the authors attributed to inhibition of NFκB activation, enhancement of p21 expression, and decreased expression of the apoptosis inhibitor, survivin. These findings are potentially important because xanthohumol appears to suppress cell proliferation through a mechanism that is distinctly different from that of imatinib, indicating that xantohumol's activity cannot be circumvented by ABL kinase mutations and thus potentially beneficial in the treatment of imatinib-resistant CML (Monteghirfo et al. 2008). By the same mechanism, Benelli and coworkers (2012) found that xanthohumol dose-dependently (0–10 μM) induced growth arrest of B-cell acute lymphocytic leukemia (B-ALL L1210) cells and it induced apoptosis in this cell line. Mice xenografted with L1210 leukemia cells develop neurological symptoms due to infiltration of the leukemia cells in the brain. When the authors of the study treated the xenografted mice with xanthohumol at an intraperitoneal dose level of 5 μg (0.2 mg/kg), 5 times per week, the mean survival time of the animals increased from 6 to 9 days while the treatment delayed the onset of neurological manifestations, indicating reduced migration of leukemia cells to the brain. To explore possible mechanisms, the authors observed that exposure of the cells to xanthohumol resulted in decreased focal adhesion kinase (FAK) and Akt phosphorylation (activation). FAK activation reduces affinity of cells to the extracellular matrix and promotes cell migration via PI3K/Akt activation. The authors also tested the hypothesis whether drug-resistant cancer cells can become sensitive to drug treatment in the presence of xanthohumol. To test that hypothesis, they exposed adriamycin-resistant Nalm-6 leukemia cells to non-toxic doses of adriamycin in the presence of xanthohumol (3.5 μM, not cytotoxic) and observed increased cell death due to apoptosis (Benelli et al. 2012). These important findings demonstrate the potential efficacy of xanthohumol therapy in drug resistant leukemia and other cancers. One possible mechanism for overcoming drug resistance is ability of prenylflavonoids to block xenobiotic efflux transporters, which Tan and coworkers (2014) have demonstrated for the efflux transporter ABCG2 in MDCKII cell monolayers. In other cell lines, xanthohumol decreased the expression of the drug efflux transporters ABCB1, ABCC1, ABBC2, and ABCC3 (Lee et al. 2007).

Lust and coworkers (2005, 2009) investigated the ex vivo effects of xanthohumol on lymphocytes obtained from patients diagnosed with chronic lymphocytic leukemia (CLL). They hypothesized that xanthohumol targets the endoplasmic reticulum (ER) thereby activating the proapoptotic arm of the unfolded protein response (UPR). Xanthohumol induced apoptosis in the CLL cells, which the authors were able to associate with ER stress and UPR. Targeting the ER has become an increasingly attractive approach to overcome resistance to chemotherapy (Bahar et al. 2019).

Extracellular stimuli can activate several mitogen activated protein kinases (MAPKs), of which ERKs, JNKs, and p38s are well known and whose activation is converted into cellular responses. MAPKs are dysregulated in a significant proportion of melanomas, papillary thyroid tumors, ovarian tumors, colorectal tumors, and leukemias. Abnormal MAPK signaling can lead to increased cell proliferation, resistance to apoptosis, and resistance to chemotherapy. The ERK/MAPK pathway is initiated by activation of the protein Ras by receptor tyrosine kinases, which, in turn, activate Raf proteins that phosphorylate the kinase MEK. Activated MEK phosphorylates ERK which can activate transcription factors involved in the expression of genes encoding proteins that regulate cell proliferation and survival (Burrows et al. 2011; Chappell et al. 2011; Cseh et al. 2014; Knight and Irving 2014; Ott and Bhardwaj 2013; Rauen 2013; Santarpia et al. 2012; Urick et al. 2011). The p38/MAPK pathway is stimulated by cytokines, activates MEKs, which, in turn, activate p38 (a 38 kDa polypeptide), leading to adaptive and physiological responses via transcriptional regulation of genes (Cuenda and Rousseau 2007). Mi and coworkers (2017) identified paraptosis induced through the p38/MAPK pathway as a mechanism by which xanthohumol inhibited proliferation of HL-60 leukemia cells. Paraptosis is characterized by cytoplasmic vacuolation, swelling of the mitochondria and the endoplasmic reticulum as well as absence of caspase activation and apoptotic morphology (Sperandio et al. 2004). Exposure of the HL-60 cells to xanthohumol did not cause cleavage of caspase-3, leading the authors to conclude that cell death was not due to apoptosis (Mi et al. 2017). In an earlier study, Delmulle and coworkers (2008) observed that xanthohumol and its derivatives, isoxanthohumol, 6- and 8-prenylnaringenin induced cell death in prostate cancer PC-3 and DU145 cells that occurred in the absence of caspase-3 activation and typical apoptotic morphological features. They observed formation of vacuoles in the PC-3 cells treated with isoxanthohumol and 6-prenylnaringenin as well as in the DU145 cells exposed to the three tested prenylated flavanones which they attributed to autophagy (Delmulle et al. 2008). It is conceivable that the observed non-apoptotic cell death induced by the prenylflavonoids has the characteristics of paraptotic cell death, similar to the observations made by Mi and co-workers (2017).

Tumor necrosis factor (TNF)-related apoptosis-inducing ligand (TRAIL) is a cytokine that functions as a ligand for death receptors (TRAIL receptors), whose stimulation results in apoptotic cell death (Wiley et al. 1995). Szliszka and coworkers (2009) examined the effects of three prenylated chalcones (xanthohumol, licochalcone A, and isobavachalcone) and two non-prenylated chalcones (chalcone and butein) on TRAIL-induced apoptosis of androgen-sensitive prostate cancer LNCaP cells at concentrations of 20 and 50 μM. All five tested chalcones enhanced TRAIL-induced apoptosis in the cells. In a subsequent study, the same research group found that the xanthohumol-enhancing pro-apoptotic effect of TRAIL is, in part, due to a positive interaction between xanthohumol and TRAIL to activate the proapoptotic caspases Bid and Bax (Kłósek et al. 2016). In addition, co-treatment of the cells with xanthohumol and TRAIL decreased the expression of the anti-apoptotic protein Bcl-xL. Synergy between TRAIL and xanthohumol to induce apoptosis was also observed in SK-N-AS neuroblastoma cells (Engelsgjerd et al. 2019). These findings are potentially important in (prostate) cancer control because cancer cells can become resistant to TRAIL-mediated apoptosis due to overexpression of anti-apoptotic proteins (Catz and Johnson 2003).

Using benign prostate hyperplasia (BPH-1) and prostate cancer (PC3, malignant androgen-independent) cells as models of prostate cancer tumorigenesis, Colgate and coworkers (Colgate et al. 2007) observed that xanthohumol exposure (2.5–20 μM) leads to inhibition of cell proliferation and induction of apoptosis. They contributed the apoptotic effect of xanthohumol to inhibition of NFκB activation. Delmulle and coworkers (2006) examined the effects of xanthohumol, *O*-desmethylxanthohumol, isoxanthohumol, 6-prenylnaringenin, and 8-prenylnaringenin on cell proliferation in the human prostate cancer PC-3 and DU145 cell lines. Xanthohumol was most potent in decreasing cell viability (IC_{50} 13 and 12 μM, resp.), followed by 6-prenylnaringenin, 8-prenylnaringenin (IC_{50} 34 and 43 μM, resp.), isoxanthohumol, and *O*-desmethylxanthohumol (IC_{50} 50 and 54 μM, resp.). The authors hypothesized that the reduced potency of *O*-desmethylxanthohumol compared to xanthohumol is due to its facile isomerization into 6- and 8-prenylnaringenin [see Stevens et al. (1999a)]. The lower potency of 8-prenylnaringenin was attributed to its activity as a weak estrogen receptor agonist (Milligan et al. 1999, 2000, 2002), which would promote cell growth and counter any anti-inflammatory effect on cell viability. Both prostate cancer cell lines express estrogen receptors α and β (Lau et al. 2000; Maruyama et al. 2000). Tronina and coworkers (2013a) generated a series of xanthohumol metabolites by incubation with fungi and bacteria; they found that α,β-dihydroxanthohumol, obtained from an incubation of xanthohumol with *Fusarium tricinctum*, had similar potencies, compared to cisplatin, with regard to antiproliferative activity against human breast cancer MCF-7 cells and against PC-3 cells. Logan and coworkers also found that xanthohumol, α,β-dihydroxanthohumol, and tetrahydroxanthohumol exerted similar antiproliferative activities in colon (HCT116, HT29) and hepatocellular (HepG2, Huh7) carcinoma cell lines (Logan et al. 2019). Deep and workers (2010) determined that the anti-proliferative and pro-apoptotic effects of xanthohumol in androgen-senstive prostate cancer LNCaP cells and androgen-insensitive PC-3 cells can be attributed to inhibition of pro-survival NFκB, Akt, and mTOR signaling. Venè and coworkers (2012) treated prostate cancer PC-3 and DU145 cells with xanthohumol and found that its anti-proliferative effect is mediated via downregulation of FAK/Akt/NFκB signaling induced by ROS. They also treated transgenic adenocarcinoma of the mouse prostate (TRAMP) transgenic mice as an in vivo model of prostate cancer and observed a reduction in the weight of the urogenital tract as well as delayed advanced tumor progression (Venè et al. 2012).

In estrogen-sensitive breast cancer, the oncoprotein brefeldin A-inhibited guanine nucleotide-exchange protein 3 (BIG3) and tumor suppressor prohibitin 2 (PHB2) form a complex. When PHB2 is released from the complex, it binds to cytoplasmic and nuclear ER-α and suppresses ER-α signaling. Yoshimaru and coworkers (2014) discovered that xanthohumol interferes with binding of BIG3 to PHB2, resulting in decreased PHB2-mediated E2 signaling in estrogen-sensitive breast cancer MCF-7 cells and in cell growth inhibition. Potentially relevant to aromatase (CYP19)-expressing breast cancer cells is the inhibition of this enzyme by the xanthohumol metabolite, 8-prenylnaringenin ($IC_{50} < 0.09$ μM), as demonstrated in the breast cancer Sk-Br-3 cell line (Monteiro et al. 2007) and in choriocarcinoma-derived JAR cells (Monteiro et al. 2006).

Expression of genes can be regulated by small organic molecules (e.g., hormones) and by macromolecules (polypeptides, proteins). In recent years, micro RNAs (mRNAs, miRs; small noncoding RNAs) have received increasing attention as regulators of gene expression relevant to tumorigenesis (Auffinger et al. 2013). Chen and coworkers (2016) studied the correlation between miRNAs and xanthohumol-mediated cell death in glioma U-87 MG cells. By conducting a miRNA microarray, miR-204-3p was significantly upregulated by exposure of the cells to xanthohumol. Subsequently, the authors implicated the ERK/MAPK pathway in XN-mediated miR-204-3p upregulation which resulted in attenuation of IGFB-2-mediated downstream pathways, including the ERK and Akt MAPK signaling, thereby reducing cell proliferation and increasing apoptosis (Chen et al. 2016). Activation of Insulin-like Growth Factor (IGF) binding proteins (IGFBPs) has been associated with tumor growth and metastasis (Yau et al. 2015) and its plasma levels have diagnostic value in predicting clinical outcomes of gliomas (Lin et al. 2009). Ho and coworkers identified miR-4725-3p as a regulator of stromal interaction protein 1 (STIM1) signaling involved in xanthohumol-mediated inhibition of glioma cell invasion (Ho et al. 2018).

10.4.3 Prenylated Flavonoids as Inhibitors of the Wnt/β-Catenin Signaling Pathway

The wnt/β-catenin pathway is an important regulatory pathway that plays a key role in cell-cell adhesion, maintaining integrity and homeostasis of epithelial tissue, and tissue regeneration after injury. It intersects with major inflammatory pathways, which is particularly relevant to inflammation of the intestine. Chronic inflammation of the intestinal mucosa, a characteristic of inflammatory bowel diseases (IBDs) such as Crohn's disease and ulcerative colitis, is a risk factor for developing colorectal cancer. In the majority of colorectal cancers, the wnt/β-catenin pathway is aberrantly stimulated by intrinsic (e.g., host genetics) and extrinsic (e.g., the gut microbiome and exposure to dietary carcinogens) factors. Dysfunction of the wnt/β-catenin pathway leads to disbalance between epithelial tissue injury and repair, and eventually to loss of epithelial barrier integrity. When degradation products of intestinal microbiota (e.g., LPS) enter intestinal tissue, an immunological response causes gut inflammation and tissue damage, upon which the clinical symptoms of IBD can become manifest. The wnt/β-catenin pathway intersects with the NFκB pathway, the MAPK signaling pathway, the Akt signaling pathway, and the STAT signaling pathway (Moparthi and Koch 2019). While many researchers have studied the antiproliferative effects of xanthohumol and related prenylated flavonoids from hops on colon cancer cells (Allsopp et al. 2013; Bartmańska et al. 2018; Cömert Önder et al. 2016; Miranda et al. 1999; Pan et al. 2005; Popłoński et al. 2018; Sastre-Serra et al. 2018; Tronina et al. 2013b), to date there are no reports on hop flavonoids showing evidence that they affect the wnt/β-catenin pathway. It is conceivable, however, that xanthohumol and related hop flavonoids exert antiproliferative effects through the wnt/β-catenin pathway because the structurally closely related prenylated chalcones, derricin and derricidin from *Longocarpus sericeus* (Fabaceae), reduced cell viability and caused cell cycle arrest in colorectal cancer HCT116 cells by negatively modulating the wnt/β-catenin pathway (Fonseca et al. 2015).

10.5 Chemotherapeutic Potential of Xanthohumol

In the foregoing discussion, multiple studies have shown that xanthohumol exerts its chemopreventive and cancer control activities by inhibiting various pro-inflammatory pathways that drive tumorigenesis, angiogenesis, and metastasis. Under certain conditions (e.g., elevated oxidative stress in cancer cells), xanthohumol can induce cell death by activating pro-inflammatory pathways to increase oxidative stress to a level that cancer cells can no longer cope with the ROS-induced damage. This cancer therapeutic potential of xanthohumol has been exemplified by several authors. Xanthohumol appears to activate the p53 MAPK pathway to induce apoptosis in HepG2 hepatoma cells (Zhao et al. 2016), Ca Ski cervical cancer cells (Yong and Abd Malek 2015), malignant gliobastoma cells, but not in normal astrocytes (Zajc et al. 2012). Xanthohumol showed cytotoxicity to A549 human non-small cell lung cancer cells but not to normal human lung fibroblast MRC-5 cells (Yong et al. 2015). The xanthohumol metabolite, 8-prenylnaringenin, was cytotoxic to U-118 MG cells but not to normal fibroblasts (Stompor et al. 2017). Festa and coworkers found that xanthohumol (20 μM) increases ROS production and activating MAPK pathways in human T98G glioblastoma cells, causing the cells to progress into apoptosis (Festa et al. 2011). In a subsequent study, Festa and coworkers (Festa et al. 2013) induced apoptosis in three glioblastoma cell lines (T98G, U87-MG, and U343) by exposing cells to xanthohumol at 20 or 50 μM for 24 or 48 h. The proportion of apoptotic cells correlated with the xanthohumol-induced expression of AnxA1 in the T98G cells but not in the other cell lines. When the T98G cells were treated with small interference RNA directed against ANXA1, the authors observed inhibition of AnxA1 expression in the presence and absence of xanthohumol. The ANXA1 gene encodes Annexin A1 (AnxA1), a phospholipid-binding protein located at the cytosolic side of the plasma membrane, which inhibits phospholipase A2 and thereby reduces the production of pro-inflammatory eicosanoids. Recent findings suggest that the actions of Annexin A1 results in resolution of inflammation and in apoptosis, overriding pro-survival signals in (cancer) cells at a site of inflammation (Sugimoto et al. 2016). Thus, by inducing the expression of AnxA1, xanthohumol appears to inhibit pro-survival pathways in T98G glioblastoma cells.

Modulation of the immune system offers potential for cancer control. The balance between T-helper 1 (Th1) and T-helper 2 (Th2) cells is thought to determine production of cytokine profiles. Th1 cells drive cellular immunity and eliminate cancerous cells. Several dietary factors and hormones influence the Th1/Th2 balance and Th1/Th2-based immunotherapies could prove useful in cancer control (Kidd 2003). Zhang and coworkers (2018) treated BALB/c-4 T1 mice, a breast cancer mouse model, with xanthohumol and found that it decreased tumor growth. Xanthohumol upregulated Th1 cytokines while it downregulated Th2 cytokines. The authors attributed the balance drift towards Th1 polarization to stimulation of the STAT4 pathway.

Although several researchers have demonstrated that xanthohumol and related prenylflavonoids have the ability to scavenge ROS in vitro (Gerhauser et al. 2002; Miranda et al. 2000b; Tronina et al. 2013b; Vogel et al. 2010), others have shown that xanthohumol can act as a pro-oxidant in cell-free systems (Schempp et al. 2010) and in cell culture to induce apoptosis at pharmacological concentrations (Blanquer-Rosselló et al. 2013; Strathmann et al. 2010). Strathmann and coworkers (2010) found that xanthohumol (1.6–25 μM) induced the production of superoxide ($O_2^{-\bullet}$) in several cell lines, which resulted in GSH (thiol) depletion, reduction of ATP levels (12.5–50 μM), release of cytochrome c, and decrease of the mitochondrial membrane potential, and ultimately apoptosis. Using mouse C2C12 myocytes, Kirkwood and coworkers (2013) also observed GSH depletion by non-toxic exposure to xanthohumol (5 μM), which the authors attributed to Michael-type addition of GSH to xanthohumol based on measurements of the resulting xanthohumol-SG conjugate. These oxidative stress-inducing effects were attenuated by pre- or co-incubation with the antioxidants MnTMPyP (Kirkwood et al. 2013; Strathmann et al. 2010) and *N*-acetylcysteine (Strathmann et al. 2010). Collectively, these activities have the characteristics of mitocans, which induce apoptosis by targeting mitochondria via ROS production (Neuzil et al. 2006).

10.6 Xanthohumol as an Inducer of the Keap1-Nrf2-Dependent ARE Signaling Pathway

Nrf2 (nuclear erythroid-2 related factor 2) is a transcription factor that regulates the cellular redox homeostasis and drives the enzymatic machinery that protects cells against oxidative stress. Nrf2 interacts with DNA's 'antioxidant response element' (ARE) to induce transcription. Transcriptional activation of ARE target genes results in the synthesis of antioxidant defense enzymes, such as GSH biosynthetic enzymes, GSH reductase, GSH peroxidase, thioredoxin, peroxiredoxins, NADPH quinone oxidoreductase, heme oxygenase-1, superoxide dismutase (SOD), glutathione *S*-transferases (GSTs), and UDP-glucuronosyltransferases (Dinkova-Kostova and Talalay 2008). Inactive Nrf2 is bound to Kelch-like ECH-associated protein 1 (Keap1) in the cytosol. Human Keap1 contains 27 cysteine residues, nine of which are reactive towards electrophiles produced, for instance, by lipid peroxidation. Under conditions of oxidative/electrophilic stress, Michael-type addition of cysteine residues (particularly Cys-151) to electrophiles induces conformational changes within Keap1 and renders Nrf2 less susceptible to degradation via ubiquitination, with the overall result that the cytosolic and nuclear concentrations of free Nrf2 increase leading to increased transcription of ARE target genes (Eggler et al. 2005, 2007). Xanthohumol, by virtue of its α,β-unsaturated keto functionality, has electrophilic properties and has been shown to form covalent bonds with Keap1 (Liu et al. 2005; Luo et al. 2007), which provides a mechanistic explanation for how it induces the ARE signaling pathway. Brodziak-Jarosz and coworkers (2016), applying an unbiased click-chemistry approach to identify protein targets of xanthohumol (using an alkyne-functionalized derivative of xanthohumol for affinity purification) in lysates of AREc32 cells (a reporter cell line derived from MCF-7 cells), confirmed that xanthohumol forms covalent adducts with Keap1. In an immunodetection approach using antibodies against xanthohumol, the flavonoid was found to associate with specific members of the histone family in MCF-7/6 cells (Wyns et al. 2012).

Consistent with xanthohumol acting as an inducer of the ARE pathway, it provided protection against cisplatin-induced nephrotoxicity in C57BL/6 mice. It attenuated the cisplatin-induced lowering of GSH, SOD activity, and ROS (Li et al. 2018). The suppressing effects of xanthohumol on cisplatin-mediated elevation of kidney interleukins (IL-6 and IL-1β) and TNFα can be explained by xanthohumol's interfering with the pro-inflammatory NFκB pathway. In an LPS-induced mouse model of lung injury, xanthohumol reduced phenotype severity and attenuated formation of ROS and malondialdehyde (a lipid peroxidation product), and it protected against GSH depletion (Lv et al. 2017).

A prominent mechanism by which cancer chemopreventive agents act to detoxify carcinogens is by inducing the transcriptional expression of ARE target genes coding for enzymes that convert carcinogens into metabolites without reactivity towards DNA bases. NAD(P)H quinone oxido reductase (NQO1), UDP-glucuronosyl transferases, sulfotransferases, and GSTs belong to this group of detoxifying enzymes. We determined that xanthohumol and 16 related prenylated flavonoids induce the expression of NQO1 in mouse Hepa 1c1c7 cells (Miranda et al. 2000a). In these cells, xanthohumol doubled the activity of NQO1 at a concentration of 2.1 μM. The most potent prenylated flavonoid was dehydrocycloxanthohumol hydrate whose concentration to double NQO1 activity was 1.8 μM (Miranda et al. 2000a). Other researchers identified xanthohumol's ability to induce NQO1 in mouse Hepa 1c1c7 cells (Gerhauser et al. 2002), human hepatocytes (Krajka-Kuzniak et al. 2013), as a mechanism to inhibit menadione-induced DNA damage in Hepa 1c1c7 cells (Dietz et al. 2005), to detoxify benzo[*a*]pyrene, IQ, and *tert*-butyl hydroperoxide in human HepG2 hepatoma cells (Plazar et al. 2007), and to protect oxidative stress-induced neuronal cell damage in the neuron-like rat pheochromocytoma cell line PC12 (Yao et al. 2015). Besides NQO1, xanthohumol (0.5 μM) also significantly induced the expression of the ARE target genes, heme oxygenase-1, thioredoxin 1, and thioredoxin reductase 1 in PC12 cells which could be attributed to increased nuclear accumulation and activation of Nrf2 (Yao et al. 2015). Using LPS to induce inflammation in mouse microglial BV2 cells, Lee and coworkers (2011) established that the anti-inflammatory effect of xanthohumol in this model involves heme oxygenase-1 and NQO1 induction as well as GSH synthesis via Nrf2-ARE signaling. Dietz and coworkers (2013) examined the effects of subcutaneously injected xanthohumol and oral administration of a hop extract on NQO1 activation in Sprague-Dawley rats. They found that xanthohumol and the hop extract induced NQO1 expression in the liver but that the hop extract treatment resulted in reduced NQO1 activity in the mammary gland. They attributed the latter effect to enrichment and estrogenic effects of 8-prenylnaringenin in breast tissue. They hypothesized that the 8-prenylnaringenin-estrogen receptor-α acts as a co-repressor of the ARE domain of DNA (Dietz et al. 2013).

10.7 Prenylflavonoids as Inducers of Apoptosis by Mild Mitochondrial Uncoupling

The previous paragraphs discuss several molecular mechanisms by which xanthohumol induces apoptosis in cancer cells but not in normal cells. This raises the question whether multiple molecular signaling pathways are initiated by a common upstream mechanism of action. Regardless of their cancer type, tumor cells have in common that they have higher nutrient, energy, and oxygen needs than their normal counterparts. They operate in a state of anabolic metabolism and secure their nutrient and oxygen needs by promoting signaling pathways that induce angiogenesis. The higher rate of metabolism leads to elevated oxidative stress and increased risk of apoptosis. Cancer cells respond by switching from oxidative phosphorylation to aerobic glycolysis (a phenomenon referred to as the Warburg effect), which reduces oxygen consumption and demand, averts apoptosis risk, and increases cell survival. These metabolic changes of the cellular microenvironment have an impact on the mitochondrial membrane potential, $\Delta\psi_m$. Within a population of proliferating colonic cancer cells, Heerdt and coworkers (2005) found subtle but distinct and stable differences among cells with regard to $\Delta\psi_m$. Cells with a higher $\Delta\psi_m$ produced more vascular endothelial growth factor (VEGF) and matrix metalloproteinase-7, two species that are known to drive tumor progression, cell invasion, and metastasis. When challenged with butyrate, colonic epithelial cells with a lower $\Delta\psi_m$ had a higher proportion of apoptotic cells in the population (Heerdt et al. 2003). These observations raise the question whether there are chemical agents that can lower the $\Delta\psi_m$ and thus would have potential as cancer chemotherapeutics by forcing cells into apoptosis. One of the most well-known agents that lowers $\Delta\psi_m$ is 2,4-dinitrophenol, which drives cells into catabolism and has found (illicit) use as an anti-obesity agent (Colman 2007). However, it was considered too toxic for consideration as a cancer chemotherapeutic. Lowering $\Delta\psi_m$ can be achieved by facilitating transport of protons from the acidic side of the mitochondrial inner membrane (the intermembrane space) to the more alkaline side (the mitochondrial matrix). Uncoupling proteins control thermogenesis by this mechanism. Chemicals whose functional groups with pK_a values within the pH range from the intermembrane space (~pH 6.8) to the matrix (~pH 7.7) and whose lipophilicty favors residence in membranes will facilitate such proton transport through a biophysical mechanism and are referred to as 'protonophores' (Fig. 10.3). By their protonophoric effect, these compounds uncouple oxygen consumption from ATP production in the electron transport chain and are therefore also referred to as mitochondrial uncouplers.

Many dietary polyphenols meet the criteria for exerting a protonophoric effect (Stevens et al. 2018). Prenylated flavonoids should be well represented in this group of polyphenols because they are more lipophilic than their non-prenylated counterparts. The most acidic hydroxyl group of xanthohumol has a pK_a value of 7.59 (Arczewska et al. 2017) and a LogP value of 4.82 (Stevens et al. 2018). Our group described the mitochondrial uncoupling effect of xanthohumol in mouse C2C12 cells (Kirkwood et al. 2013); when these cells were treated with oligomycin to block ATP synthase (complex V) and then treated with xanthohumol (5 μM), oxygen consumption increased within minutes as would be expected for a mitochondrial uncoupler. The actual lowering effect of xanthohumol on $\Delta\psi_m$ was demonstrated by de Montgolfier (2014) (Fig. 10.4). Kłósek and coworkers (2016) observed that the xanthohumol-induced loss of $\Delta\psi_m$ was associated with apoptosis induction in prostate cancer cells. Similar associations between xanthohumol-induced mitochondrial membrane depolarization and apoptosis induction were observed in the alveolar adenocarcinoma cell line A549 (Yong et al. 2015), in Ca Ski cervical cancer cells (Yong and Abd Malek 2015), and in human prostate cancer cells (Deeb et al. 2010). The hypothesis that xanthohumol can induce apoptosis by lowering $\Delta\psi_m$ is attractive, because it would provide a general mechanism for apoptosis induction and it would reduce the metastatic potential of cancer cells.

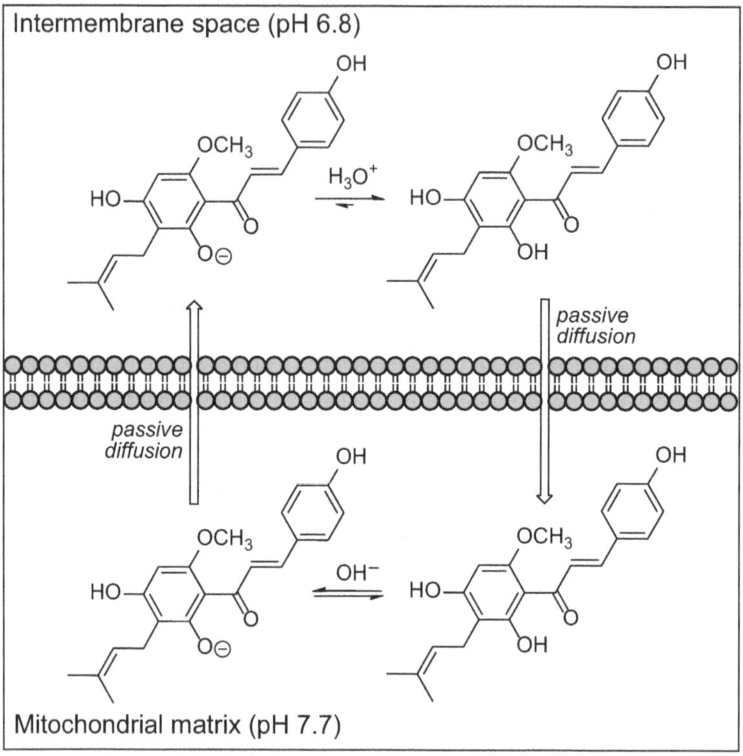

Fig. 10.3 Protonophore action of xanthohumol. Xanthohumol reaches the intermembrane space and the matrix of mitochondria by passive diffusion. In the matrix, xanthohumol deprotonates and the resulting phenolate anion diffuses back to the intermembrane space down the electrochemical gradient. The protonated and deprotonated forms of xanthohumol travel back and forth between the intermembrane space and the matrix, thereby transporting protons from the intermembrane space to the matrix. Dissipation of the mitochondrial membrane potential ($\Delta\psi_m$) ensues

10.8 Conclusions and Perspectives

Many studies have reported that xanthohumol can exert anticarcinogenic effects in cell culture and animal models. Xanthohumol appears to exert antiproliferative effects by acting as an anti-inflammatory agent to counter oxidative stress-driven cancer cell proliferation during the early stages of carcinogenesis. While pro-apoptotic pathways may involve NFκB signaling or other pro-inflammatory pathways that can be promoted by xanthohumol during the later stages of carcinogenesis, its ability to induce apoptosis by dissipation of $\Delta\psi_m$ has not received sufficient attention. This biophysical effect, however, holds promise for exploitation in cancer chemotherapy in combination with prescription drugs because cancer cells cannot develop resistance against xanthohumol's effect on $\Delta\psi_m$. Several researchers cited in this review have shown that non-toxic concentrations of xanthohumol can drive drug-resistant cancer cells into apoptosis. As the available literature on

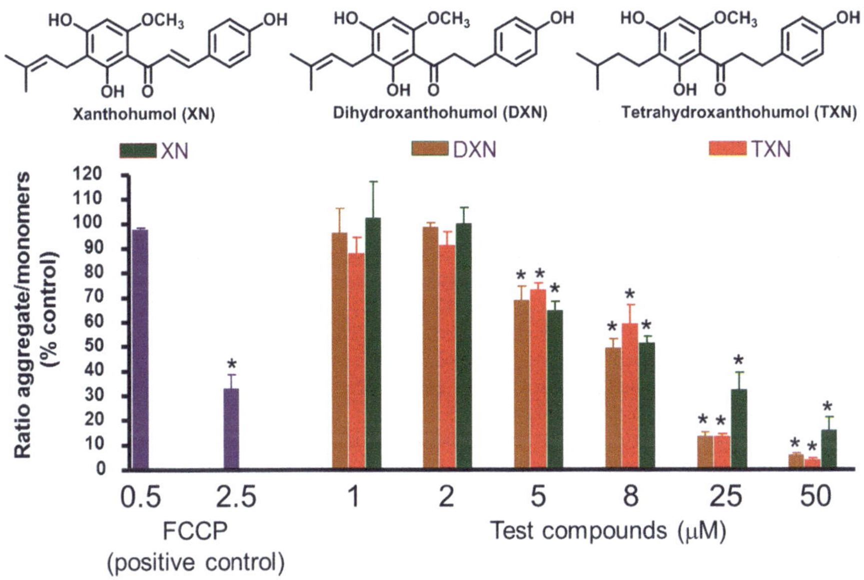

Fig. 10.4 Xanthohumol, α,β-dihydroxanthohumol, and tetrahydroxanthohumol depolarize the mitochondrial transmembrane potential ($\Delta\psi_m$) in C2C12 mouse skeletal muscle cells, measured by the JC-1 assay. With mitochondrial loss of $\Delta\psi_m$, the JC-1 dye used in the assay cannot accumulate in the mitochondria, resulting in fewer J-aggregates and a higher proportion of dye monomers. Using a single excitation wavelength, both monomers and aggregates are measured by dual wavelength fluorescence emission. FCCP (Trifluoromethoxy carbonylcyanide phenylhydrazone) is a potent uncoupler of oxidative phosphorylation and used as the positive control. *Asterisk* indicates $p < 0.05$ from the control. Adapted from de Montgolfier [Oregon State University Dissertation (de Montgolfier 2014)]

xanthohumol indicates that it is not toxic to laboratory animals and to humans, there is sufficient rationale to explore treating patients with difficult-to-treat cancers with a combination of a chemotherapeutic agent and xanthohumol. The available literature indicates that mono-therapy with xanthohumol holds little promise for treating or controlling cancer. This assessment is based on a general observation that antiproliferative effects of xanthohumol in cancer cells require very high concentrations (>25 μM) which are unlikely to be reached in tumors by oral administration. This discrepancy between in vitro and in vivo concentrations as well as its consequence for translation of in vitro data to humans is a concern (Willson and Grundmann 2017). The exception might be cancer of the colon whose cells' exposure to xanthohumol does not require intestinal absorption and tissue distribution.

Acknowledgments The author receives support for research on xanthohumol from the National Institutes of Health (NIH Grants R01AT009168 and R01AT010271).

References

Albini A, Dell'Eva R, Vene R, Ferrari N, Buhler DR, Noonan DM, Fassina G (2006) Mechanisms of the antiangiogenic activity by the hop flavonoid xanthohumol: NF-kappaB and Akt as targets. FASEB J 20:527–529

Allsopp P, Possemiers S, Campbell D, Gill C, Rowland I (2013) A comparison of the anticancer properties of isoxanthohumol and 8-prenylnaringenin using in vitro models of colon cancer. Biofactors 39:441–447

Alsaleh M, Leftley Z, Barbera TA, Sithithaworn P, Khuntikeo N, Loilome W, Yongvanit P, Cox IJ, Chamodol N, Syms RR, Andrews RH, Taylor-Robinson SD (2019) Cholangiocarcinoma: a guide for the nonspecialist. Int J Gen Med 12:13–23

Arczewska M, Kamiński DM, Gieroba B, Gagoś M (2017) Acid-base properties of xanthohumol: a computational and experimental investigation. J Nat Prod 80:3194–3202

Auffinger B, Thaci B, Ahmed A, Ulasov I, Lesniak MS (2013) MicroRNA targeting as a therapeutic strategy against glioma. Curr Mol Med 13:535–542

Bahar E, Kim JY, Yoon H (2019) Chemotherapy resistance explained through endoplasmic reticulum stress-dependent signaling. Cancers (Basel) 11. https://doi.org/10.3390/cancers11030338

Barron D, Ibrahim RK (1996) Isoprenylated flavonoids—a survey. Phytochemistry 43:924–982

Bartmańska A, Tronina T, Popłoński J, Milczarek M, Filip-Psurska B, Wietrzyk J (2018) Highly cancer selective antiproliferative activity of natural prenylated flavonoids. Molecules 23. https://doi.org/10.3390/molecules23112922

Benelli R, Venè R, Ciarlo M, Carlone S, Barbieri O, Ferrari N (2012) The AKT/NF-κB inhibitor xanthohumol is a potent anti-lymphocytic leukemia drug overcoming chemoresistance and cell infiltration. Biochem Pharmacol 83:1634–1642

Blanquer-Rosselló MM, Oliver J, Valle A, Roca P (2013) Effect of xanthohumol and 8-prenylnaringenin on MCF-7 breast cancer cells oxidative stress and mitochondrial complexes expression. J Cell Biochem 114:2785–2794

Boelsterli UA (2007) Mechanistic toxicology. CRC, Boca Raton, FL

Bolca S, Possemiers S, Maervoet V, Huybrechts I, Heyerick A, Vervarcke S, Depypere H, De Keukeleire D, Bracke M, De Henauw S, Verstraete W, Van de Wiele T (2007) Microbial and dietary factors associated with the 8-prenylnaringenin producer phenotype: a dietary intervention trial with fifty healthy post-menopausal Caucasian women. Br J Nutr 98:950–959

Bolton JL, Dunlap TL, Hajirahimkhan DA, Mbachu OC, Chen SN, Chadwick L, Nikolic D, van Breemen RB, Pauli GF, Dietz BM (2019) The multiple biological targets of hops and bioactive compounds. Chem Res Toxicol 32(8):1732

Bridgewater JA, Goodman KA, Kalyan A, Mulcahy MF (2016) Biliary tract cancer: epidemiology, radiotherapy, and molecular profiling. Am Soc Clin Oncol Educ Book 35:e194–e203

Brodziak-Jarosz L, Fujikawa Y, Pastor-Flores D, Kasikci S, Jirásek P, Pitzl S, Owen RW, Klika KD, Gerhäuser C, Amslinger S, Dick TP (2016) A click chemistry approach identifies target proteins of xanthohumol. Mol Nutr Food Res 60:737–748

Burrows N, Babur M, Resch J, Williams KJ, Brabant G (2011) Hypoxia-inducible factor in thyroid carcinoma. J Thyroid Res 2011:762905

Catz SD, Johnson JL (2003) BCL-2 in prostate cancer: a minireview. Apoptosis 8:29–37

Chappell WH, Steelman LS, Long JM, Kempf RC, Abrams SL, Franklin RA, Bäsecke J, Stivala F, Donia M, Fagone P, Malaponte G, Mazzarino MC, Nicoletti F, Libra M, Maksimovic-Ivanic D, Mijatovic S, Montalto G, Cervello M, Laidler P, Milella M, Tafuri A, Bonati A, Evangelisti C, Cocco L, Martelli AM, McCubrey JA (2011) Ras/Raf/MEK/ERK and PI3K/PTEN/Akt/mTOR inhibitors: rationale and importance to inhibiting these pathways in human health. Oncotarget 2:135–164

Chen PH, Chang CK, Shih CM, Cheng CH, Lin CW, Lee CC, Liu AJ, Ho KH, Chen KC (2016) The miR-204-3p-targeted IGFBP2 pathway is involved in xanthohumol-induced glioma cell apoptotic death. Neuropharmacology 110:362–375

Chen G, Xiao B, Chen L, Bai B, Zhang Y, Xu Z, Fu L, Liu Z, Li X, Zhao Y, Liang G (2017) Discovery of new MD2-targeted anti-inflammatory compounds for the treatment of sepsis and acute lung injury. Eur J Med Chem 139:726–740

Cho YC, Kim HJ, Kim YJ, Lee KY, Choi HJ, Lee IS, Kang BY (2008) Differential anti-inflammatory pathway by xanthohumol in IFN-gamma and LPS-activated macrophages. Int Immunopharmacol 8:567–573

Colgate EC, Miranda CL, Stevens JF, Bray TM, Ho E (2007) Xanthohumol, a prenylflavonoid derived from hops induces apoptosis and inhibits NF-kappaB activation in prostate epithelial cells. Cancer Lett 246:201–209

Colman E (2007) Dinitrophenol and obesity: an early twentieth-century regulatory dilemma. Regul Toxicol Pharmacol 48:115–117

Cömert Önder F, Ay M, Aydoğan Türkoğlu S, Tura Köçkar F, Çelik A (2016) Antiproliferative activity of Humulus lupulus extracts on human hepatoma (Hep3B), colon (HT-29) cancer cells and proteases, tyrosinase, β-lactamase enzyme inhibition studies. J Enzyme Inhib Med Chem 31:90–98

Cseh B, Doma E, Baccarini M (2014) "RAF" neighborhood: protein-protein interaction in the Raf/Mek/Erk pathway. FEBS Lett 588:2398–2406

Cuenda A, Rousseau S (2007) p38 MAP-kinases pathway regulation, function and role in human diseases. Biochim Biophys Acta 1773:1358–1375

de Montgolfier O (2014) Development of xanthohumol as mild mitochondrial uncouplers for treatment of metabolic syndrome. College of Pharmacy, vol. Master's. Oregon State University, Corvallis, p 49

Deeb D, Gao X, Jiang H, Arbab AS, Dulchavsky SA, Gautam SC (2010) Growth inhibitory and apoptosis-inducing effects of xanthohumol, a prenylated chalone present in hops, in human prostate cancer cells. Anticancer Res 30:3333–3339

Deininger M, Buchdunger E, Druker BJ (2005) The development of imatinib as a therapeutic agent for chronic myeloid leukemia. Blood 105:2640–2653

Dell'Eva R, Ambrosini C, Vannini N, Piaggio G, Albini A, Ferrari N (2007) AKT/NF-kappaB inhibitor xanthohumol targets cell growth and angiogenesis in hematologic malignancies. Cancer 110:2007–2011

Delmulle L, Bellahcène A, Dhooge W, Comhaire F, Roelens F, Huvaere K, Heyerick A, Castronovo V, De Keukeleire D (2006) Anti-proliferative properties of prenylated flavonoids from hops (*Humulus lupulus* L.) in human prostate cancer cell lines. Phytomedicine 13:732–734

Delmulle L, Vanden Berghe T, Keukeleire DD, Vandenabeele P (2008) Treatment of PC-3 and DU145 prostate cancer cells by prenylflavonoids from hop (*Humulus lupulus* L.) induces a caspase-independent form of cell death. Phytother Res 22:197–203

Dietz BM, Kang YH, Liu G, Eggler AL, Yao P, Chadwick LR, Pauli GF, Farnsworth NR, Mesecar AD, van Breemen RB, Bolton JL (2005) Xanthohumol isolated from *Humulus lupulus* Inhibits menadione-induced DNA damage through induction of quinone reductase. Chem Res Toxicol 18:1296–1305

Dietz BM, Hagos GK, Eskra JN, Wijewickrama GT, Anderson JR, Nikolic D, Guo J, Wright B, Chen SN, Pauli GF, van Breemen RB, Bolton JL (2013) Differential regulation of detoxification enzymes in hepatic and mammary tissue by hops (*Humulus lupulus*) in vitro and in vivo. Mol Nutr Food Res 57:1055–1066

Dinkova-Kostova AT, Talalay P (2008) Direct and indirect antioxidant properties of inducers of cytoprotective proteins. Mol Nutr Food Res 52(Suppl 1):S128–S138

Dixon RA, Pasinetti GM (2010) Flavonoids and isoflavonoids: from plant biology to agriculture and neuroscience. Plant Physiol 154:453–457

Dokduang H, Yongvanit P, Namwat N, Pairojkul C, Sangkhamanon S, Yageta MS, Murakami Y, Loilome W (2016) Xanthohumol inhibits STAT3 activation pathway leading to growth suppression and apoptosis induction in human cholangiocarcinoma cells. Oncol Rep 35:2065–2072

Dorn C, Weiss TS, Heilmann J, Hellerbrand C (2010) Xanthohumol, a prenylated chalcone derived from hops, inhibits proliferation, migration and interleukin-8 expression of hepatocellular carcinoma cells. Int J Oncol 36:435–441

Dorn C, Heilmann J, Hellerbrand C (2012) Protective effect of xanthohumol on toxin-induced liver inflammation and fibrosis. Int J Clin Exp Pathol 5:29–36

Eggler AL, Liu G, Pezzuto JM, van Breemen RB, Mesecar AD (2005) Modifying specific cysteines of the electrophile-sensing human Keap1 protein is insufficient to disrupt binding to the Nrf2 domain Neh2. Proc Natl Acad Sci U S A 102:10070–10075

Eggler AL, Luo Y, van Breemen RB, Mesecar AD (2007) Identification of the highly reactive cysteine 151 in the chemopreventive agent-sensor Keap1 protein is method-dependent. Chem Res Toxicol 20:1878–1884

Engelsgjerd S, Kunnimalaiyaan S, Kandil E, Gamblin TC, Kunnimalaiyaan M (2019) Xanthohumol increases death receptor 5 expression and enhances apoptosis with the TNF-related apoptosis-inducing ligand in neuroblastoma cell lines. PLoS One 14:e0213776

Fenselau C, Talalay P (1973) Is estrogenic activity present in hops? Food Cosmet Toxicol 11:597–603

Ferk F, Huber WW, Filipic M, Bichler J, Haslinger E, Misík M, Nersesyan A, Grasl-Kraupp B, Zegura B, Knasmüller S (2010) Xanthohumol, a prenylated flavonoid contained in beer, prevents the induction of preneoplastic lesions and DNA damage in liver and colon induced by the heterocyclic aromatic amine amino-3-methyl-imidazo[4,5-f]quinoline (IQ). Mutat Res 691:17–22

Ferk F, Misik M, Nersesyan A, Pichler C, Jager W, Szekeres T, Marculescu R, Poulsen HE, Henriksen T, Bono R, Romanazzi V, Al-Serori H, Biendl M, Wagner KH, Kundi M, Knasmuller S (2016) Impact of xanthohumol (a prenylated flavonoid from hops) on DNA stability and other health-related biochemical parameters: results of human intervention trials. Mol Nutr Food Res 60:773–786

Festa M, Capasso A, D'Acunto CW, Masullo M, Rossi AG, Pizza C, Piacente S (2011) Xanthohumol induces apoptosis in human malignant glioblastoma cells by increasing reactive oxygen species and activating MAPK pathways. J Nat Prod 74:2505–2513

Festa M, Caputo M, Cipolla C, D'Acunto C, Rossi A, Tecce M, Capasso A (2013) The involvement of xanthohumol in the expression of annexin in human malignant glioblastoma cells. Open Biochem J 7:1–10

Fonseca BF, Predes D, Cerqueira DM, Reis AH, Amado NG, Cayres MC, Kuster RM, Oliveira FL, Mendes FA, Abreu JG (2015) Derricin and derricidin inhibit Wnt/β-catenin signaling and suppress colon cancer cell growth in vitro. PLoS One 10:e0120919

Fu W, Chen L, Wang Z, Zhao C, Chen G, Liu X, Dai Y, Cai Y, Li C, Zhou J, Liang G (2016) Determination of the binding mode for anti-inflammatory natural product xanthohumol with myeloid differentiation protein 2. Drug Des Devel Ther 10:455–463

Gerhauser C (2005) Beer constituents as potential cancer chemopreventive agents. Eur J Cancer 41:1941–1954

Gerhäuser C, Frank N (2005) Xanthohumol, a new all-rounder? Mol Nutr Food Res 49:821–823

Gerhauser C, Alt A, Heiss E, Gamal-Eldeen A, Klimo K, Knauft J, Neumann I, Scherf HR, Frank N, Bartsch H, Becker H (2002) Cancer chemopreventive activity of Xanthohumol, a natural product derived from hop. Mol Cancer Ther 1:959–969

Guo J, Nikolic D, Chadwick LR, Pauli GF, van Breemen RB (2006) Identification of human hepatic cytochrome P450 enzymes involved in the metabolism of 8-prenylnaringenin and isoxanthohumol from hops (*Humulus lupulus* L.). Drug Metab Dispos 34:1152–1159

Guo D, Zhang B, Liu S, Jin M (2018) Xanthohumol induces apoptosis via caspase activation, regulation of Bcl-2, and inhibition of PI3K/Akt/mTOR-kinase in human gastric cancer cells. Biomed Pharmacother 106:1300–1306

Halliwell B, Gutteridge JMC (1999) Free radicals in biology and medicine. Oxford University Press, Oxford

Harikumar KB, Kunnumakkara AB, Ahn KS, Anand P, Krishnan S, Guha S, Aggarwal BB (2009) Modification of the cysteine residues in IkappaBalpha kinase and NF-kappaB (p65) by xanthohumol leads to suppression of NF-kappaB-regulated gene products and potentiation of apoptosis in leukemia cells. Blood 113:2003–2013

Heerdt BG, Houston MA, Wilson AJ, Augenlicht LH (2003) The intrinsic mitochondrial membrane potential (Deltapsim) is associated with steady-state mitochondrial activity and the extent to which colonic epithelial cells undergo butyrate-mediated growth arrest and apoptosis. Cancer Res 63:6311–6319

Heerdt BG, Houston MA, Augenlicht LH (2005) The intrinsic mitochondrial membrane potential of colonic carcinoma cells is linked to the probability of tumor progression. Cancer Res 65:9861–9867

Henderson MC, Miranda CL, Stevens JF, Deinzer ML, Buhler DR (2000) In vitro inhibition of human P450 enzymes by prenylated flavonoids from hops, *Humulus lupulus*. Xenobiotica 30:235–251

Ho KH, Chang CK, Chen PH, Wang YJ, Chang WC, Chen KC (2018) miR-4725-3p targeting stromal interacting molecule 1 signaling is involved in xanthohumol inhibition of glioma cell invasion. J Neurochem 146:269–288

Hori K, Sen A, Artavanis-Tsakonas S (2013) Notch signaling at a glance. J Cell Sci 126:2135–2140

Jamnongkan W, Thanee M, Yongvanit P, Loilome W, Thanan R, Kimawaha P, Boonmars T, Silakit R, Namwat N, Techasen A (2018) Antifibrotic effect of xanthohumol in combination with praziquantel is associated with altered redox status and reduced iron accumulation during liver fluke-associated cholangiocarcinogenesis. PeerJ 6:e4281

Jiang CH, Sun TL, Xiang DX, Wei SS, Li WQ (2018) Anticancer activity and mechanism of xanthohumol: a prenylated flavonoid from hops (*Humulus lupulus* L.). Front Pharmacol 9:530

Kaewpitoon N, Kaewpitoon SJ, Pengsaa P, Sripa B (2008) Opisthorchis viverrini: the carcinogenic human liver fluke. World J Gastroenterol 14:666–674

Kang Y, Park MA, Heo SW, Park SY, Kang KW, Park PH, Kim JA (2013) The radio-sensitizing effect of xanthohumol is mediated by STAT3 and EGFR suppression in doxorubicin-resistant MCF-7 human breast cancer cells. Biochim Biophys Acta 1830:2638–2648

Kidd P (2003) Th1/Th2 balance: the hypothesis, its limitations, and implications for health and disease. Altern Med Rev 8:223–246

Kirkwood JS, Legette LL, Miranda CL, Jiang Y, Stevens JF (2013) A metabolomics-driven elucidation of the anti-obesity mechanisms of xanthohumol. J Biol Chem 288:19000–19013

Kłósek M, Mertas A, Król W, Jaworska D, Szymszal J, Szliszka E (2016) Tumor necrosis factor-related apoptosis-inducing ligand-induced apoptosis in prostate cancer cells after treatment with xanthohumol-a natural compound present in *Humulus lupulus* L. Int J Mol Sci 17. https://doi.org/10.3390/ijms17060837

Knight T, Irving JA (2014) Ras/Raf/MEK/ERK pathway activation in childhood acute lymphoblastic leukemia and its therapeutic targeting. Front Oncol 4:160

Krajka-Kuzniak V, Paluszczak J, Baer-Dubowska W (2013) Xanthohumol induces phase II enzymes via Nrf2 in human hepatocytes in vitro. Toxicol in Vitro 27:149–156

Krajnović T, Kaluđerović GN, Wessjohann LA, Mijatović S, Maksimović-Ivanić D (2016) Versatile antitumor potential of isoxanthohumol: enhancement of paclitaxel activity in vivo. Pharmacol Res 105:62–73

Kunnimalaiyaan S, Trevino J, Tsai S, Gamblin TC, Kunnimalaiyaan M (2015) Xanthohumol-mediated suppression of Notch1 signaling is associated with antitumor activity in human pancreatic cancer cells. Mol Cancer Ther 14:1395–1403

Lau KM, LaSpina M, Long J, Ho SM (2000) Expression of estrogen receptor (ER)-alpha and ER-beta in normal and malignant prostatic epithelial cells: regulation by methylation and involvement in growth regulation. Cancer Res 60:3175–3182

Lee SH, Kim HJ, Lee JS, Lee IS, Kang BY (2007) Inhibition of topoisomerase I activity and efflux drug transporters' expression by xanthohumol. From hops. Arch Pharm Res 30:1435–1439

Lee IS, Lim J, Gal J, Kang JC, Kim HJ, Kang BY, Choi HJ (2011) Anti-inflammatory activity of xanthohumol involves heme oxygenase-1 induction via NRF2-ARE signaling in microglial BV2 cells. Neurochem Int 58:153–160

Legette L, Ma L, Reed RL, Miranda CL, Christensen JM, Rodriguez-Proteau R, Stevens JF (2012) Pharmacokinetics of xanthohumol and metabolites in rats after oral and intravenous administration. Mol Nutr Food Res 56:466–474

Legette L, Karnpracha C, Reed RL, Choi J, Bobe G, Christensen JM, Proteau RR, Purnell J, Stevens JF (2014) Human pharmacokinetics of xanthohumol, an anti-hyperglycemic flavonoid from hops. Mol Nutr Food Res 58:248–255

Li F, Yao Y, Huang H, Hao H, Ying M (2018) Xanthohumol attenuates cisplatin-induced nephrotoxicity through inhibiting NF-κB and activating Nrf2 signaling pathways. Int Immunopharmacol 61:277–282

Lin Y, Jiang T, Zhou K, Xu L, Chen B, Li G, Qiu X, Zhang W, Song SW (2009) Plasma IGFBP-2 levels predict clinical outcomes of patients with high-grade gliomas. Neuro-Oncology 11:468–476

Liu G, Eggler AL, Dietz BM, Mesecar AD, Bolton JL, Pezzuto JM, van Breemen RB (2005) Screening method for the discovery of potential cancer chemoprevention agents based on mass spectrometric detection of alkylated Keap1. Anal Chem 77:6407–6414

Liu M, Yin H, Qian X, Dong J, Qian Z, Miao J (2016) Xanthohumol, a prenylated chalcone from hops, inhibits the viability and stemness of doxorubicin-resistant MCF-7/ADR cells. Molecules 22. https://doi.org/10.3390/molecules22010036

Logan IE, Miranda CL, Lowry MB, Maier CS, Stevens JF, Gombart AF (2019) Antiproliferative and cytotoxic activity of xanthohumol and its non-estrogenic derivatives in colon and hepatocellular carcinoma cell lines. Int J Mol Sci 20. https://doi.org/10.3390/ijms20051203

Luo Y, Eggler AL, Liu D, Liu G, Mesecar AD, van Breemen RB (2007) Sites of alkylation of human Keap1 by natural chemoprevention agents. J Am Soc Mass Spectrom 18:2226–2232

Lust S, Vanhoecke B, Janssens A, Philippe J, Bracke M, Offner F (2005) Xanthohumol kills B-chronic lymphocytic leukemia cells by an apoptotic mechanism. Mol Nutr Food Res 49:844–850

Lust S, Vanhoecke B, VAN Gele M, Boelens J, VAN Melckebeke H, Kaileh M, Vanden Berghe W, Haegeman G, Philippé J, Bracke M, Offner F (2009) Xanthohumol activates the proapoptotic arm of the unfolded protein response in chronic lymphocytic leukemia. Anticancer Res 29:3797–3805

Lv H, Liu Q, Wen Z, Feng H, Deng X, Ci X (2017) Xanthohumol ameliorates lipopolysaccharide (LPS)-induced acute lung injury via induction of AMPK/GSK3β-Nrf2 signal axis. Redox Biol 12:311–324

Maemura K, Natsugoe S, Takao S (2014) Molecular mechanism of cholangiocarcinoma carcinogenesis. J Hepatobiliary Pancreat Sci 21:754–760

Maruyama S, Fujimoto N, Asano K, Ito A, Usui T (2000) Expression of estrogen receptor alpha and beta mRNAs in prostate cancers treated with leuprorelin acetate. Eur Urol 38:635–639

Mi X, Wang C, Sun C, Chen X, Huo X, Zhang Y, Li G, Xu B, Zhang J, Xie J, Wang Z, Li J (2017) Xanthohumol induces paraptosis of leukemia cells through p38 mitogen activated protein kinase signaling pathway. Oncotarget 8:31297–31304

Milligan SR, Kalita JC, Heyerick A, Rong H, De Cooman L, De Keukeleire D (1999) Identification of a potent phytoestrogen in hops (*Humulus lupulus* L.) and beer. J Clin Endocrinol Metab 84:2249–2252

Milligan SR, Kalita JC, Pocock V, Van De Kauter V, Stevens JF, Deinzer ML, Rong H, De Keukeleire D (2000) The endocrine activities of 8-prenylnaringenin and related hop (*Humulus lupulus* L.) flavonoids. J Clin Endocrinol Metab 85:4912–4915

Milligan S, Kalita J, Pocock V, Heyerick A, De Cooman L, Rong H, De Keukeleire D (2002) Oestrogenic activity of the hop phytoestrogen, 8-prenylnaringenin. Reproduction 123:235–242

Miranda CL, Stevens JF, Helmrich A, Henderson MC, Rodriguez RJ, Yang YH, Deinzer ML, Barnes DW, Buhler DR (1999) Antiproliferative and cytotoxic effects of prenylated flavonoids from hops (*Humulus lupulus*) in human cancer cell lines. Food Chem Toxicol 37:271–285

Miranda CL, Aponso GL, Stevens JF, Deinzer ML, Buhler DR (2000a) Prenylated chalcones and flavanones as inducers of quinone reductase in mouse Hepa 1c1c7 cells. Cancer Lett 149:21–29

Miranda CL, Stevens JF, Ivanov V, McCall M, Frei B, Deinzer ML, Buhler DR (2000b) Antioxidant and prooxidant actions of prenylated and nonprenylated chalcones and flavanones in vitro. J Agric Food Chem 48:3876–3884

Miranda CL, Yang YH, Henderson MC, Stevens JF, Santana-Rios G, Deinzer ML, Buhler DR (2000c) Prenylflavonoids from hops inhibit the metabolic activation of the carcinogenic heterocyclic amine 2-amino-3-methylimidazo[4, 5-f]quinoline, mediated by cDNA-expressed human CYP1A2. Drug Metab Dispos 28:1297–1302

Miranda CL, Johnson LA, de Montgolfier O, Elias VD, Ullrich LS, Hay JJ, Paraiso IL, Choi J, Reed RL, Revel JS, Kioussi C, Bobe G, Iwaniec UT, Turner RT, Katzenellenbogen BS, Katzenellenbogen JA, Blakemore PR, Gombart AF, Maier CS, Raber J, Stevens JF (2018) Non-estrogenic xanthohumol derivatives mitigate insulin resistance and cognitive impairment in high-fat diet-induced obese mice. Sci Rep 8:613

Monteghirfo S, Tosetti F, Ambrosini C, Stigliani S, Pozzi S, Frassoni F, Fassina G, Soverini S, Albini A, Ferrari N (2008) Antileukemia effects of xanthohumol in Bcr/Abl-transformed cells involve nuclear factor-kappaB and p53 modulation. Mol Cancer Ther 7:2692–2702

Monteiro R, Becker H, Azevedo I, Calhau C (2006) Effect of hop (*Humulus lupulus* L.) flavonoids on aromatase (estrogen synthase) activity. J Agric Food Chem 54:2938–2943

Monteiro R, Faria A, Azevedo I, Calhau C (2007) Modulation of breast cancer cell survival by aromatase inhibiting hop (*Humulus lupulus* L.) flavonoids. J Steroid Biochem Mol Biol 105:124–130

Moparthi L, Koch S (2019) Wnt signaling in intestinal inflammation. Differentiation 108:24–32

Negrão R, Duarte D, Costa R, Soares R (2013) Isoxanthohumol modulates angiogenesis and inflammation via vascular endothelial growth factor receptor, tumor necrosis factor alpha and nuclear factor kappa B pathways. Biofactors 39:608–622

Neuzil J, Wang XF, Dong LF, Low P, Ralph SJ (2006) Molecular mechanism of 'mitocan'-induced apoptosis in cancer cells epitomizes the multiple roles of reactive oxygen species and Bcl-2 family proteins. FEBS Lett 580:5125–5129

Niit M, Hoskin V, Carefoot E, Geletu M, Arulanandam R, Elliott B, Raptis L (2015) Cell-cell and cell-matrix adhesion in survival and metastasis: Stat3 versus Akt. Biomol Concepts 6:383–399

Nuti E, Bassani B, Camodeca C, Rosalia L, Cantelmo A, Gallo C, Baci D, Bruno A, Orlandini E, Nencetti S, Noonan DM, Albini A, Rossello A (2017) Synthesis and antiangiogenic activity study of new hop chalcone Xanthohumol analogues. Eur J Med Chem 138:890–899

Ott PA, Bhardwaj N (2013) Impact of MAPK pathway activation in BRAF(V600) melanoma on T cell and dendritic cell function. Front Immunol 4:346

Pan L, Becker H, Gerhäuser C (2005) Xanthohumol induces apoptosis in cultured 40–16 human colon cancer cells by activation of the death receptor- and mitochondrial pathway. Mol Nutr Food Res 49:837–843

Paraiso IL, Plagmann LS, Yang L, Zielke R, Gombart AF, Maier CS, Sikora AE, Blakemore PR, Stevens JF (2018) Reductive metabolism of xanthohumol and 8-prenylnaringenin by the intestinal bacterium Eubacterium ramulus. Mol Nutr Food Res 63(2):e1800923

Peluso MR, Miranda CL, Hobbs DJ, Proteau RR, Stevens JF (2010) Xanthohumol and related prenylated flavonoids inhibit inflammatory cytokine production in LPS-activated THP-1 monocytes: structure-activity relationships and in silico binding to myeloid differentiation protein-2 (MD-2). Planta Med 76:1536–1543

Pichler C, Ferk F, Al-Serori H, Huber W, Jäger W, Waldherr M, Mišík M, Kundi M, Nersesyan A, Herbacek I, Knasmueller S (2017) Xanthohumol prevents DNA damage by dietary carcinogens: results of a human intervention trial. Cancer Prev Res (Phila) 10:153–160

Pinto C, Duque AL, Rodríguez-Galdón B, Cestero JJ, Macías P (2012) Xanthohumol prevents carbon tetrachloride-induced acute liver injury in rats. Food Chem Toxicol 50:3405–3412

Plazar J, Zegura B, Lah TT, Filipic M (2007) Protective effects of xanthohumol against the genotoxicity of benzo(a)pyrene (BaP), 2-amino-3-methylimidazo[4,5-f]quinoline (IQ) and tert-butyl hydroperoxide (t-BOOH) in HepG2 human hepatoma cells. Mutat Res 632:1–8

Plazar J, Filipic M, Groothuis GM (2008) Antigenotoxic effect of Xanthohumol in rat liver slices. Toxicol in Vitro 22:318–327

Popłoński J, Turlej E, Sordon S, Tronina T, Bartmańska A, Wietrzyk J, Huszcza E (2018) Synthesis and antiproliferative activity of minor hops prenylflavonoids and new insights on prenyl group cyclization. Molecules 23

Possemiers S, Heyerick A, Robbens V, De Keukeleire D, Verstraete W (2005) Activation of proestrogens from hops (*Humulus lupulus* L.) by intestinal microbiota; conversion of isoxanthohumol into 8-prenylnaringenin. J Agric Food Chem 53:6281–6288

Possemiers S, Bolca S, Grootaert C, Heyerick A, Decroos K, Dhooge W, De Keukeleire D, Rabot S, Verstraete W, Van de Wiele T (2006) The prenylflavonoid isoxanthohumol from hops (*Humulus lupulus* L.) is activated into the potent phytoestrogen 8-prenylnaringenin in vitro and in the human intestine. J Nutr 136:1862–1867

Possemiers S, Rabot S, Espin JC, Bruneau A, Philippe C, Gonzalez-Sarrias A, Heyerick A, Tomas-Barberan FA, De Keukeleire D, Verstraete W (2008) Eubacterium limosum activates isoxanthohumol from hops (*Humulus lupulus* L.) into the potent phytoestrogen 8-prenylnaringenin in vitro and in rat intestine. J Nutr 138:1310–1316

Quintas-Cardama A, Kantarjian H, Jones D, Nicaise C, O'Brien S, Giles F, Talpaz M, Cortes J (2007) Dasatinib (BMS-354825) is active in Philadelphia chromosome-positive chronic myelogenous leukemia after imatinib and nilotinib (AMN107) therapy failure. Blood 109:497–499

Rauen KA (2013) The RASopathies. Annu Rev Genomics Hum Genet 14:355–369

Saito K, Matsuo Y, Imafuji H, Okubo T, Maeda Y, Sato T, Shamoto T, Tsuboi K, Morimoto M, Takahashi H, Ishiguro H, Takiguchi S (2018) Xanthohumol inhibits angiogenesis by suppressing nuclear factor-κB activation in pancreatic cancer. Cancer Sci 109:132–140

Santarpia L, Lippman SM, El-Naggar AK (2012) Targeting the MAPK-RAS-RAF signaling pathway in cancer therapy. Expert Opin Ther Targets 16:103–119

Sasazawa Y, Kanagaki S, Tashiro E, Nogawa T, Muroi M, Kondoh Y, Osada H, Imoto M (2012) Xanthohumol impairs autophagosome maturation through direct inhibition of valosin-containing protein. ACS Chem Biol 7:892–900

Sastre-Serra J, Ahmiane Y, Roca P, Oliver J, Pons DG (2018) Xanthohumol, a hop-derived prenylflavonoid present in beer, impairs mitochondrial functionality of SW620 colon cancer cells. Int J Food Sci Nutr 70(4):396–404

Schempp H, Vogel S, Hückelhoven R, Heilmann J (2010) Re-evaluation of superoxide scavenging capacity of xanthohumol. Free Radic Res 44:1435–1444

Shikata Y, Yoshimaru T, Komatsu M, Katoh H, Sato R, Kanagaki S, Okazaki Y, Toyokuni S, Tashiro E, Ishikawa S, Katagiri T, Imoto M (2017) Protein kinase A inhibition facilitates the antitumor activity of xanthohumol, a valosin-containing protein inhibitor. Cancer Sci 108:785–794

Sleightholm RL, Neilsen BK, Li J, Steele MM, Singh RK, Hollingsworth MA, Oupicky D (2017) Emerging roles of the CXCL12/CXCR4 axis in pancreatic cancer progression and therapy. Pharmacol Ther 179:158–170

Sperandio S, Poksay K, de Belle I, Lafuente MJ, Liu B, Nasir J, Bredesen DE (2004) Paraptosis: mediation by MAP kinases and inhibition by AIP-1/Alix. Cell Death Differ 11:1066–1075

Sripa B, Pairojkul C (2008) Cholangiocarcinoma: lessons from Thailand. Curr Opin Gastroenterol 24:349–356

Stevens JF, Page JE (2004) Xanthohumol and related prenylflavonoids from hops and beer: to your good health! Phytochemistry 65:1317–1330

Stevens JF, Taylor AW, Clawson JE, Deinzer ML (1999a) Fate of xanthohumol and related prenylflavonoids from hops to beer. J Agric Food Chem 47:2421–2428

Stevens JF, Taylor AW, Deinzer ML (1999b) Quantitative analysis of xanthohumol and related prenylflavonoids in hops and beer by liquid chromatography-tandem mass spectrometry. J Chromatogr A 832:97–107

Stevens JF, Revel JS, Maier CS (2018) Mitochondria-centric review of polyphenol bioactivity in cancer models. Antioxid Redox Signal 29(16):1589–1611

Stompor M, Uram Ł, Podgórski R (2017) In vitro effect of 8-prenylnaringenin and naringenin on fibroblasts and glioblastoma cells-cellular accumulation and cytotoxicity. Molecules 22. https://doi.org/10.3390/molecules22071092

Strathmann J, Klimo K, Sauer SW, Okun JG, Prehn JH, Gerhauser C (2010) Xanthohumol-induced transient superoxide anion radical formation triggers cancer cells into apoptosis via a mitochondria-mediated mechanism. FASEB J 24:2938–2950

Sugimoto MA, Vago JP, Teixeira MM, Sousa LP (2016) Annexin A1 and the resolution of inflammation: modulation of neutrophil recruitment, apoptosis, and clearance. J Immunol Res 2016:8239258

Sun Z, Zhou C, Liu F, Zhang W, Chen J, Pan Y, Ma L, Liu Q, Du Y, Yang J, Wang Q (2018) Inhibition of breast cancer cell survival by Xanthohumol via modulation of the Notch signaling pathway. Oncol Lett 15:908–916

Szliszka E, Czuba ZP, Mazur B, Sedek L, Paradysz A, Krol W (2009) Chalcones enhance TRAIL-induced apoptosis in prostate cancer cells. Int J Mol Sci 11:1–13

Tan KW, Cooney J, Jensen D, Li Y, Paxton JW, Birch NP, Scheepens A (2014) Hop-derived prenylflavonoids are substrates and inhibitors of the efflux transporter breast cancer resistance protein (BCRP/ABCG2). Mol Nutr Food Res 58:2099–2110

Traber MG, Stevens JF (2011) Vitamins C and E: beneficial effects from a mechanistic perspective. Free Radic Biol Med 51:1000–1013

Tronina T, Bartmańska A, Filip-Psurska B, Wietrzyk J, Popłoński J, Huszcza E (2013a) Fungal metabolites of xanthohumol with potent antiproliferative activity on human cancer cell lines in vitro. Bioorg Med Chem 21:2001–2006

Tronina T, Bartmańska A, Milczarek M, Wietrzyk J, Popłoński J, Rój E, Huszcza E (2013b) Antioxidant and antiproliferative activity of glycosides obtained by biotransformation of xanthohumol. Bioorg Med Chem Lett 23:1957–1960

Urick ME, Chung EJ, Shield WP, Gerber N, White A, Sowers A, Thetford A, Camphausen K, Mitchell J, Citrin DE (2011) Enhancement of 5-fluorouracil-induced in vitro and in vivo radiosensitization with MEK inhibition. Clin Cancer Res 17:5038–5047

Vanhoecke B, Derycke L, Van Marck V, Depypere H, De Keukeleire D, Bracke M (2005) Antiinvasive effect of xanthohumol, a prenylated chalcone present in hops (*Humulus lupulus* L.) and beer. Int J Cancer 117:889–895

Venè R, Benelli R, Minghelli S, Astigiano S, Tosetti F, Ferrari N (2012) Xanthohumol impairs human prostate cancer cell growth and invasion and diminishes the incidence and progression of advanced tumors in TRAMP mice. Mol Med 18:1292–1302

Venturelli S, Burkard M, Biendl M, Lauer UM, Frank J, Busch C (2016) Prenylated chalcones and flavonoids for the prevention and treatment of cancer. Nutrition 32:1171–1178

Verzele M (1986) 100 Years of hop chemistry and its relevance to brewing. J Inst Brew 92:32–48

Viola K, Kopf S, Rarova L, Jarukamjorn K, Kretschy N, Teichmann M, Vonach C, Atanasov AG, Giessrigl B, Huttary N, Raab I, Krieger S, Strnad M, de Martin R, Saiko P, Szekeres T, Knasmüller S, Dirsch VM, Jäger W, Grusch M, Dolznig H, Mikulits W, Krupitza G (2013) Xanthohumol attenuates tumour cell-mediated breaching of the lymphendothelial barrier and prevents intravasation and metastasis. Arch Toxicol 87:1301–1312

Vogel S, Barbic M, Jürgenliemk G, Heilmann J (2010) Synthesis, cytotoxicity, anti-oxidative and anti-inflammatory activity of chalcones and influence of A-ring modifications on the pharmacological effect. Eur J Med Chem 45:2206–2213

Walden D, Kunnimalaiyaan S, Sokolowski K, Clark TG, Kunnimalaiyaan M (2017) Antiproliferative and apoptotic effects of xanthohumol in cholangiocarcinoma. Oncotarget 8:88069–88078

Wang Y, Chen Y, Wang J, Chen J, Aggarwal BB, Pang X, Liu M (2012) Xanthohumol, a prenylated chalcone derived from hops, suppresses cancer cell invasion through inhibiting the expression of CXCR4 chemokine receptor. Curr Mol Med 12:153–162

Wiley SR, Schooley K, Smolak PJ, Din WS, Huang CP, Nicholl JK, Sutherland GR, Smith TD, Rauch C, Smith CA (1995) Identification and characterization of a new member of the TNF family that induces apoptosis. Immunity 3:673–682

Willson CM, Grundmann O (2017) In vitro assays in natural products research – a matter of concentration and relevance to in vivo administration using resveratrol, α-mangostin/γ-mangostin and xanthohumol as examples. Nat Prod Res 31:492–506

Wyns C, van Steendam K, Vanhoecke B, Deforce D, Bracke M, Heyerick A (2012) Prenylated chalcone xanthohumol associates with histones in breast cancer cells – a novel target identified by a monoclonal antibody. Mol Nutr Food Res 56:1688–1696

Yao J, Zhang B, Ge C, Peng S, Fang J (2015) Xanthohumol, a polyphenol chalcone present in hops, activating Nrf2 enzymes to confer protection against oxidative damage in PC12 cells. J Agric Food Chem 63:1521–1531

Yau SW, Azar WJ, Sabin MA, Werther GA, Russo VC (2015) IGFBP-2 - taking the lead in growth, metabolism and cancer. J Cell Commun Signal 9:125–142

Yong WK, Abd Malek SN (2015) Xanthohumol induces growth inhibition and apoptosis in ca ski human cervical cancer cells. Evid Based Complement Alternat Med 2015:921306

Yong WK, Ho YF, Malek SN (2015) Xanthohumol induces apoptosis and S phase cell cycle arrest in A549 non-small cell lung cancer cells. Pharmacogn Mag 11:S275–S283

Yoshimaru T, Komatsu M, Tashiro E, Imoto M, Osada H, Miyoshi Y, Honda J, Sasa M, Katagiri T (2014) Xanthohumol suppresses oestrogen-signalling in breast cancer through the inhibition of BIG3-PHB2 interactions. Sci Rep 4:7355

Zajc I, Filipič M, Lah TT (2012) Xanthohumol induces different cytotoxicity and apoptotic pathways in malignant and normal astrocytes. Phytother Res 26:1709–1713

Zenisek A, Bednar IJ (1960) Contribution to the identification of estrogen activity in hops. Am Perfumer Arom 75:61–62

Zhang W, Pan Y, Gou P, Zhou C, Ma L, Liu Q, Du Y, Yang J, Wang Q (2018) Effect of xanthohumol on Th1/Th2 balance in a breast cancer mouse model. Oncol Rep 39:280–288

Zhao X, Jiang K, Liang B, Huang X (2016) Anticancer effect of xanthohumol induces growth inhibition and apoptosis of human liver cancer through NF-κB/p53-apoptosis signaling pathway. Oncol Rep 35:669–675

Chapter 11
Anthocyanins and Cancer Prevention

Rasika Hudlikar, Renyi Wu, David Cheng, Dina Hsiao-Chen Kuo, Lujing Wang, Rebecca Peter, Ran Yin, Shanyi Li, and Ah-Ng Kong

Abstract Anthocyanins are a class of water-soluble flavonoids, which give the intense color to many fruits and vegetables, such as blueberries and red cabbages. Recent studies have shown that anthocyanins have a range of pharmacological properties, such as prevention of cardiovascular disease, improvement of visual functions, obesity control, and anticancer activity. Their potential anticancer effects are reported to be based on a wide variety of biological activities including anti-oxidative stress; anti-inflammation; anti-mutagenesis; induction of differentiation; inhibition of proliferation; cell cycle arrest and apoptosis; anti-invasion; anti-metastasis; anti-angiogenesis and sensitizing cancer cells to chemotherapy. This chapter summarizes the latest developments on the anticancer activities of anthocyanins and anthocyanin-rich extracts in cell culture models, animal cancer models and some clinical trials. Their chemical structures, molecular mechanisms of action in cancer prevention, and *in vivo* pharmacokinetics-pharmacodynamics (PK-PD) properties will also be discussed.

Keywords Anthocyanins · Anthocyanidins · Cyanidin · Delphinidin · Malvidin · Flavonoids · Cancer prevention · Nrf2-mediated antioxidative stress · Anti-inflammatory · Cellular signaling · Pharmacokinetics (PK)/pharmacodynamics (PD)

Rasika Hudlikar and Renyi Wu contributed equally to this work.

R. Hudlikar · R. Wu · D. Cheng · D. H.-C. Kuo · L. Wang · R. Peter · R. Yin · S. Li · A.-N. Kong (✉)
Center for Phytochemicals Epigenome Studies, Department of Pharmaceutics, Ernest Mario School of Pharmacy, Rutgers, The State University of New Jersey, Piscataway, NJ, USA
e-mail: kongt@pharmacy.rutgers.edu

J. M. Pezzuto, O. Vang (eds.), *Natural Products for Cancer Chemoprevention*,
https://doi.org/10.1007/978-3-030-39855-2_11

11.1 Introduction

Anthocyanins (from the Greek *Anthos* for flower and *kianos* for blue) are amongst the most utilized vegetable colorants in the food industry because of its water-soluble nature. They are extracted from grapes, berries, red cabbage, apples, radishes, tulips, roses and orchids. Its high dietary consumption makes it important to understand its potential biological effects on human health. The potential dietary intake of anthocyanin is among the greatest of the various classes of flavonoids (Wu et al. 2006). The potential health benefits of anthocyanin as dietary antioxidants, which help to prevent neuronal diseases, cardiovascular illnesses, diabetes, inflammation, and many other diseases including cancer (Prior and Wu 2006). Numerous anthocyanins have been identified from fruits and vegetables can interfere with several cell-signaling pathways to delay the progression of the disease.

In this chapter, we present the latest developments on research regarding potential cancer prevention mechanism of the anthocyanins, including *in vitro* cell culture and *in vivo* animal model at various organ sites, as well as data from human studies, including pharmacokinetics (PK)/pharmacodynamics (PD), bioavailability of anthocyanins. Although *in vitro* and *in vivo* animal studies using anthocyanins have provided convincing evidence about the modulation of various signaling pathways, much still needs to be done to advance the biomarker endpoints into possible human clinical trials.

11.2 Chemical Properties and Structures of Anthocyanins

Thousands of phytochemicals have been identified so far and the number is growing each day (Liu 2004). Flavonoids accounted for approximate 60% of phenolic compounds among all the phytochemicals. Anthocyanins are water-soluble polyphenolic pigments and secondary metabolites of plant products (Bunea et al. 2013). Anthocyanins are a type of flavonoid class of compounds which are found naturally in several foods that give red, purple, and blue plants their rich coloring. The anthocyanidins are the basic structures of the anthocyanins without the sugar moieties. The anthocyanidins (or aglycons) consist of an aromatic ring [A] bonded to an heterocyclic ring [C] that contains oxygen, which is also bonded by a carbon–carbon bond to a third aromatic ring [B] (Konczak and Zhang 2004). When the anthocyanidins are found in their glycoside form (bonded to a sugar moiety) they are known as anthocyanins. There is a huge variety of anthocyanins spread in nature; the most common anthocyanins are represented in Fig. 11.1. The main difference between them are the number of hydroxylated groups, the nature and the number of bonded sugars to their structure, the aliphatic or aromatic carboxylates bonded to the sugar in the molecule and the position of these bonds (Kong et al. 2003). The isolated anthocyanins are highly unstable molecules, susceptible to degradation. Their stability is affected by several factors such as pH, storage temperature, chemical structure, concentration,

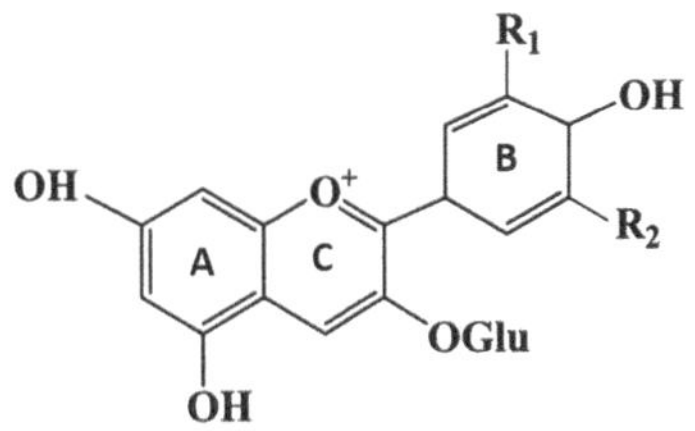

Anthocyanins	R1	R2
Cyanidin	OH	H
Malvidin	OCH_3	OCH_3
Peonidin	OCH_3	H
Delphinidin	OH	OH
Pelargonidin	H	H
Petunidin	OCH_3	OH

Fig. 11.1 Structure of most common anthocyanins [adopted and modified from Tadesse et al. (2012)]

light, oxygen, solvents, the presence of enzymes, flavonoids, proteins and metallic ions. Cyanidin, delphinidin and malvidin are three major compounds of anthocyanidins and the content of these compounds have been found mainly in berries consumed in United States (blackberries, cherries and blueberries) (Khoo et al. 2017). The range of anthocyanidins is at the 30–120 mg per 100 g of fresh weight. Numerous studies have been conducted on anthocyanidins or anthocyanins and their anticancer, antibacterial and activity in scavenging free radicals will be discussed in the following sections.

11.3 Cancer Preventive Properties of Anthocyanins

11.3.1 In Vitro *Studies*

11.3.1.1 Anti-initiation Mechanism of Anthocyanins

Cellular metabolism plays a pivotal role in the process of initiation during carcinogenesis. Xenobiotic molecules entering the cellular environment are metabolized by metabolizing [phase I (functionalization) and phase II (conjugation)] xenobiotic metabolizing enzymes (XMEs), rendering them into water-soluble compounds to make it less reactive towards different biomolecules. Hence, these XMEs could be one of the potential targets for cancer chemoprevention by anthocyanins.

Anthocyanins have demonstrated multiple anti-carcinogenic effects such as: direct scavenging of reactive oxygen species (ROS), stimulating the expression of Phase II detoxification enzymes, reducing the formation of oxidative adducts in DNA by acting as blocking agents (Maru et al. 2016). The antioxidant potential of anthocyanins is governed by scavenging ROS such as superoxide, singlet oxygen, peroxide, hydrogen peroxide, and hydroxyl radical (Wang and Jiao 2000). Anthocyanins scavenge free radicals, thereby reducing damage to the genome of normal cells by oxidative stress and the subsequent malignant transformation by gene mutation, ultimately preventing tumor formation (Shih et al. 2007; Yi et al. 2010). Yi et al. (2010) found that the antioxidant effect of anthocyanins is determined by the 3′,4′,5′-hydroxyl on the B-ring and the 3′-hydroxyl on the C-ring. Shih et al. (2007)

found that anthocyanins (cyanidin, delphinidin and malvidin) could act on antioxidant response element (ARE) through the Keap1-Nrf2 pathway and inhibit the activity of cysteinyl aspartate specific proteinase-3 (caspase-3) by regulating the expression of phase II enzymes (glutathione reductase, glutathione peroxidase, glutathione transferase and quinone oxidoreductase), thus playing a role in antioxidant protection. Although most of the protective effects of anthocyanins are attributed to their ability to scavenge ROS, they also function by chelating metals and by direct binding to proteins (Kong et al. 2003). Although modulation of cytochrome P450 activity has been observed by constituents of fruit extracts including several flavonoids, anthocyanins happened to be one of the weak inhibitors of the CYPs isozymes including 3A4 (Dreiseitel et al. 2008), and CYP2C9, CYP2A6, CYP2B6 (Srovnalova et al. 2014).

The expression of phase II enzymes is governed by a cis-acting regulatory element named the anti-oxidant response element (ARE). ARE containing genes are regulated by nuclear factor erythroid 2-related factor 2 (Nfe2l2 or Nrf2), a member of the cap 'n' collar family basic-leucine-zipper family of transcription factors via ARE. The protective effect of pelargonidin have demonstrated to decrease oxidative stress in HepG2 cells by the activation of detoxification enzyme levels through Keap1/Nrf2 signaling pathway (Sharath Babu et al. 2017). Cyanidin-3-*O*-glucoside has protective effects through the inhibition of NF-κB signaling in Caco-2 cells by activated cellular protective responses modulated by Nrf2 (Ferrari et al. 2016). Shih et al. (2007) shows that anthocyanins induction of ARE-regulated phase II enzyme expression is crucial for protecting cells against oxidative stress-induced apoptosis.

11.3.1.2 Anti-promotion Mechanism of Anthocyanins

Chronic inflammation is often a harbinger in the process of tumorigenesis (Maru et al. 2016). It is reported that anthocyanins can control the expression and secretion of inflammatory factors by inhibiting the transcription factor NF-κB, through multiple pathways to exert their anti-inflammatory function (Esposito et al. 2014). For example, cyanidin-3-glucoside (C-3-G), delphinidin-3-glucoside and petunidin-3-glucoside inhibit the activation of NF-κB induced by external stimuli (e.g., LPS or IFN-γ) by acting on the PI3K/PKB and MAPK pathways (Limtrakul et al. 2015) and can inhibit the expression of COX-2 and inducible NO synthase (iNOS), as well as the production of PGE2 and NO (Jeong et al. 2013). Treatment of JB-6 Cl 41 mouse epidermal cells with black raspberries anthocyanin resulted in down-regulation of benzopyrene diol-epoxide (BaPDE)-induced expression of NF-κB (Huang et al. 2002).

Tumor promotion involves the clonal expansion of initiated cells giving rise to tumor comprised pre-neoplastic cells. This stage is mainly characterized by two important cellular events, viz., cellular proliferation and apoptosis. Pure anthocyanins and anthocyanin-rich extracts from fruits and vegetables have exhibited anti-proliferative activity towards multiple cancer cell types *in vitro* including oral squamous cell carcinoma (Rodrigo et al. 2006), breast (MCF-7), colon (HT-29,

HCT116), and prostate (LNCaP) (Seeram et al. 2006). Interestingly, several investigations have compared the antiproliferative effects of anthocyanins on normal vs. cancer cells and found that they selectively inhibit the growth of cancer cells with relatively little or no effect on the growth of normal cells (Hakimuddin et al. 2004; Galvano et al. 2004). Miyake et al. (2012) and Burton et al. (2015) found that anthocyanins could also block the activation of STAT3 and inhibit the expression of NF-κB.

Extracts from blueberries, black currant, black chokeberries, apple, sea buckthorn, plum, lingonberries, cherries, and raspberries decreased the proliferation of both colon cancer HT29 cells and breast cancer MCF-7 cells and the effect was concentration dependent (Olsson et al. 2004). Cyanidin-3-*O*-glucoside was the most potent anthocyanin on kinase inhibition (Mazewski and Liang 2018). Standardized anthocyanin-rich extract demonstrated marked decreased Caco-2 cell proliferation, induced apoptosis by activating caspase-3 cleavage, and upregulated cyclin-dependent kinase inhibitor 1 (p21Waf/Cif1) expression in a dose-dependent manner (Anwar et al. 2016). Anthocyanin-rich grape and strawberry extracts and their generated metabolites such as hydroxyphenyl acetic acid showed apoptotic effects in HT-29 colon cancer cells (Lopez de Las Hazas et al. 2017).

Under normal conditions, cell proliferation is tightly regulated by proliferative signals. However, in transformed cells, they are over ridden to cause hyper proliferation under the influence of promotion signals. Promotion can be initiated by mitogenic stimuli like growth factors, oxidative stress, hormones, etc. Cyanidin and delphinidin have demonstrated to decrease EGFR kinase activity and phosphorylation of the transcription factor Elk-1 thereby inhibiting the activation of the GAL4-Elk-1 fusion protein in human vulva carcinoma cell line A431 (Meiers et al. 2001). Delphinidin inhibited VEGF-induced tyrosine phosphorylation of VEGFR-2, by attenuating VEGF-induced ERK phosphorylation in human umbilical vein endothelial cells (Lamy et al. 2006). Mouse skin epidermal (JB6 P+) cells can be inhibited by delphinidin at <40 μM concentration by suppressing Raf1 and MEK1 kinase activity and attenuation of (ERK), p90RSK, and MSK (Kang et al. 2008). Peonidin-3-glucoside inhibits the phospho-HER2, phospho-AKT and phopspho-p44/42MAPK levels and induces HER2-positive cells specific apoptosis (Liu et al. 2013). Malvidin-3-galactoside modulates regulation of cyclin D1, cyclin B, cyclin E, caspase-3, cleaved caspase-3, Bax, p-JNK, and p-P38. It also was demonstrated to activate phosphatase and tensin homolog deleted on chromosome ten (PTEN), accompanied by a decrease in the p-AKT level and lowering the protein expression of MMP-2 and MMP-9 in HepG2 cells (Wang et al. 2018). Overall, anthocyanins decreased carcinogen induced proliferation and induces apoptosis which have been closely linked to the modulation of the signaling kinases in the promotion phase of carcinogenesis.

11.3.1.3 Anti-progression Mechanism

Effect on Invasion and Metastasis

Tumor metastasis is one the most common causes of cancer death and various treatment strategies have targeted on preventing the occurrence of metastasis. Invasion and metastasis involve three main processes: adhesion, degradation and movement. Anthocyanins can act on some adhesion molecules and proteolytic enzymes to inhibit the adhesion and degradation of cells (Xia et al. 2009). Cyanidin 3-rutinoside and cyanidin 3-glucoside (extracted from *Morus alba L.*) exhibited a dose-dependent inhibitory effect on the migration and invasion, of highly metastatic A549 human lung carcinoma cells without any toxicity. It acts by decreasing the expressions of matrix matalloprotinase-2 (MMP-2) and urokinase-plasminogen activator (u-PA) in a dose-dependent manner and enhancing the expression of tissue inhibitor of matrix matalloprotinase-2 (TIMP-2) and plasminogen activator inhibitor (PAI) (Chen et al. 2006a). A similar effect was demonstrated by peonidin 3-glucoside and cyanidin 3-glucoside by modulating matrix metalloproteinase (MMP)-9 and urokinase-type plasminogen activator (u-PA) in SKHep-1 cells (Chen et al. 2006b) and lung cancer cells (Ho et al. 2010).

11.3.2 In Vivo *Studies*

Anthocyanins has shown to exert chemoprevention effect through an array of biological activities and signaling pathways *in vitro*. To translate to clinical research, the therapeutic efficacy, mechanism of action, and the metabolic processes are needed to be further examined in *in vivo* models. Anthocyanins isolated from diverse fruits and vegetables have been administrated to experimental animals mainly in the form of extracts or (lyophilized) powder. For delivery of the anthocyanins, diverse administrative routes were used including the oral route for esophageal, small intestine, and colon cancers, or the topical route for skin cancer models.

11.3.2.1 Gastro-intestinal Cancer

In the *N*-nitrosomethylbenzylamine (NMBA) induced esophageal cancer model, rats fed diets containing black/red raspberries, strawberries, blueberries, noni, and wolfberry demonstrated a significant reduction in multiplicity of esophageal squamous cell carcinoma by downregulation of serum cytokines (IL-5 and GRO/KC) (Stoner et al. 2007, 2010). Peiffer et al. (2016) demonstrated a novel mechanism linking the chemopreventive effect of anthocyanin rich berry powder, anthocyanins, and protocatechuic acid (metabolite of anthocyanin) to the innate immune system. The chemoprevention activity of 10% bilberry-extracted anthocyanin against colitis-associated cancers was examined by Lippert et al. (2017) in the azoxymethan

(AOM)/dextran sodium sulfate (DSS) model. The 10% anthocyanins diet significantly ($P < 0.004$) reversed the reduction of colon length (from 12.1 to 11.2 cm, average tumor number decreased by 89–91%) caused by inflammation. Lala et al. (2006) reported the chemopreventive potential of monomeric anthocyanin on the specific pathogen-free F344 male rats subcutaneously injected with AOM. Rats fed with diet containing anthocyanin from bilberry, chokeberry, or grape showed a significant reduction of AOM-mediated aberrant crypt foci by 26–29% compared with AOM only group; particularly, the aberrant crypt foci were mainly observed in the distal colon (Lala et al. 2006). Another colorectal carcinogenesis model were adopted by applying initiator, 1,2-dimethylhydrazine (DMH), and promoter, 2-amino-1-methyl-6-phenylimidazo[4,5-b]pyridine (PhIP) (Hagiwara et al. 2001; Hagiwara et al. 2002). Male F344/DuCrj rats orally administered commercial anthocyanins from purple sweet potatoes, red cabbage and purple corn have presented suppression of average number of colon tumors (both benign and malignant) by 48, 63 and 89% compared with DMH/PhIP control group. In addition to chemopreventive effect of anthocyanins on colon cancers, several small intestinal cancer studies have also shown the chemopreventive effect. APCmin mice fed with anthocyanin-rich tart cherry extract with sulindac showed a significant decrease in total small intestine tumor number and total tumor area by 22 and 20% compared with mice fed sulindac alone (Bobe et al. 2006).

11.3.2.2 Skin Cancer

Razina et al. (2016) reported in 2016 the skin cancer prevention effect of anthocyanin extract isolated from mountain ash fruit (*Fructus Sorbi aucupariae*). Injected with melanoma B-16 intramuscularly as a model of metastatic melanoma, C57Bl/6 mice administered intragastrically with anthocyanin extract have shown the inhibition in the primary melanoma growth by 35% and decrease the incidence of metastases by 25%, by inhibiting cell proliferation. Afaq et al. (2007) reported a skin carcinogenesis model using UVB as the carcinogen in female SKH-1 hairless mice. Topical application (pretreatment or post-treatment) with delphinidin onto the dorsal skin decreased the apoptotic cell numbers in the epidermis and reversed the markers of DNA damage observed in skin biopsies from mice. Similar results were observed by using DMBA- and TPA-induced two-stage skin tumorigenesis model by inhibiting ornithine decarboxylase (ODC) activity and inhibiting phosphorylation of MAPKs proteins (ERK1/2, p38 and JNK1/2) (Afaq et al. 2005). More studies including mixed exposures will help to understand the detailed mechanism of anthocyanins in inhibition of skin carcinogenesis.

11.3.2.3 Breast Cancer

Liu et al. (2014) reported the chemopreventive efficacy of anthocyanin in a human breast carcinoma xenograft model was demonstrated by subcutaneous injection of

BT474 cells, with overexpressed human epidermal growth factors receptors 2 (HER-2) and estrogen receptors (ER) into the flank region of female nude mice. Anthocyanins have been shown to decrease Ki67 and HER2 expression in the xenograft as compared to control group. HER2-positive trastuzumab-resistant BT474 xenograft were studied using female nude mice by i.p. administration of peonidin-3-glucoside. It was demonstrated that tumor volume was reduced by 88% by decreasing HER2 and Ki67 expression (Li et al. 2016). The chemopreventive effect of anthocyanin-rich extract from black rice was reported against skin cancer by injecting HER2 overexpressed MDA-MB-453 cells subcutaneously into the right axilla of female BALB/c nude mice reversing the tumor growth mediated by VEGF (Hui et al. 2010). The possible mechanism was interpreted by decreased expression of nuclear antigen Ki67, angiogenesis factors (MMP9, MMP-2, and uPA). In another study using MDA-MB-453 xenografts model on BALB/c nude mice fed with distilled water containing commercial anthocyanins have shown a significant reduction in tumor volumes and tumor weight and a significant inhibition of Ki67 positive tumor cells (Luo et al. 2014). However, more studies using breast cancer *in vivo* models and various study parameters will help to assess the chemoprevention effect and the mechanism of action of anthocyanins in breast cancers.

11.3.2.4 Lung Cancer

Cyanidin-3-glucoside (C3G) from blackberry has been shown to suppress lung tumor growth by 50% and inhibit tumor metastasis in A549 xenograft as a human lung carcinoma model (Ding et al. 2006). In another study, C57BL/6 male mice implanted with Lewis lung carcinoma cells administered orally with cyanidin-3-glucoside (C3G) or peonidine-3-glucoside (P3G)-rich anthocyanins extracted from black rice by oral gavage significantly reduced tumor volume by 52% (Chen et al. 2005). Aqil et al. (2016) also showed the chemopreventive efficacy of anthocyanins (glycones of delphinidin, cyanidin, malvidin, peonidin and petunidin) suppressed tumor volume by 42% against lung cancer xenografts using A549 and H1299. The therapeutic effects of the anthocyanins against lung cancer reported in these independent studies are promising. However, additional examination into the mechanism of action of anthocyanin or anthocyanin/polyphenolics combination in lung cancers will be valuable to achieve clinical application.

11.3.3 Human Studies

Many clinical studies investigating the impact of anthocyanins on human health have been conducted to translate whether preclinical findings have real benefit in humans (Wallace and Giusti 2015). Varying compositions of anthocyanins from different plant sources have been tested in a range of different conditions. Common conditions testing anthocyanins include but are not limited to the following:

cardiovascular disease, vision improvement, neuroprotection, diabetes, obesity, cancer chemoprevention, and inflammation (Prior and Wu 2006; Mitscher 2007; Reis et al. 2016; Pojer et al. 2013). The majority of clinical studies on anthocyanins have used extracts and mixtures enriched with anthocyanins from different sources, berries among the most common. The complex mixtures of each source and different batches from producers make direct comparisons more challenging (Pojer et al. 2013). Though many sources of anthocyanins have been tested, consumption of anthocyanins is considered relatively safe (Wallace and Giusti 2015; Pojer et al. 2013) and currently there are no specific dietary recommendations on anthocyanin intake.

While numerous clinical investigations on anthocyanins have been performed on other conditions such as cardiovascular disease (Cassidy et al. 2013; Curtis et al. 2009; Yang et al. 2017; Fairlie-Jones et al. 2017; Vetrani et al. 2018; Huang et al. 2016; Hassellund et al. 2012, 2013; Dohadwala et al. 2011), dyslipidemia (Shah and Shah 2018; Qin et al. 2009; Broncel et al. 2010; Kusunoki et al. 2015; Li et al. 2015; Zhu et al. 2011), and inflammation (Jennings et al. 2014; Martin et al. 2018; Lynn et al. 2014; Coelho Rabello Lima et al. 2015; Seymour et al. 2009; Kim et al. 2018; Lee et al. 2017; Edirisinghe et al. 2011), in comparison, limited clinical research has been done on the potential of anthocyanins for cancer chemoprevention. Most studies involving human cancer subjects and anthocyanins have primarily focused on gastrointestinal cancer prevention (Bishayee et al. 2016).

Results surrounding intake of anthocyanins and colorectal cancer (CRC) prevention have been mixed. Epidemiological evidence suggests higher intake of flavonoids such as anthocyanins can reduce CRC risk but some studies have found no support for higher anthocyanin intake and decreased CRC risk (Nimptsch et al. 2016). Though the evidence for anthocyanin intake and cancer risk is not conclusive, several studies suggest anthocyanins can decrease oxidative damage. An intervention of mixed berry juice rich in anthocyanins in healthy male volunteers showed an increase in reduced glutathione and decrease in oxidative DNA damage (Weisel et al. 2006) compared to control. A phase II study in patients with esophageal dysplastic lesions who are at higher risk for esophageal cancer received freeze-dried strawberry powder at 30 or 60 g/day. 80.6% of patients in the 60 g/day arm had lower histologic grade of precancerous esophageal lesions. Patients in the high-dose strawberry group also had significant reductions in iNOS, COX-2, p-NF-κB-p65, and pS6 protein expression, while the lower-dose groups were not significantly reduced. Cell proliferation, as measured by Ki-67, was also reduced in patients receiving 60 g/day of strawberry powder compared to baseline. In a phase I study of CRC patients, oral freeze-dried black raspberries decreased Ki-67 staining and suggest IL-8 and GM-CSF are potential indicators of response to berry-based CRC chemoprevention (Mentor-Marcel et al. 2012). Interestingly, black raspberry treatment could influence epigenetic markers in tissues with demethylation of tumor suppressor genes, possibly by decreasing DNMT1 (Wang et al. 2011). Observations of anthocyanins reducing oxidative stress and inflammation have been reported for other conditions (Li et al. 2015; Traustadottir et al. 2009; Alvarez-Suarez et al. 2014; Riso et al. 2005; Davinelli et al. 2015; Lyall et al. 2009; Kuntz et al. 2014; Kaspar et al. 2011; Seymour et al. 2014) though conflicting findings on oxidative stress have also been reported (Moller et al. 2004; Mertens-Talcott et al. 2008; Ellinger et al. 2012; Desai et al. 2018; Duthie et al. 2006). Further studies are needed to standardize preparations to anthocyanin contents and more rigorous study designs may help determine the effects of anthocyanins on cancer chemoprevention in humans.

In addition to esophageal and colorectal cancer, oral cancer prevention studies on patients with premalignant oral lesions have been conducted using freeze-dried black raspberry gel. Patients receiving topical application of raspberry gel on intraepithelial neoplasia had significant reduction in loss of heterozygosity of tumor suppressor genes and histological regression in a patient subpopulation (Shumway et al. 2008). A separate report from the same research group also observed significant reductions in epithelial COX-2 and lower but non-significant decreases in iNOS (Mallery et al. 2008). In both studies, the black raspberry gel was well-tolerated with no observed adverse effects.

Many studies have investigated the effects of anthocyanins on oxidative stress and inflammation as a possible mechanism for cancer chemoprevention. However, recent findings have suggested that the effects of black raspberries (Gu et al. 2019) and tart cherries (Mayta-Apaza et al. 2018) may be mediated by influencing the gut microbiome. Anthocyanins may impact gut microbiota to modulate inflammation (Morais et al. 2016) and control obesity (Jamar et al. 2017). In one recent study, black raspberry anthocyanins altered gut microbiota in an *in vivo* CRC mouse model and through epigenetic demethylation of SFRP2 (Chen et al. 2018). Recent advances in gut microbiome and anthocyanin interactions should be considered in future human clinical studies investigating anthocyanins in cancer chemoprevention. The influence of anthocyanins on gut microbiota may shed new insights into the chemopreventive mechanisms of dietary anthocyanins.

11.4 Pharmacokinetics (PK)/Pharmacodynamics (PD) and Metabolism of Anthocyanins, Food Source and Bioavailability

The fate of anthocyanins after oral administration follows a unique pattern as compared to the other flavonoids since they could be absorbed from the stomach as well as intestine and colon. Also, active transporters may play a role in the absorption of anthocyanins from the stomach as well as in their transport in the kidney or liver. In a cell culture study, anthocyanins were found to be able to cross MKN-28 cell monolayers (differentiated adenocarcinoma stomach cells) through glucose transporters 1 (GLUT1) and 3 (GLUT3) (Fang 2014; Oliveira et al. 2015). Many Studies of individual anthocyanins reveal their oral bioavailability is generally $<1\%$ (Milbury et al. 2010). Anthocyanins can be absorbed intact from the stomach as well as the intestine despite having different physicochemical properties including molecular size and type of sugar or acylated groups attached (Stalmach et al. 2012;

Matsumoto et al. 2001; Kurilich et al. 2005). Some factors such as glycated groups, glycine and sugar moiety (Wu et al. 2004, 2005; Tian et al. 2006; Milbury et al. 2002) can affect the absorption rate and extent of anthocyanins. Anthocyanins were found in the blood stream within minutes of consumption in human (Tian et al. 2006), suggesting that anthocyanins can be quickly absorbed from the stomach, which has also been confirmed in animal studies. Furthermore, in human studies, anthocyanins were absorbed when introduced through nasal intubation directly into the jejunum (Passamonti et al. 2009; Cai et al. 2011). Anthocyanins were absorbed efficiently after *in situ* perfusion of the jejunum and ileum in rats (Talavera et al. 2004). Another study using chamber mounted with mouse intestine sections showed that the highest absorption of anthocyanins occurred with jejunum tissue ($55.3 \pm 7.6\%$) (Matuschek et al. 2006). Minor absorption occurred with duodenal tissue ($10.4 \pm 7.6\%$), and no absorption was detected from the ileum or colon. The absorption of anthocyanin was usually influenced by their chemical structure and varied between malvidine-3-glucoside (10.7%) and cynidine-3-glucoside (22.4%).

Anthocyanins are the largest group of water-soluble pigments in the fruits and vegetables. The uptake of anthocyanins from the gastrointestinal lumen into the blood depends on the structure of the absorbed molecules (Hribar and Ulrih 2014). Research over the past decade suggested that the majority of conjugation reactions involved in the metabolism of flavonoids include glucuronidation, methylation and sulfation (Mullen et al. 2006; Hollman and Katan 1998; Donovan et al. 2001; Shimoi et al. 1998) with only 0.1–1.5% of ingested dietary anthocyanidins reported to be excreted unmetabolized (Mullen et al. 2006; Hollman et al. 1995). Glucuronide conjugation is usually regarded as the major conjugation reaction involved in flavonoid metabolism (Shimoi et al. 1998; Kuhnle et al. 2000; Oliveira et al. 2002; Spencer et al. 1999). The glucuronidation reaction is catalyzed by UDP-glucuronosyltranferases (UGT) which is found in high concentrations in the liver, intestine and kidneys. Of all these tissues, the liver has the largest capability for glucuronidation (Mojarrabi and Mackenzie 1998; Strassburg et al. 1998) but increasing evidence suggests that the intestine as being the initial and principal site for flavonoid glucuronidation in clinical trials following dietary consumption. Methylation appears as the second most significant metabolism conjugation reaction involved in flavonoids (Kuhnle et al. 2000; Williamson et al. 2000).

In human pharmacokinetic (PK) study including both male and female, it is observed that the maximum plasma concentration is achieved within 0.5–2 h after consumption of anthocyanin-rich fruits (Charron et al. 2009). The systemic bioavailability of anthocyanins is estimated to be 0.26–1.8% in animal studies (Ichiyanagi et al. 2006; Borges et al. 2007; Felgines et al. 2002, 2003). Maximum plasma concentration levels of total anthocyanins are in the range of 1–100 nmol/l following consumption of berries or grapes in human studies (Prior and Wu 2006) . Despite low bioavailability, plasma concentrations of anthocyanins appear sufficient to induce changes in signal transduction and gene expression *in vivo* (Karlsen et al. 2007; DeFuria et al. 2009) in a manner that suggests their potential effects in physiological functions and health outcomes. The absorbed anthocyanins are rapidly eliminated from the circulation. The anthocyanins are detected in the blood stream within very short time (minutes) after administration in human suggesting that its quick absorption (Milbury et al. 2002). Furthermore, when anthocyanins were introduced through nasal tubes, the anthocyanin urine concentrations were fivefold higher as opposed to stomach administration in patients (Cai et al. 2011). Many studies demonstrated that around 7.5% of ingested anthocyanins were detected in the small intestine tissue in their native form 2 h following administration of black raspberries to rats (He et al. 2009). Other study also mentioned that the cynidine-3-glucoside and its methylated and glucuronosyl-conjugated metabolites in jejunum tissue reached 605 nmol/g after administration of an anthocyanin enriched diet for 15 days in rats (Karlsen et al. 2007). Furthermore, several studies have shown that anthocyanins exhibit a complex dose-response, with decreased absorption efficiencies with increased doses (Kurilich et al. 2005; Borges et al. 2007; Charron et al. 2007). The health benefits of anthocyanins have been suggested to be associated with their oral bioavailability and other pharmacokinetic behaviors, such as peak plasma concentration (Cmax) and exposure (AUC) of anthocyanins or their metabolites at peripheral tissue (Milbury et al. 2010; Xiao et al. 2017; de Ferrars et al. 2014). The oral bioavailability of dietary anthocyanins that maintain their parent C6-C3-C6 structure has been reported to be relatively low and various dietary factors such as mixed nutrient meals may have an impact (de Ferrars et al. 2014). Future *in vivo* PKPD studies would be needed to clarify these issues.

11.5 Conclusions

The preponderance of evidence indicates that polyphenolic compounds found in fruits and vegetables have potential chemopreventive properties in various organ specific cancers. There are a significant number of studies with anthocyanins that indicate they can decrease the incidence of some cancers. Anthocyanins have been shown to exert chemopreventive effects *in vitro* on cellular differentiation/cell cycle and cellular growth, apoptosis, activation or deactivation of various enzyme systems such as the phase I biotransformation enzymes, antioxidant action, antimutagenic, antimetastatic activities, interacting with various signaling pathways or direct interaction with the carcinogen. *In vivo* studies have shown that dietary anthocyanins inhibit cancers of the gastrointestinal tract, breast, lung cancer and topically applied anthocyanins inhibited skin cancer. Along with xenograft models, carcinogen induced and patient derived xenograft (PDX) models will help to generate the relevant evidence for the chemopreventive efficacy of anthocyanins. Along with human epidemiological studies, PK-PD data indicate that the minimal absorption of anthocyanins into the bloodstream, complicate the potential efficacy in tissues other than the directly exposing the GI tract and skin. Hence, measuring tissue-bound and circulating anthocyanins would be needed to ascertain the potential chemopreventive effects of anthocyanins at various organ sites. Further studies of individual or combination of the anthocyanins at physiological concentrations and quantifying the metabolites, and the role of gut microbiome, will contribute to the overall knowledge of potential cancer chemoprevention of anthocynanins in humans.

Acknowledgements We thank all members of Professor Ah-Ng Tony Kong's lab for helpful discussions and preparation of this chapter. This work was supported in part by Institutional Funds and NIH R01 AT007065 and R01AT009152 from National Center for Complementary and Integrative Health (NCCIH), and Office of Dietary Supplements (ODS), and R01 CA200129, from the National Cancer Institute to Dr. Ah-Ng Tony Kong.

References

Afaq F, Saleem M, Krueger CG, Reed JD, Mukhtar H (2005) Anthocyanin- and hydrolyzable tannin-rich pomegranate fruit extract modulates MAPK and NF-κB pathways and inhibits skin tumorigenesis in CD-1 mice. Int J Cancer 113(3):423–433. https://doi.org/10.1002/ijc.20587

Afaq F, Syed DN, Malik A, Hadi N, Sarfaraz S, Kweon M-H, Khan N, Zaid MA, Mukhtar H (2007) Delphinidin, an anthocyanidin in pigmented fruits and vegetables, protects human HaCaT keratinocytes and mouse skin against UVB-mediated oxidative stress and apoptosis. J Invest Dermatol 127(1):222–232

Alvarez-Suarez JM, Giampieri F, Tulipani S, Casoli T, Di Stefano G, Gonzalez-Paramas AM, Santos-Buelga C, Busco F, Quiles JL, Cordero MD, Bompadre S, Mezzetti B, Battino M (2014) One-month strawberry-rich anthocyanin supplementation ameliorates cardiovascular risk, oxidative stress markers and platelet activation in humans. J Nutr Biochem 25(3):289–294. Epub 2014/01/11, PubMed PMID: 24406274. https://doi.org/10.1016/j.jnutbio.2013.11.002

Anwar S, Fratantonio D, Ferrari D, Saija A, Cimino F, Speciale A (2016) Berry anthocyanins reduce proliferation of human colorectal carcinoma cells by inducing caspase-3 activation and p21 upregulation. Mol Med Rep 14(2):1397–1403. Epub 2016/06/18, PubMed PMID: 27314273. https://doi.org/10.3892/mmr.2016.5397

Aqil F, Jeyaprakash J, Kausar H, Munagala R, Singh IP, Gupta R (2016) Lung cancer inhibitory activity of dietary berries and berry polyphenolics. J Berry Res 6(2):105–114. https://doi.org/10.3233/JBR-160120

Bishayee A, Haskell Y, Do C, Siveen KS, Mohandas N, Sethi G, Stoner GD (2016) Potential benefits of edible berries in the management of aerodigestive and gastrointestinal tract cancers: preclinical and clinical evidence. Crit Rev Food Sci Nutr 56(10):1753–1775. Epub 2015/03/18, PubMed PMID: 25781639. https://doi.org/10.1080/10408398.2014.982243

Bobe G, Wang B, Seeram NP, Nair MG, Bourquin LD (2006) Dietary anthocyanin-rich tart cherry extract inhibits intestinal tumorigenesis in APCMin mice fed suboptimal levels of sulindac. J Agric Food Chem 54(25):9322–9328. https://doi.org/10.1021/jf0612169

Borges G, Roowi S, Rouanet JM, Duthie GG, Lean ME, Crozier A (2007) The bioavailability of raspberry anthocyanins and ellagitannins in rats. Mol Nutr Food Res 51(6):714–725. Epub 2007/05/30, PubMed PMID: 17533654. https://doi.org/10.1002/mnfr.200700024

Broncel M, Kozirog M, Duchnowicz P, Koter-Michalak M, Sikora J, Chojnowska-Jezierska J (2010) Aronia melanocarpa extract reduces blood pressure, serum endothelin, lipid, and oxidative stress marker levels in patients with metabolic syndrome. Med Sci Monit 16(1):Cr28–Cr34. Epub 2009/12/29, PubMed PMID: 20037491

Bunea A, Rugina D, Sconta Z, Pop RM, Pintea A, Socaciu C, Tabaran F, Grootaert C, Struijs K, VanCamp J (2013) Anthocyanin determination in blueberry extracts from various cultivars and their antiproliferative and apoptotic properties in B16-F10 metastatic murine melanoma cells. Phytochemistry 95:436–444. Epub 2013/07/31, PubMed PMID: 23890760. https://doi.org/10.1016/j.phytochem.2013.06.018

Burton LJ, Smith BA, Smith BN, Loyd Q, Nagappan P, McKeithen D, Wilder CL, Platt MO, Hudson T, Odero-Marah VA (2015) Muscadine grape skin extract can antagonize Snail-cathepsin L-mediated invasion, migration and osteoclastogenesis in prostate and breast cancer cells. Carcinogenesis. 36(9):1019–1027. Epub 2015/06/13, PubMed PMID: 26069256, PMCID: PMC4643647. https://doi.org/10.1093/carcin/bgv084

Cai H, Thomasset SC, P-Berry D, Garcea G, Brown K, Steward WP, Gescher AJ (2011) Determination of anthocyanins in the urine of patients with colorectal liver metastases after administration of bilberry extract. Biomed Chromatogr 25(6):660–663. Epub 2010/09/03, PubMed PMID: 20812200. https://doi.org/10.1002/bmc.1499

Cassidy A, Mukamal KJ, Liu L, Franz M, Eliassen AH, Rimm EB (2013) High anthocyanin intake is associated with a reduced risk of myocardial infarction in young and middle-aged women. Circulation 127(2):188–196. Epub 2013/01/16, PubMed PMID: 23319811, PMCID: PMC3762447. https://doi.org/10.1161/CIRCULATIONAHA.112.122408

Charron CS, Clevidence BA, Britz SJ, Novotny JA (2007) effect of dose size on bioavailability of acylated and nonacylated anthocyanins from red cabbage (Brassica oleracea L. Var. capitata). J Agric Food Chem 55(13):5354–5362. https://doi.org/10.1021/jf0710736

Charron CS, Kurilich AC, Clevidence BA, Simon PW, Harrison DJ, Britz SJ, Baer DJ, Novotny JA (2009) Bioavailability of anthocyanins from purple carrot juice: effects of acylation and plant matrix. J Agric Food Chem 57(4):1226–1230. https://doi.org/10.1021/jf802988s

Chen PN, Chu SC, Chiou HL, Chiang CL, Yang SF, Hsieh YS (2005) Cyanidin 3-glucoside and peonidin 3-glucoside inhibit tumor cell growth and induce apoptosis in vitro and suppress tumor growth in vivo. Nutr Cancer 53(2):232–243. https://doi.org/10.1207/s15327914nc5302_12

Chen PN, Chu SC, Chiou HL, Kuo WH, Chiang CL, Hsieh YS (2006a) Mulberry anthocyanins, cyanidin 3-rutinoside and cyanidin 3-glucoside, exhibited an inhibitory effect on the migration and invasion of a human lung cancer cell line. Cancer Lett 235(2):248–259. Epub 2005/06/25, PubMed PMID: 15975709. https://doi.org/10.1016/j.canlet.2005.04.033

Chen PN, Kuo WH, Chiang CL, Chiou HL, Hsieh YS, Chu SC (2006b) Black rice anthocyanins inhibit cancer cells invasion via repressions of MMPs and u-PA expression. Chem Biol Interact 163(3):218–229. Epub 2006/09/15, PubMed PMID: 16970933. https://doi.org/10.1016/j.cbi.2006.08.003

Chen L, Jiang B, Zhong C, Guo J, Zhang L, Mu T, Zhang Q, Bi X (2018) Chemoprevention of colorectal cancer by black raspberry anthocyanins involved the modulation of gut microbiota and SFRP2 demethylation. Carcinogenesis 39(3):471–481. Epub 2018/01/24, PubMed PMID: 29361151. https://doi.org/10.1093/carcin/bgy009

Coelho Rabello Lima L, Oliveira Assumpcao C, Prestes J, Sergio Denadai B (2015) Consumption of cherries as a strategy to attenuate exercise-induced muscle damage and inflammation in humans. Nutr Hosp 32(5):1885–1893. Epub 2015/11/08, PubMed PMID: 26545642. https://doi.org/10.3305/nh.2015.32.5.9709

Curtis PJ, Kroon PA, Hollands WJ, Walls R, Jenkins G, Kay CD, Cassidy A (2009) Cardiovascular disease risk biomarkers and liver and kidney function are not altered in postmenopausal women after ingesting an elderberry extract rich in anthocyanins for 12 weeks. J Nutr 139 (12):2266–2271. Epub 2009/10/02, PubMed PMID: 19793846. https://doi.org/10.3945/jn.109.113126

Davinelli S, Bertoglio JC, Zarrelli A, Pina R, Scapagnini G (2015) A randomized clinical trial evaluating the efficacy of an anthocyanin-maqui berry extract (delphinol(R)) on oxidative stress biomarkers. J Am Coll Nutr 34(Suppl 1):28–33. Epub 2015/09/25, PubMed PMID: 26400431. https://doi.org/10.1080/07315724.2015.1080108

de Ferrars RM, Czank C, Zhang Q, Botting NP, Kroon PA, Cassidy A, Kay CD (2014) The pharmacokinetics of anthocyanins and their metabolites in humans. Br J Pharmacol 171 (13):3268–3282. https://doi.org/10.1111/bph.12676

DeFuria J, Bennett G, Strissel KJ, Perfield JW, 2nd, Milbury PE, Greenberg AS, Obin MS (2009) Dietary blueberry attenuates whole-body insulin resistance in high fat-fed mice by reducing adipocyte death and its inflammatory sequelae. J Nutr 139(8):1510–1516. Epub 2009/06/12, PubMed PMID: 19515743; PMCID: PMC2709302. https://doi.org/10.3945/jn.109.105155

Desai T, Bottoms L, Roberts M (2018) The effects of Montmorency tart cherry juice supplementation and FATMAX exercise on fat oxidation rates and cardio-metabolic markers in healthy humans. Eur J Appl Physiol 118(12):2523–2539. Epub 2018/09/03, PubMed PMID: 30173287. https://doi.org/10.1007/s00421-018-3978-9

Ding M, Feng R, Wang SY, Bowman L, Lu Y, Qian Y, Castranova V, Jiang BH, Shi X (2006) Cyanidin-3-glucoside, a natural product derived from blackberry, exhibits chemopreventive and chemotherapeutic activity. J Biol Chem 281(25):17359–17368. https://doi.org/10.1074/jbc.M600861200

Dohadwala MM, Holbrook M, Hamburg NM, Shenouda SM, Chung WB, Titas M, Kluge MA, Wang N, Palmisano J, Milbury PE, Blumberg JB, Vita JA (2011) Effects of cranberry juice consumption on vascular function in patients with coronary artery disease. Am J Clin Nutr 93(5):934–940. Epub 2011/03/18. PubMed PMID: 21411615, PMCID: PMC3076649. https://doi.org/10.3945/ajcn.110.004242

Donovan JL, Crespy V, Manach C, Morand C, Besson C, Scalbert A, Rémésy C (2001) Catechin is metabolized by both the small intestine and liver of rats. J Nutr 131(6):1753–1757. https://doi.org/10.1093/jn/131.6.1753

Dreiseitel A, Schreier P, Oehme A, Locher S, Hajak G, Sand PG (2008) Anthocyanins and their metabolites are weak inhibitors of cytochrome P450 3A4. Mol Nutr Food Res 52(12):1428–1433. Epub 2008/08/30, PubMed PMID: 18727015. https://doi.org/10.1002/mnfr.200800043

Duthie SJ, Jenkinson AM, Crozier A, Mullen W, Pirie L, Kyle J, Yap LS, Christen P, Duthie GG (2006) The effects of cranberry juice consumption on antioxidant status and biomarkers relating to heart disease and cancer in healthy human volunteers. Eur J Nutr 45(2):113–122. Epub 2005/07/21, PubMed PMID: 16032375. https://doi.org/10.1007/s00394-005-0572-9

Edirisinghe I, Banaszewski K, Cappozzo J, Sandhya K, Ellis CL, Tadapaneni R, Kappagoda CT, Burton-Freeman BM (2011) Strawberry anthocyanin and its association with postprandial inflammation and insulin. Br J Nutr 106(6):913–922. Epub 2011/07/09, PubMed PMID: 21736853. https://doi.org/10.1017/s0007114511001176

Ellinger S, Gordon A, Kurten M, Jungfer E, Zimmermann BF, Zur B, Ellinger J, Marx F, Stehle P (2012) Bolus consumption of a specifically designed fruit juice rich in anthocyanins and ascorbic acid did not influence markers of antioxidative defense in healthy humans. J Agric Food Chem 60(45):11292–11300. Epub 2012/10/18, PubMed PMID: 23072538. https://doi.org/10.1021/jf300719t

Esposito D, Chen A, Grace MH, Komarnytsky S, Lila MA (2014) Inhibitory effects of wild blueberry anthocyanins and other flavonoids on biomarkers of acute and chronic inflammation in vitro. J Agric Food Chem 62(29):7022–7028. Epub 2014/01/09, PubMed PMID: 24397282. https://doi.org/10.1021/jf4051599

Fairlie-Jones L, Davison K, Fromentin E, Hill AM (2017) The effect of anthocyanin-rich foods or extracts on vascular function in adults: a systematic review and meta-analysis of randomised controlled trials. Nutrients 9(8). Epub 2017/08/22, PubMed PMID: 28825651, PMCID: PMC5579701. https://doi.org/10.3390/nu9080908

Fang J (2014) Bioavailability of anthocyanins. Drug Metab Rev 46(4):508–520. https://doi.org/10.3109/03602532.2014.978080

Felgines C, Texier O, Besson C, Fraisse D, Lamaison JL, Remesy C (2002) Blackberry anthocyanins are slightly bioavailable in rats. J Nutr 132(6):1249–1253. Epub 2002/06/04, PubMed PMID: 12042441. https://doi.org/10.1093/jn/132.6.1249

Felgines C, Talavera S, Gonthier MP, Texier O, Scalbert A, Lamaison JL, Remesy C (2003) Strawberry anthocyanins are recovered in urine as glucuro- and sulfoconjugates in humans. J Nutr 133(5):1296–1301. Epub 2003/05/06, PubMed PMID: 12730413. https://doi.org/10.1093/jn/133.5.1296

Ferrari D, Speciale A, Cristani M, Fratantonio D, Molonia MS, Ranaldi G, Saija A, Cimino F (2016) Cyanidin-3-O-glucoside inhibits NF-kB signalling in intestinal epithelial cells exposed to TNF-alpha and exerts protective effects via Nrf2 pathway activation. Toxicol Lett 264:51–58. Epub 2016/10/30, PubMed PMID: 27793764. https://doi.org/10.1016/j.toxlet.2016.10.014

Galvano F, La Fauci L, Lazzarino G, Fogliano V, Ritieni A, Ciappellano S, Battistini NC, Tavazzi B, Galvano G (2004) Cyanidins: metabolism and biological properties. J Nutr Biochem 15(1):2–11. Epub 2004/01/09, PubMed PMID: 14711454

Gu J, Thomas-Ahner JM, Riedl KM, Bailey MT, Vodovotz Y, Schwartz SJ, Clinton SK (2019) Dietary black raspberries impact the colonic microbiome and phytochemical metabolites in mice. Mol Nutr Food Res 2019:e1800636. Epub 2019/02/15, PubMed PMID: 30763455. https://doi.org/10.1002/mnfr.201800636

Hagiwara A, Miyashita K, Nakanishi T, Sano M, Tamano S, Kadota T, Koda T, Nakamura M, Imaida K, Ito N, Shirai T (2001) Pronounced inhibition by a natural anthocyanin, purple corn color, of 2-amino-1-methyl-6-phenylimidazo[4,5-b]pyridine (PhIP)-associated colorectal carcinogenesis in male F344 rats pretreated with 1,2-dimethylhydrazine. Cancer Lett 171(1):17–25. https://doi.org/10.1016/S0304-3835(01)00510-9

Hagiwara A, Yoshino H, Ichihara T, Kawabe M, Tamano S, Aoki H, Koda T, Nakamura M, Imaida K, Ito N, Shirai T (2002) Prevention by natural food anthocyanins, purple sweet potato color and red cabbage color, of 2-amino-1-methyl-6-phenylimidazo[4,5-b]pyridine (PhIP)-associated colorectal carcinogenesis in rats initiated with 1,2-dimethylhydrazine. J Toxicol Sci 27(1):57–68. https://doi.org/10.2131/jts.27.57

Hakimuddin F, Paliyath G, Meckling K (2004) Selective cytotoxicity of a red grape wine flavonoid fraction against MCF-7 cells. Breast Cancer Res Treat 85(1):65–79. Epub 2004/03/25, PubMed PMID: 15039598. https://doi.org/10.1023/B:BREA.0000021048.52430.c0

Hassellund SS, Flaa A, Sandvik L, Kjeldsen SE, Rostrup M (2012) Effects of anthocyanins on blood pressure and stress reactivity: a double-blind randomized placebo-controlled crossover study. J Hum Hypertens 26(6):396–404. Epub 2011/05/06, PubMed PMID: 21544087. https://doi.org/10.1038/jhh.2011.41

Hassellund SS, Flaa A, Kjeldsen SE, Seljeflot I, Karlsen A, Erlund I, Rostrup M (2013) Effects of anthocyanins on cardiovascular risk factors and inflammation in pre-hypertensive men: a double-blind randomized placebo-controlled crossover study. J Hum Hypertens 27 (2):100–106. Epub 2012/02/18, PubMed PMID: 22336903. https://doi.org/10.1038/jhh.2012.4

He J, Wallace TC, Keatley KE, Failla ML, Giusti MM (2009) Stability of black raspberry anthocyanins in the digestive tract lumen and transport efficiency into gastric and small intestinal tissues in the rat. J Agric Food Chem 57(8):3141–3148. Epub 2009/03/26, PubMed PMID: 19317488. https://doi.org/10.1021/jf900567t

Ho ML, Chen PN, Chu SC, Kuo DY, Kuo WH, Chen JY, Hsieh YS (2010) Peonidin 3-glucoside inhibits lung cancer metastasis by downregulation of proteinases activities and MAPK pathway. Nutr Cancer 62(4):505–516. Epub 2010/05/01, PubMed PMID: 20432172. https://doi.org/10.1080/01635580903441261

Hollman PC, Katan MB (1998) Bioavailability and health effects of dietary flavonols in man. Arch Toxicol Suppl 20:237–248

Hollman PC, de Vries JH, van Leeuwen SD, Mengelers MJ, Katan MB (1995) Absorption of dietary quercetin glycosides and quercetin in healthy ileostomy volunteers. Am J Clin Nutr 62 (6):1276–1282. https://doi.org/10.1093/ajcn/62.6.1276

Hribar U, Ulrih NP (2014) The metabolism of anthocyanins. Curr Drug Metab 15(1):3–13. Epub 2013/12/18, PubMed PMID: 24329109

Huang C, Huang Y, Li J, Hu W, Aziz R, Tang MS, Sun N, Cassady J, Stoner GD (2002) Inhibition of benzo(a)pyrene diol-epoxide-induced transactivation of activated protein 1 and nuclear factor kappaB by black raspberry extracts. Cancer Res 62(23):6857–6863. Epub 2002/12/04, PubMed PMID: 12460899

Huang H, Chen G, Liao D, Zhu Y, Xue X (2016) Effects of berries consumption on cardiovascular risk factors: a meta-analysis with trial sequential analysis of randomized controlled trials. Sci Rep 6:23625. Epub 2016/03/24, PubMed PMID: 27006201, PMCID: PMC4804301. https://doi.org/10.1038/srep23625

Hui C, Bin Y, Xiaoping Y, Long Y, Chunye C, Mantian M, Wenhua L (2010) Anticancer activities of an anthocyanin-rich extract from black rice against breast cancer cells in vitro and in vivo. Nutr Cancer 62(8):1128–1136

Ichiyanagi T, Shida Y, Rahman MM, Hatano Y, Konishi T (2006) Bioavailability and tissue distribution of anthocyanins in bilberry (Vaccinium myrtillus L.) extract in rats. J Agric Food Chem 54(18):6578–6587. Epub 2006/08/31, PubMed PMID: 16939312. https://doi.org/10.1021/jf0602370

Jamar G, Estadella D, Pisani LP (2017) Contribution of anthocyanin-rich foods in obesity control through gut microbiota interactions. BioFactors (Oxford, England) 43(4):507–516. Epub 2017/05/16. PubMed PMID: 28504479. https://doi.org/10.1002/biof.1365

Jennings A, Welch AA, Spector T, Macgregor A, Cassidy A (2014) Intakes of anthocyanins and flavones are associated with biomarkers of insulin resistance and inflammation in women. J Nutr 144(2):202–208. Epub 2013/12/18, PubMed PMID: 24336456. https://doi.org/10.3945/jn.113.184358

Jeong JW, Lee WS, Shin SC, Kim GY, Choi BT, Choi YH (2013) Anthocyanins downregulate lipopolysaccharide-induced inflammatory responses in BV2 microglial cells by suppressing the NF-kappaB and Akt/MAPKs signaling pathways. Int J Mol Sci 14(1):1502–1515. Epub 2013/01/25, PubMed PMID: 23344054, PMCID: PMC3565332. https://doi.org/10.3390/ijms14011502

Kang NJ, Lee KW, Kwon JY, Hwang MK, Rogozin EA, Heo YS, Bode AM, Lee HJ, Dong Z (2008) Delphinidin attenuates neoplastic transformation in JB6 Cl41 mouse epidermal cells by blocking Raf/mitogen-activated protein kinase kinase/extracellular signal-regulated kinase signaling. Cancer Prev Res (Phila) 1(7):522–531. Epub 2009/01/14, PubMed PMID: 19139002, PMCID: PMC2832759. https://doi.org/10.1158/1940-6207.CAPR-08-0071

Karlsen A, Retterstol L, Laake P, Paur I, Bohn SK, Sandvik L, Blomhoff R (2007) Anthocyanins inhibit nuclear factor-kappaB activation in monocytes and reduce plasma concentrations of pro-inflammatory mediators in healthy adults. J Nutr 137(8):1951–1954. Epub 2007/07/20, PubMed PMID: 17634269. https://doi.org/10.1093/jn/137.8.1951

Kaspar KL, Park JS, Brown CR, Mathison BD, Navarre DA, Chew BP (2011) Pigmented potato consumption alters oxidative stress and inflammatory damage in men. J Nutr 141(1):108–111. Epub 2010/11/26, PubMed PMID: 21106930. https://doi.org/10.3945/jn.110.128074

Khoo HE, Azlan A, Tang ST, Lim SM (2017) Anthocyanidins and anthocyanins: colored pigments as food, pharmaceutical ingredients, and the potential health benefits. Food Nutr Res 61:1–21. PubMed PMID: WOS:000408042100001. https://doi.org/10.1080/16546628.2017.1361779

Kim H, Simbo SY, Fang C, McAlister L, Roque A, Banerjee N, Talcott ST, Zhao H, Kreider RB, Mertens-Talcott SU (2018) Acai (Euterpe oleracea Mart.) beverage consumption improves biomarkers for inflammation but not glucose- or lipid-metabolism in individuals with metabolic syndrome in a randomized, double-blinded, placebo-controlled clinical trial. Food Funct 9(6):3097–3103. Epub 2018/06/01, PubMed PMID: 29850709. https://doi.org/10.1039/c8fo00595h

Konczak I, Zhang W (2004) Anthocyanins-more than nature's colours. J Biomed Biotechnol 2004(5):239–240. Epub 2004/12/04, PubMed PMID: 15577183, PMCID: PMC1082903. https://doi.org/10.1155/S1110724304407013

Kong JM, Chia LS, Goh NK, Chia TF, Brouillard R (2003) Analysis and biological activities of anthocyanins. Phytochemistry 64(5):923–933. Epub 2003/10/17, PubMed PMID: 14561507

Kuhnle G, Spencer JP, Schroeter H, Shenoy B, Debnam ES, Srai SK, Rice-Evans C, Hahn U (2000) Epicatechin and catechin are O-methylated and glucuronidated in the small intestine. Biochem Biophys Res Commun 277(2):507–512. https://doi.org/10.1006/bbrc.2000.3701

Kuntz S, Kunz C, Herrmann J, Borsch CH, Abel G, Frohling B, Dietrich H, Rudloff S (2014) Anthocyanins from fruit juices improve the antioxidant status of healthy young female volunteers without affecting anti-inflammatory parameters: results from the randomised, double-blind, placebo-controlled, cross-over ANTHONIA (ANTHOcyanins in Nutrition Investigation Alliance) study. Br J Nutr 112(6):925–936. Epub 2014/08/05, PubMed PMID: 25089359. https://doi.org/10.1017/s0007114514001482

Kurilich AC, Clevidence BA, Britz SJ, Simon PW, Novotny JA (2005) Plasma and urine responses are lower for acylated vs nonacylated anthocyanins from raw and cooked purple carrots. J Agric Food Chem 53(16):6537–6542. https://doi.org/10.1021/jf050570o

Kusunoki M, Sato D, Tsutsumi K, Tsutsui H, Nakamura T, Oshida Y (2015) Black soybean extract improves lipid profiles in fenofibrate-treated type 2 diabetics with postprandial hyperlipidemia. J Med Food 18(6):615–618. Epub 2015/02/05, PubMed PMID: 25651043. https://doi.org/10.1089/jmf.2014.3234

Lala G, Malik M, Zhao C, He J, Kwon Y, Giusti MM, Magnuson BA (2006) Anthocyanin-rich extracts inhibit multiple biomarkers of colon cancer in rats. Nutr Cancer 54(1):84–93. Epub 2006/06/28, PubMed PMID: 16800776. https://doi.org/10.1207/s15327914nc5401_10

Lamy S, Blanchette M, Michaud-Levesque J, Lafleur R, Durocher Y, Moghrabi A, Barrette S, Gingras D, Beliveau R (2006) Delphinidin, a dietary anthocyanidin, inhibits vascular endothelial growth factor receptor-2 phosphorylation. Carcinogenesis 27(5):989–996. Epub 2005/11/26, PubMed PMID: 16308314. https://doi.org/10.1093/carcin/bgi279

Lee YM, Yoon Y, Yoon H, Park HM, Song S, Yeum KJ (2017) Dietary anthocyanins against obesity and inflammation. Nutrients 9(10). Epub 2017/10/05, PubMed PMID: 28974032, PMCID: PMC5691706. https://doi.org/10.3390/nu9101089

Li D, Zhang Y, Liu Y, Sun R, Xia M (2015) Purified anthocyanin supplementation reduces dyslipidemia, enhances antioxidant capacity, and prevents insulin resistance in diabetic patients. J Nutr 145(4):742–748. Epub 2015/04/04, PubMed PMID: 25833778. https://doi.org/10.3945/jn.114.205674

Li X, Xu J, Tang X, Liu Y, Yu X, Wang Z, Liu W (2016) Anthocyanins inhibit trastuzumab-resistant breast cancer in vitro and in vivo. Mol Med Rep 13(5):4007–4013. Epub 2016/03/18, PubMed PMID: 26985659. https://doi.org/10.3892/mmr.2016.4990

Limtrakul P, Yodkeeree S, Pitchakarn P, Punfa W (2015) Suppression of inflammatory responses by black rice extract in RAW 264.7 macrophage cells via downregulation of NF-kB and AP-1 signaling pathways. Asian Pac J Cancer Prev 16(10):4277–4283. Epub 2015/06/02, PubMed PMID: 26028086

Lippert E, Ruemmele P, Obermeier F, Goelder S, Kunst C, Rogler G, Dunger N, Messmann H, Hartmann A, Endlicher E (2017) Anthocyanins prevent colorectal cancer development in a mouse model. Digestion 95(4):275–280. Epub 2017/05/12, PubMed PMID: 28494451. https://doi.org/10.1159/000475524

Liu RH (2004) Potential synergy of phytochemicals in cancer prevention: mechanism of action. J Nutr 134(12 Suppl):3479S–3485S. PubMed PMID: 15570057. https://doi.org/10.1093/jn/134.12.3479S

Liu W, Xu J, Wu S, Liu Y, Yu X, Chen J, Tang X, Wang Z, Zhu X, Li X (2013) Selective anti-proliferation of HER2-positive breast cancer cells by anthocyanins identified by high-throughput screening. PLoS One 8(12):e81586. Epub 2013/12/07, PubMed PMID: 24312561, PMCID: PMC3849376. https://doi.org/10.1371/journal.pone.0081586

Liu W, Xu J, Liu Y, Yu X, Tang X, Wang Z, Li X (2014) Anthocyanins potentiate the activity of trastuzumab in human epidermal growth factor receptor 2-positive breast cancer cells in vitro and in vivo. Mol Med Rep 10(4):1921–1926. Epub 2014/07/30, PubMed PMID: 25070704. https://doi.org/10.3892/mmr.2014.2414

Lopez de Las Hazas MC, Mosele JI, Macia A, Ludwig IA, Motilva MJ (2017) Exploring the colonic metabolism of grape and strawberry anthocyanins and their in vitro apoptotic effects in HT-29 colon cancer cells. J Agric Food Chem 65(31):6477–6487. Epub 2016/10/30, PubMed PMID: 27790915. https://doi.org/10.1021/acs.jafc.6b04096

Luo L-P, Han B, Yu X-P, Chen X-Y, Zhou J, Chen W, Zhu Y-F, Peng X-L, Zou Q, Li S-Y (2014) Anti-metastasis activity of black rice anthocyanins against breast cancer: analyses using an ErbB2 positive breast cancer cell line and tumoral xenograft model. Asian Pac J Cancer Prev 15(15):6219–6225

Lyall KA, Hurst SM, Cooney J, Jensen D, Lo K, Hurst RD, Stevenson LM (2009) Short-term blackcurrant extract consumption modulates exercise-induced oxidative stress and lipopolysaccharide-stimulated inflammatory responses. Am J Physiol Regul Integr Comp Physiol 297(1):R70–R81. Epub 2009/05/01, PubMed PMID: 19403859. https://doi.org/10.1152/ajpregu.90740.2008

Lynn A, Mathew S, Moore CT, Russell J, Robinson E, Soumpasi V, Barker ME (2014) Effect of a tart cherry juice supplement on arterial stiffness and inflammation in healthy adults: a randomised controlled trial. Plant Foods Hum Nutr 69(2):122–127. Epub 2014/02/27, PubMed PMID: 24570273. https://doi.org/10.1007/s11130-014-0409-x

Mallery SR, Zwick JC, Pei P, Tong M, Larsen PE, Shumway BS, Lu B, Fields HW, Mumper RJ, Stoner GD (2008) Topical application of a bioadhesive black raspberry gel modulates gene expression and reduces cyclooxygenase 2 protein in human premalignant oral lesions. Cancer Res 68(12):4945–4957. Epub 2008/06/19. PubMed PMID: 18559542, PMCID: PMC2892791. https://doi.org/10.1158/0008-5472.CAN-08-0568

Martin KR, Burrell L, Bopp J (2018) Authentic tart cherry juice reduces markers of inflammation in overweight and obese subjects: a randomized, crossover pilot study. Food Funct 9 (10):5290–5300. Epub 2018/09/27, PubMed PMID: 30255184. https://doi.org/10.1039/c8fo01492b

Maru GB, Hudlikar RR, Kumar G, Gandhi K, Mahimkar MB (2016) Understanding the molecular mechanisms of cancer prevention by dietary phytochemicals: from experimental models to clinical trials. World J Biol Chem 7(1):88–99. Epub 2016/03/17, PubMed PMID: 26981198, PMCID: PMC4768127. https://doi.org/10.4331/wjbc.v7.i1.88

Matsumoto H, Inaba H, Kishi M, Tominaga S, Hirayama M, Tsuda T (2001) Orally administered delphinidin 3-rutinoside and cyanidin 3-rutinoside are directly absorbed in rats and humans and appear in the blood as the intact forms. J Agric Food Chem 49(3):1546–1551

Matuschek MC, Hendriks WH, McGhie TK, Reynolds GW (2006) The jejunum is the main site of absorption for anthocyanins in mice. J Nutr Biochem 17(1):31–36. Epub 2005/08/16, PubMed PMID: 16098729. https://doi.org/10.1016/j.jnutbio.2005.04.005

Mayta-Apaza AC, Pottgen E, De Bodt J, Papp N, Marasini D, Howard L, Abranko L, Van de Wiele T, Lee SO, Carbonero F (2018) Impact of tart cherries polyphenols on the human gut microbiota and phenolic metabolites in vitro and in vivo. J Nutr Biochem 59:160–172. Epub 2018/07/29, PubMed PMID: 30055451. https://doi.org/10.1016/j.jnutbio.2018.04.001

Mazewski C, Liang K, Gonzalez de Mejia E (2018) Comparison of the effect of chemical composition of anthocyanin-rich plant extracts on colon cancer cell proliferation and their potential mechanism of action using in vitro, in silico, and biochemical assays. Food Chem 242:378–388. Epub 2017/10/19, PubMed PMID: 29037704. https://doi.org/10.1016/j.foodchem.2017.09.086

Meiers S, Kemeny M, Weyand U, Gastpar R, von Angerer E, Marko D (2001) The anthocyanidins cyanidin and delphinidin are potent inhibitors of the epidermal growth-factor receptor. J Agric Food Chem 49(2):958–962. Epub 2001/03/23, PubMed PMID: 11262056

Mentor-Marcel RA, Bobe G, Sardo C, Wang LS, Kuo CT, Stoner G, Colburn NH (2012) Plasma cytokines as potential response indicators to dietary freeze-dried black raspberries in colorectal cancer patients. Nutr Cancer 64(6):820–825. Epub 2012/07/25. PubMed PMID: 22823889, PMCID: PMC3427773. https://doi.org/10.1080/01635581.2012.697597

Mertens-Talcott SU, Rios J, Jilma-Stohlawetz P, Pacheco-Palencia LA, Meibohm B, Talcott ST, Derendorf H (2008) Pharmacokinetics of anthocyanins and antioxidant effects after the consumption of anthocyanin-rich acai juice and pulp (Euterpe oleracea Mart.) in human healthy volunteers. J Agric Food Chem 56(17):7796–7802. Epub 2008/08/13, PubMed PMID: 18693743. https://doi.org/10.1021/jf8007037

Milbury PE, Cao G, Prior RL, Blumberg J (2002) Bioavailablility of elderberry anthocyanins. Mech Ageing Dev 123(8):997–1006. Epub 2002/06/05, PubMed PMID: 12044949

Milbury PE, Vita JA, Blumberg JB (2010) Anthocyanins are bioavailable in humans following an acute dose of cranberry juice. J Nutr 140(6):1099–1104. https://doi.org/10.3945/jn.109.117168

Mitscher LA (2007) Traditional medicines. In: Taylor JB, Triggle DJ (eds) Comprehensive medicinal chemistry II. Elsevier, Amsterdam, pp 405–430

Miyake S, Takahashi N, Sasaki M, Kobayashi S, Tsubota K, Ozawa Y (2012) Vision preservation during retinal inflammation by anthocyanin-rich bilberry extract: cellular and molecular mechanism. Lab Invest 92(1):102–109. Epub 2011/09/07, PubMed PMID: 21894150. https://doi.org/10.1038/labinvest.2011.132

Mojarrabi B, Mackenzie PI (1998) Characterization of two UDP glucuronosyltransferases that are predominantly expressed in human colon. Biochem Biophys Res Commun 247(3):704–709. https://doi.org/10.1006/bbrc.1998.8843

Moller P, Loft S, Alfthan G, Freese R (2004) Oxidative DNA damage in circulating mononuclear blood cells after ingestion of blackcurrant juice or anthocyanin-rich drink. Mutat Res 551 (1-2):119–126. Epub 2004/07/01, PubMed PMID: 15225586. https://doi.org/10.1016/j.mrfmmm.2004.02.020

Morais CA, de Rosso VV, Estadella D, Pisani LP (2016) Anthocyanins as inflammatory modulators and the role of the gut microbiota. J Nutr Biochem 33:1–7. Epub 2016/06/05, PubMed PMID: 27260462. https://doi.org/10.1016/j.jnutbio.2015.11.008

Mullen W, Edwards CA, Crozier A (2006) Absorption, excretion and metabolite profiling of methyl-, glucuronyl-, glucosyl- and sulpho-conjugates of quercetin in human plasma and urine after ingestion of onions. Br J Nutr 96(01):107. https://doi.org/10.1079/BJN20061809

Nimptsch K, Zhang X, Cassidy A, Song M, O'Reilly EJ, Lin JH, Pischon T, Rimm EB, Willett WC, Fuchs CS, Ogino S, Chan AT, Giovannucci EL, Wu K (2016) Habitual intake of flavonoid subclasses and risk of colorectal cancer in 2 large prospective cohorts. Am J Clin Nutr 103 (1):184–191. Epub 2015/11/06, PubMed PMID: 26537935, PMCID: PMC4691672. https://doi.org/10.3945/ajcn.115.117507

Oliveira EJ, Watson DG, Grant MH (2002) Metabolism of quercetin and kaempferol by rat hepatocytes and the identification of flavonoid glycosides in human plasma. Xenobiotica 32 (4):279–287. https://doi.org/10.1080/00498250110107886

Oliveira H, Fernandes I, Bras NF, Faria A, De Freitas V, Calhau C, Mateus N (2015) Experimental and theoretical data on the mechanism by which red wine anthocyanins are transported through a human MKN-28 gastric cell model. J Agric Food Chem 63(35):7685–7692. Epub 2015/04/11, PubMed PMID: 25858301. https://doi.org/10.1021/acs.jafc.5b00412

Olsson ME, Gustavsson KE, Andersson S, Nilsson A, Duan RD (2004) Inhibition of cancer cell proliferation in vitro by fruit and berry extracts and correlations with antioxidant levels. J Agric Food Chem 52(24):7264–7271. Epub 2004/11/26, PubMed PMID: 15563205. https://doi.org/10.1021/jf030479p

Passamonti S, Terdoslavich M, Franca R, Vanzo A, Tramer F, Braidot E, Petrussa E, Vianello A (2009) Bioavailability of flavonoids: a review of their membrane transport and the function of bilitranslocase in animal and plant organisms. Curr Drug Metab 10(4):369–394. Epub 2009/06/13, PubMed PMID: 19519345

Peiffer DS, Wang L-S, Zimmerman NP, Ransom BWS, Carmella SG, Kuo C-T, Chen J-H, Oshima K, Huang Y-W, Hecht SS, Stoner GD (2016) Dietary consumption of black raspberries or their anthocyanin constituents alters innate immune cell trafficking in esophageal cancer. Cancer Immunol Res 4(1):72. https://doi.org/10.1158/2326-6066.CIR-15-0091

Pojer E, Mattivi F, Johnson D, Stockley CS (2013) The case for anthocyanin consumption to promote human health: a review. Compr Rev Food Sci Food Saf 12(5):483–508. https://doi.org/10.1111/1541-4337.12024

Prior RL, Wu X (2006) Anthocyanins: structural characteristics that result in unique metabolic patterns and biological activities. Free Radic Res 40(10):1014–1028. Epub 2006/10/04, PubMed PMID: 17015246. https://doi.org/10.1080/10715760600758522

Qin Y, Xia M, Ma J, Hao Y, Liu J, Mou H, Cao L, Ling W (2009) Anthocyanin supplementation improves serum LDL- and HDL-cholesterol concentrations associated with the inhibition of cholesteryl ester transfer protein in dyslipidemic subjects. Am J Clin Nutr 90(3):485–492. Epub 2009/07/31, PubMed PMID: 19640950. https://doi.org/10.3945/ajcn.2009.27814

Razina T, Zueva E, Ulrich A, Rybalkina OY, Chaikovskii A, Isaikina N, Kalinkina G, Zhdanov V, Zyuz'kov G (2016) Antitumor effects of Sorbus aucuparia L. extract highly saturated with anthocyans and their mechanisms. Bull Exp Biol Med 162(1):93–97

Reis JF, Monteiro VV, de Souza GR, do Carmo MM, da Costa GV, Ribera PC, Monteiro MC (2016) Action mechanism and cardiovascular effect of anthocyanins: a systematic review of animal and human studies. J Transl Med 14(1):315. Epub 2016/11/17. PubMed PMID: 27846846, PMCID: PMC5111351. https://doi.org/10.1186/s12967-016-1076-5

Riso P, Visioli F, Gardana C, Grande S, Brusamolino A, Galvano F, Galvano G, Porrini M (2005) Effects of blood orange juice intake on antioxidant bioavailability and on different markers related to oxidative stress. J Agric Food Chem 53(4):941–947. Epub 2005/02/17, PubMed PMID: 15713002. https://doi.org/10.1021/jf0485234

Rodrigo KA, Rawal Y, Renner RJ, Schwartz SJ, Tian Q, Larsen PE, Mallery SR (2006) Suppression of the tumorigenic phenotype in human oral squamous cell carcinoma cells by an ethanol extract derived from freeze-dried black raspberries. Nutr Cancer 54(1):58–68. Epub 2006/06/28, PubMed PMID: 16800773, PMCID: PMC2392889. https://doi.org/10.1207/s15327914nc5401_7

Seeram NP, Adams LS, Zhang Y, Lee R, Sand D, Scheuller HS, Heber D (2006) Blackberry, black raspberry, blueberry, cranberry, red raspberry, and strawberry extracts inhibit growth and stimulate apoptosis of human cancer cells in vitro. J Agric Food Chem 54(25):9329–9339. Epub 2006/12/07, PubMed PMID: 17147415. https://doi.org/10.1021/jf061750g

Seymour EM, Lewis SK, Urcuyo-Llanes DE, Tanone II, Kirakosyan A, Kaufman PB, Bolling SF (2009) Regular tart cherry intake alters abdominal adiposity, adipose gene transcription, and inflammation in obesity-prone rats fed a high fat diet. J Med Food 12(5):935–942. Epub 2009/10/28, PubMed PMID: 19857054. https://doi.org/10.1089/jmf.2008.0270

Seymour EM, Warber SM, Kirakosyan A, Noon KR, Gillespie B, Uhley VE, Wunder J, Urcuyo DE, Kaufman PB, Bolling SF (2014) Anthocyanin pharmacokinetics and dose-dependent plasma antioxidant pharmacodynamics following whole tart cherry intake in healthy humans. J Funct Foods 11:509–516. https://doi.org/10.1016/j.jff.2014.08.007

Shah K, Shah P (2018) Effect of anthocyanin supplementations on lipid profile and inflammatory markers: a systematic review and meta-analysis of randomized controlled trials. Cholesterol 2018:8450793. Epub 2018/06/01. PubMed PMID: 29850238, PMCID: PMC5937577. doi: https://doi.org/10.1155/2018/8450793

Sharath Babu GR, Anand T, Ilaiyaraja N, Khanum F, Gopalan N (2017) Pelargonidin modulates Keap1/Nrf2 pathway gene expression and ameliorates citrinin-induced oxidative stress in HepG2 cells. Front Pharmacol 8:868. Epub 2017/12/13, PubMed PMID: 29230174, PMCID: PMC5711834. https://doi.org/10.3389/fphar.2017.00868

Shih PH, Yeh CT, Yen GC (2007) Anthocyanins induce the activation of phase II enzymes through the antioxidant response element pathway against oxidative stress-induced apoptosis. J Agric Food Chem 55(23):9427–9435. Epub 2007/10/16, PubMed PMID: 17935293. https://doi.org/10.1021/jf071933i

Shimoi K, Okada H, Furugori M, Goda T, Takase S, Suzuki M, Hara Y, Yamamoto H, Kinae N (1998) Intestinal absorption of luteolin and luteolin 7-O-beta-glucoside in rats and humans. FEBS Lett 438(3):220–224

Shumway BS, Kresty LA, Larsen PE, Zwick JC, Lu B, Fields HW, Mumper RJ, Stoner GD, Mallery SR (2008) Effects of a topically applied bioadhesive berry gel on loss of heterozygosity indices in premalignant oral lesions. Clin Cancer Res 14(8):2421–2430. Epub 2008/04/17. PubMed PMID: 18413833, PMCID: PMC3498466. https://doi.org/10.1158/1078-0432.CCR-07-4096

Spencer JP, Chowrimootoo G, Choudhury R, Debnam ES, Srai SK, Rice-Evans C (1999) The small intestine can both absorb and glucuronidate luminal flavonoids. FEBS Lett 458(2):224–230

Srovnalova A, Svecarova M, Zapletalova MK, Anzenbacher P, Bachleda P, Anzenbacherova E, Dvorak Z (2014) Effects of anthocyanidins and anthocyanins on the expression and catalytic activities of CYP2A6, CYP2B6, CYP2C9, and CYP3A4 in primary human hepatocytes and human liver microsomes. J Agric Food Chem 62(3):789–797. Epub 2014/01/07, PubMed PMID: 24387788. https://doi.org/10.1021/jf404643w

Stalmach A, Edwards CA, Wightman JD, Crozier A (2012) Gastrointestinal stability and bioavailability of (poly)phenolic compounds following ingestion of Concord grape juice by humans. Mol Nutr Food Res 56(3):497–509. https://doi.org/10.1002/mnfr.201100566

Stoner GD, Wang LS, Zikri N, Chen T, Hecht SS, Huang C, Sardo C, Lechner JF (2007) Cancer prevention with freeze-dried berries and berry components. Semin Cancer Biol 17(5):403–410. https://doi.org/10.1016/j.semcancer.2007.05.001

Stoner GD, Wang LS, Seguin C, Rocha C, Stoner K, Chiu S, Kinghorn AD (2010) Multiple berry types prevent N-nitrosomethylbenzylamine-induced esophageal cancer in rats. Pharm Res 27 (6):1138–1145. Epub 2010/03/17, PubMed PMID: 20232121, PMCID: PMC3016717. https://doi.org/10.1007/s11095-010-0102-1

Strassburg CP, Nguyen N, Manns MP, Tukey RH (1998) Polymorphic expression of the UDP-glucuronosyltransferase UGT1A gene locus in human gastric epithelium. Mol Pharmacol 54(4):647–654

Tadesse S, Abebe A, Chebude Y, Garcia IV, Yohannes T (2012) Natural dye-sensitized solar cells using pigments extracted from *Syzygium guineense*. J Photonics Energy 2(1):027001. https://doi.org/10.1117/1.JPE.2.027001

Talavera S, Felgines C, Texier O, Besson C, Manach C, Lamaison JL, Remesy C (2004) Anthocyanins are efficiently absorbed from the small intestine in rats. J Nutr 134(9):2275–2279. Epub 2004/08/31, PubMed PMID: 15333716. https://doi.org/10.1093/jn/134.9.2275

Tian Q, Giusti MM, Stoner GD, Schwartz SJ (2006) Urinary excretion of black raspberry (Rubus occidentalis) anthocyanins and their metabolites. J Agric Food Chem. 54(4):1467–1472. https://doi.org/10.1021/jf052367z

Traustadottir T, Davies SS, Stock AA, Su Y, Heward CB, Roberts LJ, 2nd, Harman SM (2009) Tart cherry juice decreases oxidative stress in healthy older men and women. J Nutr 139 (10):1896–1900. Epub 2009/08/21. PubMed PMID: 19692530, PMCID: PMC3151016. doi: https://doi.org/10.3945/jn.109.111716

Vetrani C, Vitale M, Bozzetto L, Della Pepa G, Cocozza S, Costabile G, Mangione A, Cipriano P, Annuzzi G, Rivellese AA (2018) Association between different dietary polyphenol subclasses and the improvement in cardiometabolic risk factors: evidence from a randomized controlled clinical trial. Acta Diabetol 55(2):149–153. Epub 2017/11/21, PubMed PMID: 29151225. https://doi.org/10.1007/s00592-017-1075-x

Wallace TC, Giusti MM (2015) Anthocyanins. Adv Nutr 6(5):620–622. Epub 2015/09/17, PubMed PMID: 26374184, PMCID: PMC4561837. https://doi.org/10.3945/an.115.009233

Wang SY, Jiao H (2000) Scavenging capacity of berry crops on superoxide radicals, hydrogen peroxide, hydroxyl radicals, and singlet oxygen. J Agric Food Chem 48(11):5677–5684. Epub 2000/11/23, PubMed PMID: 11087538

Wang LS, Arnold M, Huang YW, Sardo C, Seguin C, Martin E, Huang TH, Riedl K, Schwartz S, Frankel W, Pearl D, Xu Y, Winston J, 3rd, Yang GY, Stoner G (2011) Modulation of genetic and epigenetic biomarkers of colorectal cancer in humans by black raspberries: a phase I pilot study. Clin Cancer Res 17(3):598–610. Epub 2010/12/03. PubMed PMID: 21123457, PMCID: PMC3076314. https://doi.org/10.1158/1078-0432.CCR-10-1260

Wang YH, Lin J, Tian J, Si X, Jiao X, Zhang W, Gong E, Li B (2018) Blueberry malvidin-3-galactoside suppresses hepatocellular carcinoma by regulating apoptosis, proliferation, and metastases pathways in vivo and in vitro. J Agric Food Chem. Epub 2018/12/28, PubMed PMID: 30586992. https://doi.org/10.1021/acs.jafc.8b06209

Weisel T, Baum M, Eisenbrand G, Dietrich H, Will F, Stockis JP, Kulling S, Rufer C, Johannes C, Janzowski C (2006) An anthocyanin/polyphenolic-rich fruit juice reduces oxidative DNA damage and increases glutathione level in healthy probands. Biotechnol J 1(4):388–397. Epub 2006/08/08, PubMed PMID: 16892265. https://doi.org/10.1002/biot.200600004

Williamson G, Day AJ, Plumb GW, Couteau D (2000) Human metabolic pathways of dietary flavonoids and cinnamates. Biochem Soc Trans 28(2):16–22

Wu X, Pittman HE, Prior RL (2004) Pelargonidin is absorbed and metabolized differently than cyanidin after marionberry consumption in pigs. J Nutr 134(10):2603–2610. https://doi.org/10.1093/jn/134.10.2603

Wu X, Pittman HE, McKay S, Prior RL (2005) Aglycones and sugar moieties alter anthocyanin absorption and metabolism after berry consumption in weanling pigs. J Nutr 135 (10):2417–2424. https://doi.org/10.1093/jn/135.10.2417

Wu X, Beecher GR, Holden JM, Haytowitz DB, Gebhardt SE, Prior RL (2006) Concentrations of anthocyanins in common foods in the United States and estimation of normal consumption. J Agric Food Chem 54(11):4069–4075. Epub 2006/05/25, PubMed PMID: 16719536. https://doi.org/10.1021/jf060300l

Xia M, Ling W, Zhu H, Ma J, Wang Q, Hou M, Tang Z, Guo H, Liu C, Ye Q (2009) Anthocyanin attenuates CD40-mediated endothelial cell activation and apoptosis by inhibiting CD40-induced MAPK activation. Atherosclerosis 202(1):41–47. Epub 2008/05/23, PubMed PMID: 18495129. https://doi.org/10.1016/j.atherosclerosis.2008.04.005

Xiao D, Sandhu A, Huang Y, Park E, Edirisinghe I, Burton-Freeman BM (2017) The effect of dietary factors on strawberry anthocyanins oral bioavailability. Food Funct 8(11):3970–3979. https://doi.org/10.1039/C7FO00885F

Yang L, Ling W, Yang Y, Chen Y, Tian Z, Du Z, Chen J, Xie Y, Liu Z, Yang L (2017) Role of purified anthocyanins in improving cardiometabolic risk factors in chinese men and women with prediabetes or early untreated diabetes—a randomized controlled trial. Nutrients 9(10). Epub 2017/10/11, PubMed PMID: 28994705, PMCID: PMC5691720. https://doi.org/10.3390/nu9101104

Yi L, Chen CY, Jin X, Mi MT, Yu B, Chang H, Ling WH, Zhang T (2010) Structural requirements of anthocyanins in relation to inhibition of endothelial injury induced by oxidized low-density lipoprotein and correlation with radical scavenging activity. FEBS Lett 584(3):583–590. Epub 2009/12/17, PubMed PMID: 20004199. https://doi.org/10.1016/j.febslet.2009.12.006

Zhu Y, Xia M, Yang Y, Liu F, Li Z, Hao Y, Mi M, Jin T, Ling W (2011) Purified anthocyanin supplementation improves endothelial function via NO-cGMP activation in hypercholesterolemic individuals. Clin Chem 57(11):1524–1533. Epub 2011/09/20, PubMed PMID: 21926181. https://doi.org/10.1373/clinchem.2011.167361

Chapter 12
Grape Chemopreventive Agents Against Angiogenesis and Metastasis

Chandra K. Singh, Gagan Chhabra, Charlotte A. Mintie, and Nihal Ahmad

Abstract Recent advances in the identification of efficient diagnostic means, novel targets and therapeutics, have resulted in a significant decline in cancer mortality. However, based on recent estimates from the American Cancer Society, 1,762,450 new cancer cases and 606,880 cancer-deaths are projected to occur in the United States, in the year 2019. Therefore, an expedition for more efficient means of cancer management continues. Cancer cells cannot prosper without an adequate supply of blood through angiogenesis, a process of forming new blood vessels. Angiogenesis is a multistep process controlled by several proangiogenic and antiangiogenic factors. Dysregulated angiogenesis contributes to unlimited growth and metastasis of cancer, with fatal consequences. In a quest for novel agents/drugs to curtail metastatic spread of cancer, the dietary agents are being actively investigated. Grapes are, arguably, one of the most valuable fruits, containing more than 1600 phytochemicals. Among these, resveratrol, catechin, epicatechin, peonidin, cyanidin, malvidin, kaempferol, isorhamnetin, taxifolin, and quercetin are the top ten compounds that account for more than 70% of the grape polyphenols. These grape constituents alone, in combinations, or as whole grape products, have been shown to have anticancer activities. In this chapter, we have discussed the mechanistic action(s) of grape agents against angiogenesis and metastasis, both of which are crucial requirements for cancer survival and progression. Studies have shown how grape chemopreventive agents are proficient at challenging the proangiogenic and antiangiogenic factors necessary for tumor angiogenesis and metastasis. This makes grape antioxidants very promising in cancer management.

C. K. Singh · G. Chhabra · C. A. Mintie
Department of Dermatology, University of Wisconsin-Madison, Madison, WI, USA

N. Ahmad (✉)
Department of Dermatology, University of Wisconsin-Madison, Madison, WI, USA

William S. Middleton VA Medical Center, Madison, WI, USA
e-mail: nahmad@wisc.edu

J. M. Pezzuto, O. Vang (eds.), *Natural Products for Cancer Chemoprevention*,
https://doi.org/10.1007/978-3-030-39855-2_12

Keywords Cancer · Angiogenesis · Metastasis · Chemopreventive agents · Whole grape · Grape extracts · Grape antioxidants · Resveratrol · Quercetin · Kaempferol · Isorhamnetin · Taxifolin · Catechin · Epicatechin · Proanthocyanidins · Anthocyanins · Peonidin · Cyanidin · Malvidin

12.1 Introduction

Angiogenesis and metastasis are linked processes involved in cancer progression and expansion. Angiogenesis is a multistep process promoting the growth of blood vessels from the existing vasculature that has been considered essential for tumor cell proliferation and viability, and represents as an essential component of the metastatic spread of the tumor. Angiogenesis is controlled by several proangiogenic and antiangiogenic factors and is considered to be crucial in the growth and progression of most tumors (Hanahan and Weinberg 2000, 2011). Distant organ metastasis, which is dependent on angiogenesis, is the major reason for cancer-fatalities. The word 'metastasis' stems from a Greek word meaning 'displacement', and represents a process when cancerous cells move from the primary tumor site (where the cells initially transformed) to other distant organs of the body. Metastasis is also a multistep process encompassing several inefficient steps including, (1) penetration of tumor cells deeper into surrounding tissues, (2) migration into the vessels, also known as 'intravasation', and (3) survival of the motile cells into the circulatory system and to distant organs where they can colonize and develop into a secondary lesion (Hanahan and Weinberg 2000, 2011; van Zijl et al. 2011). The capability of cancer cells to conquer and metastasize is extraordinarily complicated and one of the strategic symbols of cancer progression. In fact, primary carcinomas (except for lung and liver) hardly cause patient death, whereas most of the cancer-related mortality occurs due to complications linked to metastasis (van Zijl et al. 2011). The beginning of tumor metastasis includes invasion, which is facilitated by epithelial-mesenchymal transition (EMT), an event through which epithelial cells lose their cell-cell adherence and gain mesenchymal characteristics, resulting in increased migration potential and invasiveness of cancer. Hence, tumor angiogenesis and metastasis have been considered as pivotal points in tumor progression (Hanahan and Weinberg 2000, 2011; Singh et al. 2018), and thus, blocking these two phenomena of cancer could be useful in cancer management. Figure 12.1 outlines the key factors involved in tumor angiogenesis and metastasis.

As angiogenesis is one of the required critical events for cancer metastasis, it has been found that angiogenesis inhibitors would, therefore, avert or halt the growth of tumors. Several drugs are being used in the clinic that targets angiogenesis and metastasis. The Food and Drug Administration (FDA) has approved several antiangiogenic agents including monoclonal antibodies, proteasome inhibitors, tyrosine kinase inhibitors (TKIs) and mTOR inhibitors, such as Bevacizumab (Avastin), Bortezomib (Velcade), Gefitinib and Temsirolimus, respectively (Feng et al. 2010; Samant and Shevde 2011). The first case of successful antiangiogenic treatment was

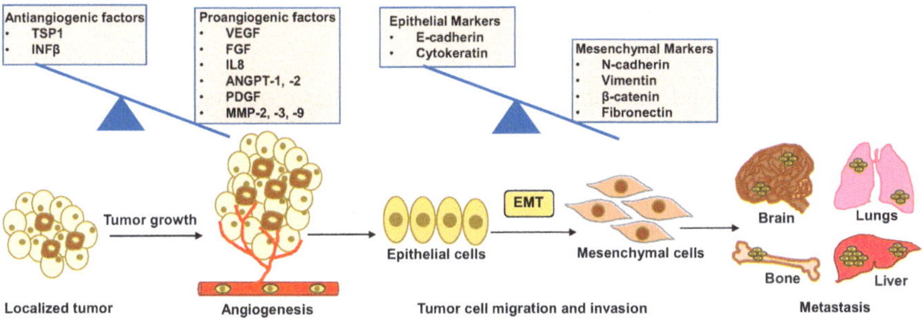

Fig. 12.1 Schematic diagram showing factors involved in tumor angiogenesis and metastasis

reported in 1989 when the drug interferon alfa-2a, a recombinant interferon possessing antiviral, immunomodulatory and antitumor characteristics, was used to suppress angiogenesis. This drug suppressed angiogenesis by inhibiting the production of two key angiogenic factors vascular endothelial growth factor (VEGF) and basic fibroblast growth factor (bFGF) (Feng et al. 2010). A monoclonal antibody that has been approved to curtail angiogenesis is Bevacizumab, which was approved in 2004 as a VEGF blocker to treat metastatic colorectal cancer, ovarian cancer, and breast cancer (Samant and Shevde 2011). TKIs, such as Sorafenib, Sunitinib, Gefitinib, and Erlotinib have also been developed to treat cancer by blocking angiogenesis pathways (Feng et al. 2010). However, these drugs present some unwanted adverse effects that may complicate the treatment. For example, although Bevacizumab has been shown to increase the survival of cancer patients, it is also associated with risks of diarrhea, hypertension, leucopenia, thrombosis, fatal hemorrhage and visceral perforation (reviewed in Sagar et al. 2006). In some cases, during a course of radiotherapy, tumors increase their angiogenic activity (Ansiaux et al. 2005). Resistance to antiangiogenic therapy also occurs frequently and constitutes a critical barrier in the inhibition of tumor growth. Additionally, the efficacy of antiangiogenic compounds varies from one tumor to another. If the angiogenic activity of a tumor is initiated primarily by only one or two factors, then blocking the activity of one factor may be enough to inhibit tumor growth. For example, expressions of VEGF and epidermal growth factor receptor (EGFR) correlate with the metastatic characteristics of human colon cancer, and therefore, targeting VEGF or EGFR may be beneficial (Iqbal and Lenz 2004). However, if several factors mediate the angiogenic activity in a particular tumor, additional intervention strategy may be required. Interestingly, grapes contain a range of compounds that may have synergistic or additive anti-proliferative activity against cancer (Singh et al. 2015a, 2016). Because of their pleiotropic mechanistic actions, these grape antioxidants may inhibit angiogenesis by interacting with multiple pathways and by affecting cell signaling that modulates other relevant processes such as apoptosis and the interaction of cells with the immune system. This chapter is dedicated to discussing the action(s) of grape compounds on mechanistic pathways relevant to angiogenesis and metastasis.

12.2 Tumor Angiogenesis

In order to understand how the process of angiogenesis occurs, it is essential to describe the origin of blood vessels, as they are pivotal in understanding this process. The cardiovascular system is one of the preliminary systems that develop in the embryo and is needed for supporting the nutritional requirements. Within the cardiovascular system are the endothelial cells, lining the surfaces of vascular structures (Risau 1997). These vascular endothelial cells play an important role in various processes such as tissue homeostasis, blood-tissue exchange, and blood cell activation. The vascular system forms by two processes, angiogenesis and vasculogenesis. Vasculogenesis is the formation of new vessels, whereas angiogenesis is the growth of vessels from pre-existing vessels. Angiogenesis begins during embryo formation and is necessary for the normal growth of embryonic and post-natal tissues, as well as for wound healing. It also contributes to the sprouting of vessels in organs that arc avascular (i.e., kidney) and remodeling of the capillary networks to form smaller and larger vessels, as well (Risau 1997).

However, during cancer progression, cancer cells hijack this process for their growth. Unlike normal blood vessels, the blood vessels formed within tumors are dilated with uneven shapes. The process of tumor angiogenesis was first noticed by Judah Folkman, who hypothesized and demonstrated in 1971 that tumor growth is angiogenesis-dependent (Folkman 1971). Realizing that understanding the mechanism(s) of angiogenesis could lead to cancer therapies enthused intensive research in this field, as can be appreciated that there are over 55,000 manuscripts dealing with angiogenesis in cancer research (PubMed search; keywords 'angiogenesis and cancer'; June 2019). Cancer cells instigate angiogenesis quite early during the development of a tumor. The angiogenesis is characterized by oncogene-driven tumor expression of pro-angiogenic proteins. Angiogenesis plays a crucial task in the progression of most solid tumors, including those of bladder, brain, breast, cervix, colon, lung, and prostate. An increasing density of tumor vasculature raises the probability that the tumor will metastasize (Bielenberg and Zetter 2015).

Although the process of angiogenesis is quite complex, one critical growth factor very important in this process is the vascular endothelial growth factor (VEGF) (Carmeliet and Jain 2011). VEGF is one of the most well-studied growth factors involved in angiogenesis. With the loss of a single VEGF allele, there is a link to embryonic vascular defects (Carmeliet 2003). Also known as VEGF-A, VEGF stimulates the process of angiogenesis by signaling through another component VEGF receptor-2 (VEGFR2) (Lee et al. 2015b). A high level of VEGF is associated with poor disease outcome in a wide array of malignancies. VEGF accelerates the proliferation and migration of endothelial cells and stimulates the levels of plasminogen and metalloproteinases. In several animal models, overexpression of VEGF in tumor cells enhances tumor growth and metastasis by stimulating vascularization (Risau 1997). Expression of VEGF mRNA is upregulated by many oncogenes (including H-RAS, K-RAS, SRC, and C-JUN) and growth factors [including epidermal growth factor (EGF), transforming growth factor (TGF)-α and -β, insulin-like growth factor-1 (IGF1), and platelet-derived growth factors (PDGF) (Hanahan and Weinberg 2000; Lee et al. 2015b)].

Another key group of molecules that are important in angiogenesis is the PDGF family of proteins, which consists of TGF-β and angiopoietins. TGF-β has shown to be an important signaling pathway in angiogenesis. This family of molecules consists of several structurally similar growth factors that play important roles in embryonic and postnatal angiogenesis. The PDGF signaling pathway has some parallels to the VEGF system (Thurston and Daly 2012). Angiopoietins (ANGPTs), a family of four proteins, are extracellular ligands that bind to endothelial cell-specific tyrosine kinase receptor TIE2 (Fagiani and Christofori 2013). Two of these, ANGPT1 and ANGPT2, are well studied and described for its role in angiogenesis. ANGPT1 is known to be crucial for vessel growth, adhesion, migration, and survival. ANGPT2 is generally limited to endothelial cells and known to stimulate cell death and disrupts vascularization. However, in conjunction with VEGF, ANGPT2 supports neo-vascularization, suggesting that it may be useful together with anti-VEGF treatments against cancer (Fagiani and Christofori 2013).

Fibroblast growth factor (FGF) family has also been shown to play a pivotal role in the process of angiogenesis. In fact, basic fibroblast growth factor (bFGF) also known as FGF2 is one of the first angiogenic factors to be discovered (Carmeliet and Jain 2011). Another commonly studied form of FGF is acidic fibroblast growth factor (aFGF), also known as FGF1. FGF1 and FGF2, like other FGF family members, possess mitogenic and cell survival activities, and play a crucial role in tumor growth and invasion (Beenken and Mohammadi 2009). FGFs are known to stimulate fibroblast growth factor receptors (FGFRs) on endothelial cells as well as trigger angiogenesis by producing angiogenic factors from other cell types. In tumors, aberrant FGF signaling has been noted to promote angiogenesis. However, the development of anti-FGF treatments are lagging as 22 members FGF family are structurally related and show biologically substantial redundancy (Beenken and Mohammadi 2009; Ucuzian et al. 2010).

During the process of wound healing, the eruption of angiogenesis must be stopped once the newly developed capillaries have reached a certain density. Therefore, a homeostatic equilibration of proangiogenic and antiangiogenic factors is very crucial for normal cells. The development and progression of many cancers are associated with lack of the endogenous angiogenesis inhibitors. For example, a potent inhibitor of angiogenesis, interferon beta (INFβ) works by blocking interleukin-8 (IL8) (Oliveira et al. 1992), bFGF (Singh et al. 1995) and collagenase type V (Gohji et al. 1994), which all are angiogenic factors aiding in tumor development and invasiveness. Tumor cells also halt production of angiogenesis inhibitor thrombospondin-1 (TSP1), which is regulated by tumor suppressor protein P53 (Grant et al. 1998). Interestingly, P53 loss is frequently noticed in more than 50% of the cancers. Currently, antiangiogenic therapies are being used to manage malignancies, while proangiogenic therapies are being investigated to handle cardiovascular diseases. Some of the angiogenic factors and their regulation is shown in Figs. 12.1 and 12.2 (Bashir et al. 2002; Hanahan and Weinberg 2000, 2011).

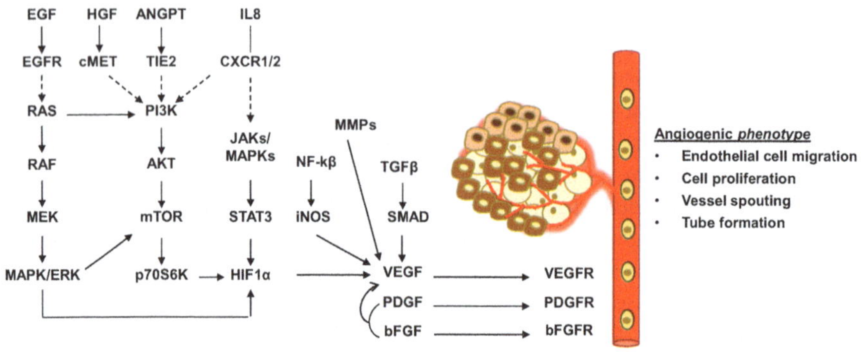

Fig. 12.2 Key mediators involved in tumor angiogenesis

12.3 Tumor Invasion and Metastasis

Tumor invasion is the direct extension and penetration of cancer cells into adjacent tissues, while metastasis is the expansion of cancer cells through the circulatory or lymphatic system to distant sites. Metastasis is of crucial importance in cancer progression because most cancer-related deaths are due to metastatic spread to cancer cells affecting organs secondary to original tumor locale (Hanahan and Weinberg 2000, 2011; van Zijl et al. 2011). Commonly, tumor metastases occur in lungs, liver, brain, and bones after localization to the lymph nodes. Metastasis is an important factor in deciding the staging of cancer, depending on the extent to which cancer has spread. Interestingly, metastatic tumors shed ~1 million cancer cells per gram of tumor in the blood circulation each day, and out of them, ~0.01% cells possess the characteristics of metastatic progenitor cells, which is also studied as one of the key targets for metastatic prevention (Chang et al. 2000; Langley and Fidler 2011; Payen et al. 2017).

Epithelial-mesenchymal transition (EMT) has been progressively recognized as a key event in tumor metastasis. EMT is characterized by loss of epithelial markers (E-) cadherin (ECAD), which is a crucial component of adherence junctions, and cytokeratin (CK1), which is a key component of intermediate filaments. Loss of ECAD by the transcriptional repressors SNAIL, SLUG, ZEB2 or TWIST leads to the dismantling of adherence junctions and translocation of membrane-bound β-catenin (CTNNB) to the cell nucleus (Thiery et al. 2009; van Zijl et al. 2011). EMT is also characterized by concurrent gain of mesenchymal markers such as vimentin (VIM) and N-cadherin (NCAD). This change from E- to N-cadherin expression, termed cadherin-switch, leads to enhanced motility of EMT-transformed cells (van Zijl et al. 2011; Yilmaz and Christofori 2010). The molecular machinery of EMT process has been a target of anti-cancer drug development as well as for their potential use as biomarkers of cancer progression.

The molecular mechanism of metastasis involves several critical molecular events. The genes responsible for metastasis are mostly developmentally non-essential stress response genes that, if expressed, physiologically facilitate the homing of immune cells. Two key proteins involved in this progression are CD44, a cell-surface glycoprotein involved in cell-cell interactions, cell adhesion, and migration, and osteopontin (OPN), which facilitates the linking of osteoclasts to the mineralized bone matrix (reviewed in Weber 2008). CD44 is expressed on macrophages and lymphocytes and contains ten exons that are prone to alternative splicing. The presence of CD44, though not essential for early transformation and growth, has been demonstrated to be a key regulator of metastasis (Weber 2008; Weber et al. 2002). Recent studies have shown the characterization of two isoforms of CD44, which are standard CD44 (CD44s) and variant CD44 (CD44v). CD44v overexpressed in metastasized tumors, and the interplay of CD44v and CD44s has been suggested to play a role in regulating EMT (reviewed in Chen et al. 2018a). The crucial other protein, OPN, is essential in macrophage filtration during stimuli responses. Interestingly, macrophages in the tumor microenvironment have been suggested to promote tumor invasion and metastasis via epidermal growth factor (EGF) and EGF receptor (EGFR). Additionally, OPN is overexpressed in several cancers and has been correlated with poor prognosis in patients (Anborgh et al. 2010). OPN is also a mediator that protects against pathogens. Both CD44 and OPN, are stress response proteins known to be involved in physiological defenses (Weber 2008). The manipulation of plasma or tumor tissue-specific levels of CD44 and OPN has been suggested as a useful strategy to manage cancer metastasis. Figure 12.3 outlines the major signaling mediators involved in EMT and metastasis.

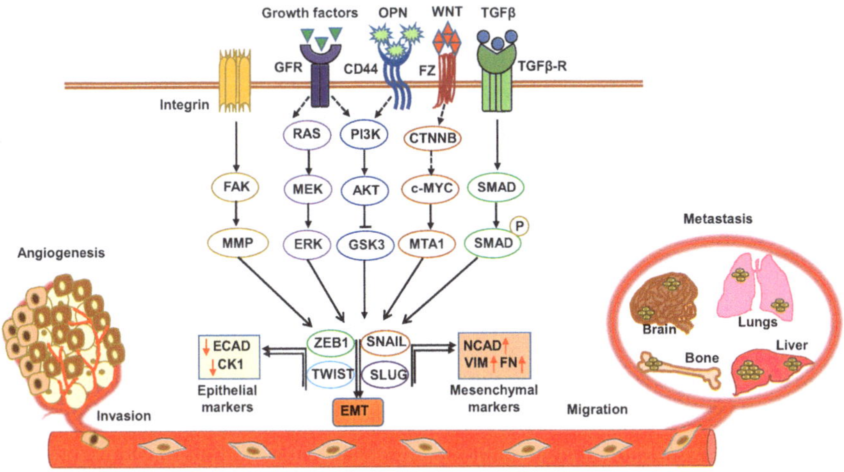

Fig. 12.3 Signaling mediators involved in EMT and metastasis

12.4 Grape Antioxidants Against Angiogenesis and Metastasis

Historically, plant-derived agents (including herbs, fruits and vegetable, and their individual constituents) have been widely investigated and used for achieving health benefits and in the management of a variety of disease conditions (Greenwell and Rahman 2015). Grape (*Vitis vinifera*) is probably one of the most valuable fruits, in terms of availability of health-beneficial phytochemical constituents. In two recent publications, we have discussed how grape constituents, in its natural combination in whole grape or in certain specific combination may be useful in the management of diseases including cancer (Singh et al. 2015a, 2016). Grapes are very rich in antioxidants and contain a number of phytochemicals including stilbenes, phenolic acids, and flavonoids. The actual composition of these phytochemicals varies greatly among different grape varieties. The medicinal use of grape/grape constituents dates back to ancient time. For example, traditional Ayurvedic tonic called Drakshasava, which is very popular in the Indian subcontinent is made from fermented grapes. Drakshasava is used to manage a variety of health issues including lethargy, weakness, and heart-health. Chromatographic assessment of Drakshasava established the presence of numerous polyphenols, including resveratrol and pterostilbenes (Paul et al. 1999). In the early 1990s, red wine derived from grapes gained popularity as a reason for the "French Paradox", which accounts for the somewhat paradoxical epidemiological observation that French population have a relatively lower risk of certain heart diseases despite the high-fat diet, owing to the consumption of red wine (Renaud and de Lorgeril 1992). Since then, hundreds of compounds have been identified in grapes that have been linked with a variety of health benefits (Pezzuto 2008). As discussed in a recent study from our laboratory, where we assessed the effect of grape powder against UVB-mediated skin carcinogenesis in SKH-1 hairless mice, the top ten antioxidants of the grape powder are resveratrol, catechin, epicatechin, peonidin, cyanidin, malvidin, kaempferol, isorhamnetin, taxifolin, and quercetin (Singh et al. 2019). Individually, these agents, are widely reported for their anticancer activities. Here, we have discussed the studies suggesting that these grape-based individual chemopreventive agents alone or, in combinations, including extracts, are promising against angiogenesis and metastasis.

12.4.1 Grape Stilbene Resveratrol

Resveratrol, a well-known grape antioxidant, is a phytoalexin produced by plants to prevent parasitic growth. Chemically, resveratrol (3,5,4′-trihydroxystilbene), a stilbenoid that exists in *trans*- and *cis*-configuration. The *trans*-resveratrol is known to photo-isomerizes to cis-resveratrol in the presence of ultraviolet irradiation (Figueiras et al. 2011). Resveratrol has been characterized as one of the most important active agents of the grape powder (0.69–1.01 mg/kg) (Singh et al. 2019) and grape-derived products such as red wine (concentrations of 0.1–14.3 mg/L) (Mukherjee et al. 2010). In fact, the resveratrol in red wine has been touted as a major reason behind the so-called *French Paradox* (Catalgol et al. 2012). Though bioavailability of resveratrol is somewhat low (~0.5%) due to immediate hepatic glucuronidation and sulfation (Walle et al. 2004), it has been shown to elicit broader biological effects against various health conditions including cancer, aging, diabetes, cardiovascular diseases, etc. (Singh et al. 2015b). This has been explained because of a number of reasons; including the regeneration of resveratrol from an intracellular pool of resveratrol sulfates (Patel et al. 2013), and the fact that some resveratrol metabolites like resveratrol 3-sulfate are known to possess their own biological activity (Hoshino et al. 2010).

The effect of resveratrol against cancer in multiple animal models has shown to be mostly protective with some exceptions of no effect depending on cancer types and resveratrol dose and route of administration. Similar results have been seen in the clinical trials, except one case where some adverse events were noticed in multiple myeloma patients (Berman et al. 2017; Popat et al. 2013). Interestingly, no adverse events were found when the same formulation was used in other studies (Popat et al. 2013; Singh et al. 2015b). In the recent past, we have reviewed the issues and questions which hinder the clinical translation of resveratrol for cancer management (Singh et al. 2015b). To understand the challenges that need to be overcome for the success of resveratrol to the clinic, it's important to examine the key signaling molecules/pathways known to be affected by resveratrol in cancer. The effect of resveratrol against key cancer signaling molecules/pathways is well documented in multiple cell culture experiments and animal studies. For example, resveratrol has been found to inhibit key cancer-promoting pathways, e.g., IGF-1R/AKT/WNT, PI3K/AKT/mTOR and NF-κB signaling pathways, which are known to be associated with tumor growth and progression (reviewed in Berman et al. 2017).

The effect of resveratrol against angiogenesis has been widely studied. Resveratrol has been found to inhibit angiogenesis and tumor growth in human breast cancer xenografts as well as reduce levels of VEGF in MDA-MB-231 breast cancer cells (Garvin et al. 2006). Yu et al. have shown the inhibitory effect of resveratrol on VEGF and angiogenesis in hepatocellular carcinoma partly via inhibiting NF-κB signaling (Yu et al. 2010). Resveratrol has been found to inhibit tumor growth in rat RT-2 gliomas and angiogenesis in the glioma cells (Tseng et al. 2004). Resveratrol-mediated inhibition of rat glioma has been shown to be associated with the suppression of macroscopic and microscopic angiogenesis (Chen et al. 2006). Hu et al. have found modulation of several important angiogenic factors such as VEGF, bFGF, matrix metallopeptidase-2 and -9 (MMP2 and MMP9) in exerting the antimyeloma effects of resveratrol (Hu et al. 2007). The antiangiogenic effect of resveratrol in human ovarian cancer cells has shown to be mediated via inhibition of VEGF as well as hypoxia-inducible factor 1α (HIF1α), which plays a key role in tumor progression (Cao et al. 2004; Park et al. 2007). The antiangiogenic activity of resveratrol has also been demonstrated by modulation of TSP1, which is a downstream target of P53 and known to inhibit angiogenesis naturally. In this study, Trapp et al. have shown the correlation of antiangiogenic effects of resveratrol with increased P53 and TSP1, and decreased HIF1α and VEGF levels (Trapp et al. 2010).

Similarly, resveratrol's antimetastatic potential has been demonstrated in various model systems. Wu et al. have investigated the antimetastatic potential of resveratrol under normoxia and hypoxia conditions, and found that resveratrol restricts the cell migration, adhesion, and invasion in colon carcinoma cells. This was mediated by a reduced level of VEGF, MMP2, and MMP9 under normoxia and hypoxia, and reduced HIF1α under hypoxia (Wu et al. 2008). Resveratrol has also been shown to modulate key EMT-related markers that are crucial for cancer cell motility, invasiveness, and metastasis. Wang and colleagues have shown resveratrol as an inhibitor of TGF-β1-induced EMT, where resveratrol was found to inhibit cell adhesion, migration, and invasion of A549 lung cancer cells. In this study, resveratrol was found to increase epithelial marker ECAD and represses mesenchymal markers, fibronectin (FN) and VIM, inhibits expression of EMT-inducing transcription factors SNAIL and SLUG (Wang et al. 2013). Resveratrol has also been shown to inhibit characteristics of pancreatic cancer stem cells (CSCs) originated from human primary tumors as well as in KRAS(G12D) transgenic mice by inhibiting self-renewal capacity and EMT transcriptional regulators ZEB1, SLUG, and SNAIL (Shankar et al. 2011). Resveratrol treatment of human tongue squamous cell carcinoma cell line CAL-27 showed decreased cell migration, invasion by inhibiting the EMT-inducing transcription factors (Kim et al. 2018). Resveratrol has been shown to inhibit invasion and metastasis in gastric cancer cells via inhibiting hedgehog signaling and EMT (Gao et al. 2015). In a study by Sheth et al., resveratrol administration has been found to inhibit prostate tumor growth as well as lung metastasis by inhibiting the AKT/MicroRNA-21 pathway (Sheth et al. 2012). Figure 12.4 outlines the molecular actions of resveratrol against angiogenesis and metastasis.

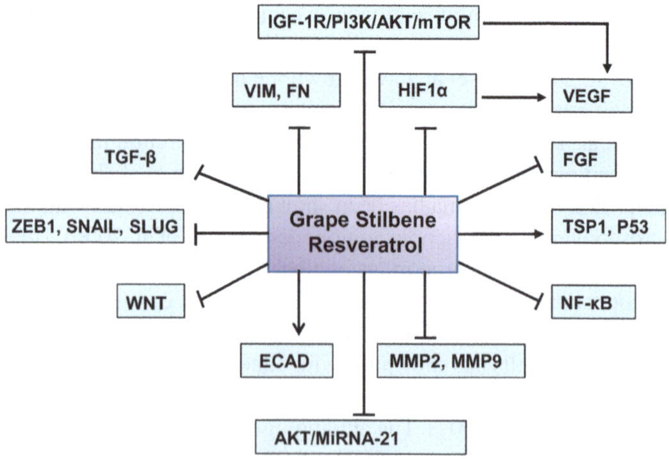

Fig. 12.4 Molecular actions of resveratrol against angiogenesis and metastasis

12.4.2 Grape Flavonols (Quercetin, Kaempferol, Isorhamnetin, Taxifolin)

Flavonols are a class of flavonoids that are known to act as antioxidants to reduce oxidative stress and also can serve as anti-inflammatory agents (Cook and Samman 1996). Flavonols are known to inhibit CYP2C9 and CYP3A4 enzymes, which metabolize most drugs in the body (Sprouse and van Breemen 2016). Although many flavonols are present in dietary grape, the four most common are quercetin, kaempferol, isorhamnetin and taxifolin (Singh et al. 2019), all of which have been individually evaluated among many diseases and disorders demonstrating beneficial effects.

Quercetin (chemically, 5,7,3′,4′-flavon-3-ol) has been shown to prevent low-density lipoprotein from oxidizing, modify eicosanoid biosynthesis (anti-inflammatory responses), prevent platelet accumulation, and promote relaxation of cardiac smooth muscle (Formica and Regelson 1995). Quercetin is a powerful antioxidant, which has been shown to have potential in cancer management. Quercetin possesses anti-inflammatory functions, which are mainly attributed to its inhibitory effect on inflammatory mediators like nitric oxide, catalase, and pro-inflammatory cytokines (Ward et al. 2018). In addition, quercetin exerts an apoptotic effect in tumor cells and can block cancer progression. Quercetin has demonstrated cancer chemopreventive effects in multiple models (Gibellini et al. 2011). Quercetin has been shown to inhibit angiogenesis in several models through multiple mechanisms, including interaction with the cyclooxygenase-2 (COX2) and lipoxygenase-5 enzymes, EGFR, the HER2 intracellular signaling pathway, and the NF-κB nuclear transcription protein (reviewed in Sagar et al. 2006). In ascite cells of Dalton's lymphoma-bearing mice, quercetin attenuated levels of VEGF-A, COX2, iNOS and NO (Maurya and Vinayak 2017). The treatment of breast cancer cells with gold nanoparticles carrying quercetin demonstrated inhibited angiogenesis, EMT, and metastasis of mammary tumors in Sprague-Dawley rats (Balakrishnan et al. 2016). Treatment with the quercetin inhibited EGFR-mediated AKT signaling and reduced migration in human pancreatic cells and human head and neck squamous cell carcinomas (Chan et al. 2016; Lee et al. 2015a). In oral cancer, quercetin-induced growth inhibition has been found to be associated with inhibition of EGFR/AKT activation with simultaneous activation of Forkhead Box O1 (FOXO1) (Huang et al. 2013), which is one of four members of FOXO transcription factors and known to inhibit angiogenesis in certain cancers (Kim et al. 2016).

Quercetin also demonstrates the ability to inhibit angiogenesis in prostate cancer through the VEGFR2 pathway, by regulation of the AKT/mTOR/P70S6K signaling pathways both in vitro and in vivo (Pratheeshkumar et al. 2012). Quercetin has been shown to prevent EGF-induced EMT via inhibition of EGFR/PI3K/AKT/ERK1/2 pathway as well as by suppressing transcriptional repressors SNAIL, SLUG and TWIST in prostate cancer cells. As per this pathway, quercetin may prevent cancer metastasis by targeting EMT (Bhat et al. 2014). Additionally, in prostate cancer, the anticancer effects of quercetin combined with tamoxifen enhanced antiangiogenesis effects (Ma et al. 2004). A study by Igura et al. examining the effects of resveratrol and quercetin on angiogenesis found decreased growth of bovine aorta endothelial (BAE) cells in a concentration-dependent manner in vitro. The migration of BAE was substantially inhibited by resveratrol, but only weakly inhibited by quercetin (Igura et al. 2001).

Another potentially therapeutic flavonal, kaempferol (chemically 3,4′,5,7-tetrahydroxyflavone), is known to act as modulators of EMT markers (NCAD, ECAD, SLUG, and SNAIL) and metastasis marker MMP2 (reviewed in Imran et al. 2019). In ovarian cancer cell lines, kaempferol works against angiogenesis through multiple pathways including the HIF-dependent (AKT/HIF) and HIF-independent estrogen-related receptor alpha (ESRRA) pathways, (Luo et al. 2009) and by impairing VEGF synthesis through the ERK/NF-κB/cMYC/P21 pathway (Luo et al. 2012). Reduction of VEGF secretion was also noted in human MDA breast cancer cells upon kaempferol treatment (Schindler and Mentlein 2006). Another breast cancer study demonstrated that kaempferol treatment did not affect secretion, but did significantly inhibit the activity of MMP3 accompanied by a blockage of MDA-MB-231 cell migration (Phromnoi et al. 2009). Reduced migratory effects in prostate cancer cells after kaempferol treatment was suggested to be due to the inhibitory effects of kaempferol on EGFR, and further SRC, AKT and ERK related survival, migration, and invasion (Lee and Kim 2016). Medulloblastoma cell line migration was also decreased upon treatment with kaempferol or quercetin, suggestively through a reduction of hepatocyte growth factor (HGF)-mediated activation of AKT (Labbé et al. 2009).

Limited information is available regarding the potential anti-cancer effects of grape flavonols isorhamnetin and taxifolin. Isorhamnetin is a 3′-methoxylated derivative of quercetin and known for its anticancer properties demonstrated in certain cancers. For example, isorhamnetin has shown to suppress colon cancer cell growth by inhibiting the PI3K/AKT/mTOR pathway (Li et al. 2014). Likewise, taxifolin (5,7,3′,4′-flavan-on-ol), also identified as dihydroquercetin, has been suggested to exert chemopreventive activity by modulating antioxidant response element (ARE) mediated gene regulation (Lee et al. 2007). Although there is a general lack of studies of these two flavonols, implications of the antiangiogenic and antimigratory effects suggest the potential basis of anti-cancer effects of these agents. In a Lewis lung cancer mouse model, isorhamnetin treatment reduced VEGF protein expression, metastatic lesions, and tumor cell density. The results were enhanced further when isorhamnetin was combined with cisplatin (Zhu et al. 2017). In MDA breast carcinoma cells, the downregulation of MMP2 and MMP9 suggest that isorhamnetin may act to suppress p38 MAPK and STAT3 to inhibit invasion (Li et al. 2015). Isorhamnetin also reduced EMT and pulmonary fibrosis in a murine model (Zheng et al. 2019). Similar to other grape flavonols, taxifolin reduces AKT, as well as represses cell migration and invasion of osteosarcoma cells (Chen et al. 2018b). In skin scar cell carcinoma (SSCC), the inhibited invasion SSCC cells were associated with downregulation of MMP2 and MMP9 by taxifolin (Zhou et al. 2019). However, taxifolin, compared to kaempferol and quercetin, does not possess a strong cytotoxic effect in reducing VEGF in human ovarian cancer cells (Luo et al. 2008). Figure 12.5 outlines the molecular actions of grape flavonols against angiogenesis and metastasis.

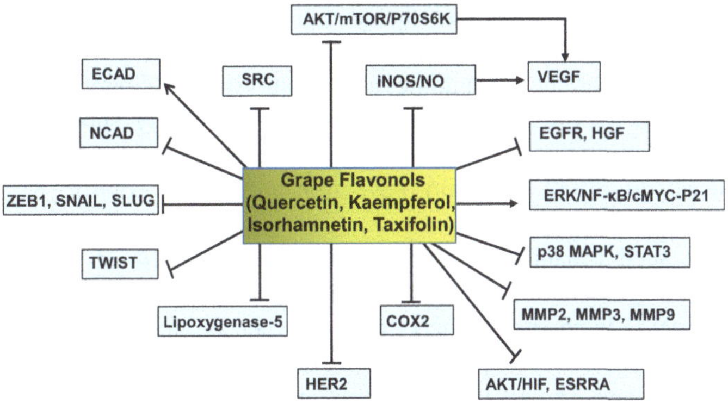

Fig. 12.5 Molecular actions of grape flavonols against angiogenesis and metastasis

12.4.3 Grape Catechins (Catechin, Epicatechin)

Catechin and epicatechin have been quantified as two major components of the top ten compounds of the grape powder (Singh et al. 2019). These are epimers, with D-catechin and L-epicatechin being the commonly occurring optical isomers in nature. Catechins fall into the flavonoid family and give rise to other oligomeric compounds including proanthocyanidins (or condensed procyanidins) that yield cyanidin when depolymerized under oxidative conditions. Catechin is the major monomeric polyphenol in whole grape or its products such as red wine. In addition to other observed mechanisms of action that lead to an antiproliferative effect in various cancer, catechin has been shown to inhibit angiogenesis in certain cancers. Ebeler et al. have shown that dietary supplementation of catechin delayed tumor onset in a linear dose-dependent manner in a transgenic mice model of neurofibromatosis. It was also found that the plasma levels of catechin and its metabolite 3′-*O*-methylcatechin (3′MC) were positively associated with the delay in tumor onset, without obvious adverse effects in mice (Ebeler et al. 2002). In another study, Payen and colleagues demonstrated that catechins inhibited cancer cell migration in vitro in a model of super-invasive human cervix cancer cells SiHa-F3. Further, (+)-catechin: lysine complexes (1:2) were shown to prevent metastasis of B16F10 melanoma cells to the lungs of C57BL/6JRj male mice (Payen et al. 2017).

Grape seed extract (GSE) obtained from Palieri grape cultivar that contained 6.2 mg/g catechins and 5.6 mg/g procyanidins were assessed for their effects against MDA-MB231 breast cancer cell migration and invasion (Dinicola et al. 2014). GSE at a sub-lethal concentration (25 μg/ml) strongly inhibited cell migration and invasion ability of MDA-MB231 cells. This was accompanied by a decrease in urokinase-type plasminogen activator (uPA), MMP2 and MMP9 activities, as well as in a down-regulation of CTNNB, fascin (FSCN1) and NF-κB expression (Dinicola et al. 2014). Another study was performed on procyanidin B2-3,3″-di-*O*-gallate (B2G2), a component of grape seed extract, where it was shown to inhibit the motility and invasiveness of human umbilical vein endothelial cells (HUVECs) and human prostate microvascular endothelial cells (HPMECs). Mechanistic studies have shown that B2G2 targets VEGFR2/PI3K/AKT and integrin signaling molecules, which are important for endothelial cells survival, proliferation, tube formation, and motility (Kumar et al. 2015). Overall, this study showed that B2G2 inhibited several attributes of angiogenesis in cell culture and warrants future studies for the efficacy of B2G2 for angio-prevention and cancer control (Kumar et al. 2015).

The grape seed proanthocyanidins (GSP) are composed of dimers, trimers, tetramers, and oligomers of monomeric catechins or epicatechins (Shi et al. 2003). Feng et al. (2014) have shown the effects of grape proanthocyanidins on tumor angiogenesis in liver cancer (hepatocellular carcinoma or HCC) xenograft models. In this study, they have shown that grape proanthocyanidins inhibited tumor cells growth and metastasis by exerting antiangiogenesis effects via inhibition of microvessel density (MVD), which is a quantitative index of tumor angiogenesis. It is related to the supply of nutrition and oxygen to tumors towards proliferation, invasion, growth, and metastasis of tumor cells (Zhao et al. 2006). MVD is calculated by labeling cells with an anti-CD34 antibody specific to vascular endothelial cells in the tumor tissues followed by counting the number of microvessels per unit area to reflect the degree of angiogenesis in tumor tissues. In this study, a gradual reduction in MVD was observed with increasing concentration of grape proanthocyanidins including a significant positive correlation between MVD and the expression of angiogenesis marker VEGF. Tumor angiogenesis involves various types of growth factors, out of which VEGF is the most prevailing and a potent inducer of capillary growth into a tumor. VEGF, a hexose-modified multifunctional protein, specifically acts on vascular endothelial cells, inducing micro-angiogenesis and causing tumor invasion and metastasis. It was also suggested that grape proanthocyanidins may exhibit the antiangiogenic activity by inhibition of vascular endothelial cell proliferation (Feng et al. 2014).

Further, grape seed proanthocyanidin extract containing 5000 ppm resveratrol (GSPE) has been shown to facilitate oxidant-induced VEGF expression in keratinocytes. Using a ribonuclease protection assay (RPA), GSPE has been shown to regulate oxidant-induced changes in several angiogenesis-related genes. Further, pretreatment of HaCaT keratinocytes with GSPE upregulated both hydrogen peroxide (H_2O_2) and TNFα-induced VEGF expression and release. The results of the study suggested that GSPE might have beneficial therapeutic effects in promoting dermal wound healing and other related skin disorders (Khanna et al. 2001). Similarly, Luan et al. investigated the anti-vasculogenic mimicry (VM) activity of grape seed proanthocyanidins in human triple negative breast cancer (TNBC). This study demonstrated that highly aggressive TNBC cells HCC1937 formed vasculogenic-like network structures when cultured on a three-dimensional matrix compared to aggressive MCF-7 cells that were unable to form the patterned networks with the same conditions. Interestingly, grape seed proanthocyanidins inhibited proliferation of HCC1937 cells significantly and suppressed tubular-like structures. Therefore, this study suggests that grape seed proanthocyanidins may be a potential anti-VM agent for human TNBC (Luan et al. 2015).

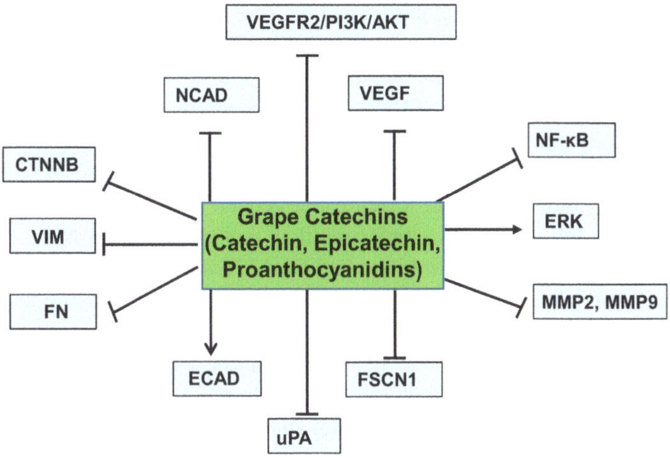

Fig. 12.6 Molecular actions of grape catechins against angiogenesis and metastasis

Further, Sun et al. assessed the chemotherapeutic effects of GSP on the invasion potential of human head and neck cutaneous squamous cell carcinoma (SCC) cells. The results obtained from this study suggested that GSP has the ability to inhibit the invasion of head and neck cutaneous SCC cells by targeting the EGFR expression and reversing the process of EMT (Sun et al. 2011). Further, GSP treatment of SCC13 cells showed the down-regulation of mesenchymal biomarkers, such as VIM, FN and NCAD while up-regulated the expression of the epithelial biomarker ECAD. These data suggested that inhibition of EMT by GSP may also be one of the possible mechanisms through which it reduces the invasiveness of cutaneous head and neck SCC cells and that lead to inhibition of invasion ability of SCC13 cells (Sun et al. 2011). Figure 12.6 shows the molecular actions of grape catechins against angiogenesis and metastasis.

12.4.4 Grape Anthocyanins (Cyanidin, Peonidin, Malvidin)

Anthocyanins belong to a group of flavonoids and are known for their antioxidant, anti-inflammatory and anticancer effects. Cyanidin, peonidin, and malvidin are the top thee anthocyanins characterized in grape powder (Singh et al. 2019) or, grape powder extract (van Breemen et al. 2016). Anthocyanins isolated from fruits of *Vitis coignetiae* Pulliat, a variety of wild grape called meoru in Korea and is used in Korean folk medicine, has been investigated against angiogenesis and metastasis. Compositional analysis of this anthocyanins identified the presence of the highest amount of cyanidin along with other anthocyanins peonidin, malvidin, delphinidin and petunidin (Lu et al. 2017). Lu et al. have demonstrated that the anthocyanins extract inhibited cancer cell proliferation, invasion, and angiogenesis in human lung cancer A549 cells. In this study, anthocyanins have been shown to suppress migration and invasion of cancer cells by inhibiting MMP2 and MMP9 expression as well as adhesion and angiogenesis by inhibiting intercellular adhesion molecule 1 (ICAM1) and VEGF (Lu et al. 2017). In another study, Lu et al. investigated the effects of anthocyanins on cellular responses and molecular changes intricate in cancer invasion and EMT in EGF or TGF-β treated human lung cancer cells. This extracted anthocyanin was found to repress glycogen synthase kinase-3β (GSK3β) phosphorylation and CTNNB expression that is involved in EMT. This study demonstrated that anthocyanin inhibited PI3K/AKT and EGFR pathway independently in a dual repression mode as well as inhibited invasion and migration at least in part by suppressing EMT (Lu et al. 2014). Anthocyanins have also been shown to inhibit invasion and EMT markers in human uterine cervical cancer HeLa cells. Treatment with anthocyanins suppressed mesenchymal markers VIM, NCAD, and CTNNB expression and induced epithelial marker ECAD as well as suppressed expression of SNAIL, a transcriptional regulator of EMT (Lu et al. 2013). Furthermore, Burton and colleagues have shown that anthocyanin comprising muscadine grape skin extract inhibited SNAIL and pSTAT3, and abolished SNAIL-mediated cathepsin L (CTSL) activity, migration, invasion, and osteoclastogenesis in the breast (MCF-7) and prostate (LNCaP, ARCaP-E) cancer cells (Burton et al. 2015). In conclusion, these studies suggest that grape anthocyanins have antiangiogenesis and antimetastatic activities.

Further, there is limited literature available assessing the effects of anthocyanins individually against cancer, showing their anti-angiogenic and/or anti-metastatic potential. In one study, cyanidin-3-glucoside (C3G) was found to inhibit UVB-mediated oxidative damage and inflammation in SKH-1 hairless mice. Specifically, C3G inhibited glutathione depletion, lipid peroxidation, myelo-peroxidation and pro-inflammatory cytokines (IL6 and TNFα) in mouse skin. Further, C3G supplementation modulated UVB-induced MAP kinase and NF-κB signaling pathways (Pratheeshkumar et al. 2014). Liu and colleagues have shown that C3G, as well as peonidin-3-glucoside (P3G), inhibited the phosphorylation of human epidermal growth factor receptor-2 (HER2), which is known to be overexpressed in breast cancer as well as known to upregulate angiogenesis at different levels in cells (Alameddine et al. 2013; Liu et al. 2013). The antiproliferative effect of P3G and C3G were shown to be related to inhibited p-AKT and induced apoptosis in HER2-positive breast cancer cells (Liu et al. 2013). Moreover, in HER2-positive MDA-MB-453 xenografted mouse supplemented with P3G or, C3G, at a dose of 6 mg/kg, were found to reduce tumor growth (Liu et al. 2013). Importantly, in a clinical trial, assessing the bioavailability of isotopically labeled C3G (500 mg), has found relatively more bioavailable and metabolites were noticed in the circulation for $\leq$48 h after ingestion (Czank et al. 2013). Like cyanidin and peonidin, malvidin has been shown to inhibit TNFα-induced inflammatory response in endothelial cells, indicating its possible role in preventing atherosclerosis and cancer. Specifically, malvidin has been shown to inhibit TNFα-induced increase in monocyte chemotactic protein-1 (MCP1), vascular cell adhesion molecule-1 (VCAM1), intercellular adhesion molecule-1 (ICAM1), IκBα degradation and NF-κB p65 nuclear translocation

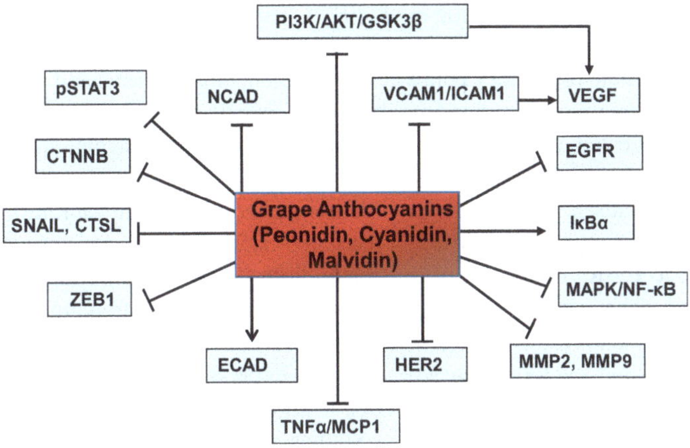

Fig. 12.7 Molecular actions of grape anthocyanins against angiogenesis and metastasis

(Huang et al. 2014). All these studies suggest direct/indirect effects of anthocyanins against tumor angiogenesis and metastasis. Figure 12.7 shows the molecular actions of grape anthocyanins against angiogenesis and metastasis.

12.4.5 Whole Grape Powder Against Angiogenesis and Metastasis

A limited number of studies have assessed the effects of whole grape powder against angiogenesis and metastasis, in certain models. Liu and colleagues tested the antiangiogenic activity of four grape varieties, Concord, Niagara, Chardonnay, and Pinot noir, and demonstrated that those with the highest total phenolics and flavonoids possess the highest antiangiogenic activity (Liu et al. 2010). Recently, we used freeze-dried grape powder, which was comprised of fresh black, green, and red grapes of both seeded and seedless varieties [provided from the California Table Grape Commission (CTGC)]. Phytochemical analysis of this grape powder showed a considerable amount of total polyphenols (3260 mg/kg in gallic acid equivalents). Dietary supplementation of this grape powder was found to protect against UVB-mediated skin carcinogenesis in female SKH-1 hairless mice (Singh et al. 2019). Moreover, the grape powder was found to improve DNA damage repair, decreased cell proliferation, increased apoptosis, and modulations in several genes involved in antioxidant function, metabolism of reactive oxygen species (ROS), superoxide metabolism and oxidative stress response (Singh et al. 2019). Additionally, proteomics analysis of tumor samples of mice supplemented with grape powder identified modulation of several proteins whose interactions and cumulative actions were linked to reduced oxidative stress through increased ROS metabolism and reduced quantity of H_2O_2 (Mintie et al. 2019). This is an important finding as ROS, H_2O_2 and other free radicals are often produced at elevated levels in tumors and known to modulate regulatory pathways involved in angiogenesis and metastasis. In fact, targeting the redox-regulated mechanisms for antiangiogenic anticancer therapy has been suggested to overcome the limitations of single-agent antiangiogenic treatments (reviewed in Tertil et al. 2010).

Earlier, Hanausek and Spears have demonstrated significant inhibition of 7,12-dimethylbenz(*a*)anthracene (DMBA)-mediated skin tumorigenesis in SENCAR (SENsitive to CARcinogenesis) mice treated with grape powder and grape-derived antioxidants. The authors found that simultaneous dietary supplementation with grape powder and topical treatment with resveratrol reduced DMBA-induced tumor burden and cyclooxygenase-2 (COX2) expression (Hanausek et al. 2011). It's important to mention here that COX2 is an enzyme associated with inflammation, angiogenesis, and tumorigenesis. Studies in primary tumors have suggested that COX2 inhibition is a potent mechanism to reduce angiogenesis. Yao et al. have demonstrated how COX2 play roles in angiogenesis of gastric cancer via modulation of VEGF, FLT1, FLK1/KDR, ANGPT1, TIE2, MMP2, and OPN (Yao et al. 2011).

Interestingly, limited clinical studies have been done, despite the promising in vitro and in vivo studies, on the anticancer activities of grape and grape constituents. Low dose resveratrol or resveratrol-containing freeze-dried grape powder treatment to patients with colon cancer was found to inhibit WNT target genes in the normal colonic mucosa, but no change in cancer tissue (Nguyen et al. 2009). The WNT signaling pathway plays an essential role in cellular proliferation, survival, apoptosis, and angiogenesis (Olsen et al. 2017). In several clinical trials, the effect of grape powder has been assessed in multiple diseases showing beneficial effects and well tolerability (reviewed in Singh et al. 2015a). In the future, more clinical trials are needed and expected to determine the beneficial effects of grape powder in cancer patients. Figure 12.8 outlines the molecular actions of grape powder against angiogenesis and metastasis.

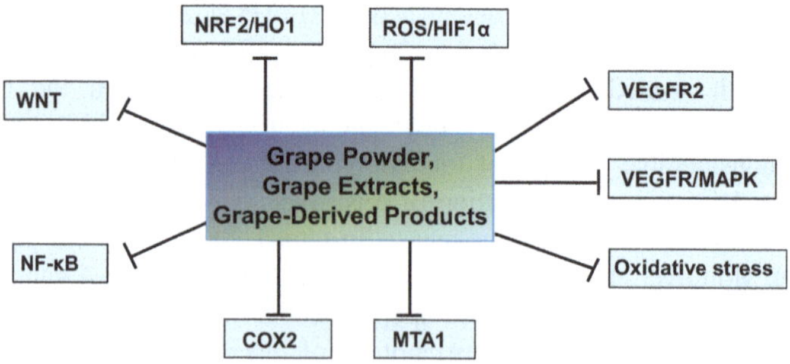

Fig. 12.8 Molecular actions of grape powder, grape extracts/grape-derived products against angiogenesis and metastasis

12.4.6 Grape Extracts/Grape-Derived Products Against Angiogenesis and Metastasis

Several forms of grape extracts have also been evaluated against multiple cancers. An extract of grape powder (obtained from the California Table Grape Commission) was prepared and standardized by Dr. Richard van Breemen (van Breemen et al. 2016). A photochemical analysis of this extract shows almost the same composition as of the grape powder (Singh et al. 2019; van Breemen et al. 2016). Kumar et al. (2018) have used this preparation and demonstrated the anticancer effects of grape powder extract (GPE) on cell viability, proliferation, and metastatic capability against prostate cancer cells in vitro. Upon molecular analysis, GPE, like resveratrol and pterostilbene, was found to downregulate metastasis-associated protein 1 (MTA1), which is a vital downstream target of c-MYC oncoprotein, and known to regulate EMT and metastasis (Kumar et al. 2018; Zhang et al. 2005).

Grape seed extract (GSE) has also been shown to inhibit VEGF via modulating HIF1α protein (Lu et al. 2009). Filip et al. sought to understand the protective effects of red grape seed extract against UVB-induced damages in female SKH-1 hairless mice. Topically applied GSE, before or after each UVB exposure, was found to effectively reduce cyclobutane pyrimidine dimers (CPDs), hyperplasia, cytokine release, and oxidative stress while increasing antioxidant response (Filip et al. 2011). As discussed above with grape powder, this again indicates the possibility of inhibition of angiogenesis via inhibiting oxidative stress manifested by tumor cells.

GSE has also been found to inhibit the kinase activity of purified VEGFR2, and VEGFR/MAPK-mediated signaling in endothelial cells (Wen et al. 2008). Moreover, GSE has been shown to inhibit tumor growth and angiogenesis of MDA-MB-231 tumors in mice (Wen et al. 2008). In the United States, GSE is marketed as a dietary supplement owing to their powerful protective properties against free radicals and oxidative stress.

Certain other grape-derived products, such as red wine, have also shown to affect angiogenesis. Baron-Menguy et al. have demonstrated the effects of low and high doses of red wine polyphenolic compounds (RWPC) in vivo on postischemic neovascularization in rats. Treatment with low and high doses RWPC showed pro- and anti-angiogenic properties, respectively, suggesting high dose may be beneficial against tumor angiogenesis via inhibiting VEGF expression (Baron-Menguy et al. 2007). Utilizing an uncommon part of the grape, Che et al. demonstrated that topical treatment with grape stem extracts reversed skin damage induced by the UVB radiation via decreasing lipid peroxidation, neutrophil, and mast cell infiltrations, and reducing the expressions levels of COX2, NRF2, and HO1 (Che et al. 2017). Figure 12.8 outlines the molecular actions of grape extracts/grape-derived products against angiogenesis and metastasis.

Overall, these studies suggest that grape and grape antioxidants may have strong potential towards developing complementary and alternative approaches for the inhibition of invasion/metastasis as well as angiogenesis. Therefore, further exploration and clinical evaluation of these agents alone or in combination with the established treatment regimen is needed for the effective management of cancers.

12.5 Concluding Remarks

Cancer incidence is still on the rise, probably due to lifestyle changes and increasing longevity. Although significant advancements have been made in cancer management, there is a need for further improvement in several respects. Many harsh treatments such as radiation and chemotherapy pose severe adverse side effects and produce both short- and long-term consequences, which place further strain on the quality of life. Interestingly, grape contains a range of complex natural agents that appear to inhibit angiogenesis and metastasis by interacting with multiple pathways and by reducing tumor burden by multiple mechanisms. Considering the fact that most of the current antiangiogenesis agents, approved for clinical use or being tested in clinical trials, are associated with several adverse effects; grape or grape components as a dietary supplement appear to be an inexpensive inhibitor of angiogenesis and metastasis. Therefore, further investigations in this direction are warranted.

References

Alameddine RS, Otrock ZK, Awada A, Shamseddine A (2013) Crosstalk between HER2 signaling and angiogenesis in breast cancer: molecular basis, clinical applications and challenges. Curr Opin Oncol 25:313–324

Anborgh PH, Mutrie JC, Tuck AB, Chambers AF (2010) Role of the metastasis-promoting protein osteopontin in the tumour microenvironment. J Cell Mol Med 14:2037–2044

Ansiaux R, Baudelet C, Jordan BF, Beghein N, Sonveaux P, De Wever J et al (2005) Thalidomide radiosensitizes tumors through early changes in the tumor microenvironment. Clin Cancer Res 11:743–750

Balakrishnan S, Bhat FA, Raja Singh P, Mukherjee S, Elumalai P, Das S et al (2016) Gold nanoparticle-conjugated quercetin inhibits epithelial-mesenchymal transition, angiogenesis and invasiveness via EGFR/VEGFR-2-mediated pathway in breast cancer. Cell Prolif 49:678–697

Baron-Menguy C, Bocquet A, Guihot AL, Chappard D, Amiot MJ, Andriantsitohaina R et al (2007) Effects of red wine polyphenols on postischemic neovascularization model in rats: low doses are proangiogenic, high doses anti-angiogenic. FASEB J 21:3511–3521

Bashir R, Vale PR, Isner JM, Losordo DW (2002) Angiogenic gene therapy: pre-clinical studies and phase I clinical data. Kidney Int 61:S110–S114

Beenken A, Mohammadi M (2009) The FGF family: biology, pathophysiology and therapy. Nat Rev Drug Discov 8:235–253

Berman AY, Motechin RA, Wiesenfeld MY, Holz MK (2017) The therapeutic potential of resveratrol: a review of clinical trials. NPJ Precis Oncol 1

Bhat FA, Sharmila G, Balakrishnan S, Arunkumar R, Elumalai P, Suganya S et al (2014) Quercetin reverses EGF-induced epithelial to mesenchymal transition and invasiveness in prostate cancer (PC-3) cell line via EGFR/PI3K/Akt pathway. J Nutr Biochem 25:1132–1139

Bielenberg DR, Zetter BR (2015) The contribution of angiogenesis to the process of metastasis. Cancer J 21:267–273

Burton LJ, Smith BA, Smith BN, Loyd Q, Nagappan P, McKeithen D et al (2015) Muscadine grape skin extract can antagonize Snail-cathepsin L-mediated invasion, migration and osteoclastogenesis in prostate and breast cancer cells. Carcinogenesis 36:1019–1027

Cao Z, Fang J, Xia C, Shi X, Jiang BH (2004) Trans-3,4,5′-trihydroxystibene inhibits hypoxia-inducible factor 1alpha and vascular endothelial growth factor expression in human ovarian cancer cells. Clin Cancer Res 10:5253–5263

Carmeliet P (2003) Angiogenesis in health and disease. Nat Med 9:653–660

Carmeliet P, Jain RK (2011) Molecular mechanisms and clinical applications of angiogenesis. Nature 473:298–307

Catalgol B, Batirel S, Taga Y, Ozer NK (2012) Resveratrol: French paradox revisited. Front Pharmacol 3:141

Chan CY, Lien CH, Lee MF, Huang CY (2016) Quercetin suppresses cellular migration and invasion in human head and neck squamous cell carcinoma (HNSCC). Biomedicine (Taipei) 6:15

Chang YS, di Tomaso E, McDonald DM, Jones R, Jain RK, Munn LL (2000) Mosaic blood vessels in tumors: frequency of cancer cells in contact with flowing blood. Proc Natl Acad Sci USA 97:14608–14613

Che DN, Xie GH, Cho BO, Shin JY, Kang HJ, Jang SI (2017) Protective effects of grape stem extract against UVB-induced damage in C57BL mice skin. J Photochem Photobiol B 173:551–559

Chen JC, Chen Y, Lin JH, Wu JM, Tseng SH (2006) Resveratrol suppresses angiogenesis in gliomas: evaluation by color Doppler ultrasound. Anticancer Res 26:1237–1245

Chen C, Zhao S, Karnad A, Freeman JW (2018a) The biology and role of CD44 in cancer progression: therapeutic implications. J Hematol Oncol 11:64

Chen X, Gu N, Xue C, Li BR (2018b) Plant flavonoid taxifolin inhibits the growth, migration and invasion of human osteosarcoma cells. Mol Med Rep 17:3239–3245

Cook NC, Samman S (1996) Flavonoids—chemistry, metabolism, cardioprotective effects, and dietary sources. J Nutr Biochem 7:66–76

Czank C, Cassidy A, Zhang Q, Morrison DJ, Preston T, Kroon PA et al (2013) Human metabolism and elimination of the anthocyanin, cyanidin-3-glucoside: a (13)C-tracer study. Am J Clin Nutr 97:995–1003

Dinicola S, Pasqualato A, Cucina A, Coluccia P, Ferranti F, Canipari R et al (2014) Grape seed extract suppresses MDA-MB231 breast cancer cell migration and invasion. Eur J Nutr 53:421–431

Ebeler SE, Brenneman CA, Kim GS, Jewell WT, Webb MR, Chacon-Rodriguez L et al (2002) Dietary catechin delays tumor onset in a transgenic mouse model. Am J Clin Nutr 76:865–872

Fagiani E, Christofori G (2013) Angiopoietins in angiogenesis. Cancer Lett 328:18–26

Feng X, Ofstad W, Hawkins D (2010) Antiangiogenesis therapy: a new strategy for cancer treatment. US Pharm 35(7)(oncology suppl):4–9

Feng LL, Liu BX, Zhong JY, Sun LB, Yu HS (2014) Effect of grape procyanidins on tumor angiogenesis in liver cancer xenograft models. Asian Pac J Cancer Prev 15:737–741

Figueiras TS, Neves-Petersen MT, Petersen SB (2011) Activation energy of light induced isomerization of resveratrol. J Fluoresc 21:1897–1906

Filip A, Daicoviciu D, Clichici S, Bolfa P, Catoi C, Baldea I et al (2011) The effects of grape seeds polyphenols on SKH-1 mice skin irradiated with multiple doses of UV-B. J Photochem Photobiol B 105:133–142

Folkman J (1971) Tumor angiogenesis: therapeutic implications. N Engl J Med 285:1182–1186

Formica JV, Regelson W (1995) Review of the biology of quercetin and related bioflavonoids. Food Chem Toxicol 33:1061–1080

Gao Q, Yuan Y, Gan HZ, Peng Q (2015) Resveratrol inhibits the hedgehog signaling pathway and epithelial-mesenchymal transition and suppresses gastric cancer invasion and metastasis. Oncol Lett 9:2381–2387

Garvin S, Ollinger K, Dabrosin C (2006) Resveratrol induces apoptosis and inhibits angiogenesis in human breast cancer xenografts in vivo. Cancer Lett 231:113–122

Gibellini L, Pinti M, Nasi M, Montagna JP, De Biasi S, Roat E et al (2011) Quercetin and cancer chemoprevention. Evid Based Complement Alternat Med 2011:591356

Gohji K, Fidler IJ, Tsan R, Radinsky R, von Eschenbach AC, Tsuruo T et al (1994) Human recombinant interferons-beta and -gamma decrease gelatinase production and invasion by human KG-2 renal-carcinoma cells. Int J Cancer 58:380–384

Grant SW, Kyshtoobayeva AS, Kurosaki T, Jakowatz J, Fruehauf JP (1998) Mutant p53 correlates with reduced expression of thrombospondin-1, increased angiogenesis, and metastatic progression in melanoma. Cancer Detect Prev 22:185–194

Greenwell M, Rahman PK (2015) Medicinal plants: their use in anticancer treatment. Int J Pharm Sci Res 6:4103–4112

Hanahan D, Weinberg RA (2000) The hallmarks of cancer. Cell 100:57–70

Hanahan D, Weinberg RA (2011) Hallmarks of cancer: the next generation. Cell 144:646–674

Hanausek M, Spears E, Walaszek Z, Kowalczyk MC, Kowalczyk P, Wendel C et al (2011) Inhibition of murine skin carcinogenesis by freeze-dried grape powder and other grape-derived major antioxidants. Nutr Cancer 63:28–38

Hoshino J, Park EJ, Kondratyuk TP, Marler L, Pezzuto JM, van Breemen RB et al (2010) Selective synthesis and biological evaluation of sulfate-conjugated resveratrol metabolites. J Med Chem 53:5033–5043

Hu Y, Sun CY, Huang J, Hong L, Zhang L, Chu ZB (2007) Antimyeloma effects of resveratrol through inhibition of angiogenesis. Chin Med J (Engl) 120:1672–1677

Huang CY, Chan CY, Chou IT, Lien CH, Hung HC, Lee MF (2013) Quercetin induces growth arrest through activation of FOXO1 transcription factor in EGFR-overexpressing oral cancer cells. J Nutr Biochem 24:1596–1603

Huang WY, Wang J, Liu YM, Zheng QS, Li CY (2014) Inhibitory effect of Malvidin on TNF-alpha-induced inflammatory response in endothelial cells. Eur J Pharmacol 723:67–72

Igura K, Ohta T, Kuroda Y, Kaji K (2001) Resveratrol and quercetin inhibit angiogenesis in vitro. Cancer Lett 171:11–16

Imran M, Rauf A, Shah ZA, Saeed F, Imran A, Arshad MU et al (2019) Chemo-preventive and therapeutic effect of the dietary flavonoid kaempferol: a comprehensive review. Phytother Res 33:263–275

Iqbal S, Lenz HJ (2004) Integration of novel agents in the treatment of colorectal cancer. Cancer Chemother Pharmacol 54(Suppl 1):S32–S39

Khanna S, Roy S, Bagchi D, Bagchi M, Sen CK (2001) Upregulation of oxidant-induced VEGF expression in cultured keratinocytes by a grape seed proanthocyanidin extract. Free Radic Biol Med 31:38–42

Kim SY, Ko YS, Park J, Choi Y, Park JW, Kim Y et al (2016) Forkhead transcription factor FOXO1 inhibits angiogenesis in gastric cancer in relation to SIRT1. Cancer Res Treat 48:345–354

Kim SE, Shin SH, Lee JY, Kim CH, Chung IK, Kang HM et al (2018) Resveratrol induces mitochondrial apoptosis and inhibits epithelial-mesenchymal transition in oral squamous cell carcinoma cells. Nutr Cancer 70:125–135

Kumar R, Deep G, Wempe MF, Agarwal R, Agarwal C (2015) Procyanidin B2 3,3″-di-O-gallate inhibits endothelial cells growth and motility by targeting VEGFR2 and integrin signaling pathways. Curr Cancer Drug Targets 15:14–26

Kumar A, D'Silva M, Dholakia K, Levenson AS (2018) In vitro anticancer properties of table grape powder extract (GPE) in prostate cancer. Nutrients 10:1804

Labbé D, Provençal M, Lamy S, Boivin D, Gingras D, Béliveau R (2009) The flavonols quercetin, kaempferol, and myricetin inhibit hepatocyte growth factor-induced medulloblastoma cell migration. J Nutr 139:646–652

Langley RR, Fidler IJ (2011) The seed and soil hypothesis revisited—the role of tumor-stroma interactions in metastasis to different organs. Int J Cancer 128:2527–2535

Lee J, Kim JH (2016) Kaempferol inhibits pancreatic cancer cell growth and migration through the blockade of EGFR-related pathway in vitro. PLoS One 11:e0155264

Lee SB, Cha KH, Selenge D, Solongo A, Nho CW (2007) The chemopreventive effect of taxifolin is exerted through ARE-dependent gene regulation. Biol Pharm Bull 30:1074–1079

Lee J, Han SI, Yun JH, Kim JH (2015a) Quercetin 3-O-glucoside suppresses epidermal growth factor-induced migration by inhibiting EGFR signaling in pancreatic cancer cells. Tumour Biol 36:9385–9393

Lee SH, Jeong D, Han YS, Baek MJ (2015b) Pivotal role of vascular endothelial growth factor pathway in tumor angiogenesis. Ann Surg Treat Res 89:1–8

Li C, Yang X, Chen C, Cai S, Hu J (2014) Isorhamnetin suppresses colon cancer cell growth through the PI3KAktmTOR pathway. Mol Med Rep 9:935–940

Li CL, Yang D, Zhao YW, Qiu Y, Cao X, Yu YY et al (2015) Inhibitory effects of isorhamnetin on the invasion of human breast carcinoma cells by downregulating the expression and activity of matrix metalloproteinase-2/9. Nutr Cancer 67:1191–1200

Liu M, Liu RH, Song BB, Li CF, Lin LQ, Zhang CP et al (2010) Antiangiogenetic effects of 4 varieties of grapes in vitro. J Food Sci 75:T99–T104

Liu W, Xu J, Wu S, Liu Y, Yu X, Chen J et al (2013) Selective anti-proliferation of HER2-positive breast cancer cells by anthocyanins identified by high-throughput screening. PLoS One 8: e81586

Lu J, Zhang K, Chen S, Wen W (2009) Grape seed extract inhibits VEGF expression via reducing HIF-1alpha protein expression. Carcinogenesis 30:636–644

Lu JN, Lee WS, Yun JW, Kim MJ, Kim HJ, Kim DC et al (2013) Anthocyanins from *Vitis coignetiae* Pulliat inhibit cancer invasion and epithelial-mesenchymal transition, but these effects can be attenuated by tumor necrosis factor in human uterine cervical cancer HeLa cells. Evid Based Complement Alternat Med 2013:503043

Lu JN, Lee WS, Kim MJ, Yun JW, Jung JH, Yi SM et al (2014) The inhibitory effect of anthocyanins on Akt on invasion and epithelial-mesenchymal transition is not associated with the anti-EGFR effect of the anthocyanins. Int J Oncol 44:1756–1766

Lu JN, Panchanathan R, Lee WS, Kim HJ, Kim DH, Choi YH et al (2017) Anthocyanins from the fruit of *Vitis coignetiae* Pulliat inhibit TNF-augmented cancer proliferation, migration, and invasion in A549 cells. Asian Pac J Cancer Prev 18:2919–2923

Luan YY, Liu ZM, Zhong JY, Yao RY, Yu HS (2015) Effect of grape seed proanthocyanidins on tumor vasculogenic mimicry in human triple-negative breast cancer cells. Asian Pac J Cancer Prev 16:531–535

Luo HT, Jiang BH, King SM, Chen YC (2008) Inhibition of cell growth and VEGF expression in ovarian cancer cells by flavonoids. Nutr Cancer 60:800–809

Luo H, Rankin GO, Liu L, Daddysman MK, Jiang BH, Chen YC (2009) Kaempferol inhibits angiogenesis and VEGF expression through both HIF dependent and independent pathways in human ovarian cancer cells. Nutr Cancer 61:554–563

Luo H, Rankin GO, Juliano N, Jiang BH, Chen YC (2012) Kaempferol inhibits VEGF expression and in vitro angiogenesis through a novel ERK-NFkappaB-cMyc-p21 pathway. Food Chem 130:321–328

Ma ZS, Huynh TH, Ng CP, Do PT, Nguyen TH, Huynh H (2004) Reduction of CWR22 prostate tumor xenograft growth by combined tamoxifen-quercetin treatment is associated with inhibition of angiogenesis and cellular proliferation. Int J Oncol 24:1297–1304

Maurya AK, Vinayak M (2017) Quercetin attenuates cell survival, inflammation, and angiogenesis via modulation of AKT signaling in murine T-cell lymphoma. Nutr Cancer 69:470–480

Mintie CA, Singh CK, Ndiaye MA, Barrett-Wilt GA, Ahmad N (2019) Identification of molecular targets of dietary grape-mediated chemoprevention of ultraviolet B skin carcinogenesis: a comparative quantitative proteomics analysis. J Proteome Res 18(10):3741–3751

Mukherjee S, Dudley JI, Das DK (2010) Dose-dependency of resveratrol in providing health benefits. Dose Response 8:478–500

Nguyen AV, Martinez M, Stamos MJ, Moyer MP, Planutis K, Hope C et al (2009) Results of a phase I pilot clinical trial examining the effect of plant-derived resveratrol and grape powder on Wnt pathway target gene expression in colonic mucosa and colon cancer. Cancer Manag Res 1:25–37

Oliveira IC, Sciavolino PJ, Lee TH, Vilcek J (1992) Downregulation of interleukin 8 gene expression in human fibroblasts: unique mechanism of transcriptional inhibition by interferon. Proc Natl Acad Sci U S A 89:9049–9053

Olsen JJ, Pohl SO, Deshmukh A, Visweswaran M, Ward NC, Arfuso F et al (2017) The role of Wnt signalling in angiogenesis. Clin Biochem Rev 38:131–142

Park SY, Jeong KJ, Lee J, Yoon DS, Choi WS, Kim YK et al (2007) Hypoxia enhances LPA-induced HIF-1alpha and VEGF expression: their inhibition by resveratrol. Cancer Lett 258:63–69

Patel KR, Andreadi C, Britton RG, Horner-Glister E, Karmokar A, Sale S et al (2013) Sulfate metabolites provide an intracellular pool for resveratrol generation and induce autophagy with senescence. Sci Transl Med 5:205ra133

Paul B, Masih I, Deopujari J, Charpentier C (1999) Occurrence of resveratrol and pterostilbene in age-old darakchasava, an ayurvedic medicine from India. J Ethnopharmacol 68:71–76

Payen VL, Porporato PE, Danhier P, Vazeille T, Blackman M, May BH et al (2017) (+)-Catechin in a 1:2 complex with lysine inhibits cancer cell migration and metastatic take in mice. Front Pharmacol 8:869

Pezzuto JM (2008) Grapes and human health: a perspective. J Agric Food Chem 56:6777–6784

Phromnoi K, Yodkeeree S, Anuchapreeda S, Limtrakul P (2009) Inhibition of MMP-3 activity and invasion of the MDA-MB-231 human invasive breast carcinoma cell line by bioflavonoids. Acta Pharmacol Sin 30:1169–1176

Popat R, Plesner T, Davies F, Cook G, Cook M, Elliott P et al (2013) A phase 2 study of SRT501 (resveratrol) with bortezomib for patients with relapsed and or refractory multiple myeloma. Br J Haematol 160:714–717

Pratheeshkumar P, Budhraja A, Son YO, Wang X, Zhang Z, Ding S et al (2012) Quercetin inhibits angiogenesis mediated human prostate tumor growth by targeting VEGFR-2 regulated AKT/mTOR/P70S6K signaling pathways. PLoS One 7:e47516

Pratheeshkumar P, Son YO, Wang X, Divya SP, Joseph B, Hitron JA et al (2014) Cyanidin-3-glucoside inhibits UVB-induced oxidative damage and inflammation by regulating MAP kinase and NF-kappaB signaling pathways in SKH-1 hairless mice skin. Toxicol Appl Pharmacol 280:127–137

Renaud S, de Lorgeril M (1992) Wine, alcohol, platelets, and the French paradox for coronary heart disease. Lancet 339:1523–1526

Risau W (1997) Mechanisms of angiogenesis. Nature 386:671–674

Sagar SM, Yance D, Wong RK (2006) Natural health products that inhibit angiogenesis: a potential source for investigational new agents to treat cancer-Part 1. Curr Oncol 13:14–26

Samant RS, Shevde LA (2011) Recent advances in anti-angiogenic therapy of cancer. Oncotarget 2:122–134

Schindler R, Mentlein R (2006) Flavonoids and vitamin E reduce the release of the angiogenic peptide vascular endothelial growth factor from human tumor cells. J Nutr 136:1477–1482

Shankar S, Nall D, Tang SN, Meeker D, Passarini J, Sharma J et al (2011) Resveratrol inhibits pancreatic cancer stem cell characteristics in human and KrasG12D transgenic mice by inhibiting pluripotency maintaining factors and epithelial-mesenchymal transition. PLoS One 6:e16530

Sheth S, Jajoo S, Kaur T, Mukherjea D, Sheehan K, Rybak LP et al (2012) Resveratrol reduces prostate cancer growth and metastasis by inhibiting the Akt/MicroRNA-21 pathway. PLoS One 7:e51655

Shi J, Yu J, Pohorly JE, Kakuda Y (2003) Polyphenolics in grape seeds-biochemistry and functionality. J Med Food 6:291–299

Singh RK, Gutman M, Bucana CD, Sanchez R, Llansa N, Fidler IJ (1995) Interferons alpha and beta down-regulate the expression of basic fibroblast growth factor in human carcinomas. Proc Natl Acad Sci U S A 92:4562–4566

Singh CK, Liu X, Ahmad N (2015a) Resveratrol, in its natural combination in whole grape, for health promotion and disease management. Ann N Y Acad Sci 1348:150–160

Singh CK, Ndiaye MA, Ahmad N (2015b) Resveratrol and cancer: challenges for clinical translation. Biochim Biophys Acta 1852:1178–1185

Singh CK, Siddiqui IA, El-Abd S, Mukhtar H, Ahmad N (2016) Combination chemoprevention with grape antioxidants. Mol Nutr Food Res 60:1406–1415

Singh CK, Chhabra G, Ahmad N (2018) Chapter 7: Resveratrol and cancer cell biology. In Wu JM, Hsieh T-c (eds) Resveratrol: state of the art science and health applications. Actionable targets and mechanisms of resveratrol. World Scientific, Singapore, pp 183–207

Singh CK, Mintie CA, Ndiaye MA, Chhabra G, Dakup PP, Ye T et al (2019) Chemoprotective effects of dietary grape powder on UVB radiation-mediated skin carcinogenesis in SKH-1 hairless mice. J Invest Dermatol 139:552–561

Sprouse AA, van Breemen RB (2016) Pharmacokinetic interactions between drugs and botanical dietary supplements. Drug Metab Dispos 44:162–171

Sun Q, Prasad R, Rosenthal E, Katiyar SK (2011) Grape seed proanthocyanidins inhibit the invasive potential of head and neck cutaneous squamous cell carcinoma cells by targeting EGFR expression and epithelial-to-mesenchymal transition. BMC Complement Altern Med 11:134

Tertil M, Jozkowicz A, Dulak J (2010) Oxidative stress in tumor angiogenesis—therapeutic targets. Curr Pharm Des 16:3877–3894

Thiery JP, Acloque H, Huang RY, Nieto MA (2009) Epithelial-mesenchymal transitions in development and disease. Cell 139:871–890

Thurston G, Daly C (2012) The complex role of angiopoietin-2 in the angiopoietin-tie signaling pathway. Cold Spring Harb Perspect Med 2:a006550

Trapp V, Parmakhtiar B, Papazian V, Willmott L, Fruehauf JP (2010) Anti-angiogenic effects of resveratrol mediated by decreased VEGF and increased TSP1 expression in melanoma-endothelial cell co-culture. Angiogenesis 13:305–315

Tseng SH, Lin SM, Chen JC, Su YH, Huang HY, Chen CK et al (2004) Resveratrol suppresses the angiogenesis and tumor growth of gliomas in rats. Clin Cancer Res 10:2190–2202

Ucuzian AA, Gassman AA, East AT, Greisler HP (2010) Molecular mediators of angiogenesis. J Burn Care Res 31:158–175

van Breemen RB, Wright B, Li Y, Nosal D (2016) Burton T standardized grape powder for basic and clinical research. In: Pezzuto JM (ed) Grapes and health. Springer, Cham, pp 17–26

van Zijl F, Krupitza G, Mikulits W (2011) Initial steps of metastasis: cell invasion and endothelial transmigration. Mutat Res 728:23–34

Walle T, Hsieh F, DeLegge MH, Oatis JE Jr, Walle UK (2004) High absorption but very low bioavailability of oral resveratrol in humans. Drug Metab Dispos 32:1377–1382

Wang H, Zhang H, Tang L, Chen H, Wu C, Zhao M et al (2013) Resveratrol inhibits TGF-beta1-induced epithelial-to-mesenchymal transition and suppresses lung cancer invasion and metastasis. Toxicology 303:139–146

Ward AB, Mir H, Kapur N, Gales DN, Carriere PP, Singh S (2018) Quercetin inhibits prostate cancer by attenuating cell survival and inhibiting anti-apoptotic pathways. World J Surg Oncol 16:108

Weber GF (2008) Molecular mechanisms of metastasis. Cancer Lett 270:181–190

Weber GF, Bronson RT, Ilagan J, Cantor H, Schmits R, Mak TW (2002) Absence of the CD44 gene prevents sarcoma metastasis. Cancer Res 62:2281–2286

Wen W, Lu J, Zhang K, Chen S (2008) Grape seed extract inhibits angiogenesis via suppression of the vascular endothelial growth factor receptor signaling pathway. Cancer Prev Res (Phila) 1:554–561

Wu H, Liang X, Fang Y, Qin X, Zhang Y, Liu J (2008) Resveratrol inhibits hypoxia-induced metastasis potential enhancement by restricting hypoxia-induced factor-1 alpha expression in colon carcinoma cells. Biomed Pharmacother 62:613–621

Yao L, Liu F, Hong L, Sun L, Liang S, Wu K et al (2011) The function and mechanism of COX-2 in angiogenesis of gastric cancer cells. J Exp Clin Cancer Res 30:13

Yilmaz M, Christofori G (2010) Mechanisms of motility in metastasizing cells. Mol Cancer Res 8:629–642

Yu HB, Zhang HF, Zhang X, Li DY, Xue HZ, Pan CE et al (2010) Resveratrol inhibits VEGF expression of human hepatocellular carcinoma cells through a NF-kappa B-mediated mechanism. Hepatogastroenterology 57:1241–1246

Zhang XY, DeSalle LM, Patel JH, Capobianco AJ, Yu D, Thomas-Tikhonenko A et al (2005) Metastasis-associated protein 1 (MTA1) is an essential downstream effector of the c-MYC oncoprotein. Proc Natl Acad Sci U S A 102:13968–13973

Zhao HC, Qin R, Chen XX, Sheng X, Wu JF, Wang DB et al (2006) Microvessel density is a prognostic marker of human gastric cancer. World J Gastroenterol 12:7598–7603

Zheng Q, Tong M, Ou BQ, Liu CZ, Hu CP, Yang Y (2019) Isorhamnetin protects against bleomycin-induced pulmonary fibrosis by inhibiting endoplasmic reticulum stress and epithelial-mesenchymal transition. Int J Mol Med 43:117–126

Zhou W, Liu ZM, Wang M, Chen DY, Zhou L, Guo L (2019) Taxifolin inhibits the development of scar cell carcinoma by inducing apoptosis, cell cycle arrest, and suppression of PI3K/AKT/mTOR pathway. J Buon 24:853–858

Zhu YC, Sun LN, Zhang HJ, Li Y, Lai ST (2017) Effects of isorhamnetin on protein expression of VEGF, MMP-2 and endostatin in Lewis lung cancer mouse. Int J Clin Exp Med 10:11488–11495

Chapter 13
Punica granatum L. Constituents for Cancer Prevention, Chemosensitisation and Therapeutic Treatment

Julio César Rodríguez González, René Delgado Hernández, and Wim Vanden Berghe

Abstract Cancer is still a major public health burden because its incidence and mortality continue to increase worldwide. The limited treatment options for patients with advanced stages, the severe toxicity, the onset of multiple drug resistance and the high costs of current anticancer therapies favor poor prognosis and high mortality rates. Thus, the identification and development of preventive and cost effective therapeutic strategies to reverse cancer-associated morbidity and mortality are needed. Vegetable and fruit consumption is associated with decreased risk of cancer because of its chemopreventive and chemotherapeutic effects. The use of *Punica granatum* preparations has a long ethnomedical history and preclinical research has reported many pharmacological activities, including chemopreventive, chemosensitisation and chemotherapeutic effects. Many of these health beneficial effects are related to its complex chemical composition and synergistic interactions of its colonic microbial metabolites including ellagic acid, ellagitannins, punicic acid, flavonoids, anthocyanidins, anthocyanins, and estrogenic flavonols. This chapter summarizes the scientific evidence supporting anticancer effects of pomegranate constituents, focusing on its molecular targets and anticancer mechanisms of action, along with a critical evaluation of pomegranate polyphenols as future anticancer agents.

J. C. Rodríguez González
Genotoxicology and Antitumor Research Laboratory, Center for Pharmaceutical Research and Development (CIDEM), BioCubaFarma, Havana, Cuba
e-mail: jcesar.rodriguez@cidem.cu

R. Delgado Hernández
Center for Research and Drug Biological Evaluation, Institute of Food and Pharmacy, University Havana, Havana, Cuba
e-mail: rdelgado@infomed.sld.cu

W. Vanden Berghe (✉)
Laboratory of Protein Chemistry, Proteomics and Epigenetic Signaling (PPES), Department of Biomedical Sciences, University of Antwerp (UA), Antwerp, Belgium
e-mail: Wim.vandenberghe@uantwerpen.be

J. M. Pezzuto, O. Vang (eds.), *Natural Products for Cancer Chemoprevention*,
https://doi.org/10.1007/978-3-030-39855-2_13

Keywords Pomegranate · *Punica granatum* L. · Natural product · Polyphenols · Cancer · Chemoprevention · Chemotherapeutic

Abbreviations

[B(a)P]	benzo(a)pyrene
27HC	27-hydroxycholesterol
5-FU	5-fluorouracil
8-OHdG	8-hydroxy-2-deoxyguanosine
AA	Arachidonic acid
ACF	Aberrant cryptic foci
ADR	Adriamycin
AKT	Serine-threonine kinase B
ALDH	Aldehyde dehydrogenase
AOM	Azoxymethane
APC	Adenomatous polyposis coli
Bax	Bcl-2 associated X protein
BCa	Breast cancer
Bcl-2	Protein B Cell Lymphoma-2
Bcl-xL	B cell lymphoma-extralarge
BCR	Biochemical recurrent
BIP/GRP78	Binding-immunoglobulin protein
CASP	Caspase
CDDP	Cisplatin
Cdk	Cyclin-dependent kinase
c-MYC	v-myc avian myelocytomatosis viral oncogene homolog
COX-2	Cyclooxygenase 2
CP	Cyclophosphamide
CRC	Colorectal cancer
CSCs	Cancer stem cells
CXCL	C-X-C motif chemokine ligand
CXCR4	Chemokine receptor 4
CYP	Cytochrome P450
CYP1A1	Cytochrome P450 1A1
CYP1B1	Cytochrome P450 1B1
DENA	Diethylnitrosamine
DMBA	7,12-dimethylbenz[a]anthracene
DMH	1,2-dimethylhydrazine dihydrochloride
DSB	DNA double strand break
DTX	Docetaxel
E2	Estradiol
EA	Ellagic acid
ERE	Estrogen response elements
ERK	Extracellular signal-regulated kinase

ERS	Endoplasmic reticulum stress
ER-α	Estrogen receptor alpha
ER-β	Estrogen receptor beta
ETs	Ellagitannins
FGF	Fibroblast growth factor
G-CSF	Granulocyte colony-stimulating factor
GST	Glutathione S-transferase
HBMEC	Human brain microvascular endothelial cells
HGF	Hepatocyte growth factor
HIF-1α	Hypoxia inducible factor 1 alpha
HMMR	Hyaluronan-mediated motility receptor
HO	Heme oxygenasse
HR	Homologous recombination
ICAM1	Intercellular adhesion molecule 1
IFO	Ifosfamide
IGF-1	Insulin-like growth factor-1
IGFBP7	Insulin-like growth factor binding protein 7
IKKα	Inhibitor of NF-κB kinase subunit-α
IL-15	Interleukin 15
INPP5	Inositol polyphosphate-5-phosphatase
IκBα	Inhibitor of κB-α
JNK	c-Jun N-terminal kinases
LC3-II	Microtubule-associated protein light chain 3
LDH	Lactate dehydrogenase
LOX	Lipoxygenase
MAPKs	Mitogen-activated protein kinases
MARCKS	Myristoylated alanine-rich protein kinase C
MCP-1	Monocyte chemoattractant protein-1
MIF	Migration inhibitory factor
MIP-1α	Macrophage inflammatory proteins 1 alpha
miRNAs	Microribonucleic acids
MM	Multiple myeloma
MMPs	Metalloproteinases
MnSOD	Manganese superoxide dismutase
mTOR	Mammalian target of rapamycin
MTX	Methotrexate
NF-κB	Nuclear factor kappa B
NO	Nitric oxide
NOS2	Nitric oxide synthase 2
NQO1	NAD(P)H: quinone oxido-reductase 1
Nrf2	Hepatic nuclear factor E2-related factor 2
NTCU	*N*-nitroso-trischloroethylurea
ODC	Ornithine decarboxylase
OPG	Osteoprotegerin

p70S6	Phosphorylated ribosomal protein S6
PARP	Poly-ADP-ribose polymerases
PC	Punicalagin
PCa	Prostate cancer
PCNA	Proliferating cell nuclear antigen
Pes	Pomegranate extracts
PFE	Pomegranate fruit extract
PFJ	Pomegranate fermented juice
PGE2	Prostaglandin E2
PgLE	Punica granatum leaves extract
PI3K	Phosphoinositide 3-kinase
PJ	Pomegranate juice
PJEs	Pomegranate juice extracts
PKC	Protein kinase C
PLA2	Phospholipase A2
PPAR	Peroxisome proliferator-activated receptor
PPE	Pomegranate peel extract
PR	Progesterone receptor
PSA	Prostatic antigen
PSADT	PSA doubling time
PSO	Pomegranate seed oil
PuA	Punicic acid
RA	Retinoic acid
ROS	Reactive oxygen species
SA-β-Gal	Senescence-associated β-galactosidase
SHBG	Sex hormone binding globulin
Sp	Specificity protein
STAT3	Signal transducer and activator of transcription 3
TAM	Tamoxifen
TCa	Thyroid cancer
TCF4/LEF1	T cell factor/lymphoid enhancer binding protein
TGF	Transforming growth factor
TIMPs	Tissue inhibitors of metalloproteinase
TNF-α	Tumor necrosis factor alpha
TPA	12-*O*-tetradecanoylphorbol-13-acetate
TRAMP	Transgenic adenocarcinoma mouse prostate
UBUC	Urinary bladder urothelial carcinoma
UDP	Uridine diphosphate
UGT	Glucuronosyl-transferase
Uro-A	Urolithin A
Uro-B	Urolithin B
Uro-C	Urolithin C
VCAM-1	Vascular cell adhesion molecule 1
VEGF	Vascular endothelial growth factor

13.1 Introduction

Today, cancer has become a major public health burden because its incidence and mortality continue to increase worldwide (Torre et al. 2015; Siegel et al. 2016). It is estimated that there will be virtually 20 million cancer patients by the year 2025 (Siegel et al. 2016), and by 2030 the number of new cancer cases will increase by 70% worldwide due to demographic changes and environmental risk factors (Siegel et al. 2011). The limited availability of effective diagnostic tools for early detection of several tumors, the limited treatment options for patients with advanced stages and the onset of multiple drug resistance result in poor prognosis and high mortality rates. The limited therapeutic improvement of survival, the severe toxicity profile, and the high costs of many current anticancer therapies clearly show the urgent need of novel innovative, preventive as well as therapeutic strategies to reduce cancer-associated morbidity and mortality.

Cancer is a genomic and epigenetic disease associated with multiple risk factors and is widely accepted as a lifestyle disease (Weinberg and Robert 2011; Pogribny and Rusyn 2013). Therefore, prevention strategies have also been gaining importance as an effective strategy for the management of cancer since two-thirds of cancer-related deaths may be prevented through lifestyle variation, mostly through dietary means (Khan et al. 2010; Key et al. 2004; Barnard 2004; Anand et al. 2008; DiMarco-Crook and Xiao 2015). Several medicinal systems support consumption of vegetables to prevent/treat diseases, hence, creating awareness of the potential of phytochemicals as promising cancer chemopreventive/chemotherapeutic drugs. Currently, over half of the anticancer drugs used today are derived from natural resources (Newman and Cragg 2007). Various medicinal plants are becoming increasingly popular among medical science researchers for characterization of novel anticancer drug lead compounds to treat proliferation and metastasis of cancer cells (Huang et al. 2010). However, the pathways through which various anticancer phytochemicals act on neoplastic cells remain poorly characterized.

One popular hypothesis that involves oxidative stress as an inducer of various cancer, has led to the application of antioxidant therapy for prevention and cure of cancer (Valko et al. 2006; Khan et al. 2008). Research databases have concluded that the incidence of cancer progression is low in persons that daily consume a diet rich antioxidants contained in fruits and vegetables, and have revealed that some of the dietary forms are associated with low risk of cancer (Liu 2003; Boeing et al. 2012; Van Ryswyk et al. 2016). Thus, it is clear that natural products can serve as potential source of lead compounds that show direct anticancer properties, augment conventional anticancer therapeutic responses, possess low toxicity and generally target multiple signaling pathways (DiMarco-Crook and Xiao 2015; Khan et al. 2008; Gordaliza 2007).

In the last two decades, *Punica granatum* L. preparations have received growing interest as a nutraceutical or dietary supplement, including multi-component herbal formulations for cancer prevention and treatment. In the current review, we summarize scientific evidence for human health beneficial effects, molecular targets, and mechanisms of action of *Punica granatum* L. extracts and its major bioactive constituents as potential dietary agents in cancer prevention and treatment.

13.2 *Punica granatum* L.

Punica granatum L. (pomegranate) is a fruit-bearing deciduous shrub that belongs to the *Punicaceae* family, and with a unique biochemistry since the seeds contain a rare *trans* 18 carbon fatty acid (punicic acid, PuA), specific of genus *Punica* (Lansky and Newman 2007; Longtin 2003; Jurenka 2008; Bhandari 2012; Faria and Calhau 2011). Also, it is one of the only plants in nature known to contain in its seed oil the highest botanical concentration of the sex steroid estrone (Bhandari 2012; Faria and Calhau 2011). The pomegranate has been cultivated in many parts of the world since it grows in a wide range of climatic conditions and different soils. It is native from the Himalayas to Iran but has been naturalized over the entire Mediterranean region. It is also found in Middle East, Southeast Asia, China, Japan, Russia, tropical Africa, drier regions of the United States, and in tropical and subtropical regions of Latin America (Jurenka 2008; Bhandari 2012; Faria and Calhau 2011; Shaygannia et al. 2016).

The pomegranate contains high amounts of seeds (arils) separated by white and membranous pericarp, and each is surrounded by small amounts of a translucent tart red juice-containing sac. Thus, the fruit itself gives rise to three parts: the seeds, about 3% of the weight of the fruit, containing about 20% oil; the juice, accounting for approximately 30% total fruit weight; and pericarp, including skin and inner membranous walls, accounting for approximately 67% total fruit weight (Lansky and Newman 2007; Longtin 2003; Jurenka 2008; Bhandari 2012; Faria and Calhau 2011; Shaygannia et al. 2016; Rahimi et al. 2012).

Punica granatum L. has a long ethnomedical tradition and represents a phytochemical reservoir of heuristic medicinal value. Pomegranate has been described as nature's power fruit for its pleasant taste and excellent health benefiting properties (Lansky and Newman 2007; Longtin 2003). Interestingly, its remedial purposes and nutraceutical properties are not limited to its edible part. In fact, the non-edible fractions of fruit and tree, although considered as waste, contain even higher amounts of nutritionally valuable and biologically active components (Akhtar et al. 2015; Orgil et al. 2014). Pomegranate has been used in medical Ayurvedic system, which regards pomegranate as a 'pharmacy unto itself', and the Unani system of medicine for treatment of dysentery, diarrhea, helminthiasis, acidosis, hemorrhage, aphthae, gallbladder diseases, ulcers, respiratory pathologies, cholera, stomach disorders, and several other uses (Jurenka 2008; Shaygannia et al. 2016; Arun and Singh 2012; Viuda-Martos et al. 2010; Lansky et al. 1997). Fresh or dried root bark or ethanol extracts of pomegranate are used to remove intestinal parasites due to the alkaloid substances (Jurenka 2008; Bhandari 2012; Faria and Calhau 2011). In traditional Cuban medicine, pomegranate fruits have been used to treat acidosis, dysentery, microbial infections, diarrhea, helminthiasis, hemorrhage and respiratory pathologies (Roig 1974; Seoane 1984; Fuentes and Expósito 1995).

Over the last two decades, investigations have laid a scientific basis for some of pomegranate ethnomedical uses (Lansky and Newman 2007; Longtin 2003; Jurenka 2008; Bhandari 2012; Faria and Calhau 2011; Shaygannia et al. 2016). All parts of the *Punica granatum* L. have been shown to possess preventive and attenuating activities that suggest therapeutic activity against numerous chronic and health/life threatening maladies. Several pharmacological effects have been reported such as antimicrobial and antiparasitic, antidiarrhoeal, free radical scavenging and antioxidant capability, anti-inflammatory, antinociceptive, immunostimulant, antimutagenic, antitumorigenic and anticancer, antiulcer, hepatoprotective, nephroprotective, neuroprotective, cardioprotective, dermoprotective, wound healing, antiaging, anti-urolithiatic, estrogenic activity, and several others. Also, it is effective in prevention and treatment of osteoporosis, osteoarthritis, erectile dysfunction, male infertility, neonatal hypoxic-ischemic brain injury, Alzheimer's disease, inflammatory dental conditions, help to decrease the anemic symptoms; and many other uses (Lansky and Newman 2007; Jurenka 2008; Bhandari 2012; Faria and Calhau 2011; Shaygannia et al. 2016; Arun and Singh 2012; Viuda-Martos et al. 2010; Lansky et al. 1997). The numerous reported functional properties and healthy profits of pomegranate make it a unique fruit (Lansky and Newman 2007) to include in the diet (2013).

The wide range of health-promoting biological activities of pomegranate are related to the synergistic presence of a unique and complex phytochemical composition (Table 13.1) (Seeram et al. 2005; Lansky et al. 2005a, b; Nainwani et al. 2013; Prakash and Prakash 2011). The major source of dietary pomegranate phytochemicals is the whole fruit. It is rich in polyphenols, mainly the flavonoids, anthocyanins, hydrolysable tannins, and organic acids alone and conjugated as esters of glucose, which account for 92% of the antioxidant activity of the whole fruit (Gil et al. 2000; Tezcan et al. 2009). More than 120 different phytochemicals can be found in pomegranate fruit (Akhtar et al. 2015). Nearly 50 phenolic compounds have been identified in pomegranate peel but, interestingly, pomegranate peel contains the most promising pool of phenolics, mainly those from hydrolysable tannins (Faria and Calhau 2011; Akhtar et al. 2015). Hydrolyzable tannins are divided into gallotannins and ellagitannins (ETs), since their hydrolysis yields gallic acid and ellagic acid (EA), respectively (Arapitsas 2012). Amongst ETs there is a unique group named gallagyl esters, such as the main hydrolyzable tannin known as punicalagin (PC) which is unique to promeganate (Nainwani et al. 2013; Prakash and Prakash 2011; Gil et al. 2000; Tezcan et al. 2009; Arapitsas 2012). The peel has the highest antioxidant activity, which is in line with its high content of polyphenols (Faria and Calhau 2011; Prakash and Prakash 2011; Gil et al. 2000; Tezcan et al. 2009). Pomegranate juice (PJ) was reported to be comprised of 85.4% water, 10.6% total sugars, 1.4% pectin, 0.2–1.0% polyphenols (Prakash and Prakash 2011). During the juice processing, the ETs are released into PJ in significant levels and they are the most antioxidants in the PJs (Prakash and Prakash 2011; Gil et al. 2000). PC is a major antioxidant polyphenol from PJ, however, whole PJ has more antioxidant

Table 13.1 *Punica granatum* L. parts and its chemical constituents

Plant component	Chemical constituents
Pomegranate fruit juice	*Anthocyanins*: delphinidin, cyanidin, and pelargonidin, all conjugated to glucose at −3 and −5 position *Ellagitannins*: punicalagin, punicallin, punicacortein, punigluconin, galloylpunicalin corilagin, casuarinin, gallagyldilacton, gallagic acid *Flavon-3-ols/flavonoids and their glycosides*: catechin, epicatechin, epigallocatechin gallate, querticin, rutin *Hydroxybezoic acids/Cyclitol carboxylic*: ellagic acid, gallic acid, quinic acid *Hydroxycinnamic acids*: caffeic acid, chlorogenic acid, *p*-coumaric acid *Organic acids*: ascorbic acid, citric acid, malic acid, tartaric acid, fumaric acid, succinic acid *Amino acids*: proline, valine, methionine, glutamic, aspartic acid *Sugars*: glucose, fructose, sucrose *Fatty acids*: conjugated linoleic acid, linoleic acid, punicic acid and eleostearic acid *Indoleamines*: tryptamine, serotonin, melatonin *Vitamins*: B complex like B_1 and B_2, C and E vitamins *Minerals*: particularly Fe, and Ca, Ce, Cl, Co, Cr, Cs, Cu, K, Mg, Mn, Mo, Na, Rb, Sc, Se, Sn, Sr, and Zn *Others*: coenzyme Q10, peptin, sterols, triterpenoids, α-tocopherol
Pomegranate pericarp (peel, rind)	*Anthocyanins*: delphinidin, cyanidin, and pelargonidin, all conjugated to glucose at −3 and −5 position *Ellagitannins*: punicallin, punicalagin, corilagin, casuarinin, gallagyldilacton, pedunculagin, tellimagrandin I, granatin A, granatin B, gallagic acid *Ellagitannin oligomers*: pomegraniins A (7, tetramer) and B (8, pentamer) (Gil et al. 2000) *Gallotannins* (condensed tannins or proanthocyanidins) *Flavon-3-ols/flavonoids and their glycosides*: catechin, epicatechin, epigallocatechin-3-gallate, quercetin, kaempferol and its derivatives, luteolin, rutin, naringin, naringenin *Hydroxybezoic acids/Cyclitol carboxylic*: gallic acid, ellagic acid, quinic acid, ferrulic acid *Hydroxycinnamic acids*: caffeic acid, chlorogenic acid, p-coumaric acid, cinnamic acid *Alkaloids*: pelletierine, isopelletierine methylpelletierine, pseudopelletierine *Minerals*: N, Ca, K, P, Mn, and Na *Others*: hydroxy protocatechuic acid, ferulic acid, ergot alkaloid, saponins, triterpenes potassium, and complex polysaccharides, pomegralignan (glucose ester of neolignan)
Pomegranate seed (oil, matrix)	*Oil* *Fatty acids*: omega-5 long chain polyunsaturated fatty acid (C18:3, *cis*-9, *trans*-11, *cis*-13 such as punicic acid), non-conjugated fatty acids (n-3): linolenic acid and linolenic acid isomers; and other fatty acids such as oleic acid, palmitic acid, stearic acid *Triterpenes*: ursolic acid, oleanolic acid *Tocopherols*: α-tocopherol, γ-tocopherol *Sterols*: cholesterol, stigmasterol, β-sitosterol, daucosterol,

(continued)

Table 13.1 (continued)

Plant component	Chemical constituents
	campesterol and coumestrol (phytoestrogen) *Steroids*: 17-α-estradiol, estrone, testosterone, estriol) *Cerebrosides* *Hydroxybezoic acids*: ellagic acid, 3,3′-Di-O-methylellagic acid, 3,3′.4′-Tri-O-methylellagic acid *Matrix* *Anthocyanins*: delphinidin-3-glucoside, cyanidin-3-glucoside, delphinidin-3,5-diglucoside, cyanidin-3,5-diglucoside, pelargonidin-3,5-diglucoside and pelargoni-din-3-glucoside (Tezcan et al. 2009) *Lignins/lignin Phenyl aliphatic glycosides derivatives*: coniferyl-9-*O*-[β-dapiofuranosyl(1 → 6)-*O*-β-*D*-glucopyranoside,sinapyl-9-*O*-[β-*D*-apiofuranosyl (1→6)-*O*-β-*D*-glucopyranoside, phenylethyl rutinoside, icariside D1 *Hydroxybenzoic/cinnamic acids*, *isoflavones* (genistein, daidzein), *proteins*, *vitamins*, *minerals*, *peptin*, *sugars* and *crude fibers* and fusion products of cell wall components
Pomegranate leaves	*Tannins*: punicalin and punicafolin *Flavone glycosides*: luteolin and apigenin (flavone with progestinic and anxiolytic properties) *Apophine alkaloids*: anonaine, roemerine, corydine, isocorydine *Minerals*: N, K, Ca, and Fe
Pomegranate flower	*Polyphenols*: gallic acid, ellagic acid and ethyl brevifolin-carboxylate *Coumarin derivatives* *Hydrolyzable tannin* (punicatannin C) *Triterpinoids*: ursolic acid, maslinic acid, oleanolic acid and asiatic acid
Pomegranate roots and bark	*Ellagitannins*: punicalin and punicalagin *Piperidine alkaloids*

Note: The compilation of the major chemical constituents from *Punica granatum* L. parts was obtained from the references (Gil et al. 2000; Lansky and Newman 2007; Longtin 2003; Jurenka 2008; Bhandari 2012; Faria and Calhau 2011; Shaygannia et al. 2016; Rahimi et al. 2012; Akhtar et al. 2015; Arun and Singh 2012; Viuda-Martos et al. 2010; Nainwani et al. 2013; Prakash and Prakash 2011; Arapitsas 2012; Ito et al. 2014; Sreekumar et al. 2014)

activity than any of its individual constituents (Prakash and Prakash 2011). Pomegranate seed oils are rich in fatty acids (over 95% of the oil), of which 99% are triacylglycerols (Lansky and Newman 2007; Longtin 2003; Jurenka 2008; Bhandari 2012; Faria and Calhau 2011). The oil consists of approximately 80% conjugate doctadecatrienoic fatty acids, with a high content of *cis* 9, *trans* 11, *cis* 13 acid, synthesized in situ from nonconjugated octadecadienoic fatty acid, linoleic acid.

Factors such as cultivars, environmental conditions, the fruit's stage of maturity, cultivation practice, storage and postharvest treatments, contribute to the chemical changes of *Punica granatum* L. components (Gil et al. 2000; Kalaycıoğlu and Bedia 2017). Also, the antioxidant capability is affected by the fruit development as the highest antioxidant activity was observed in newly formed fruits. Likewise, antioxidant activity varies among different varieties of pomegranate plant (Gil et al. 2000; Kalaycıoğlu and Bedia 2017). Some studies reported that the antioxidant activity of pomegranate extracts (PEs) surpasses that of vitamins, red wine, green tea, tomatoes and several fruits such as apples, blueberries, canberries, kiwi, grape, oranges and some others (Lansky and Newman 2007; Nainwani et al. 2013; Prakash and Prakash 2011).

Although the health benefits attributed to pomegranate have been associated with its high content antioxidant polyphenols, their bioavailability is however very low (Gil et al. 2000). It is well established that ETs and EA absorption is very low and that the unabsorbed compounds are further metabolized to urolithins, mainly urolithin A (Uro-A), urolithin B (Uro-B) and urolithin C (Uro-C) and EA metabolites, in conjugated and free forms, that are much better absorbed by the gut microbiota in the colon (Seeram et al. 2004, 2006; Cerdá et al. 2003, 2004, 2005; Tomás-Barberán et al. 2006; Mertens-Talcott et al. 2006). On the other hand, urolithins can reach systemic organs, with high levels accumulating in prostate, colon, gall bladder, urine bladder and other intestinal tissues (Espín et al. 2007; Seeram et al. 2007; González-Sarrías et al. 2010; Nuñez-Sánchez et al. 2014a). Also, urolithins circulate in plasma as glucuronide and sulfate conjugates at low concentrations (Espín et al. 2013). The poor bioavailability and the extensive gut catabolism suggest that urolithins rather than ETs or EA may be the actual bioactive molecules. It is therefore conceivable that the health effects of ETs-containing products can be associated with these gut-produced urolithins (Tomás-Barberán et al. 2006, 2009; Espín et al. 2013). It is important to emphasize that the metabolite profile strongly varies among subjects, probably due to differences in colonic microflora composition (Cerdá et al. 2003, 2004; Espín et al. 2007). This indicate that the health effects observed after the intake of pomegranates and other ETs-containing diet can be modulated by the occurrence of specific microbiota to produce urolithins (Selma et al. 2009).

13.3 Potential Anticancer Activities of *Punica granatum* L. Extracts and Its Chemical Constituents

A significant body of literature supports preclinical (Table 13.2) and clinical (Table 13.3) use of *Punica granatum* L. products for chemoprevention and treatment of cancer. Extensive mechanistic studies of its phytochemicals have demonstrated that the antioxidant capacity depends on their direct radical scavenging and iron chelation activity (Lansky and Newman 2007; Longtin 2003; Jurenka 2008; Bhandari 2012; Faria and Calhau 2011; Shaygannia et al. 2016; Rahimi et al. 2012; Akhtar et al. 2015; Orgil et al. 2014; Arun and Singh 2012; Viuda-Martos et al. 2010; Lansky et al. 1997). The well-known anti-inflammatory capacity represents another important feature of *Punica granatum* L. products to its chemopreventive and antitumor activities (Lansky and Newman 2007; Longtin 2003; Jurenka 2008; Bhandari 2012; Faria and Calhau 2011; Shaygannia et al. 2016; Rahimi et al. 2012; Akhtar et al. 2015; Orgil et al. 2014; Arun and Singh 2012; Viuda-Martos

Table 13.2 Preventive and therapeutic anticancer activity of *Punica granatum* L. forms and its bioactive chemical compounds

Cancer type	*Punica g.* form and its chemical compounds	Cancer model	Effect	Molecular mechanism(s)/cellular target(s)	References
Prostate	Pomegranate juice extract and ellagic acid	In vivo TRAMP model Cancer cell lines	Antiproliferative and antimetastatic. Inhibition of doubling the overall survival time. Inhibition of PSA, T, DHT, DHEA, androstenedione, androsterone, pregnenolone	Inhibition of PI3K/AKT/mTOR and IGF-1)/AKT/mTOR pathways	Adhami et al. (2012)
		LNCaP, PC3, DU145 and TRAMP model	Reduction of serum steroids levels Decrease in lipid peroxidation levels Suppress of prostate carcino-genesis and induced apoptosis	Increase of cdk2, p21, p27, cyclin E Decrease of cdk1 and cyclin D1 Increase Bax/(Bcl-2) ratio and CASP-3 activation	Naiki-Ito et al. (2015)
	Punica granatum extracts and ellagic acid, caffeic acid, luteolin, and punicic acid (alone or in combination)	Subcutaneous and orthotopic xenograft in vivo mice models LNCaP, CWR22Rv PC3, DU145, LAPC4	Antiproliferative (G1-phase arrest). Pro-apoptotic Antiangiogenic Antimetastatic (inhibition of chemotaxis processes and cell migration) Anti-invasive	Modulation of cdk by upregulation of p21 and p27, cyclin D1, 2, cyclin E, cdk2, cdk4, and cdk6, PARP, inhibition of Bcl-2. Increase of cleaved of PARP and Bax. Decrease of Bcl-2PLA2/AA/PGE2/PI3K/AKT pathway, COX-2, LOX, HMMR and modulation of hyaluronan signaling pathway, CXCL2, CXCR4 and CXCL12/CXCR4, Gα 13, PI3K, and p-AKT Downregulation of type I collagen, tenascin C, and chimerin 1. Upregulation of E-cadherin, ICAM1, MARCKS, anti-invasive miRNAs, COL1A1. Downregulation of pro-invasive miRNAs and MARCKS. Downregulation of MMPs-1-2-3-7-9 and upregulation TIMPs	Lansky et al. (2005a), Lansky et al. (2005b) Albrecht et al. (2004) Malik et al. (2005) Rettig et al. (2008) Wang and Martins-Green (2014) Deng et al. (2017)

(continued)

Table 13.2 (continued)

Cancer type	*Punica g.* form and its chemical compounds	Cancer model	Effect	Molecular mechanism(s)/cellular target(s)	References
	Pomegranate extracts and juice	LNCaP-AR cells overexpressing the androgen receptor	Anti-androgenic	Downregulation of 3β-hydroxysteroid dehydrogenase type II and steroid 5α reductase type I. Downregulation of androgen receptor	Hong et al. (2008)
	Ethanolic pomegranate extract	In vitro and in vivo cancer murine knockout model (PTEN)	Tumor growth inhibition. Reduction of production of T, DHT, DHEA, and pregnenolone. Inhibition of the expression and serum levels of PSA		Ming et al. (2014)
	Pomegranate extract	Metastatic castration-resistant prostate cancer cells (C4–2, PC3 and ARCaPM) C4–2-induced skeletal metastases in athymic nude mice. PC3 cell-transplanted BALB/c nu/nu mice. LAPC4 cell-transplanted in severe combined immuno-deficient mice (SCID)	Antiproliferative. Enhances the in vivo efficacy of docetaxel	Reduction of survivin protein and gene expression, and modulate survivin pathway by STAT3 phosphorylation inhibition, inactivation of STAT3-dependent transcription of survivin	Wang et al. (2014)
	Pomegranate extract	LAPC4 tumor and normal endothelial HUVEC cell lines. LAPC4 cell-xeno-transplanted SCID mice	Antiproliferative, pro-apoptotic and anti-angiogenic. Retarded the growth of LAPC4 androgen-independent tumor and microvessel density	Inhibition of NF-κB. Downregulation of VEGF and HIF-1α expression and protein levels	Rettig et al. (2008), Sartippour et al. (2008)
	Pomegranate fruit juice	DU145 cells	Anti-angiogenic	Downregulation of prolidase gene expression	(Lee et al. (2012)

	Ellagic acid	LNCaP cell line	Antiproliferative and differentiating Anti-angiogenic	Decrease of VEGF, FGF, G-CSF, HGF, IL-15. Inhibits the expression of CYP450 epoxygenases isoforms (CYP2J2, CYP4F2 and CYPA22), epoxydation of AA and its hydroxylation with the subsequent inhibition of CYP450-derived eicosanoids	Vanella et al. (2013a), Vanella et al. (2013b)
	Ellagic acid	Japanese prostate cancer patients with bone metastasis	Anti-angiogenic and antimetastatic with reduction of bone metastatic spread	Decrease serum levels of OPG and the expressions of HO-1 and HO-2	Kamiya et al. (2011)
	Punicalagin.	PC3 and LNCaP cells Normal BPH-1 cells	Antiproliferative, pro-apoptotic and antiangiogenic. Antitumor specific action	Increase in expression of CASP-3 and -8 (in PC3 cells)	Adaramoye et al. (2017)
	β-sitosterol	LNCaP cells	Antiproliferative and pro-apoptotic	Activation of sphingomyelin cycle	von Holtz et al. (1998)
			Antiproliferative (arrest cells at G2/M phse) Pro-apoptotic	Antimitotic mechanism (affect tubulin microtubule assembly). Inhibition of Bcl-2 and PI3K/Akt signaling pathways	Moon et al. (2008)
	γ-Tocopherol	Prostate cancer cells Normal prostate epithelial cell	Antiproliferative. Antitumor specific action	Inhibition of sphingolipid synthesis de novo Inhibited COX activity in macrophages and epithelial cells	Jiang et al. (2004), Kasimsetty et al. (2009)
	Urolithins (Uro-A and Uro-B).	22Rv1 prostate cancer cells	Anticarcinogenic	Inhibition CYP1B1 and CYP1A1 activities. Inhibition of CYP1B1 expression	Paller et al. (2017)
Breast	Pomegranate fermented juice, pericarp and oil polyphenols	7,12-dimethylbenz-[a]-anthracene (DMBA)-induced mammary carcinogenesis model	Anticarcinogenic	Inhibition of endogenous active estrogen biosynthesis with subsequent inhibition of aromatase activity	Mehta and Lansky (2004)
	Pomegranate and its constituents		Anticarcinogenic Pro-apoptotic Anti-angiogenic (ellagic acid)	Inhibition of COX, decrease of PGE2 and downregulation of aromatase expression (anti-oestrogenic mechanisms)	Sturgeon and Ronnenberg (2010)
	Pomegranate emulsion formulation from the whole fruit	DMBA-induced mammary tumorigenesis	Anticarcinogenic Antiporliferative Pro-apoptotic	Upregulation of Bax, downregulation of Bcl-2, intratumor ER-α and ER-β expressions and lower ER-α: ER-β ratio. Decrease the expression,	Bishayee et al. (2016), Mandal and

(continued)

Table 13.2 (continued)

Cancer type	*Punica g.* form and its chemical compounds	Cancer model	Effect	Molecular mechanism(s)/cellular target(s)	References
				cytoplasmic accumulation, and nuclear translocation of β-catenin. Suppression the expression of cyclin D1	Bishayee (2015)
	Pomegranate constitu-ents, fermented juice and peel extracts	HUVEC, MCF-10A and MCF-7, MDA-MB-231 cells Chicken chorioallan-toic membrane	Anti-angiogenic Antimigration Antimetastatic	Downregulation of VEGF and PPAR. Upregulation of MIF	Toi et al. (2003) Dana et al. (2016)
	Polyphenols from fermented and fresh pomegranate juice Pomegranate seed oil	ER^+-MCF-7, ER^--MDA-MB-231, MDA-MB-435 human tumor and normal human breast MCF-10A cell lines	Antiproliferative Anti-invasive Anti-angiogenic	Retard prostaglandin synthesis Modulation of Bcl-2 proteins, upregulation of p27 and p21, and downregulation of cyclin-cdk network	Kim et al. (2002) Jeune et al. (2005) Bhandari (2012)
	Aqueous methanol extract of pomegranate seed oil (rich in punicic acid and its congeners)	MCF-7 and MDA-MB-231 cells	Antiproliferative and cytotoxic (cell cycle arrest at G0/G1 phase) Anti-inflammatory Anti-oxidant	Decreased the levels of VEGF and pro-inflammatory cytokines (IL-2, IL-6, IL-12, IL-17, CXCL10, MIP-1α (or CCL3), MIP-1β, MCP-1 and TNF-α. Inactivation of NF-κB and STAT1, and modulation of NOS2 and NO production	Costantini et al. (2014)
	Ellagic acid	MCF-7 cells	Antiproliferative (cell cycle arrest at G0/G1 phase)	Modulation of TGF-β)/SMAD proteins signaling pathway	Chen et al. (2015)
	Ellagitannin-derived compounds		Antiproliferative Anti-aromatase activity		Adams et al. (2010)
	Pomegranate seed linolenic acid isomers (punicic acid and α-eleostearic acid)	MCF-7 and MDA-MB-231 cells	Antiproliferative Anti-estrogenic specific effects	Selective ER modulators	Tran et al. (2010)
	Pomegranate juice or combinations of its com-ponents (luteolin, ellagic acid and punicic acid)	MCF-7 and MDA-MB-231 cells	Antimetastatic specific action (increase cancer cell adhesion and decrease cancer cell	Inhibition of CXCL-12. Inhibition of pro-inflammatory cytokines/chemokines	Rocha et al. (2012)

			migration and chemotaxis. Inhibition of epithelial-to-meshenchymal transitions		
	Methanolic extract of pomegranate pericarp	MCF-7 cells	Antiproliferative by anti-estrogenicity selectivity action without being agonistic in the uterine endometrium	Decrease pS2 protein levels and downregulation of ERE-mediated transcription	Sreeja et al. (2012)
	Pomegranate extract	MCF-7 cells	Antiproliferative (cell cycle arrest at G2/M) Pro-apoptotic	Downregulation of genes associated with mitosis, chromosome organization, RNA processing, DNA replication and DNA repair: DSB repair by HR. Increase levels of miR-183 and miR-24 Upregulation of genes involved in regulation of apoptosis and cell proliferation	Banerjee et al. (2012)
	Pomegranate extract	BT-474 and MDA-MB-231 cells Non-cancer MCF-10F and MCF-12F cells Subcutaneous and xenograft with BT474 cells in nude mice	Antiproliferative specific antitumor effect Anti-inflammatory	Decrease Sp1, Sp3, and Sp4 and miR-27a, miRNA-155, and inhibition of PI3K-dependent phosphorylation of AKT. Increase expression of the transcriptional repressor *ZBTB10* and *INPP5* expression. Overall, disruption of both miR-27a-ZBTB10 and miR-155-INPP5	Dai et al. (2010)
	Pomegranate extract (Pomella) and its phytochemicals: ellagic acid, ursolic acid and luteolin	WA4 cells (cancer stem cells characteristics)	Antiproliferative (cell cycle arresting at G0/G1 phase) Proapoptotic	Induction through CASP-3 activity	Larrosa et al. (2006a)
	Pomegranate ellagitannin-derived compounds and urolithins A and B	MCF-7aro (overexpress aromatase)	Antiproliferative	Anti-aromatase activity	Van Elswijk et al. (2004)
	Pomegranate components: luteolin, kaempferol, quercetin, and naringenin			Anti-estrogenic activity	Qasim et al. (2013)

(continued)

Table 13.2 (continued)

Cancer type	*Punica g.* form and its chemical compounds	Cancer model	Effect	Molecular mechanism(s)/cellular target(s)	References
Colorectal	Ellagitannin-rich fruit extracts, urolitinins, and ellagic acid	293 T cell line with luciferase reporter of Wnt pathway-mediated transcriptional activation		Inhibition Wnt signalling pathway	Sharma et al. (2010)
	Standardized pomegranate extract, urolitinin-A, and ellagic acid	1,2-dimethylhydrazine dihydrochloride (DMH)-induced male Wistar albino rat colon carcinogenesis model	Anticarcinogenic (Inhibition of tumor incidence and minimise all the aberrant alterations DMH-induced in colon tissues) Normalization of survival rate and a reduction of serum tumour marker carcinoembryonic antigen level	Modulate the expression pattern of the main key players in Wnt signalling: down-regulation of *Wnt5a*, frizzled receptor *(FRZ)-8*, *β-catenin*, T cell factor/lymphoid enhancer binding protein (*TCF4/LEF1*), *c-myc* and *cyclin D1* and up-regulation of adenomatous polyposis coli (APC) and axin1	Sadik and Shaker (2013)
	Pomegranate juice derived ellagitannins (punicalagin and ellagic acid), and urolithins	HT-29 human tumor cells	Antiproliferative (cell-cycle arrest by a block in S phase by ET, and cell-cycle block in G2/M phase by urolithins Anticlonogenic Pro-apoptotic by a selective action	Apoptotic intrinsic pathway by activation of CASP-3, -9, release of cytochrome c, and the downregulation of Bcl-xL (PC and EA). Ellagitannins promote downregulation of cyclins A and B1, with activation of cyclin E. Urolithins modulate the MAPKs	Kasimsetty et al. (2010)
	Pomegranate juice	Colon carcinogenesis induced by azoxymethane (AOM) in to F344 rats	Anticarcinogenic (reduction of the number of ACF and large crypts). Increase in weight gain and feed intake (anticachexia) Anti-oxidantive	Increase GST levels	Boateng et al. (2007)
	Pomegranate juice	In vivo model of AOM-treated male Sprague-Dawley rats	Anticarcinogenic (suppresse the number of ACF) Anti-inflammatory	Down-regulation of mRNA and protein expressions of iNOS, COX-2, IGF, NF-κB and VCAM-1. Inhibition of PI3K/AKT activation and mTOR	Banerjee et al. (2013)

				expression and increased the expression of miR-126 and targeting miR-126-regulated pathways	
	Pomegranate seed oil extract	Colon carcinogenesis induced by AOM in F344 rats	Anticarcinogenic		Kohno et al. (2004)
	Pomegranate peel extract	AOM-induced oxidative stress and carcinogenesis in male Sprague-Dawley rat colon	Antioxidant activity Anticarcinogenic	Down-regulation of myeloperoxidase and up-regulation of GSH/GSSC ratio, total antioxidant concentration and antioxidant enzymes activity	Waly et al. (2012, 2014)
	Pomegranate juice and its constituents (total pomegranate tannin extract, ellagic acid, and punicalagin)	In vitro cell lines (HT29, HCT116, SW460 and SW620)	Antiproliferative Pro-apoptotic		Seeram et al. (2005)
	Pomegranate juice and its components	HT-29 cell line	Anti-inflammatory	Suppress the TNFα-induced COX-2 protein expression, and downregulated the TNFα-induced AKT activation required for NF-κB activity, and inhibited phosphorylation and binding of the p65 subunit to the NF-κB response element	Adams et al. (2006)
	Punicalagin and ellagic acid	Caco-2 cell line	Antiproliferative (EA arrest the cell cycle in S phase) Pro-apoptotic	Downregulation of cyclins A and B1 and upregulation of cyclin E Bcl-XL downregulation, mitochondrial release of cytochrome c, and activation of initiator CASP-9 and effector CASP-3	Larrosa et al. (2006b)
	Pomegranate peel extracts	HCT-116 cells	Anti-proliferative Anti-oxidantive		Campbell et al. (2006)
	γ-tocopherol	Human colon cancer cell lines		Reduction levels of C-reactive protein, inhibition of neoplastic transformation, suppression of ras p-21, inhibition of COX-2 activity, down-regulation of cyclins, and upregulation of PPAR –γ	Nuñez-Sánchez et al. (2016)
	Urolithins and ellagic acid in two different mixture	Models of colon cancer stem cells: Caco-2 cells and primary tumour cells from a patient with CRC	Inhibited the number and size of colonospheres	Inhibit phenotypic and molecular colon cancer stem cell features Inhibition of ALDH activity	Nuñez-Sánchez et al. (2014b)
Lung	Pomegranate fruit extract	Non-small lung cell carcinoma (NSLC) human	Antiproliferative (cell cycle arrest at G0/G1	Upregulation of p21 (WAF1/CIP1) and cdk inhibitor 1B (KIP1/p27)	Khan et al. (2007a)

(continued)

Table 13.2 (continued)

Cancer type	*Punica g.* form and its chemical compounds	Cancer model	Effect	Molecular mechanism(s)/cellular target(s)	References
		cells A549 Normal human bronchial epithelial cells Athymic mice xenotransplanted with A549 cells	phase) specific effect Prolongs the latency period for tumor appearance	Downregulation of the expression cyclins D1, D2, and E, and cdk2, cdk4, and cdk6 Downregulation of Ki-67, PCNA. Inhibition of MAPK, PI3K/AKT, and NF-κB/p65	
	Pomegranate fruit extract	Mouse lung tumor induced by benzo(a) pyrene [B(a)P] N-nitroso-trischloro-ethyl-urea (NTCU) mouse lung tumor induced by in A/J mice	Anticarcinogenic	Inhibition of NF-κB, MAPK, Ki-67, PCNA, VGEF, PI3K/AKT signaling, and mTOR phosphorylation	Khan et al. (2007b)
	Methanolic extract of pomegranate peel Punicalagin and ellagic acid	A459 cells	Antiproliferative		Modaeinama et al. (2015)
	Punicalagin and ellagic acid	Ames Salmonella assay B(a)P induced DNA adducts in mice A459 and H1299 lung cancer cells	Antimutagenic against mutagens and promutagens Anticarcinogenic Antiproliferative		Zahin et al. (2014)
	Pomegranate seed ethanolic extract	Lung large cell carci-noma COR-L23	Antiproliferative		Lucci et al. (2015)
	Methanolic extract of seeds	A549 cells	Antiproliferative		Seidi et al. (2016)
	Punica granatum leaves extract	A459 and H1299 human lung cancer cells Mouse Lewis lung carci-noma cell line LL/2	Antiproliferative effect (cell cycle arrest at G2/M phase in H1299 cells) with high selectivity index	Decrease ROS production and the mitochondrial membrane potential (ΔYm) Reduction of MMP-2 and MMP-9 expression	Li et al. (2016a)

		HEK293, LO2 and Vero normal cells	Pro-apoptotic Antioxidant Antimigration and anti-invasive		
Skin	Pomegranate fruit extract	Human epidermal keratinocyte cells	Anticarcinogenic (inhibit the appearance of erythemas, hyperplasia)	Inhibition of solar UVB-induced phosphorylation of MAPK pathway signaling proteins (STAT3, ERK-1/2, JNK1/2, p38 protein and AKT1). Inhibition of UVB-dependent activation of NF-κB. Inhibition of ODC activity	Afaq et al. (2005a)
		Human skin fibroblasts	Protective	Inhibition of NF-κB activation, downregulation of CASP-3, and increase G0/G1phase associated with DNA repair. Decrease UV-induced ROS levels and increase intracellular antioxidant capacity	Lisbeth et al. (2008)
	Pomegranate fruit extract	Normal human epidermal keratinocytes	Photochemopreventive against UVA	Inhibited UVA-mediated phosphorylation of STAT3, AKT, ERK1/2, mTOR, p70S6K and NF-κB activation	Syed et al. (2006)
	Standardized pomegranate polyphenolic extract	Human skin fibroblasts	Photochemopreventive against ultraviolet light		Pacheco-Palencia et al. (2008)
	Polyphenols from pomegranate juice (anthocyanins and tannins) Pomegranate oil extract and its constituents	Human reconstituted skin (EpiDermTM FT-200)	Photochemopreventive (quench the effects of ultraviolet rays) and protective effect against UVB-mediated damage	Inhibition of protein oxidation and PCNA and metalloprotein like collagenase, gelatinase, stromelysin, marilysin, elastase and tropoelastin expressions. Inhibition UVB-induced expressions of MMP-2 and MMP-9 activity. Inhibition in the number of cyclobutane primidine dimers and 8-OHdG positive cells	Zaid et al. (2007)
	Pomegranate fruit extract	SKH-1-Elite-Hr hairless mice	Photochemopreventive. Inhibited UVB-induced skin edema, hyperplasia, infiltration of leukocytes	Inhibition of lipid peroxidation, hydrogen peroxide generation, ODC activity and expression, COX-2 and PCNA protein expression. Enhance repair of UVB-mediated formation of cyclobutane pyrimidine dimers and 8-oxo-7-OHdG, 8-OHdG. Enhanced UVB-mediated increase in tumor suppressor p53 and p21. Inhibition of UVB-mediated	Afaq et al. (2010)

(continued)

Table 13.2 (continued)

Cancer type	*Punica g.* form and its chemical compounds	Cancer model	Effect	Molecular mechanism(s)/cellular target(s)	References
				nuclear translocation of NF-κB, activation of IKKα, and phosphorylation and degradation of inhibitor of IκBα	
	Pomegranate fruit extract	12-*O*-tetra-decanoyl-phorbol-13-acetate (TPA)-induced skin-cancer	Chemopreventive (inhibition of skin edema and hyperplasia)	Inhibition of several markers of skin tumor promotion including, epidermal ODC activity and protein expression, and suppression of COX-2, MAPKs, NF-κB	Afaq et al. (2005b)
	Ellagic acid-rich pomegranate peel extract	Melanoma tumors	Photopreventive and growth suppression effects	Supression of tyrosinase activity and UV-induced pigmentation	Yoshimura et al. (2005)
	Pomegranate seed oil (rich in punicic acid)	CD1 mice	Chemopreventive	Inhibition of ODC, prostaglandin biosynthesis, inhibiting upstream eicosanoid enzyme, and PLA2	Hora et al. (2003)
	Pomegranate seed ethanolic extract (rich punic acid)	Human amelanotic melanoma C32 and malignant melanoma A375 cell lines	Antiproliferative		Lucci et al. (2015)
Liver	Pomegranate emulsion	Diethylnitrosamine (DENA)-induced rat hepatocarcinogenesis	Chemoprevention of hepato-carcinogenesis (reduces the number and area of γ-glutamyl transpeptidase positive hepatic foci Antioxidant activity Antiproliferative Pro-apoptotic Anti-inflammatory	Inhibition of DENA-induced hepatic lipid peroxidation and protein oxidation. Upregulation of the gene expression of hepatic antioxidants, carcinogen detoxifying enzymes: GST, NAD(P)H: quinone oxido-reductase 1 (NQO1), and uridine diphosphate (UDP)-glucuronosyl-transferase (UGT) and protein and mRNA expression of Nrf2. Upregulation of Bax and downregulation of Bcl-2. Decrease hepatic expressions of iNOS, 3-nitrotyrosine, HSP70 and HSP90, COX-2 and NF-κB	Bishayee et al. (2011, 2013)
	Pomegranate peel extract	DENA-induced rat hepatocarcinogenesis	Prophylactic effect against neoplastic changes in the liver by	Decrease liver index, Bcl-2 and the increase of GSH. Decrease expression of cyclin D1 and β-catenin gene	El-Ashmawy et al. (2016), Takigawa

			decrease of tumor size Anti-oxidant, antiproliferative, and pro-apoptotic		and Brown (2008)
	Pomegranate constituents		Anti-proliferative Pro-apoptotic	Inhibition of canonical NF-κB and Wnt/β-catenin pathways	Bhatia et al. (2013)
Pancreatic	Pomegranate whole-fruit extract and its chemical compounds	PANC-1 and AsPC-1 human pancreatic cancer cells	Antiproliferative Alteration of cell phenotype	Down-regulation of CD44 and CD24 expressions	Nair et al. (2011)
Leukemia	Pomegranate seed oil	Human monocytic leukemia cells			Suzuki et al. (2001)
	Flavonoid-rich polyphenols from fresh, fermented juice and aqueous extracts of pomegranate pericarp	Human promyelocytic leukemia HL-60 cells	Promote the cell differentiation Anti-proliferative		Kawaii and Lansky (2004)
	Ellagic acid and quercetin	Human leukemia cells	Anti-proliferative Pro-apoptotic		Mertens-Talcott and Percival (2005)
	Pomegranate juice extract	Lymphoid (Jurkat, MOLT-3, SUP-B15, and CCRF-CEM) and myeloid (HL-60, THP-1, K562, and KG1a) human leukemia cell lines and non-tumor hematopoietic stem cells	Anti-proliferative (cell cycle arrest at S phase in lymphoblastic cells and G0/G1 phase in myeloblastic cells). Pro-apoptotic Induction of senescence in myeloblastic cells		Dahlawi et al. (2012)
	Acetonitrile fraction of pomegranate juice extract (rich in ellagitannins and ellagic acid)	CCRF-CEM, MOLT-3, HL-60, and THP-1 lukemia cell lines	Anti-proliferative (block in S phase with a concomitant decrease of cells in G0/G1 phase in	Decrease ATP levels Induction of CASP-3	Dahlawi et al. (2013)

(continued)

Table 13.2 (continued)

Cancer type	*Punica g.* form and its chemical compounds	Cancer model	Effect	Molecular mechanism(s)/cellular target(s)	References
			all cell lines) Pro-apoptotic		
	Ellagic acid	Human promyelocytic leukemia HL-60 cells	Anti-proliferative (S phase cell-cycle arrest) Pro-apoptotic	Induction of CASP-3	Hagiwara et al. (2010)
	Crude pomegranate peels etanolic 80% v/v extract	Human chronic myeloid leukemia K562 cells	Anti-proliferative (cell cycle arrest at G2/M phase) Pro-apoptotic	Upregulation of Bax, Bcl-2, CASP-9, cytochrome c, p21 and p53 regulatory proteins	Asmaa et al. (2015)
Bladder and urothelial	Standardized pomegranate rind extract rich in polyphenols	EJ bladder tumor cells and normal rat urinary bladder epithelial cells EJ xenograft in Balb/c nude mice	Anti-proliferative Pro-apoptotic tumor specific action	Induction of CASP-3 and CASP-8 expresssions Inhibition of c-Jun, increase p53 protein expression, and enhance miR-34a expression mediated by p53 in pomegranate-induced apoptosis. miR-34a selectively suppresse the c-Myc and CD44	Zhou et al. (2015)
	Pomegranate ethanol extract	Urinary bladder urothelial carcinoma cells T24 and J82	Antiproliferative (cell cycle arrest at S phase) Pro-apoptotic	Increase cyclin A protein level and a decrease the expression of ckd1. Activation of pro-CASP-3, pro-CASP-8, pro-CASP-9 but also increase Bax/Bcl-2 ratio	Lee et al. (2013)
	Pomegranate fruit juice ethanol extract	T24 cells	Pro-apoptotic Antiproliferative Antimigration	Differential expression of 20 proteins (19 up-regulated and 1 down-regulated proteins) involved in apoptosis, cytoskeleton regulation, AKT/mTOR signaling, cell proliferation, proteasome activity and aerobic glycolysis. The antiproliferative effect is through restriction of PTEN/AKT/mTOR complex 1 pathway via profilin 1 up-regulation. The apoptosis through DIABLO overexpression and inhibition of cell migration	Wu et al. (2016)
	Pomegranate whole fruit and peel extracts (enriched in selected	T24 cells	Anti-oxidative Antiproliferative		Masci et al. (2016)

	polyphenols like ellagic acid and/or punicalagins)				
Brain	Punicalagin	U87MG glioma cells	Antiproliferative Proapoptotic Autophagic cell death	Increase cyclin E level and decrease cyclin B and cyclin A levels. Induction of cleavage of PARP, activation of CASP-9, and increase of CASP-3 and CASP-9 activities in the cells. Induction of autophagic mechanisms by increase the expression level of phosphor-AMPK and phosphor-p27 and increased LC3-II cleavage in the cells	Wang et al. (2013)
Fibro-sarcoma	Pomegranate ethanol extract	Mouse fibrosarcoma cell line WEHI-164	Antiproliferative Pro-apoptotic	Increase nucleosome production from apoptotic cells and decreases of pro-CASP-3 and Bcl-2 proteins	Sepehr et al. (2014)
Multiple myeloma	Polypenolic-rich extract from non-endible parts of *Punica granatum* L	Multiple myeloma cancer cells U266	Antiproliferative Pro-apoptotic	Increases in loss of mitochondrial membrane potential (leaves and stem extracts). The flower extract resulted in slight increases in loss of MMPs	Kiraz et al. (2016)
	Pomegranate juice	Human multiple myeloma cell lines (KMS26, MM1S and U266). Healthy lymphocytes and monocytes. Human brain microvascular endothelial cells (HBMEC). Microvessel outgrowth in ex vivo rabbit aorting ring assay	Antiproliferative tumor specific effect (cell cycle arrest at G0/G1) Antiproliferative Anti-angiogenic	Up-regulation of PPAR-γ Inhibition of VEGF-A induced tube formation, both tube length and number of branch Obstruction of new vessel sprouting of endothelial tubes from aorta rings induced by VEGF and VEGF-A Decrease endothelial cell migration and invasion induced by VEGF and VEGF-A Downregulation of several angiogenic genes	Tibullo et al. (2016)
Ovarian	Methanolic extract of pomegranate peel Methanolic pomegranate seed extract	SKOV3 ovarian cancer cells	Antiproliferative		Modaeinama et al. (2015) Seidi et al. (2016)
	Punicalagin	Human A2780 ovarian cancer cells	Antiproliferative and pro-apoptotic (cell cycle	Upregulation of Bax and down-regulation of Bcl-2. Increase the expressions of TIMP-2 and TIMP-3, decreased the activities of MMP-2 and MMP-9, and	Tang et al. (2016)

(continued)

Table 13.2 (continued)

Cancer type	*Punica g.* form and its chemical compounds	Cancer model	Effect	Molecular mechanism(s)/cellular target(s)	References
			arrest in G1/S phase) Antimetastatic	inhibited cell migration. Supression of β-catenin pathway and its downstream factors including cyclin D1 and survivin	
Cervix	Pomegranate seed ethanolic extract rich mainly punic acid	Cervical adenocarcinoma cell line HeLa	Antiproliferative		Lucci et al. (2015)
	Fruit parts (peel, flesh, seeds, juices and leaves) of pomegranate		Antiproliferative		Li et al. (2016b)
	Ellagic acid from pomegranate peel extract	HeLa cells	Antiproliferative and anti-invasive	Upregulation of IGFBP7. Downregulation of AKT and mTOR mRNA and protein expressions	Guo et al. (2016)
Renal	Pomegranate seed ethanolic extract rich mainly punic acid	Renal adenocarcinoma ACHN cells	Antiproliferative		Lucci et al. (2015)
Thyroid	Punicalagin	BCPAP cells	Antiproliferative by autophagic cell death Induction of senescent phenotype	Increases LC3-II conversion, upregulation of beclin-1 expression, and increases p62/SQSTM1 degradation. Activation of MAPK by ERK1/2 and p38 phosphorylation, and inhibition of mTOR signaling pathways through the inhibition of p70S6, and 4EBP1 protein levels Inhibition of NF-κB	Cheng et al. (2016) Cheng et al. (2018)

Table 13.3 Clinical trials with *Punica granatum* L. extracts, and its chemical constituents in cancer

Cancer	Design	Target population	Intervention	Dose	Mean duration	Outcome	References
Prostate	Open-label, single-arm, uncontrolled, two-stage optimal flexible design[a]	BCR (n = 46)	Fermented pomegranate juice (POM Wonderful)	8 oz. per day (570 mg per day GAE)	33 months (two stages)	Mean PSADT increased (15–54 months) post-treatment ($p = 0.01$). No patients developed metastases. A 40% reduction in serum oxidative state. No serious AEs and the treatment was well-tolerated	Pantuck et al. (2006) NCT00060086
	Multi-center, randomized, double-blind, two-dose Low dose (45) versus high dose (47)[a]	BCR (n = 92) patients without metastases with rising PSA levels	Standardized pomegranate polyphenol powdered extract	1000 versus 3000 mg per day (755–2265 mg per day GAE)	18 months	Median PSADT increased (11.9–18.5 months, $p = 0.001$) in the low-dose group and in the high-dose group (12.2–17.5) months, without significant difference ($p = 0.92$) between the effects of the two doses. No patient developed metastases and few AEs; high dose showed greater incidence of diarrhea (14 vs. 8%)	Paller et al. (2013a) NCT01220817
	Multisite, randomized, double blind, placebo-controlled Eextract (36) versus placebo (33)[a]	Neoadjuvant (n = 69, prior to prostatectomy)	Powdered pomegranate extract (POMx pills)	1000 mg per day (600 mg per day GAE)	4 weeks	Significant increase in urolithin A detection (34–64%, $p = 0.031$) and non-significant 16% reduction ($p = 0.095$) in 8-OHdG	Freedland et al. (2013) NCT00719030

(continued)

Table 13.3 (continued)

Cancer	Design	Target population	Intervention	Dose	Mean duration	Outcome	References
						in the treatment arm. A strong trend between higher Uro-A levels in prostate tissues and lower 8-OHdG levels was found. No serious AEs and the treatment was well tolerated	
	Double-blinded, randomized placebo-controlled[a,b]	Metastatic prostate cancer (n = 97), CRPC 65% BCR 35% (PSA ≥ 5 ng/ml)	Juice blend (27.5% Pomegranate) plus pear puree, white tea, agave concentrate, aronia berry juice	500 mL per day (1147 mg per day GAE) 250 mL daily (573.5 mg per day GAE)	4 weeks 4 weeks	No difference between groups on PSA progression (38% treatment, 41% placebo, $p = 0.83$); no difference in pain scores ($p = 0.49$). No serious AEs	Stenner-Liewen et al. (2013)
	Double-blind, placebo-controlled randomized[a]	AS 60% BCR 40% (WW) following previous interventions (n = 199) Pill (134) versus placebo (65)	Pomi-T: capsule conteing a blend of pomegranate, broccoli, and tumeric, each 100 mg, and 20 mg of green tea extract	Pomegranate extract (300 mg per day) (GAE not reported)	6 months	AS: significantly slower increases in median PSA levels (78.5% in placebo group vs. 14.7% in supplement group); (−0.1% vs. 47.0%, $p = 0.001$). BCR: significantly lower PSA rise in treatment arm versus placebo (8.8% vs. 80.3%, $p = 0.001$). No serious AEs	Thomas et al. (2014) NCRN 11/EE/0314

	Double-blind, placebo-controlled multi-center study Liquid extract (102), standard juice (17) versus placebo (64)[c]	BCR (rising PSA levels after primary therapy, n = 183)	Liquid pomegranate extract and standard juice	8 oz. per day (776 mg per day GAE)	10 months	Median PSADT increased for each group: placebo 4.5 months, liquid extract 1.6 months, and juice 7.6 months. No significant change between groups ($p > 0.05$); larger increase in median PSADT change in MnSOD AA subgroup on liquid extract arm (12 months, $p = 0.03$) versus on placebo 1.8 months ($p = 0.22$), p for difference between arms not reported). No serious drug-related AEs	Pantuck et al. (2015)
	3-arm randomized controlled[a]	Neoadjuvant (n = 75, prior to radiation or prostatectomy) Tomato juice (26) versus blend (25) versus placebo (24)	Tomato juice (tomato based lycopene-rich) or a combination of tomato/grape juice/pomegranate/green/black teas/selenium/omega-3/soy (Tomato plus)	330 ml per day of pomegranate juice in tomato+ group	3 weeks	No significant differences were seen in PSA values between the placebo patients and either of the treatment groups, for example: tomato/grape juice/pomegranate/green/black teas/selenium/omega-3/soy group versus placebo (0.28 vs. 0.45 ng ml^{-1}, $p = 0.094$). No serious AEs	Paur et al. (2017) NCT00433797

(continued)

Table 13.3 (continued)

Cancer	Design	Target population	Intervention	Dose	Mean duration	Outcome	References
Breast	Cohort study, prospective randomized controlated	Mastectomy women (n = 50) Control group (n = 30), tamoxifen group (n = 20), pomegranate oil + tamoxifen combination (n = 20)	Tamoxifen Pomegranate seed oil	3 tablets (10 mg/day) (tablets 1 g/day)	3 months 3 months	CA 15-3 breast tumor marker, aromatase enzyme, cholesterol, and LDH levels were significantly decreased in pomegranate-tamoxifen combination while aromatase enzyme and cholesterol levels in tamoxifen group remains unchanged, both compared with breast cancer group. TG leve in both pomegranate and tamoxifen group and tamoxifen group does not show significant change compared with breast cancer group	Qasim et al. (2013)
	Randomized controlled	Healthy natural postmenopausal women (n = 64) Intervention group (n = 33) Control group (n = 31)	100% commercial pomegranate juice (POM Wonderful) to intervention group 100% apple juice (Stop and Shop 100% Unsweetened	8 oz. daily (4 oz. in the morning and 4 oz. in the early evening) for both juices	3 weeks	There were no significant differences in changes in serum estrone, E2, T, and SHBG levels between the intervention and control groups. There was a small decline in serum estrone levels in the pomegranate juice	Kapoor et al. (2015)

			Apple Juice) to control group			group compared to the control group, but the decline was statistically non-significant. Normal weight women in the pomegranate juice intervention group had a significant decrease in serum estrone and T levels compared to similar women in the control group. Among overweight/obese women, no statistically significant difference was observed between the two groups	
Colorectal	Randomized, controlled clinical trial	Patients (n = 52) with resectable CRC (normal and malignant CRC tissues) control group (n = 19) (PE-1; n = 17, completed n = 16), (PE-2; n = 16, completes n = 10)	Pomegranate extracts with different ellagitannins/ ellagic acid ratio low (PE-1) and high (PE-2) punicalagin:EA ratio PE-1: 72 mg/g punicalagin, 2 mg/g punicalin and 294 mg/g EA derivatives PE-2: 155 mg/g	900 mg/day in capsules (two hard plant-based capsules containing 450 mg of either PE-1 or PE-2	15 days The last dose was administered approximately 10–12 h before surgery	Twenty-three metabolites, but no ellagitannins, were detected in urine, plasma, normal or malignant colon tissues. The occurrence of free ellagic acid, 5 ellagic acid-conjugates, gallic acid, and 12 urolithins with higher levels in normal tissues than in malignant tissues. Moreover, higher urolithins formation	Nuñez-Sánchez et al. (2014b) Spanish National Research Project AGL2011–22447, protocol reference 03/2011 NCT01916239

(continued)

Table 13.3 (continued)

Cancer	Design	Target population	Intervention	Dose	Mean duration	Outcome	References
			punicalagin, 5.4 mg/g punicalin and 28 mg/g EA derivatives			after intake of the extract with higher free ellagic acid was evident High punicalagin content (PE-2) hampered urolithins formation	
	Randomized, double-blind, controlled trial	CRC patients (n = 35) Control group (n = 10)	Pomegranate extract	900 mg daily before surgery	15 days The last dose was administered approximately 10–12 h before surgery	Significant levels of ellagic acid derivatives and urolithins were found in surgical colon tissues from CRC patients. Moderate modulation of various miRNAs following the pomegranate extract intake was also found. Significant differences for specific miRNAs between malignant and normal tissues were obtained	Nuñez-Sánchez et al. (2017)
	Randomized controlled	CRC patients (n = 35), normal and cancerous surgical tissue samples (*post-PE intake*), and biopsies samples (*baseline*) (*previous to PE intake*) (n = 35) PE-1 group	ETs-containing pomegranate extract (PE-1 and PE-2)	900 mg daily before surgery	13.6 ± 7.5 days (range: 5–35 days) The last dose was administered approximately 10–12 h before surgery	The consumption of the PE was significantly associated with a counterbalance effect in the expression of *CD44*, *CTNNB1*, *CDKN1A*, *EGFR* and *TYMs*. These effects were not associated with the individuals' capacity to produce specific	González-Sarrías et al. (2016) NCT01916239

		(n = 19) and PE-2 (n = 16) Control patients (n = 10)				urolithins or the levels of urolithins and EA in the colon tissues	
Skin	Epidemiological multicenter hospital-based case-control	SCC patients (n = 409), BCC patients (n = 602) and CMM (n = 360) control persons (n = 1550)	Pomegranate	Regular consumption (more than three times per week) of pomegranate		Pomegranate was modestly associated with reduced risk of BCC, SCC and CMM in multivariate analysis, but this association remained significant only after correction for multiple. Also, was observe a potential protective effect to SCC	El-Ashmawy et al. (2016) EPIDERM (Project No. 2007101)

BCR biochemical recurrent prostate cancer, for example, men experiencing rising PSA following definitive local therapy, *GAE* gallic acid equivalents (polyphenols), *AEs* adversed effects, *PSA* prostatic antigen, *PSADT* PSA doubling time, 8-OHdG, 8-hydroxy-2-deoxyguanosine, *CRPC* castration-resistant prostate cancer, *AS* active surveillance (observation only, no local treatment planned), *WW* watchful waiting, *MnSOD AA* manganese superoxide dismutase AA genotype, *NCRN, UK* National Cancer Research Network, *CA 15–3* cell antigen 15–3 (breast cancer tumor marker), *LDH* lactate dehydrogenase, *TG* triglyceride, *E2* estradiol, *T* testosterone, *SHBG* sex hormone binding globulin, *CRC* colorectal cancer, *PE* pomegranate extract, *EA* ellagic acid, *PE-1* and *PE-2* pomegranate extract of low (PE-1) and high (PE-2) punicalagin:EA ratio, *miRNAs* micro-ribonucleic acids, *ET* ellagitannins, CD44, Hermes antigen (also known as H-CAM or pgp-1 antigen) *CTNNB1* Catenin β-1, *CDKN1A* cyclin-dependent kinase inhibitor 1A (p21), *EGFR* epidermal growth factor receptor, *TYM* thymidine synthetase, *SCC* squamous cell carcinoma, *BCC* basal cell carcinoma, *CMM* basal cell carcinoma

[a]Phase II clinical trial

[b]During the study, patients had to continue their baseline treatment

[c]Phase III clinical trial

et al. 2010; Lansky et al. 1997). *Punica granatum* L. products target a broad spectrum of genes and proteins to target multiple signaling pathways involved in cancer development, growth and progression, including inflammation, cellular differentiation and transformation, initiation of tumorigenesis, tumor cell proliferation, angiogenesis, migration, invasion, and metastasis; both in a chemopreventive and/or chemotherapeutic approach (Fig. 13.1). The pomegranate constituents are shown to modulate transcription factors, pro- and anti-apoptotic proteins, cell cycle regulator molecules, protein kinases, cell adhesion molecules, pro-inflammatory mediators, growth factors, and other targets in various cancers (Lansky and Newman 2007; Longtin 2003; Jurenka 2008; Bhandari 2012; Faria and Calhau 2011; Shaygannia et al. 2016; Rahimi et al. 2012; Akhtar et al. 2015; Orgil et al. 2014; Arun and Singh 2012; Viuda-Martos et al. 2010; Lansky et al. 1997), as discussed further in more detail.

13.3.1 Prostate Cancer

Prostate cancer (PCa) is the second-leading cause of cancer-related deaths in men in the world (Torre et al. 2015; Siegel et al. 2016). Various chemopreventive and therapeutic PCa effects have been described for pomegranate extracts in vitro and in vivo (Table 13.2).

Preclinical Studies It has been found that pomegranate juice extracts (PJEs) and EA have chemopreventive effects by inhibition of PCa growth and its metastasis and doubling the overall survival time using a transgenic adenocarcinoma mouse prostate (TRAMP) model (Adhami et al. 2012; Naiki-Ito et al. 2015). Likewise, the levels of prostatic antigen (PSA), testosterone, dihydrotestosterone, and other androgens were significantly inhibited and serum steroids reduced after 10 weeks of treatment (Adhami et al. 2012). The possible mechanisms include inhibition of phosphoinositide 3-kinase (PI3K)/serine-threonine kinase B (AKT)/mammalian target of rapamycin (mTOR) and insulin-like growth factor-1 (IGF-1)/AKT/mTOR signaling pathways (Adhami et al. 2012). In addition, in vitro assays were performed using different human PCa cell lines such as the androgen-dependent and non-aggressive LNCaP cells, the androgen-independent and highly invasive, strongly metastatic PC3 and the highly proliferative but moderate metastatic DU145. Both EA and PJ suppressed the progression of prostate carcinogenesis modulating cyclin-dependent kinases (cdk), cell cycle cyclins and induced apoptosis (Table 13.2) (Naiki-Ito et al. 2015).

It has been shown that different fractions of *Punica granatum* L. extracts and its respective polyphenols, alone or in combination, promote cell death of androgen dependent and independent cells and induced tumor regression in either subcutaneous and orthotopic xenografts in in vivo PCa models into immunocompromised mice via antiproliferative, apoptotic, antiangiogenic, antimetastatic, anti-invasive and antitumor mechanisms (Table 13.2) (Albrecht et al. 2004; Malik et al. 2005;

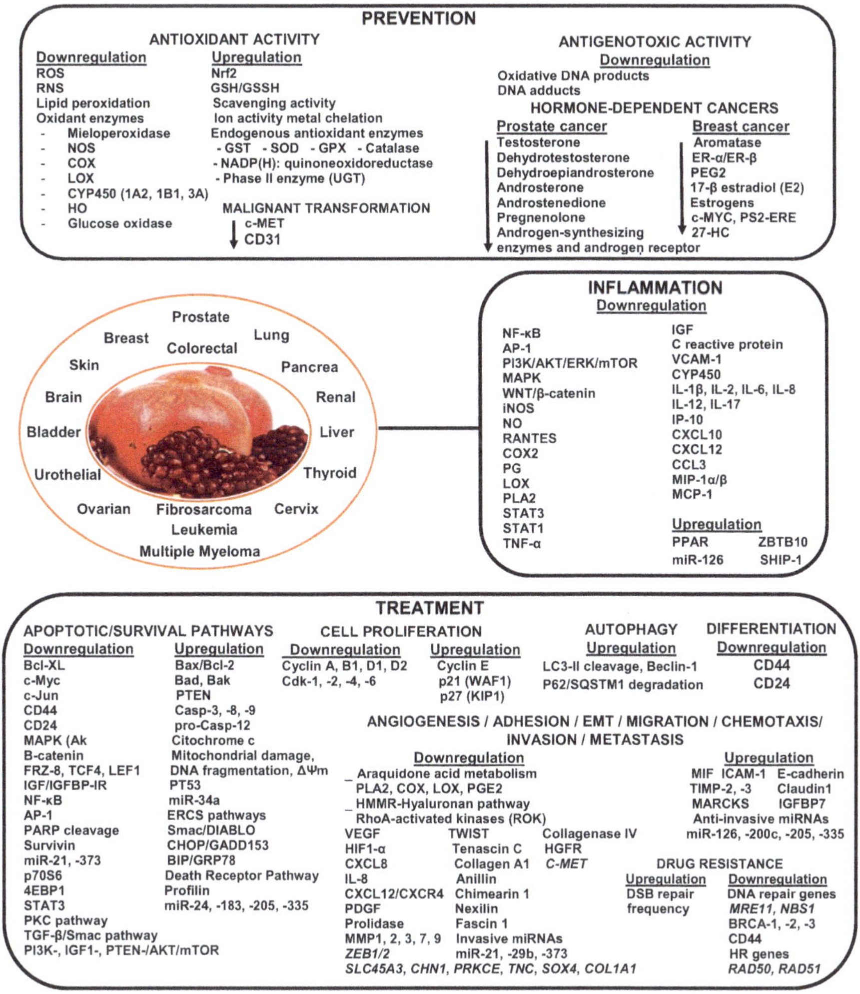

Fig. 13.1 Molecular processes and cellular targets of *Punica granatum* L

Rettig et al. 2008; Wang and Martins-Green 2014; Malik and Mukhtar 2006; Deng et al. 2017). The molecular targets and pathways by which *Punica granatum* L. extracts and its polyphenols show anticancer effects involve modulation of cdk, blocking G1–S phase transition, causing G1-phase arrest, upregulation of pro-apoptotic proteins, and downregulation of pro-apoptotic Bcl-2 protein, changes in phospholipase A2 (PLA2), Arachidonic Acid (AA), prostaglandin E2 (PGE2), cyclooxygenase (COX)-2, lipoxygenase (LOX) and PI3K/AKT pathways (Lansky et al. 2005a; Wang and Martins-Green 2014), modulation of the hyaluronan-mediated motility receptor (HMMR) and the hyaluronan signaling pathway (Wang and Martins-Green 2014). Antimetastatic effects are mediated by inhibition of chemotaxis processes through inhibition of the C-X-C motif chemokine ligand

(CXCL)-12, chemokine receptor 4 (CXCR4) axis (Wang and Martins-Green 2014). Pomegranate peel extract (PPE) and PJEs and its phytochemicals also suppressed invasion by downregulation of matrix metalloproteinases (MMPs) -1, -2, -3, -7 and -9 and upregulation of tissue inhibitors of metalloproteinase (TIMPs) (Wang and Martins-Green 2014; Deng et al. 2017). Furthermore PJ and a combination of luteolin, PuA, and EA reduced cell migration through the modulation of cell adhesion by downregulation of *type I collagen*, *tenascin C*, and *chimerin 1* in PC3 cells (Malik and Mukhtar 2006). Besides, PJ and the combinations upregulated genes involved in cell adhesion: *E-cadherin*, *intercellular adhesion molecule 1* (ICAM1) and *myristoylated alanine-rich protein kinase C* (MARCKS) in PC3 cells. In hormone-refractory PCa cells, PEs also enhances cell adhesion and reduces cell migration by modulating the expression and/or activation of molecules that modify the cytoskeleton (Malik et al. 2005; Wang and Martins-Green 2014), and the cell adhesion machinery (Bhandari 2012). Finally, PJ induced upregulation of anti-invasive micro-ribonucleic acids (miRNAs) including miR-335, miR-205, miR-200, miR-126; and downregulated proinvasive miRNAs such as miR-21 and miR-373 in DU145 cells, which adds another layer of posttranscription-translational control to suppression of invasive-metastic protein expression (Wang and Martins-Green 2014).

The reduction of circulating levels of androgens and suppression of androgen receptor are crucial for the treatment of PCa (Heinlein and Chang 2004; Attard et al. 2006; McCarty et al. 2014). In this sense, anti-androgenic effects of PEs and juice were shown to reduce the expression level of key androgen-synthesizing enzyme genes (*3β-hydroxysteroid dehydrogenase type II, steroid 5α reductase type I*), and *androgen receptor* in LNCaP-AR cells (Hong et al. 2008). More recently, an ethanolic PE reduced the production of several androgens, and pregnenolone, with tumor growth inhibition and significant decrease in the expression and serum levels of PSA (Ming et al. 2014). In metastatic castration-resistant PCa cells (C4-2, PC3 and $ARCaP_M$), a standardized PE exhibited potent in vitro cytotoxicity and in athymic nude mice, the extract retarded C4-2 skeletal metastases (Wang et al. 2014). Besides, it reduced survivin protein and gene expression by inhibition of signal transducer and activator of transcription (STAT)-3 phosphorylation (Wang et al. 2014). Furthermore, PE induced apoptosis, retarded cell growth and inhibited survivin in PC3 cell-transplanted BALB/c nu/nu mice (Wang et al. 2014) as well as LAPC4 cells implanted in severe combined immunodeficient mice (Wang et al. 2014). Similarly, Rettig et al. showed that PE retarded the growth of LAPC4 androgen-independent tumor by inhibition of nuclear factor kappa B (NF-κB) (Rettig et al. 2008). PE also exhibited antiproliferative and antiangiogenic activity in LNCaP in hypoxic environments (Sartippour et al. 2008). A proteomic study demonstrated a significant downregulation of prolidase gene expression by PJ on PCa cells DU145 (Lee et al. 2012). Prolidase can induce the expression of hypoxia inducible factor 1 alpha (HIF-1α) and vascular endothelial growth factor (VEGF) and is, therefore, involved in the angiogenic process. Taken together, these observations suggest that the inhibition of prolidase might contribute to the inhibition of angiogenesis and invasion mediated by PEs (Lee et al. 2012).

Vanella et al. showed a reversion of PCa cell lines from a proliferating to a differentiated state induced by EA, which resulted in antiproliferative effects on LNCaP cells (Vanella et al. 2013a). EA treatment induced a significant decrease of VEGF, fibroblast growth factor (FGF), granulocyte colony-stimulating factor (G-CSF), hepatocyte growth factor (HGF) and interleukin 15 (IL-15) levels (Vanella et al. 2013b). Also, this study evidenced, for the first time, the ability of EA to decrease the expression of Heme oxygenases (HO)-1 and HO-2, which are involved in tumor angiogenesis- (Alaoui-Jamali et al. 2009). HO-2 is constitutively active in all tissues, whereas selective inhibition of HO-2 by siRNA increases reactive oxygen species (ROS) and activates CASPs inducing apoptotic cell death (He et al. 2010). Moreover, this study demonstrated that EA also inhibits the expression of cytochrome P (CYP)-450 epoxygenases isoforms, the epoxidation and hydroxylation of AA, and CYP450-derived eicosanoids that can enhance angiogenesis and promote cancer growth and metastasis (Vanella et al. 2013b). Also, EA showed decreased levels of osteoprotegerin (OPG), a reliable marker in detecting bone metastatic spread and a predictor of mortality from PCa (Kamiya et al. 2011). These results support the hypothesis that EA treatment contributes to reduce tumor-related angiogenesis and metastasis.

A recent study showed that PC induces growth inhibition and apoptosis in PC3 and LNCaP cells, whereas normal BPH-1 cells remain unaffected. Also, PC led to the inhibition of vascular network; thus, demonstrating a direct inhibitory effect of PC on angiogenesis (Adaramoye et al. 2017).

β-Sitosterol is a major plant sterol present in pomegranate (Jiménez-Escrig et al. 2006) which is effective at killing LNCaP cells (von Holtz et al. 1998). Moon et al. demonstrated that β-sitosterol can arrest cells at G2/M and affect tubulin microtubule assembly (Moon et al. 2008). Recently, a binding interaction of β-sitosterol with tubulin was reported distinct from the colchicine site, which stabilizes microtubule assembly (Mahaddalkar et al. 2015). γ-Tocopherol is one of the most important constituents of pomegranate seed oil (PSO) that is responsible for anticancer activity. Jiang et al. showed that γ-tocopherol inhibits proliferation of PCa cells by inhibition of de novo sphingolipid synthesis but appears to have no effect on the growth of normal prostate cells (Jiang et al. 2004). Also, they showed that γ-tocopherol inhibited COX activity (Jiang et al. 2000). Urolithins have anticarcinogenic actions through the inhibition CYP1B1 and CYP1A1 (Kasimsetty et al. 2009).

Collectively, the above preclinical results clearly suggest that PEs and its bioactive components inhibit the development and dissemination of PCa in in vitro and in vivo models through several pathways that participate in cell proliferation, survival and death, angiogenesis, migration, invasion, metastasis, inflammation and cellular adhesion.

Clinical Trials A launch of ten clinical trials in PCa patients have been carry out; from these, only seven trials (Table 13.3) have been conducted and published to evaluate PEs and/or PJ (Paller et al. 2017). Between a 25% and 50% of PCa patients use complementary alternative medicine, in addition to standard treatments, with only modest preclinical or clinical evidence of efficacy (Bishop et al. 2011). The

National Cancer Institute website lists PJ and PJE as one of the nine dietary supplements commonly consumed by PCa patients (National Cancer Institute 2016). Pomegranate products have been tested in PCa patients in six phase II clinical trials (Pantuck et al. 2006; Paller et al. 2013a; Freedland et al. 2013; Stenner-Liewen et al. 2013; Thomas et al. 2014; Paur et al. 2017) and one phase III trial (Pantuck et al. 2015), with outcomes measured by changes in PSA doubling time (PSADT), in PSA levels, and in 8-hydroxy-2-deoxyguanosine (8-OHdG), a marker of oxidation in PCa tissue.

The two first studies (Pantuck et al. 2006; Paller et al. 2013a) demonstrated statistically significant prolongation in PSADT without metastatic progression. A major disadvantage of these trials was the absence of a proper placebo control group. The third trial (Freedland et al. 2013) suggested the need for larger, longer duration studies and higher doses in the future. A study conducted in castration-resistant PCa patients with metastasis (Stenner-Liewen et al. 2013), concluded that daily pomegranate intake had no impact on PSA levels. This conclusion was based on an inadequate amount of coactive ingredients in pomegranate mixture, suboptimal duration of treatment and the daily dose was too low for successful anticancer treatment and to produce a clinical effect (Vlachojannis et al. 2015). Other trials included pomegranate in blenders like Pomi-T (Thomas et al. 2014) and Tomato plus (Paur et al. 2017). The first intervention study suggested the great potential of the food supplement to prevent PCa progression. However, two aspects of this trial make it difficult to interpret the results to estimate the anti-cancer efficacy of pomegranate in recurrent PCa. At one hand, the product was primarily composed of polyphenol-rich compounds other than pomegranate; at the other hand, no changes were observed related to PSADT. This suggests that in future trials, additional clinical effects and markers of disease progression should be included (Paller et al. 2017). On the second intervention study (Paur et al. 2017), no significant changes in PSA levels were detected. In one phase III clinical trial the effects of PJ and PJE on PSADT were compared in subjects with rising PSA levels after primary therapy (Pantuck et al. 2015). Additional objectives were to evaluate the safety of PJ and PJE, and to determine the gene–nutrient interaction involving the manganese superoxide dismutase (MnSOD) gene (AA genotype), and antioxidant status. The trial concluded that PEs did not significantly prolong PSADT in PCa patients. Also, men with the MnSOD AA genotype may represent a group that is more sensitive to the effects of pomegranate on PSADT (Li et al. 2005); however, this finding requires additional testing and validation (Pantuck et al. 2015).

Though widely recognized as an important prognostic and surrogate biomarker for PCa mortality in men with rising PSA after primary treatment failure (D'Amico et al. 2003; Freedland et al. 2005), PSADT is controversial when used as an end point in clinical trials (Paller et al. 2013b). Others have argued for the use of other endpoints such as progression-free survival (Scher et al. 2008). A systematic review of randomized trials for the efficacy and safety of phytotherapeutic interventions in the management of BCR-PCa found that serum PSA levels stabilize, decrease or rise more slowly in a significant number of men, and three studies reported stabilizing or lengthening of PSADT (van Die et al. 2016). Although, the studies were generally of good quality and phytotherapeutic interventions were safe and well tolerated, sample sizes were predominantly small, and treatment durations short. The authors concluded that there is limited evidence that these phytoterapeutics can affect PSA dynamics, and no recommendation could be made for the use of these agents in managing PCa morbidity and mortality. Furthermore, recommendations were made for improving reproducibility and translation of findings (van Die et al. 2016). In complete agreement with this point of view are the conclusions derived of a systematic review of dietary, nutritional, and physical activity interventions for the prevention of PCa progression and mortality (Hackshaw-McGeagh et al. 2015; Iguchi et al. 2015). In a recent review by Paller et al. (2017), critical considerations were made in relation with measurements of biomarkers and metabolites, drug–drug interaction concerns, target population selection and type of clinical trial to demonstrate clinical effectiveness of pomegranate products in the treatment of prostate cancer.

13.3.2 Breast Cancer

Breast cancer (BCa) is the most common diagnosed cancer and the primary cause of cancer-associated deaths in women worldwide (Torre et al. 2015; Siegel et al. 2011, 2016). In recent years, the link between dietary factors and BCa risk has been a significant area of research. Studies have shown the beneficial effects of pomegranate in BCa (Table 13.2).

Preclinical Studies Epidemiological studies have demonstrated that elevated serum levels of estrogens and lower levels of sex hormone binding globulin (SHBG) after menopause increased the risk of BCa (Lazzeroni and DeCensi 2013). The chemopreventive role for pomegranate in BCa was first demonstrated in mouse mammary organ culture with $\geq 75\%$ of accuracy of predicting in vivo mammary carcinogenesis (Mehta and Lansky 2004). Pomegranate fermented juice (PFJ) polyphenols inhibited 7,12-dimethylbenz[*a*]anthracene (DMBA)-induced precancerous mammary lesions (Mehta and Lansky 2004). Polyphenols from PFJ, pericarp and oil were shown to inhibit endogenous active estrogen biosynthesis with subsequent inhibition of aromatase activity (Mehta and Lansky 2004). Sturgeon et al., showed that pomegranate and its constituents prevent BCa progress by anti-oestrogenic mechanisms. Also, EA seems to exhibit apoptosis, anti-inflammatory and anti-angiogenesis effects (Sturgeon and Ronnenberg 2010). Bishayee et al., reported that pomegranate reduced the incidence, total burden and weight of mammary tumors in DMBA-induced mammary tumorigenesis (Bishayee et al. 2016). Also, a downregulation of the expression of intratumor estrogen receptor (ER)-α and ER-β and lower ER-α: ER-β ratio were observed. Likewise, pomegranate promotes inhibition of WNT/β-catenin pathway, and suppressed the expression of cyclin D1. Both studies indicate that concurrent disruption of ER and Wnt/β-catenin signaling pathways contributes to antiproliferative and proapoptotic effects of pomegranate-mediated chemoprevention of DMBA-mammary tumorigenesis (Bishayee et al. 2016; Mandal and Bishayee 2015).

Pomegranate constituents, PFJ and PPE inhibited angiogenesis, migration and metastatic capability of BCa cells via downregulation of VEGF and peroxisome proliferator-activated receptor (PPAR) in HUVEC, normal human breast cells MCF-10A and MCF-7 tumor cells, and migration inhibitory factor (MIF) was upregulated in MDA-MB-231 tumor cells. These results were confirmed by inhibition of vessel formation in an in vivo angiogenesis model of chicken chorioallantoic membrane cells (Toi et al. 2003; Dana et al. 2016). Moreover, PEs inhibited invasiveness (Kim et al. 2002), growth and induced apoptosis (Faria and Calhau 2011; Jeune et al. 2005). Pomegranate linolenic fatty acid has cytotoxic effects on MCF-7 and induced apoptosis of the MDA-MB-435 human BCa cells (Bhandari 2012), which has been attributed to the antiangiogenic properties of PSO as well as its ability to retard prostaglandin synthesis (Bhandari 2012). PuA inhibited the cell growth, induced apoptosis and disrupted cellular mitochondrial membrane of both on an estrogen insensitive (MDA-MB-231) and an estrogen sensitive cell line (MDA-ERa7). The PuA inhibitor properties are dependent on lipid peroxidation and the protein kinase C (PKC) pathway (Grossmann et al. 2010). Recently, it was reported that an extract rich in PuA and its congeners decreased cell viability of MCF-7 and MDA-MB-231 cells by cell cycle arrest at G0/G1 phase (Costantini et al. 2014). Also, this extract showed anti-inflammatory, anti-angiogenenic and antimigration properties (Table 13.2).

Recently, Chen HS et al. demonstrated that EA inhibits the proliferation of MCF-7 cells by arresting cell cycle in the G0/G1 phase, and a gene expression profiling identified 2547 downregulated and 2191 upregulated genes (Chen et al. 2015). Furthermore, the changes of 16 genes, which belong to transforming growth factor (TGF)-β)/SMAD proteins signaling pathway, were confirmed (Chen et al. 2015). In another study, ETs-derived compounds inhibited aromatase activity as well as cell proliferation (Adams et al. 2010).

Tran et al., evaluated pomegranate seed linolenic acid isomers as selective estrogen receptor modulators in vitro (Tran et al. 2010). PuA and α-eleostearic acid inhibited the IC_{50} ER-α and ER-β. PuA acted as agonist at lower concentrations and as antagonist at higher concentrations for both receptors. Both acids were effective to inhibit cell proliferation on MCF-7 and MDA-MB-231 cells, and are selective ER modulators (Tran et al. 2010). Rocha et al. showed that in addition to inhibiting growth of MCF-7 and MDA-MB-231 cells, PJ or a combination of its components luteolin, EA and PuA increase cancer cell adhesion and decrease cancer cell migration and chemotaxis to bone but do not affect normal cells (Rocha et al. 2012). In addition, they found that a gene important in epithelial-to-meshenchymal transitions is decreased. Also, pro-inflammatory cytokines/chemokines are significantly reduced, thereby having the potential to decrease inflammation (Rocha et al. 2012). Sreeja et al. showed, with in vitro assays, that the antiproliferative effect and antiestrogenic selectivity action of PPE were supported by its ER-binding properties, downregulation of v-myc avian myelocytomatosis viral oncogene homolog (c-Myc) gene expression and pS2 estrogen response elements (ERE)-mediated transcription specifically through ER-α but without being agonistic in the uterine endometrium (not affecting uterine weight unlike E2 or tamoxifen) (Sreeja et al. 2012; Vini and

Sreeja 2015). Besides, the extract antagonized the activity of 27-hydroxycholesterol (27HC), an endogenous selective estrogen receptor modulator that can act through ER-mediated mechanisms, and reduced 27HC-induced proliferation of MCF-7 cells, being the first report describing this pomegranate effect and its possible role on the direct relationship between obesity and BCa (Vini et al. 2016).

In recent work, PE was found to inhibit cell growth by inducing cell cycle arrest in G2/M followed by the induction of apoptosis. In contrast, antioxidants, at doses containing equivalent antioxidant activity as the extract, did not affect cell growth, suggesting that growth inhibition by extract cannot solely be attributed to its high antioxidant potential (Shirode et al. 2014). Furthermore, downregulated genes associate with mitosis, chromosome organization, RNA processing, DNA replication and DNA repair—DNA double strand break (DSB) repair by homologous recombination (HR)—whereas upregulated genes are involved in regulation of apoptosis and cell proliferation (Shirode et al. 2014). Downregulation of HR genes correlated with increased levels of their predicted target miRNAs, miR-183 and miR-24, suggesting that PE may regulate miRNAs involved in DNA repair processes (Shirode et al. 2014). As a consequence, PE increased the frequency of DSBs. These data suggest that pomegranate downregulates HR which sensitizes cells to DSBs, growth inhibition and apoptosis, and may be exploited for sensitization of tumors to anticancer drugs such as bortezomib, imatinib, and histone deacetylase inhibitors that target HR.

PE inhibited growth of BT-474 and MDA-MB-231 cells, but not the non-cancer MCF-10F and MCF-12F cells, decreasing expression of specificity protein (Sp)-1, -3, and -4 as well as miR-27a, and increasing expression of the transcriptional repressor ZBTB10 in both cell lines. PE also induced inositol polyphosphate-5-phosphatase (INPP5) expression, and downregulation of miRNA-155 and inhibition of PI3K-dependent phosphorylation of AKT (Banerjee et al. 2012). These results were confirmed in nude mice bearing BT474 cells. The effects of antagonists and knockdown of INPP5 by RNA interference confirmed that the anti-inflammatory and cytotoxic effects of PE were partly due to the disruption of both miR-27a-ZBTB10 and miR-155-INPP5 (Banerjee et al. 2012).

Cancer stem cells (CSCs) offer a novel paradigm for cancer treatment by dietary polyphenols. PE (Pomella) inhibited the proliferation of WA4 cells derived from mouse MMTV-Wnt-1 mammary tumors, which have CSCs characteristics, by cell cycle arresting at G0/G1 phase (Dai et al. 2010). Also, the extract was cytotoxic to quiescent WA4 cells by apoptosis induction through CASP-3 activity increase. Individual phytochemicals, mainly ursolic acid, caused reduction of cell proliferation and viability, suggesting that they contribute to the inhibitory effect of extract (Dai et al. 2010).

Pomegranate ETs-derived compounds and urolithins, mainly uro-B, have been shown to possess antiproliferative and antiaromatase activity, in human BCa cells overexpressing aromatase (MCF-7aro) (Adams et al. 2010; Larrosa et al. 2006a). The marked efficacy of uro-B might be due to its better absorption in cells (Mehta and Lansky 2004). When pomegranate polyphenols were tested together, a higher antiaromatase inhibition was found, suggesting a synergistic effect. Many pomegranate components, such as luteolin, kaempferol, quercetin, and naringenin, possess antiestrogenic action through competitive binding to ER cooperating synergistically with anti-estrogenic activity of PEs (Van Elswijk et al. 2004).

Clinical Trials The effects of pomegranate and tamoxifen combination on BCa tumor antigen marker CA 15-3, aromatase enzyme, triglyceride, cholesterol, and lactate dehydrogenase (LDH) in mastectomy women was carried out (Table 13.3) (Qasim et al. 2013). This study suggested at least an additive interaction when a supplementation of pomegranate along with tamoxifen to BCa mastectomy patients was applied. This reduced the serum levels of CA 15-3, aromatase, and LDH, thereby offering better cancer prognosis by decreasing the risk of developing cancer recurrence and metastasis (Qasim et al. 2013).

To validate preclinical studies which suggest that polyphenols may exert BCa preventive effects through modulation of endogenous sex hormone levels, a clinical study was performed by Kapoor et al. (2015) (Table 13.3). Overall, women in the intervention group did not experience any significant decline in serum sex hormones or SHBG compared to the control group. However, a subgroup analyses restricted to 38 normal weight women in the intervention group compared to control group showed a significant decline in estrone and testosterone levels. The authors concluded that the results should be considered preliminary by several study limitations. In addition, longer intervention period trials with potentially higher levels of intake of PJ would be needed to determine effects in normal versus overweight/obese women (Kapoor et al. 2015).

13.3.3 Colorectal Cancer

Colorectal cancer (CRC) is the third most common type of cancer worldwide and a leading cause of cancer death (Torre et al. 2015; Siegel et al. 2016). The exact cause of CRC is not known, but certain lifestyle risk factors are strongly linked to the disease, including diet, tobacco smoking and heavy alcohol use (Vargas and Thompson 2012). Frequently, CRC patients are for the first time diagnosed in advanced stages when distant metastases are already present. At these advanced stages, patients might be unresponsive to any form of treatment (Saltz 2007).

Most studies of PE and its pholyphenols in CRC models have mainly focused on chemoprevention whereas therapeutic approaches, in particular modulating cancer cell death and proliferation, are currently receiving a growing interest (Table 13.2).

Preclinical Studies In experimental and human carcinogenesis, including CRC, a deregulation of Wnt signaling by activating mutations is implicated (Khan and Mukhtar 2010; Barker and Clevers 2006). Sharma et al. showed that urolitinins, EA and ETs-rich fruit extracts inhibit Wnt signalling pathway at physiologically relevant concentrations in a human embryonic kidney 293T cell line using a luciferase gene reporter assay (Sharma et al. 2010). Sadik et al. showed that a diet supplemented with 3% (w/w) standardized PE modulated the expression pattern of the main key players in Wnt signalling in a 1,2-dimethylhydrazine dihydrochloride (DMH)-induced male Wistar albino rat colon carcinogenesis model (Table 13.2) (Sadik and Shaker 2013). The extract totally inhibited tumor incidence and minimized all the aberrant alterations in colonic tissues following DMH treatment. Besides, EA and Uro-A also inhibit Wnt signaling (Sadik and Shaker 2013). Kasimsetty et al., has demonstrated that PJ derived ETs induce cell-cycle arrest in S phase, downregulation of cyclins A and B1, with activation of cyclin E in HT-29 cells. The urolithins induced a cell-cycle block in G2/M phase, possibly related to its modulation of mitogen-activated protein kinases (MAPKs) (Kasimsetty et al. 2010). The proapoptotic activity of PC and EA was Fas and CASP-8-independent, whereas the activation of CASP-3 and CASP-9, the release of cytochrome c in the cytosol, and the downregulation of B-cell-lymphoma-extralarge (Bcl-xL) confirmed the involvement of the apoptotic intrinsic pathway. Of note, the proapoptotic effect of PC and EA was not recorded in normal colon cells, thus suggesting a selective action (Kasimsetty et al. 2010). Boateng et al. revealed that PJ reduced the number of aberrant cryptic foci (ACF) by 91%, in AOM treated F344 rats (Boateng et al. 2007). Increase in weight gain and feed intake was observed in PJ-fed rats, suggesting a possible protective effect against cancer cachexia (Boateng et al. 2007). In another study, PJ suppressed the number of ACF and significantly lowered proliferation of mucosa cells from AOM-treated Sprague-Dawley rats (Banerjee et al. 2013). PJ significantly downregulated mRNA and protein expression of nitric oxide synthase-2 (NOS2), COX-2, IGF, NF-κB and vascular cell adhesion molecule 1 (VCAM-1). Likewise, it inhibited phosphorylation of PI3K/AKT and mTOR expression, and increased the expression of miR-126. In vitro, the involvement of miR-126 was confirmed using the antagomiR for miR-126, where PJ reversed the effects of the antagomiR on the expression of miR-126, VCAM-1 and PI3K p85β. The therapeutic potential of pomegranate in colon tumorigenesis is due in part to targeting miR-126-regulated pathways, which contribute in the underlying anti-inflammatory mechanisms (Banerjee et al. 2013). Moreover, PSO, PPE, and its constituents show chemopreventive activity. Administration of PSO has been associated with a reduced incidence of chemically induced colon carcinogenesis in F344 rat, and expression of PPAR in the colonic mucosa (Kohno et al. 2004). The chemopreventive activity of PPE against AOM-induced oxidative stress and carcinogenesis in Sprague-Dawley rat colon has been related to its antioxidant activity by improving the redox status of colonic cells (Table 13.2) (Waly et al. 2012, 2014).

PJ and its constituents revealed in vitro antiproliferative and apoptotic ability on colon cancer cell lines (HT29, HCT116, SW480 and SW620) (Seeram et al. 2005). The greatest antiproliferative activity was observed for the PJ (Seeram et al. 2005). Again, this underlies the synergistic action of pomegranate polyphenols. Adams et al. showed in HT-29 cells that inflammatory enzymes were inhibited by PJ and its components (Table 13.2), demonstrating that these chemicals could play a major role in modifying the inflammatory signaling. The effects were attributed to synergistic activity of other bioactive polyphenols such as anthocyanins and flavonols (Adams et al. 2006). In another study, Larrosa et al. showed that both PC and EA induced apoptosis via mitochondrial pathway in Caco-2 cells but not in normal colon cells, demonstrating its specific action (Table 13.2) (Larrosa et al. 2006b). The peel extracts of egyptian pomegranate showed the highest antioxidant activity, as well as a pronounced anticancer activity against HCT-116 CRC cells (Motaal and Shaker 2011). In another study, γ-tocopherol showed chemopreventive properties by reducing levels of C-reactive protein, inhibition of neoplastic transformation, inhibition of COX-2 activity, downregulation of cyclins and upregulation of PPAR γ (Campbell et al. 2006).

Polyphenol-derived colon metabolites, specifically, EA and urolithins, have the potential to interact and affect colon CSCs (Nuñez-Sánchez et al. 2016). Two different mixtures containing urolithins and low levels of EA inhibited the number and size of colonospheres and aldehyde chemoresistance associated dehydrogenase (ALDH) activity (Nuñez-Sánchez et al. 2016).

Clinical Trials Nuñez-Sánchez et al. (2014b) studied the metabolic profiling of pomegranate phenolics and its metabolites in both normal and malignant CRC tissues as well as in blood and urine from 52 patients with resectable CRC upon consumption of PEs in a randomized, controlled clinical trial (Table 13.3). Significant levels of EA derivatives and urolithins are found in colon tissues from CRC patients. Overall, the results suggest that the anticancer properties of pomegranate might be exerted by these metabolites (Nuñez-Sánchez et al. 2014b). The same team also identified various changes in miRNA transcription (Table 13.3) following PE intake, in surgical colon biopsies from CRC patients (Nuñez-Sánchez et al. 2015). The clinical relevance of these miRNA changes deserve further research (Nuñez-Sánchez et al. 2015). In a complementary study, gene expression changes in colon tissue were evaluated in the first clinical trial (Nuñez-Sánchez et al. 2014b, 2015, 2017) and compared with in vitro in colon normal and cancer cultured cells exposed to the urolithins and EA (González-Sarrías et al. 2016) (Table 13.3). The results revealed a large interindividual variability and impact of the experimental protocol on the expression of the genes investigated (Nuñez-Sánchez et al. 2017).

13.3.4 Lung Cancer

In vitro and in vivo studies showed that pomegranate fruit extract (PFE) has chemopreventive/therapeutic potential against lung cancer (LCa) models (Table 13.2) (Khan et al. 2008). Treatment of human non-small lung cell carcinoma (NSLC) A549 cells with PFE from edible seeds decreased cell viability at the highest concentration (Khan et al. 2007a). Furthermore, the extract induced a strong arrest of cells in G0/G1 phase by induction of cdk inhibitors p21 and p27, inhibition of cyclins D1, D2, E and cdk2, cdk4, and cdk6 gene expression. Moreover, it decreased expression of Ki-67 proliferating cell nuclear antigen (PCNA), inhibited MAPK, PI3K/AKT, and NF-κB/p65. Only minimal effects were observed on normal human bronchial epithelial cells. This effect was confirmed in vivo in athymic mice xenografted with A549 cells (Khan et al. 2007a). The effect of oral consumption of a human achievable dose of PFE 0.2% (w/v) in drinking water on tumor growth, progression and signaling pathways was studied in two mouse lung tumor protocols induced by benzo(*a*)pyrene [B(a)P] and *N*-nitroso-trischloroethylurea (NTCU) in A/J mice (Khan et al. 2007b). Mice treated with PFE and exposed to B(a)P and NTCU had statistically significant tumor reduction and lower lung tumor metastases than mice treated with carcinogens only. PFE treatment resulted in inhibition of NF-κB, MAPK, Ki-67, PCNA, VGEF, PI3K/AKT signaling, and mTOR phosphorylation (Khan et al. 2007b). In another study, Modaeinama et al. showed an antiproliferative effect of a methanolic PPE at low doses with A459 LCa cells (Modaeinama et al. 2015). Moreover, PPE compounds like PC and EA had antimutagenic properties, protective effect against B(a)P induced DNA adducts and antiproliferative activity against LCa cells (A459 and H1299) (Zahin et al. 2014). Lucci et al. recently showed that PSO extract has antiproliferative effect on lung large cell carcinoma (COR-L23) (Lucci et al. 2015). The antiproliferative properties of a PSO was shown in A549 cells, even at the lowest doses, and its IC_{50} was determined at doses below 5 μg/ml (Seidi et al. 2016).

Li et al. evaluated the in vitro anticancer effects of *Punica granatum* leaf extract (PgLE) on two NSCLC cells A549 and H1299, and mouse Lewis LCa cell line LL/2, and explored its mechanisms of action (Li et al. 2016a). The extract affected cell survival by arresting cell cycle at G2/M phase and induced apoptosis in H1299 cells, but not in normal cells (HEK293, LO2 and Vero), showing high selectivity (Li et al. 2016a). Moreover, PgLE could also decrease ROS and the mitochondrial membrane potential ($\Delta\psi_m$), indicating that mitochondria-mediated apoptotic pathway was involved (Li et al. 2016a). Furthermore, H1299 cell migration and invasion processes were inhibited, and the reduction of MMP-2 and MMP-9 expression were also observed. Taken together, PE holds promise as an effective and safe chemopreventive and chemotherapeutic agent in NSCLC treatment (Li et al. 2016a).

13.3.5 Skin Cancer

The increase in incidence of skin cancer (SCa) has also promoted therapeutic research and chemoprevention studies (Gupta and Mukhtar 2002; Richmond and Viner 2003). PFE pretreatment inhibits cell proliferation, differentiation, and survival processes induced by UVB-induced activation of NF-κB MAPK pathway signaling proteins like STAT3, extracellular signal-regulated kinase (ERK)-1/2, c-Jun N-terminal kinases (JNK)1/2, p38 protein and AKT1 in human normal epidermal keratinocyte cells (Afaq et al. 2005a). PE treatment of the skin before exposure to a carcinogenic agent inhibits the appearance of erythemas, hyperplasia and the activity of epithelial ornithine decarboxylase (ODC) (Lisbeth et al. 2008). Besides, PE protects human skin fibroblasts from cell death following UV exposure by inhibition of NF-κB activation, downregulation of proapoptotic CASP-3, and increased DNA repair. However, decreased levels of UV-induced ROS levels and increase intracellular antioxidant capacity was only achieved at higher concentrations (Lisbeth et al. 2008). Syed et al. has reported a photochemopreventive effects of PFE against UVA using human keratinocytes (Syed et al. 2006). Pretreatment with the extract inhibited UVA-mediated activation of STAT3, AKT, ERK1/2, mTOR, p70S6K and NF-κB pathways (Syed et al. 2006). Also, a protective effect of standardized PE in ultraviolet-irradiated human skin fibroblasts was demonstrated (Pacheco-Palencia et al. 2008).

The pretreatments of human reconstituted skin (EpiDermTM FT-200) with polyphenols contained in the juice, especially anthocyanins and tannins, were capable to quench the effects of ultraviolet rays, as well as inhibited protein oxidation and PCNA protein expression (Zaid et al. 2007). Pretreatment of EpiDermTM with PJ, oil or by-product resulted in marked inhibition in the number of cyclobutane primidine dimers and 8-OHdG positive cells, showing a protective effect against UVB-mediated DNA damage. Also, the components of pomegranate were able to inhibit UVB-induced expressions of MMP-2 and MMP-9 activity (Zaid et al. 2007). Oral feeding of PFE by 140 days before a single UVB inhibited UVB-induced skin edema, hyperplasia, infiltration of leukocytes, lipid peroxidation, hydrogen peroxide generation, ODC activity and expression, COX-2 and PCNA protein expression in photocarcinogenesis SKH-1-Elite-Hr hairless mice model (Afaq et al. 2010). Furthermore, it enhanced repair of UVB-mediated formation of cyclobutane pyrimidine dimers and 8-oxo-7-OHdG, and 8-OHdG oxidative damage. Also, the treatment synergized with UVB-induction of tumor suppressor p53 and p21. Additionally, PE inhibited UVB-mediated nuclear translocation of NF-κB, activation of inhibitor of NF-κB kinase subunit-α (IKKα), and phosphorylation and degradation of inhibitor of κB-α (IκBα) (Afaq et al. 2010). Along the same lines, topical treatment with PFE of skin cancer initiated by the 12-*O*-tetradecanoylphorbol-13-acetate (TPA) carcinogen, showed a significant reduction of skin tumors, edema and hyperplasia, epidermal ODC activity and protein expression by suppression of inflammation (COX-2, MAPKs, NF-κB) (Afaq et al. 2005b). Taken together, PFE consumption or topic application provides substantial (photo)protection from the adverse skin carcinogenic effects of UVB and UVA radiation.

Yoshimura et al. have shown that growth suppression by an EA-rich PPE is mediated through changes in tyrosinase activity and UV-induced pigmentation on skin melanoma tumors (Yoshimura et al. 2005). PSO treatment, being rich in PuA, did not delay the appearance of tumors, but significantly decreased the rate of tumor development and skin tumor numbers. Also, it exerts in vivo chemopreventive effects against SCa through inhibition of ODC, prostaglandin biosynthesis and inhibition of upstream eicosanoid enzyme, and PLA2 (Hora et al. 2003). Recently, in an in vitro study using two kinds of SCa cell lines, human amelanotic melanoma C32 and malignant melanoma A375, Lucci et al. showed that a PSE rich in bioactive lipid compounds, mainly PuA, has an antiproliferative effect (Lucci et al. 2015).

Clinical Trials With the aim of investigate environmental and personal characteristics associated with SCa risk, a multicenter hospital-based case-control study was performed in eight countries from Europe, including 409 patients with squamous cell carcinoma (SCC), 602 with basal cell carcinoma (BCC), 360 with cutaneous malignant melanoma (CMM) and 1550 control persons (Table 13.3). Pomegranate was evaluated as protective SCa development food agent considering its antioxidant, anti-inflammatory and pro-epidermal differentiation capabilities. The consumption of pomegranate was found to be modestly associated with reduced risk of BCC, SCC and CMM in multivariate analysis (de Vries et al. 2012).

13.3.6 Other Cancer Types

13.3.6.1 Liver Cancer

Globally, liver cancer is the second most common cause of cancer death (Marquardt et al. 2015). Hepatocellular carcinoma (HCC) is the fifth most common cancer and the third leading cause of cancer-related mortality and has shown an alarming rise in incidence and mortality worldwide (El-Ashmawy et al. 2016). Oxidative stress and inflammation primarily predispose to hepatocarcinogenesis (Zhou et al. 2016). Furthermore, problems such as hepatotoxicity, recurrence, drug resistance, and other adverse effects of current therapeutics urge researchers to find alternative treatments (Table 13.2). As the pomegranate has powerful antioxidant properties, investigators have examined the chemopreventive potential of pomegranate extract against diethylnitrosamine (DENA)-induced rat hepatocarcinogenesis that mimics human HCC (Bishayee et al. 2011). Pomegranate extract significantly reduces the number and area of γ-glutamyl transpeptidase positive hepatic foci. Also, it inhibited DENA-induced hepatic lipid peroxidation and protein oxidation. Pomegranate extract further elevates the gene expression and protein levels of hepatic antioxidants, carcinogen detoxifying enzymes, and mRNA expression of the hepatic nuclear factor E2-related factor 2 (Nrf2) (Bishayee et al. 2011). In addition, the extract dose dependently suppresses hepatic expression of NOS2, 3-nitrotyrosine, heat shock protein 70 and 90, Wnt/β-catenin pathways, inflammatory COX-2 and NF-κB pathways upon pomegranate treatment of DENA-exposed rat livers (Table 13.2) (Bishayee et al. 2011, 2013; Takigawa and Brown 2008; Bhatia et al. 2013). A prophylactic effect of PPE against neoplastic changes in the liver was supported by the decrease of tumor size, liver index, and Bcl-2 and the increase of GSH (El-Ashmawy et al. 2016). Also, decreased expression of cyclin D1 and β-catenin genes could be observed (El-Ashmawy et al. 2016).

13.3.6.2 Pancreatic Cancer

PFE was evaluated as an antitumor agent using PANC-1 and AsPC-1 human pancreatic cancer cells. PFE induced cell cycle arrest and inhibited cell proliferation in PANC-1 cells. Moreover, PFE decreased the proportion of tumor-initiating cells lacking CD44 and CD24 expression. Pomegranate was more effective in inhibiting the proliferation of PANC-1 cells than the clinically used dose of paclitaxel. Similar results were obtained in the AsPC-1 cell line. Individual pomegranate phytochemicals were only modestly effective in inhibiting cell proliferation and suggests synergy between pomegranate constituents (Nair et al. 2011).

13.3.6.3 Leukemia

Suzuki et al. characterized the cytotoxic effect of PSO in mouse tumors and human monocytic leukemia cells (Suzuki et al. 2001). Flavonoid-rich polyphenols from PFJ and PPE strongly promoted cellular differentiation when compared to fresh juice, and all had similar inhibitory effects on proliferation of human promyelocytic leukemia HL-60 cells (Kawaii and Lansky 2004). Synergistic effects found were demonstrated for combination treatment of EA and quercetin with resveratrol in human leukemia cells (Mertens-Talcott and Percival 2005).

PJE promotes apoptosis in lymphoid (Jurkat, MOLT-3, SUP-B15, and CCRF-CEM) and myeloid (HL-60, THP-1, K562, and KG1a) leukemia cells and to much less extent in non-tumor hematopoietic stem cells (HSCs) (Dahlawi et al. 2012). Pomegranate extract caused a significant S phase arrest in all leukemia cell lines, with the exception of HL-60 and KG-1a, where a small percent of cells were blocked in the G0/G1 phase, suggesting cell type specific therapeutic effects (Dahlawi et al. 2012; Renneville et al. 2008). The different sensitivity to PJE between lymphoblastic and myeloblastic leukemia cells is reasonable by the different molecular pathways altered in those two types of leukemia. Upon bioactivity based screening of PJE fractions, ETs and EA were identified as the most potent bioactives, by blocking S phase (Dahlawi et al. 2013), whereas EA was found to promote CASP-3-dependent apoptosis (Hagiwara et al. 2010). Finally, Asmaa et al. reported that in addition to PJE, PPE promotes apoptosis in chronic myeloid leukemia cells K562 (Table 13.2) (Asmaa et al. 2015).

13.3.6.4 Bladder and Urothelial Cancers

Urinary bladder urothelial carcinoma (UBUC) represents the most frequent cancer affecting the urinary system worldwide (Siegel et al. 2014). In bladder cancer, p53 is recognized as being abnormally inactivated in more than 50% of carcinogenesis (Hilton and Svatek 2012). A miRNA (miR-34a) was found to be a direct target of p53 and subsequently mediated effects on cell cycle and apoptosis regulation (Hermeking 2012). Recently, Zhou et al. investigated the antiproliferative, proapoptotic effects, and functional mechanism of the p53/miR-34a axis on EJ cell bladder cancer induced by a standardized PPE rich in polyphenols (Zhou et al. 2015). The extract promotes EJ apoptosis without affecting normal rat urinary bladder epithelial cells. It inhibited c-JUN, increased p53 protein expression, and enhanced miR-34a expression mediated by p53 with subsequent inhibition of c-MYC and CD44 (Zhou et al. 2015). The in vitro results could be confirmed in vivo. PPE also inhibited EJ tumor growth in Balb/c nude mice through increase of miR-34a levels, p53 activation and inhibition of cancer proliferation (Zhou et al.

2015). The anticancer effect of PE was further shown with UBUC cells (T24 and J82) of high-grade malignancy and invasiveness (Lee et al. 2013). PE promoted cell cycle arrest at S phase by an increase in cyclin A protein level and a decrease in the expression of ckd1, and cell death by apoptosis with both cell types (Table 13.2) (Lee et al. 2013). In addition, PE activates pro-CASP-12 and enhanced expression of the transcription factor CHOP/GADD153, binding-immunoglobulin protein (BIP/GRP78), and endoplasmic reticulum stress (ERS) marker (Lee et al. 2013). A comparative proteomic study of PJ ethanol extract-treated T24 cells characterized various changes in protein expression levels related to apoptosis, cytoskeleton regulation, cell proliferation, proteasome activity and aerobic glycolysis (Table 13.2) (Wu et al. 2016). Furthermore, the antiproliferative activity and antioxidant capacity of different PFE and PPE extracts in T24 cells was proved to be directly related to the phenolic content and the presence of EA, respectively (Masci et al. 2016). In another study, apoptosis induced by PPE in T24 and J82 UBUC cells and in xenograft-induced bladder tumor in nude mice was related to up-regulation of DR4 and DR5 gene expression and activation of CASP-8 (Chang et al. 2018).

13.3.6.5 Brain Cancer

Gliomas are the most frequent brain tumors which are characterized by their poor prognosis due to resistance to surgical and medical treatments. Wang et al. has shown that PC inhibits the cell viability of human U87MG glioma cells by modulation of cell cycle cyclins levels and induction of apoptosis. Besides, PC treatment also increases phospho-AMPK and phospho-p27 levels and promotes microtubule-associated protein light chain 3 (LC3-II) cleavage in the cells. Both mechanisms are associated with the induction of autophagy and could be suppressed by chloroquine treatment, a suppressor of autophaghy (Wang et al. 2013).

13.3.6.6 Fibrosarcoma

Sepehr et al. showed that an ethanolic PFE increases nucleosome production and decreases pro-CASP-3 and Bcl-2 proteins to induce apoptosis in the mouse fibrosarcoma cell line WEHI-164 (Sepehr et al. 2014).

13.3.6.7 Multiple Myeloma

(MM) is a hematological malignancy, which remains incurable because most patients eventually relapse or become refractory to current treatments. So novel effective therapies to overcome therapy resistance are needed. Kiraz et al. recently demonstrated antiproliferative and apoptotic effects of different polyphenol-rich extract from non-edible parts of *Punica granatum* L. with U266 MM cancer cells (Kiraz et al. 2016). Tibullo et al. revealed the anti-proliferative potential of PJE in human MM cell lines (KMS26, MM1S and U266) by its ability to induce G0/G1 cell cycle block and upregulate PPAR-γ in a dose-dependent manner (Tibullo et al. 2016). Of note, in healthy lymphocytes and monocytes, the PJ treatment did not show any effect.

13.3.6.8 Ovarian Cancer

A methanolic PPE has antiproliferative effects in SKOV3 ovarian cancer (OCa) cells with IC_{50} values below 5 μg/ml (Modaeinama et al. 2015; Seidi et al. 2016). Tang et al. (2016) showed in vitro antitumor effect of PC with human A2780 OCa cells. PC induced cell cycle arrest in G1/S phase transition, inhibition of cell migration and apoptosis. In addition, the β-catenin pathway was suppressed as shown by the down-regulation of β-catenin and its downstream factors including cyclin D1 and surviving (Table 13.2) (Tang et al. 2016).

13.3.6.9 Cervical Cancer

Lucci et al. have shown that an ethanolic PSE rich in PuA has an antiproliferative effect on cervical adenocarcinoma cell line (HeLa) (Lucci et al. 2015). Li et al. (2016b) tested the antiproliferative effect of different fruit parts (peel, flesh, seeds, juices) and leaves of *Punica granatum* L. on HeLa cells. Peels and flesh extract significantly inhibited the proliferation compared to the other fruit parts. Guo et al. confirmed the antiproliferative and anti-invasive properties of EA from PPE with HeLa cells (Guo et al. 2016). Dose-dependent effects were associated with increased expression of insulin-like growth factor binding protein 7 (IGFBP7) and downregulation of AKT and mTOR expression (Guo et al. 2016).

13.3.6.10 Renal Cancer

Lucci et al. have shown that pomegranate seed ethanolic extract has an antiproliferative effect on renal adenocarcinoma ACHN cells, with an IC_{50} value of 26.5 μg/ml, as compared to vinblastine (IC_{50} 22.7 μg/ml) (Lucci et al. 2015).

13.3.6.11 Thyroid Cancer

Thyroid cancer (TCa) is the most common endocrine carcinoma and its incidence worldwide steadily increased threefold in the past decade (Davies et al. 2015). The most common type of TCa is papillary thyroid cancer (PTC) which generally has a good prognosis (Niedziela 2014). However, there are still a subset of patients with PTC, mainly those patients harboring *BRAF* mutations and *TERT* promoter mutation, who have poorer clinic-pathological outcomes and higher risk of recurrence

(Melo et al. 2015). Cheng et al. has demonstrated that 24 h PC treatment of BCPAP cells derived from a human PTC with BRAF and TERT mutations, resulted in marked increase of autophagy induction. This effect was associated with upregulation of markers for autophagy (i.e., LC3-II conversion, beclin-1 expression, and polyubiquitin-binding protein p62/SQSTM1) (Cheng et al. 2016) and decrease of the autophagy inhibitor 3-methyladenine. Moreover, PC activates MAPK by ERK1/2 and p38 kinase phosphorylation and inhibits the mTOR signaling pathway to promote the process of autophagy. This result is in agreement with in vitro evidence that revealed that PC induced both apoptosis and autophagy in U87 glioma cells (Wang et al. 2013). Later, the same group showed that PC generated a senescent phenotype with BCPAP cells, characterized by an altered morphology, increased cell granularity and senescence-associated β-galactosidase (SA-β-Gal) staining. Senesence was further associated with cell cycle arrest and upregulation of the cyclin-dependent kinase inhibitor p21 (Cheng et al. 2018).

13.4 Protective Effects of *Punica granatum* L. Against Adverse Chemotherapy-Induced Side Effects

In addition to anticancer properties of pomegranate constituents, protective effects to chemotherapy-induced adverse effects have been reported. Most of the protective effects of derivatives of *Punica granatum* L. are based on its powerful antioxidant capacity and free radical scavenger activity that counteract the cellular oxidative stress generated by cytostatics due to their cellular unspecific action. In Table 13.4 we have summarized the protective effects of different extracts and derivatives of *Punica granatum* L. against adverse side effects induced by cytostatics. Intake of dietary supplement in patients receiving chemotherapy medications should not exceed daily dose recommended by the Dietary Reference Intakes (Frenkel et al. 2013; Norman et al. 2003). Furthermore, the American Institute for Cancer Research (AICR) and Cancer Resource Advisory Council rather recommends consumption of fruits and vegetables in the diet rather than relying on large amounts of a multivitamin-multimineral supplements (Norman et al. 2003).

13.5 Chemosensitising Effects of *Punica granatum* L. in Combinatory Treatments with Conventional Chemotherapy

Unfortunately, due to the plasticity of signaling processes, epigenetic heterogeneity and genetic mutations which favor clonal selection and survival of tumor cells, intrinsic and acquired resistance to chemotherapeutic agents frequently occurs. Therefore, inhibition of any pathway by a single drug has modest long-term effects

Table 13.4 Protective effects of *Punica granatum* L. forms and its chemical compounds to chemotherapy-induced toxicity

Punica granatum forms and its chemical compounds	Cytostatic	Effect	References
Fruit rinds extract	Doxorubicin (DOX)	Co-treatment protocol promotes reduction of RNA-damage by formation of complexes with DOX or its interaction with the intracellular formation of reactive substances, electrophiles as well as free radicals, and protection of nucleophilic sites in RNA	Fimognari et al. (2008)
Whole fruit extract	DOX	Cardioprotective against DOX-induced toxicity with significant decrease in CK-MB, LDH	Hassanpour Fard et al. (2011)
Whole fruit extract	Methotrexate (MTX)	Protective against methotrexate-induced oxidative bone marrow damage by increase of white blood cell count, hemoglobin, hematocrit and platelet count	Sen et al. (2014)
Fruit extract (40% of ellagic acid) from GNC Herbal Plus® Standardized	MTX	Neuroprotective effects by significant inhibition of oxidative stress and inflammmatory response by decrease MDA, IL-1β and TNF-α levels	Çelik et al. (2013)
Fruit extract (POMX; POM Wonderful)	MTX	Suppression of MTX-induced cell death, reversed methotrexate-induced oxidative stress and apoptosis in hepatocytes by modulating Nrf2-NF-κ B pathways	Mukherjee et al. (2013)
Fruit juice	MTX	Prevents mucosal injury and improves intestinal recovery following MTX injury, supported by significant decrease in enterocyte apoptosis in ileum and associated with a decrease in caspase 3 protein expression as well as increased cell proliferation, which was correlated with elevated p-ERK protein levels	Shaoul et al. (2018)
Seed extract	Cisplatin (CDDP)	Protective effect against oxidative stress caused by CDDP injury of the kidneys and liver in rats, because of of its antioxidant, radical-scavenging, and antiapoptotic effects	Cayır et al. (2011)

(continued)

Table 13.4 (continued)

Punica granatum forms and its chemical compounds	Cytostatic	Effect	References
Seed oil	CDDP	Nephroprotective action by reduction of urinary protein, glucose, and serum urea and creatinine concentration, renal MDA, and increase in thiol content induced by CDDP	Boroushaki et al. (2015)
Seed extract	CDDP	Hepatoprotective effect against CDDP-induced liver damage by reduction in liver function enzyme activities and tissue MDA levels	Yildirim et al. (2013)
Fruit extract treated enzymatically with pectinase	CDDP	Protection against cisplatin-induced hearing loss by functional hearing evaluation of distortion product-evoked otoacoustic emission average amplitudes and histopathological analysis of cochlear bone capsule	Yazici et al. (2012)
Ellagic acid	CDDP	Protection against CDDP-induced negative changes in epididymal sperm characteristics and the histologic structure of testis and prostate associated with oxidative stress by suppressing of oxidative stress (reduction of MDA level and increased GPX, catalase and GSH levels, and activities of plasma, sperm, and testicular tissue)	Turk et al. (2008)
Fruit and leaf ethanolic extracts	Cyclophosphamide (CP)	Dose-dependent protection against CP-induced oxidative DNA damage with absence of mutagenic effects	Valadares et al. (2010)
Seed extract (tablets) Source naturals, Inc. Canada	Ifosfamide (IFO)	Protection against the damage actions of the IFO on sperm shape by potent anti-oxidative effect decrease in MDA level, by product of lipid peroxidation, and marked increases in GSH, GPx and CAT activities of plasma and sperm samples	Yaseen and Mustafa Al-Attar (2014)
Fruit extract	Adriamycin (ADR)	Protection against ADR-induced oxidative stress by suppression of the reduction in body weight, volume of amniotic fluid (AF), and increase in embryo gross	Kishore et al. (2009)

(continued)

Table 13.4 (continued)

Punica granatum forms and its chemical compounds	Cytostatic	Effect	References
		morphological deformities and significant changes in the levels of biochemical parameters in AF induced by ADR	
Punicalagin-rich pomegranate ellagitannins extract	5-Fluorouracil (5-FU)	Counteracts 5-FU-induced intestinal mucositis in rats evidenced by a reduction in the number of apoptotic cells per crypt	Chen et al. (2018)

on cell viability, tumor growth, patient survival, and may be insufficient to achieve tumor recession. As such, a complicated pathology as cancer may require multi-targeted therapy (Kawasaki et al. 2008; Petrelli and Giordano 2008). Given the diversity, structural complexity and pleiotropic activity of natural products, their future use for cancer therapy probably lies in synergistic combinations. In this role, they act as modifiers of biologic response, potentially enhancing the efficacy and efficiency of current cancer polychemotherapy regimens, mitigating the phenomenon of multidrug resistance and reducing the possibility of episodes of recurrence and secondary malignancies (Petrelli and Giordano 2008; Vinod et al. 2013).

So far, only limited synergistic anticancer combinations have been reported for PE constituents with conventional antitumor therapeutic agents. Antitumor action of retinoic acid (RA) was enhanced by EA through induction of leukemic HL-60 cell differentiation towards granulocytic phenotype (Hagiwara et al. 2010). Thus, RA-EA combination therapy might be a promising strategy to reduce RA cardiorespiratory toxicity (Fenaux et al. 2001). Tamoxifen (TAM) is often used against ER+ breast cancer and acts as an ER modulator in hormone therapy for BCa ER-α(+) and Her2/neu(−) oncoprotein (Banerjee et al. 2011). Unfortunately, TAM induced adverse effects and risk to develop therapy resistance limits its use at high doses. PFEs chemosensitizes TAM-dependent suppression of estrogen dependent cell growth and apoptosis in ER(+)-MCF-7 cells under E2 stimulation or non-estrogenic conditions. Furthermore, PFE restored sensitivity to TAM of TAM-resistant MCF-7 cells (Banerjee et al. 2011). Of note, PFE is able to reverse the cancer promoting effects of estrogen through the dysregulation of proliferation and apoptosis related genes in ER(+) cells. These results suggest that pomegranate combined with tamoxifen may represent a novel and a powerful approach to enhance and sensitize tamoxifen action (Banerjee et al. 2011). These results were further supported in vivo by a clinical trial where mastectomy women were treated using a combination of PSO and TAM (Qasim et al. 2013). Standard, docetaxel (DTX) treatment is the only first-line chemotherapy with a survival benefit in metastatic castration-resistant PCa. Nonetheless, most patients become DTX resistant and inevitably progress with no cure (Attard et al. 2006; McCarty et al. 2014). Remarkably, PE (POMx) increased the efficacy of DTX in C4-2 human PCA cell-transplanted BALB/c nu/nu mice (Wang et al. 2014). These results provide the first preclinical evidence that POMx may be effective in treating metastatic castration-resistant PCa and enhance the efficacy of DXT. The downregulation of HR by pomegranate reported before on MCF-7 BCa cells (Shirode et al. 2014) was recently exploited for sensitization of tumors to anticancer drugs that target HR such as bortezomib (Dahlawi et al. 2013; Tibullo et al. 2016).

In another study, ETs from pomegranate induced synergistic cytotoxicity against HT-29 CRC in combination with 5-FU treatment (Chen et al. 2018). A recent report demonstrates that pomegranate downregulates survivin mRNA as well as its protein (Banerjee et al. 2012). Survivin is associated with chemotherapy resistance and specifically with MRP1/P-gp overexpression (Vini and Sreeja 2015). Thus, this might be an indicatory result to highlight the importance of PEs pertaining to chemotherapy resistance. The pomegranate constituent quercetin is known to reverse adriamycin (ADR) resistance in MCF-7 ADR-resistant human BCa cells, via inhibition of P-gp (Vini and Sreeja 2015). In the same way, kaempferol present in the pericarp of pomegranate is reported to be a P-gp inhibitor in P-gp-overexpressing KB-C2 cells (Vini and Sreeja 2015).

Collectively, the above mentioned studies suggest that the pomegranate constituents are promising phytochemical drugs for synergistic combination therapy with conventional cancer drugs.

13.6 Nanotechnological Drug Delivery Systems of Pomegranate Extracts and Its Bioactive Constituents

The advent of nanomedicine marks an unparalleled opportunity to advance cancer treatment with unprecedented safety and efficiency, superior to conventional cancer therapies (Dawidczyk et al. 2014; Xu et al. 2015; Sanna et al. 2014). A change of drug delivery nanotechnologic systems-disease treatments is occurring from a single therapeutic agent in one particle (single nanodelivery) (Sanna et al. 2014) to the delivery of more than a single agent in one particle, often in an optimized ratio for synergistic effect (combinatorial nanodelivery) (Xu et al. 2015). Then, multiple cancer pathways may be targeted with one particle.

As mentioned above, pomegranate polyphenols have low bioavailability and a short half-life. Pomegranate polyphenol encapsulation into biodegradable sustained release nanoparticles may circumvent these limitations. PEGylated nanoformulations with PE and polyphenols (PC and EA) were efficiently taken up into MCF-7 and Hs578T BCa cells, and had a 2- to 12-fold enhanced effect on cell growth inhibition compared to their free counterparts. PC nanoparticles were the most potent nanoprototype, while void nanoparticles did not affect cell growth (Shirode et al. 2015). Moreover, a nanoformulation with paclitaxel and EA has been developed (Vasudev et al. 2012). Also, PFE has been added as reducing and stabilizing agent to a mixture of gold nanoparticles which showed an excellent cytotoxic result against the HeLa cancer cell line (Lokina et al. 2014). Physiologically stable and biocompatible mono-dispersed gold nanoparticles with PPE and functionalizated with folic acid and 5-FU required much lower amount of 5-FU to achieve 50% of growth of inhibition of MCF-7 BCa cells when compared to free 5-FU (Ganeshkumar et al. 2013). Very recently, the use of PSO oil phase component in drug delivery nanosystems was reported (Ferreira et al. 2015). Lu et al. demonstrated synergistic therapeutic outcomes for combination of PSO with a *trans*-resveratrol-loaded self-nanoemulsifying drug delivery system and holds promise for further clinical development (Lu et al. 2015).

13.7 Future Challenges

Because of its well established health effects, pomegranate extract in Ayurveda is considered as a "pharmacy of bioactives" (Jurenka 2008), and "nature's power fruit" (Longtin 2003; No Authors 2013; Fu et al. 2011). Many studies report that the extracts are more beneficial than its purified ingredients. This suggests the existence of a chemical synergy promoting inhibition of multiple targets, and thus greater likelihood for producing robust anticancer effects. Various molecular and cellular studies have provided new insights into pomegranate-based strategies for cancer prevention and treatment (Adhami et al. 2009; Syed et al. 2013). However, pomegranate health effects against cancer development show high interindividual variation to its bioactive ingredients, as systemic concentrations of its metabolites can be quite different between individuals (van Die et al. 2016; Hackshaw-McGeagh et al. 2015; Núñez-Sánchez et al. 2015). Recent studies suggest that pomegranate metabolites may also contribute to its therapeutic effects by stimulation of probiotic bacteria, thus enhancing their beneficial effects (Nuñez-Sánchez et al. 2014a; Espín et al. 2013). Therefore, gut microflora seem to contribute in pomegranate therapeutic activities in CRC patients (Núñez-Sánchez et al. 2015). Further (pre) clinical studies are needed to identify interindividual variation of in vivo metabolites in chemopreventive interventions or chemotherapeutic treatment of CRC (Núñez-Sánchez et al. 2015). Another level of variation has been attributed to differences in pomegranate polyphenol bioavailability between clinical trial studies (Seeram et al. 2004, 2006; Adhami et al. 2009). Moreover, genetic polymorphisms in enzymes involved in absorption, bioavailability, biodistribution, and metabolism of pomegranate bioactive compounds further increase interindividual variation (Seeram et al. 2004; Mertens-Talcott et al. 2006; Turrini et al. 2015; Basu and Penugonda 2009). Structure function activity analysis of different PG plasmatic metabolites or gut microbiota-derived metabolites, such as urolithins, may further improve our understanding of variable responses in intervention studies (Nuñez-Sánchez et al. 2014a; Seeram et al. 2008; Klempner and Bubley 2012).

Furthermore, it is essential to define the toxicological properties of pomegranate herbal preparations, because chemopreventive interventions are designed at healthy populations at high risk of cancer development. Although moderate consumption of pomegranate does not result in major adverse health effects (Vlachojannis et al. 2015), the combinatory effect of pomegranate with other compounds has been sparsely examined so far as well as potential food-drug interactions that may alter the bioavailability, effectiveness and toxicity of pomegranate and its bioactive constituents as well as of pharmacological drugs (Srinivas 2013).

Another aspect is the need to demonstrate efficacy of pomegranate formulations in clinical trials. Natural products share some mechanisms with chemotherapy drugs, but the lack of long-term clinical trials prevent the validation of natural products as possible adjuvants in cancer management. One reason may be the difficulty of achieving approval of the hospital ethic committees and/or oncologists for administration of high concentrations of *Punica granatum* L. adjuvants in patients undergoing chemotherapy. One problem is the dogmatic view of some oncologists toward natural products as "simple antioxidants", with the subsequent concern for a non-effective oxidative stress-mediated chemotherapeutic treatments (Syed et al. 2013; Núñez-Sánchez et al. 2015). Thus, more randomized clinical trials are needed to evaluate the role of *Punica granatum* L. products as adjuvants in the evolution of the disease, concomitant with chemotherapy, as was reported by Braumann et al. (Braumann et al. 2009) and Hoensch et al. (van Die et al. 2016; Hackshaw-McGeagh et al. 2015; Hoensch et al. 2008). One of the major challenges in clinical studies investigating the preventive effect of pomegranate is how to show the absence or reduced incidence of a specific disease endpoint. Such intervention studies have to be long term and, therefore, will be costly. In addition, new biomarkers have to be identified, developed and verified to analyze the long-term chemopreventive benefits of pomegranate herbal preparations or combinatory pharmaceutical formulations of its chemical constituents.

In conclusion, we have summarized scientific evidence of anticancer effects of pomegranate constituents. We focused on its molecular targets and anticancer mechanisms of action along with a critical evaluation of pomegranate polyphenols as future anticancer nutraceuticals, which await further validation in randomized clinical trials.

References

Adams LS, Seeram NP, Aggarwal BB, Takada Y, Heber D (2006) Pomegranate juice, total pomegranate ellagitannins, and punicalagin suppress inflammatory cell signaling in colon cancer cells. J Agric Food Chem 54:980–985

Adams LS, Zhang Y, Seeram NP, Heber D, Chen S (2010) Pomegranate ellagitannin-derived compounds exhibit antiproliferative and antiaromatase activity in breast cancer cells in vitro. Cancer Prev Res (Phila) 3:108–113

Adaramoye O, Erguen B, Nitzsche B, Höpfner M, Jung K, Rabien A (2017) Punicalagin, a polyphenol from pomegranate fruit, induces growth inhibition and apoptosis in human PC-3 and LNCaP cells. Chem Biol Interact 274:100–106

Adhami VM, Khan N, Mukhtar H (2009) Cancer chemoprevention by pomegranate: laboratory and clinical evidence. Nutr Cancer 6:811–815
Adhami VM, Siddiqui IA, Syed DN, Lall RK, Mukhtar H (2012) Oral infusion of pomegranate fruit extract inhibits prostate carcinogenesis in the tramp model. Carcinogenesis 33:644–651
Afaq F, Malik A, Syed D, Maes D, Matsui MS, Mukhtar H (2005a) Pomegranate fruit extract modulates UV-B mediated phosphorylation of mitogen-activated protein kinases and activation of nuclear factor kappa B in normal human epidermal keratinocytes. Photochem Photobiol 81:38–45
Afaq F, Saleem M, Krueger CG, Reed JD, Mukhtar H (2005b) Anthocyaninand hydrolyzable tannin-rich pomegranate fruit extract modulates MAPK and NF-kappaB pathways and inhibits skin tumorigenesis in CD-1 mice. Int J Cancer 113:423–433
Afaq F, Khan N, Syed DN, Mukhtar H (2010) Oral feeding of pomegranate fruit extract inhibits early biomarkers of UVB radiation-induced carcinogenesis in SKH-1 hairless mouse epidermis. Photochem Photobiol 86:1318–1326
Akhtar S, Ismail T, Fraternale D, Sestile P (2015) Pomegranate peel and peel extracts: chemistry and food features. Food Chem 174:417–425
Alaoui-Jamali MA, Bismar TA, Gupta A, Szarek WA, Su J, Song W et al (2009) A novel experimental heme oxygenase-1-targeted therapy for hormone-refractory prostate cancer. Cancer Res 69:8017–8024
Albrecht M, Jiang W, Kumi-Diaka J, Lansky EP, Gommersall LM, Patel A et al (2004) Pomegranate extracts potently suppresses proliferation, xenograft growth, and invasion of human prostate cancer cells. J Med Food 7:274–283
Anand P, Kunnumakkara AB, Sundaram C, Harikumar KB, Tharakan ST, Lai OS et al (2008) Cancer is a preventable disease that requires major lifestyle changes. Pharm Res 25:2097–2116
Arapitsas P (2012) Hydrolyzable tannin analysis in food. Food Chem 135:1708–1717
Arun N, Singh DP (2012) *Punica granatum*: a review on pharmacological and therapeutic properties. IJPSR 3:1240–1245
Asmaa MJ, Ali AJH, Farid JM, Azman S (2015) Growth inhibitory effects of crude pomegranate peel extract on chronic myeloid leukemia, K562 cells. Int J App Basic Med Res 5:100–105
Attard G, Sarker D, Reid A, Molife R, Parker C, de Bon JS (2006) Improving the outcome of patients with castration-resistant prostate cancer through rational drug development. Br J Cancer 95:767–774
Banerjee S, Kambhampati S, Banerjee SK, Haque I (2011) Pomegranate sensitizes tamoxifen action in ER-α positive breast cancer cells. J Cell Commun Signal 5:317–324
Banerjee N, Talcott S, Safe S, Mertens-Talcott SU (2012) Cytotoxicity of pomegranate polyphenolics in breast cancer cells in vitro and vivo: potential role of miRNA-27a and miRNA-155 in cell survival and inflammation. Breast Cancer Res Treat 136:21–34
Banerjee N, Kim H, Talcott S, Mertens-Talcott S (2013) Pomegranate polyphenolics suppressed azoxymethane-induced colorectal aberrant crypt foci and inflammation: possible role of miR-126/VCAM-1 and miR-126/PI3K/AKT/mTOR. Carcinogenesis 34:2814–2822
Barker N, Clevers H (2006) Mining the Wnt pathway for cancer therapeutics. Nat Rev Drug Discov 5:997–1014
Barnard RJ (2004) Prevention of cancer through lifestyle changes. Evid Based Complement Altern Med 1:233–239
Basu A, Penugonda K (2009) Pomegranate juice: a heart-healthy fruit juice. Nutr Rev 67:49–56
Bhandari PR (2012) Pomegranate (*Punica granatum L*). Ancient seeds for modern cure? Review of potential therapeutic applications. Int J Nutr Pharmacol Neurol Dis 2:171–184
Bhatia D, Thoppil RJ, Mandal A, Samtani KA, Darvesh AS, Bishayee A (2013) Pomegranate bioactive constituents suppress cell proliferation and induce apoptosis in an experimental model of hepatocellular carcinoma: role of Wnt/β-catenin signaling pathway. Evid Based Complement Alternat Med 2013, 371813, 15 p. https://doi.org/10.1155/2013/371813. Epub 2013 Mar 28

Bishayee A, Bhatia D, Thoppil RJ, Darvesh AS, Nevo E, Lansky EP (2011) Pomegranate-mediated chemoprevention of experimental hepatocarcinogenesis involves Nrf2-regulated antioxidant mechanisms. Carcinogenesis 32:888–896

Bishayee A, Thoppil RJ, Darvesh AS, Ohanyan V, Meszaros JG, Bhatia D (2013) Pomegranate phytoconstituents blunt the inflammatory cascade in a chemically induced rodent model of hepatocellular carcinogenesis. J Nutr Biochem 24:178–187

Bishayee A, Mandal A, Bhattacharyya P, Bhatia D (2016) Pomegranate exerts chemoprevention of experimentally induced mammary tumorigenesis by suppression of cell proliferation and induction of apoptosis. Nutr Cancer 68:120–130

Bishop FL, Rea A, Lewith H, Chan YK, Saville J, Prescott P et al (2011) Complementary medicine use by men with prostate cancer: a systematic review of prevalence studies. Prostate Cancer Prostatic Dis 14:1–13

Boateng J, Verghese M, Shackleford L, Walker LT, Khatiwada J, Ogutu S et al (2007) Selected fruits reduce azoxymethane (AOM)-induced aberrant crypt foci (ACF) in fisher 344 male rats. Food Chem Toxicol 45:725–732

Boeing H, Bechthold A, Bub A, Ellinger S, Haller D, Kroke A et al (2012) Critical review: vegetables and fruit in the prevention of chronic diseases. Eur J Nutr 51:637–663

Boroushaki MT, Rajabian A, Farzadnia M, Hoseini A, Poorlashkari M, Taghavi A et al (2015) Protective effect of pomegranate seed oil against cisplatin-induced nephrotoxicity in rat. Ren Fail 37:1338–1343

Braumann C, Guenther N, Loeffler LM, Dubiel W (2009) Liver metastases after colonic carcinoma—palliative chemotherapy plus curcumin. Int J Color Dis 24:859–860

Campbell SE, Stone WL, Lee S, Whaley S, Yang H, Qui M et al (2006) Comparative effects of RRR-alpha- and RRR-gamma-tocopherol on proliferation and apoptosis in human colon cancer cell lines. BMC Cancer 6:13. https://doi.org/10.1186/1471-2407-6-13

Cayır K, Karadeniz A, Simşek N, Yıldırım S, Karakuş E, Kara A et al (2011) Pomegranate seed extract attenuates chemotherapy-induced acute nephrotoxicity and hepatotoxicity in rats. J Med Food 14:1254–1262

Çelik F, Gocmez C, Bozkurt M, Kaplan I, Kamasak K, Akil E et al (2013) Neuroprotective effects of carvacrol and pomegranate against methotrexate induced toxicity in rats. Eur Rev Med Pharmacol Sci 17:2988–2993

Cerdá B, Llorach R, Cerón JJ, Espín JC, Tomás-Barberán FA (2003) Evaluation of the bioavailability and metabolism in the rat of punicalagin, an antioxidant polyphenol from pomegranate juice. Eur J Nutr 42:18–28

Cerdá B, Espín JC, Parra S, Martinez P, Tomás-Barberán FA (2004) The potent in vitro antioxidant ellagitannins from pomegranate juice are metabolised into bioavailable but poor antioxidant hydroxy-6H-dibenzopyran-6-one derivatives by the colonic microflora of healthy humans. Eur J Nutr 43:205–220

Cerdá B, Periago P, Espín JC, Tomás-Barberán FA (2005) Identification of urolithin A as a metabolite produced by human colon microflora from ellagic acid and related compounds. J Agric Food Chem 53:5571–5576

Chang C-P, Chan Y-Y, Li C-F, Chien L-H, Lee S-T, Wu T-F (2018) Deciphering the molecular mechanism underlying the inhibitory efficacy of Taiwanese local pomegranate peels against urinary bladder urothelial carcinoma. Nutrients 10(5):E543. https://doi.org/10.3390/nu10050543

Chen HS, Bai MH, Zhang T, Li GD, Liu M (2015) Ellagic acid induces cell cycle arrest and apoptosis through TGF-β/Smad3 signaling pathway in human breast cancer MCF-7 cells. Int J Oncol 46:1730–1738

Chen XX, Lam KH, Feng Y, Xu K, Sze SCW, Tang CW et al (2018) Ellagitannins from pomegranate ameliorates 5-fluorouracil-induced intestinal mucositis in rats while enhancing its chemotoxicity against HT-29 colorectal cancer cells through intrinsic apoptosis induction. J Agric Food Chem 66:7054–7064. https://doi.org/10.1021/acs.jafc.8b02458

Cheng X, Gao Y, Yao X, Yu H, Bao J, Guan H et al (2016) Punicalagin induces apoptosis-independent autophagic cell death in human papillary thyroid carcinoma BCPAP cells. RSC Adv 6:72. https://doi.org/10.1039/C6RA13431A

Cheng X, Yaob X, Xua S, Panb J, Yua H, Baoa J et al (2018) Punicalagin induces senescent growth arrest in human papillary thyroid carcinoma BCPAP cells via NF-κB signaling pathway. Biomed Pharmacother 103:490–498. https://doi.org/10.1016/j.biopha.2018.04.074

Costantini S, Rusolo F, De Vito V, Moccia S, Picariello G, Capone F et al (2014) Potential anti-inflammatory effects of the hydrophilic fraction of pomegranate (*Punica granatum* L.) seed oil on breast cancer cell lines. Molecules 19:8644–8660

D'Amico AV, Moul JW, Carroll PR, Sun L, Lubeck D, Chen MH (2003) Surrogate end point for prostate cancer-specific mortality after radical prostatectomy or radiation therapy. J Natl Cancer Inst 95:1376–1383

Dahlawi H, Jordan-Mahy N, Clench MR, LeMaitre CL (2012) Bioactive actions of pomegranate fruit extracts on leukemia cell lines in vitro hold promise for new therapeutic agents for leukemia. Nutr Cancer 64:100–110

Dahlawi H, Jordan-Mahy N, Clench M, McDougall GJ, Maitre CL (2013) Polyphenols are responsible for the proapoptotic properties of pomegranate juice on leukemia cell lines. Food Sci Nutr 2:196–208

Dai Z, Nair V, Khan M, Ciolino HP (2010) Pomegranate extract inhibits the proliferation and viability of MMTV-Wnt-1 mouse mammary cancer stem cells in vitro. Oncol Rep 24:1087–1091

Dana N, Javanmard SH, Rafiee L (2016) Role of peroxisome proliferator-activated receptor alpha and gamma in antiangiogenic effect of pomegranate peel extract. Iran J Basic Med Sci 19:106–110

Davies L, Morris LG, Haymart M, Chen AY, Goldenberg D, Morris J et al (2015) American Association of Clinical Endocrinologists and American College of Endocrinology Disease state clinical review: the increasing incidence of thyroid cancer. Endocr Pract 21:686–696

Dawidczyk CM, Russell LM, Searson PC (2014) Nanomedicines for cancer therapy: state-of-the-art and limitations to pre- clinical studies that hinder future developments. Front Chem 2:69. https://doi.org/10.3389/fchem.2014.00069

de Vries E, Trakatelli M, Kalabalikis D, Ferrandiz L, Ruiz-de-Casas A, Moreno-Ramirez D et al (2012) Known and potential new risk factors for skin cancer in European populations: a multicentre case-control study. Br J Dermatol 167(Suppl 2):1–13. https://doi.org/10.1111/j.1365-2133.2012.11081.x

Deng Y, Li Y, Yang F, Zeng A, Yang S, Luo Y et al (2017) The extract from *Punica granatum* (pomegranate) peel induces apoptosis and impairs metastasis in prostate cancer cells. Biomed Pharmacother 93:976–984

DiMarco-Crook C, Xiao H (2015) Diet-based strategies for cancer chemoprevention: the role of combination regimens using dietary bioactive components. Annu Rev Food Sci Technol 6:505–552

El-Ashmawy NE, Khedr EG, El-Bahrawy HA, Abd El-Fattah EE (2016) Effect of pomegranate hull extract on liver neoplastic changes in rats: more than an antioxidant. Nutr Cancer 68:1044–1051

Espín JC, González-Barrio B, Cerdá B, López-Bote C, Rey AI, Tomás-Barberán FA (2007) Iberian pig as a model to clarify obscure points in the bioavailability and metabolism of ellagitannins in humans. J Agric Food Chem 55:10476–10485

Espín JC, Larrosa M, García-Conesa M T, Tomás-Barberán FA (2013) Biological significance of urolithins, the gut microbial ellagic acid-derived metabolites: the evidence so far. Evid Based Complement Altern Med 270418, 15 p. https://doi.org/10.1155/2013/270418

Faria A, Calhau C (2011) The bioactivity of pomegranate: impact on health and disease. Crit Rev Food Sci Nutr 51:626–634

Fenaux P, Chomienne C, Degos L (2001) All-trans retinoic acid and chemotherapy in the treatment of acute promyelocytic leukemia. Semin Hematol 38:13–25

Ferreira LM, Cervi VF, Gehrcke M, da Silveira EF, Azambuja JH, Braganhol E et al (2015) Ketoprofen-loaded pomegranate seed oil nanoemulsion stabilized bypullulan: selective antiglioma formulation for intravenous administration. Colloids Surf B: Biointerfaces 130:272–277

Fimognari C, Sestili P, Lenzi M, Bucchini A, Cantelli-Forti G, Hrelia P (2008) RNA as a new target for toxic and protective agents. Mutat Res 648:15–22

Freedland SJ, Humphreys EB, Mangold LA, Eisenberger M, Dorey FJ, Walsh PC et al (2005) Risk of prostate cancer–specific mortality following biochemical recurrence after radical prostatectomy. JAMA 294:433–439

Freedland SJ, Carducci M, Kroeger N, Partin A, Rao JY, Jin Y et al (2013) A double-blind, randomized, neoadjuvant study of the tissue effects of POMx pills in men with prostate cancer before radical prostatectomy. Cancer Prev Res 6:1120–1127

Frenkel M, Abrams DI, Ladas EJ, Deng G, Hardy M, Capodice JL et al (2013) Integrating dietary supplements into cancer care. Integr Cancer Ther 12:369–384

Fu L, Xu BT, Xu XR, Gan RY, Zhang Y, Xia EQ et al (2011) Antioxidant capacities and total phenolic contents of 62 fruits. Food Chem 129:345–350

Fuentes VR, Expósito A (1995) Las encuestas etnobotánicas sobre plantas medicinales en Cuba. Rev Jard Bot Nac 16:77–144

Ganeshkumar M, Sathishkumar M, Ponrasu T, Dinesh MG, Suguna L (2013) Spontaneous ultrafast synthesis of gold nanoparticles using *Punica granatum* for cancer targeted drug delivery. Colloids Surf B Biointerfaces 106:208–216

Gil MI, Tomas-Barberan FA, Hess-Pierce B, Holcroft DM, Kader AA (2000) Antioxidant activity of pomegranate juice and its relationship with phenolic composition and processing. J Agric Food Chem 48:4581–4589

González-Sarrías A, Giménez-Bastida JA, García-Conesa MT, Gómez-Sánchez MB, García-Talavera NV, Gil-Izquierdo A et al (2010) Occurrence of urolithins, gut microbiota ellagic acid metabolites and proliferation markers expression response in the human prostate gland upon consumption of walnuts and pomegranate juice. Mol Nutr Food Res 54:311–322

González-Sarrías A, Núñez-Sánchez MA, Tomé-Carneiro J, Tomás-Barberán FA, García-Conesa MT, Espín JC (2016) Comprehensive characterization of the effects of ellagic acid and urolithins on colorectal cancer and key associated molecular hallmarks: microRNA-cell specific induction on CDKN1A (p21) as a common mechanism involved. Mol Nutr Food Res 60:701–716

Gordaliza M (2007) Natural products as leads to anticancer drugs. Clin Trans Oncol 9:767–776

Grossmann ME, Mizuno NK, Schuster T, Cleary MP (2010) Punicic acid is an omega-5 fatty acid capable of inhibiting breast cancer proliferation. Int J Oncol 36:421–426

Guo H, Zhang D, Fu Q (2016) Inhibition of cervical cancer by promoting IGFBP7 expression using ellagic acid from pomegranate peel. Med Sci Monit 22:4881–4886

Gupta S, Mukhtar H (2002) Chemoprevention of skin cancer: current status and future prospects. Cancer Metast Rev 21:363–380

Hackshaw-McGeagh LE, Perry RE, Leach VA, Qandil S, Jeffreys M, Martin RM et al (2015) A systematic review of dietary, nutritional, and physical activity interventions for the prevention of prostate cancer progression and mortality. Cancer Causes Control 26:1521–1550

Hagiwara Y, Kasukabe T, Kaneko Y, Niitsu N, Okabe-Kado J (2010) Ellagic acid, a natural polyphenolic compound, induces apoptosis and potentiates retinoic acid-induced differentiation of human leukemia HL-60 cells. Int J Hematol 92:136–143

Hassanpour Fard M, Ghule AE, Bodhankar SL, Dikshit M (2011) Cardioprotective effect of whole fruit extract of pomegranate on doxorubicin-induced toxicity in rat. Pharm Biol 49:377–382

He JZ, Ho JJ, Gingerich S, Courtman DW, Marsden PA, Ward ME (2010) Enhanced translation of heme oxygenase-2 preserves human endothelial cell viability during hypoxia. J Biol Chem 285:9452–9461

Heinlein CA, Chang C (2004) Androgen receptor in prostate cancer. Endocr Rev 25:276–308

Hermeking H (2012) MicroRNAs in the p53 network: micromanagement of tumour suppression. Nat Rev Cancer 12:613–626
Hilton WM, Svatek RS (2012) Words of wisdom. Re: phase III study of molecularly targeted adjuvant therapy in locally advanced urothelial cancer of the bladder based on p53 status. Eur Urol 61:1062–1063
Hoensch H, Groh B, Edler L, Kirch W (2008) Prospective cohort comparison of flavonoid treatment in patients with resected colorectal cancer to prevent recurrence. World J Gastroenterol 14:2187–2193
Hong MY, Seeram NP, Heber D (2008) Pomegranate polyphenols down-regulate expression of androgen-synthesizing genes in human prostate cancer cells overexpressing the androgen receptor. J Nutr Biochem 19:848–855
Hora JJ, Maydew ER, Lansky EP, Dwivedi C (2003) Chemopreventive effects of pomegranate seed oil on skin tumor development in CD1 mice. J Med Food 6:157–161
Huang WY, Cai YZ, Zhang Y (2010) Natural phenolic compounds from medicinal herbs and dietary plants: potential use for cancer prevention. Nutr Cancer 62:1–20
Iguchi T, Wang CY, Delongchamps NB, Kato M, Tamada S, Yamasaki T et al (2015) Association of MnSOD AA genotype with the progression of prostate cancer. PLoS One 10:e0131325
Ito H, Li P, Koreishi M, Nagatomo A, Nishida N, Yoshida T (2014) Ellagitannin oligomers and a neolignan from pomegranate arils and their inhibitory effects on the formation of advanced glycation end products. Food Chem 152:323–330
Jeune MAL, Kumi-Diaka J, Brown J (2005) Anticancer activities of pomegranate extracts and genistein in human breast cancer cells. J Med Food 8:469–475
Jiang Q, Elson-Schwab I, Courtemanche C, Ames BN (2000) γ-Tocopherol and its major metabolite, in contrast to α-tocopherol, inhibit cyclooxygenase activity in macrophages and epithelial cells. Proc Nat Acad Sci 97:11494–11499
Jiang Q, Wong J, Fyrst H, Saba JD, Ames BN (2004) γ-Tocopherol or combinations of vitamin E forms induce cell death in human prostate cancer cells by interrupting sphingolipid synthesis. Proc Nat Acad Sci 101:17825–17830
Jiménez-Escrig A, Santos-Hidalgo AB, Saura-Calixto F (2006) Common sources and estimated intake of plant sterols in the Spanish diet. J Agric Food Chem 54:3462–3471. https://doi.org/10.1021/jf053188k
Jurenka JMT (2008) Therapeutic applications of pomegranate (*Punica granatum* L.): a review. Altern Med Rev 13:123–144
Kalaycıoğlu Z, Bedia EF (2017) Total phenolic contents, antioxidant activities, and bioactive ingredients of juices from pomegranate cultivars worldwide. Food Chem 221:496–507
Kamiya N, Suzuki H, Endo T, Takano M, Yano M, Naoi M et al (2011) Significance of serum osteoprotegerin and receptor activator of nuclear factor κB ligand in Japanese prostate cancer patients with bone metastasis. Int J Clin Oncol 16:366–372
Kapoor R, Ronnenberg A, Puleo E, Chatterton RT Jr, Dorgan JF, Seeram NP et al (2015) Effects of pomegranate juice on hormonal biomarkers of breast cancer risk. Nutr Cancer 67:1113–1119
Kasimsetty SG, Bialonska D, Reddy MK, Thornton CK, Willett L, Ferreira D (2009) Effects of pomegranate chemical constituents/intestinal microbial metabolites on CYP1B1 in 22Rv1 prostate cancer cells. J Agric Food Chem 57:10636–10644
Kasimsetty SG, Bialonska D, Reddy MK, Ma G, Khan SI, Ferreira D (2010) Colon cancer chemopreventive activities of pomegranate ellagitannins and urolithins. J Agric Food Chem 58:2180–2187
Kawaii S, Lansky EP (2004) Differentiation-promoting activity of pomegranate fruit extracts in HL-60 human promyelocytic leukemia cells. J Med Food 7:13
Kawasaki BT, Hurt EM, Mistree T, Farrar WL (2008) Targeting cancer stem cells with phytochemicals. Mol Interv 8:174–184
Key TJ, Schatzkin A, Willett WC, Allen NE, Spencer EA, Travis RC (2004) Diet, nutrition and the prevention of cancer. Public Health Nutr 7:187–200

Khan N, Mukhtar H (2010) Cancer chemoprevention. In: McQueen CA (ed) Comprehensive toxicology, pp 417–431

Khan N, Handi N, Afaq F, Syed DN, Kweon MH, Mukhtar H (2007a) Pomegranate fruit extracts inhibits prosurvival pathways in human A549 lung carcinoma cells and tumor growth in athymic nude mice. Carcinogenesis 28:163–173

Khan N, Afaq F, Kweon MH, Kim K, Mukhtar H (2007b) Oral consumption of pomegranate fruit extract inhibits growth and progression of primary lung tumors in mice. Cancer Res 67:3475–3482

Khan N, Afaq F, Mukhtar H (2008) Cancer chemoprevention through dietary antioxidants: progress and promise. Antioxid Redox Signal 10:475–510

Khan N, Afaq F, Mukhtar H (2010) Lifestyle as risk factor for cancer: evidence from human studies. Cancer Lett 293:133–143

Kim ND, Mehta R, Yu W, Neeman I, Livney T, Amichay A et al (2002) Chemopreventive and adjuvant therapeutic potential of pomegranate (*Punica granatum*) for human breast cancer. Breast Cancer Res Treat 71:203–217

Kiraz Y, Neergheen-Bhujun VS, Rummun N, Baran Y (2016) Apoptotic effects of non-edible parts of *Punica granatum* on human multiple myeloma cells. Tumour Biol 37:1803–1815

Kishore RK, Sudhakar D, Parthasarathy PR (2009) Embryo protective effect of pomegranate (*Punica granatum* L.) fruit extract in adriamycin-induced oxidative stress. Indian J Biochem Biophys 46:106–111

Klempner SJ, Bubley G (2012) Complementary and alternative medicine in prostate cancer: from bench to bedside? Oncologist 17:830–837

Kohno H, Suzuki R, Yasui Y, Hosokawa M, Miyashita K, Tanaka T (2004) Pomegranate seed oil rich in conjugated linolenic acid suppresses chemically induced colon carcinogenesis in rats. Cancer Sci 95:481–486

Lansky EP, Newman RA (2007) *Punica granatum* (pomegranate) and its potential for prevention and treatment of inflammation and cancer. J Ethnopharmacol 109:177–206

Lansky EP, Shubert S, Neeman I (1997) Pharmacological and therapeutic of pomegranate. Ciham Options Mediterr 5:231–235

Lansky EP, Jiang W, Mo H, Bravo L, Froom P, Yu W et al (2005a) Possible synergistic prostate cancer suppression by anatomically discrete pomegranate fractions. Investig New Drugs 23:11–20

Lansky EP, Harrison G, Froom P, Jiang WG (2005b) Pomegranate (*Punica granatum*) pure chemicals show possible synergistic inhibition of human PC-3 prostate cancer cell invasion across matrigel™. Investig New Drugs 23:121–122

Larrosa M, González-Sarrías A, García-Conesa MT, Tomás-Barberán FA, Espín JC (2006a) Urolithins, ellagic acid derived metabolites produced by human colonic microflora, exhibit estrogenic and antiestrogenic activities. J Agric Food Chem 54:1611–1620

Larrosa M, Tomás-Barberán FA, Espín JC (2006b) The dietary hydrolysable tannin punicalagin releases ellagic acid that induces apoptosis in human colon adenocarcinoma Caco-2 cells by using the mitochondrial pathway. J Nutr Biochem 17:611–625

Lazzeroni M, DeCensi A (2013) Breast cancer prevention by antihormones and other drugs: where do we stand? Hematol Oncol Clin North Am 27:657–672

Lee S-T, Wu Y-L, Chien L-H, Chen S-T, Tzeng Y-K, Wu T-F (2012) Proteomic exploration of the impacts of pomegranate fruit juice on the global gene expression of prostate cancer cell. Proteomics 12:3251–3262

Lee ST, Lu MH, Chien LH, Wu TF, Huang LC, Liao GI (2013) Suppression of urinary bladder urothelial carcinoma cell by the ethanol extract of pomegranate fruit through cell cycle arrest and apoptosis. BMC Complement Altern Med 13:364. https://doi.org/10.1186/1472-6882-13-364

Li H, Kantoff P, Giovannucci E, Leitzmann MF, Gaziano JM, Stampfer MJ et al (2005) Manganese superoxide dismutase polymorphism, prediagnostic antioxidant status, and risk of clinically significant prostate cancer risk. Cancer Res 65:2498–2504

Li Y, Yang F, Zheng W, Hu M, Wang J, Ma S et al (2016a) *Punica granatum* (pomegranate) leaves extract induces apoptosis through mitochondrial intrinsic pathway and inhibits migration and invasion in non-small cell lung cancer in vitro. Biomed Pharmacother 80:227–235

Li R, Chen XG, Jia K, Liu ZP, Peng HY (2016b) A systematic determination of polyphenols constituents and cytotoxic ability in fruit parts of pomegranates derived from five Chinese cultivars. Springerplus 5:914–922

Lisbeth A, Noratto G, Hingorani L, Talcott ST, Mertens-Talcott SU (2008) Protective effects of standardized pomegranate (*Punica granatum* L.) polyphenolic extract in ultraviolet-irradiated human skin fibroblasts. J Agric Food Chem 56:8434–8441

Liu RH (2003) Health benefits of fruit and vegetables are from additive and synergistic combinations of phytochemicals. Am J Clin Nutr 78:517S–520S

Lokina S, Suresh R, Giribabu K, Stephen A, Lakshmi Sundaram R, Narayanan V (2014) Spectroscopic investigations, antimicrobial, and cytotoxic activity of green synthesized gold nanoparticles. Spectrochim Acta A Mol Biomol Spectrosc 129:484–490

Longtin R (2003) The pomegranate: Nature's power fruit? J Natl Cancer Inst 95:346–348

Lu LY, Liu Y, Zhang ZF, Gou XJ, Jiang JH, Zhang JZ et al (2015) Pomegranate seed oil exerts synergistic effects with trans-resveratrol in a self-nanoemulsifying drug delivery system. Biol Pharm Bull 38:1658–1662

Lucci P, Pacetti D, Loizzo MR, Frega NG (2015) *Punica granatum* cv. *Dente di Cavallo* seed ethanolic extract: antioxidant and antiproliferative activities. Food Chem 167:475–483

Mahaddalkar T, Suri C, Naik PK, Lopus M (2015) Biochemical characterization and molecular dynamic simulation of β-sitosterol as a tubulin-binding anticancer agent. Eur J Pharmacol 760:154–162

Malik A, Mukhtar H (2006) Prostate cancer prevention through pomegranate fruit. Cell Cycle 5:371–373

Malik A, Afaq F, Sarfaraz S, Adhami VM, Syed DN, Mukhtar H (2005) Pomegranate fruit juice for chemoprevention and chemotherapy of prostate cancer. Proc Natl Acad Sci USA 102:14813–14818

Mandal A, Bishayee A (2015) Mechanism of breast cancer preventive action of pomegranate: disruption of estrogen receptor and Wnt/β-catenin signaling pathways. Molecules 20:22315–22328

Marquardt JU, Andersen JB, Thorgeirsson SS (2015) Functional and genetic deconstruction of the cellular origin in liver cancer. Nat Rev Cancer 15:653–667

Masci A, Coccia A, Lendaro E, Mosca L, Paolicelli P, Cesa S (2016) Evaluation of different extraction methods from pomegranate whole fruit or peels and the antioxidant and antiproliferative activity of the polyphenolic fraction. Food Chem 202:59–69

McCarty MF, Hejazi J, Rastmanesh R (2014) Beyond androgen deprivation: ancillary integrative strategies for targeting the androgen receptor addiction of prostate cancer. Integr Cancer Ther 13:386–395

Mehta R, Lansky EP (2004) Breast cancer chemopreventive properties of pomegranate (*Punica granatum*) fruit extracts in a mouse mammary organ culture. Eur J Cancer Prev 13:345–348

Melo M, da Rocha AG, Vinagre J, Sobrinho-Simoes M, Soares P (2015) Coexistence of TERT promoter and BRAF mutations in papillary thyroid carcinoma: added value in patient prognosis? J Clin Oncol 33:667–668

Mertens-Talcott SU, Percival SS (2005) Ellagic acid and quercetin interact synergistically with resveratrol in the induction of apoptosis and cause transient cell cycle arrest in human leukemia cells. Cancer Lett 218:141–151

Mertens-Talcott SU, Jilma-Stohlawetz P, Rios J, Hingorani L, Derendorf H (2006) Absorption, metabolism, and antioxidant effects of pomegranate (*Punica granatum* L.) polyphenols after ingestion of a standardized extract in healthy human volunteers. J Agric Food Chem 54:8956–8961

Ming DS, Pham S, Deb S, Chin MY, Kharmate G, Adomat H et al (2014) Pomegranate extracts impact the androgen biosynthesis pathways in prostate cancer models in vitro and in vivo. J Steroid Biochem Mol Biol 143c:19–28

Modaeinama S, Abasi M, Abbasi MM, Jahanban-Esfahlan R (2015) Antitumoral properties of *Punica granatum* (pomegranate) peel extract on different human cancer cells. Asian Pac J Cancer Prev 16:5697–5701

Moon DO, Kim MO, Choi YH, Kim GY (2008) beta-Sitosterol induces G2/M arrest, endoreduplication, and apoptosis through the Bcl-2 and PI3K/Akt signaling pathways. Cancer Lett 264:181–191. https://doi.org/10.1016/j.canlet.2008.01.032

Motaal AA, Shaker S (2011) Anticancer and antioxidant activities of standardized whole fruit, pulp, and peel extracts of Egyptian pomegranate. Open Conf Proc J 2:41–45

Mukherjee S, Ghosh S, Choudhury S, Adhikary A, Manna K, Dey S et al (2013) Pomegranate reverses methotrexate-induced oxidative stress and apoptosis in hepatocytes by modulating Nrf2-NF-κB pathways. J Nutr Biochem 24:2040–2050. https://doi.org/10.1016/j.jnutbio.2013.07.005

Naiki-Ito A, Chewonarin T, Tang M, Pitchakarn P, Kuno T, Ogawa K et al (2015) Ellagic acid, a component of pomegranate fruit juice, suppresses androgen-dependent prostate carcinogenesis via induction of apoptosis. Prostate 75:151–160

Nainwani R, Singh D, Soni PK, Gupta A, Gautam R (2013) Chemical constituents of various parts of *Punica granatum* and their anti-inflammatory activity: a review. Asian J Pharm Res Dev 1:48–53

Nair V, Dai Z, Khan M, Ciolino HP (2011) Pomegranate extract induces cell cycle arrest and alters cellular phenotype of human pancreatic cancer cells. Anticancer Res 31:2699–2704

National Cancer Institute. Prostate Cancer, Nutrition, and Dietary Supplements (PDQ®)–Health Professional Version. (2016). Retrieved from http://www.cancer.gov/about-cancer/treatment/cam/hp/prostate-supplements-pdq

Newman DJ, Cragg GM (2007) Natural products as sources of new drugs over the last 25 years. J Nat Prod 70:461–477

Niedziela M (2014) Thyroid nodules. Best Pract Res Clin Endocrinol Metab 28:245–277

No Authors (2013) I've been reading about the potential benefits of pomegranates. Should I add this fruit to my diet? Johns Hopkins Med Lett Health After 50 25:7

Norman HA, Butrum RR, Feldman E, Heber D, Nixon D, Picciano MF et al (2003) The role of dietary supplements during cancer therapy. J Nutr 133:3794S–3799S

Nuñez-Sánchez MA, García-Villalba R, Monedero-Saiz T, García-Talavera NV, Gómez-Sánchez MB, Sánchez-Álvarez C et al (2014a) Targeted metabolic profiling of pomegranate polyphenols and urolithins in plasma, urine and colon tissues from colorectal cancer patients. Mol Nutr Food Res 58:1199–1211

Nuñez-Sánchez MA, García-Villalba R, Monedero-Saiz T, García-Talavera NV et al (2014b) Targeted metabolic profiling of pomegranate polyphenols and urolithins in plasma, urine and colon tissues from colorectal cancer patients. Mol Nutr Food Res 58:1199–1211

Nuñez-Sánchez MA, Dávalos A, González-Sarrías A, Casas-Agustench P, Visioli F, Monedero-Saiz T et al (2015) MicroRNAs expression in normal and malignant colon tissues as biomarkers of colorectal cancer and in response to pomegranate extracts consumption: critical issues to discern between modulatory effects and potential artefacts. Mol Nutr Food Res 59:1973–1986

Núñez-Sánchez MA, González-Sarrías A, Romo-Vaquero M, García-Villalba R, Selma MV, Tomás-Barberán FA, Garcia-Conesa MT, Espín JC (2015) Dietary phenolics against colorectal cancer—from promising preclinical results to poor translation into clinical trials: pitfalls and future needs. Mol Nutr Food Res 59:1274–1291

Nuñez-Sánchez MA, Karmokar A, González-Sarrías A, García-Villalba R, Tomás-Barberán FA, García-Conesa MT et al (2016) In vivo relevant mixed urolithins and ellagic acid inhibit phenotypic and molecular colon cancer stem cell features: a new potentiality for ellagitannin metabolites against cancer. Food Chem Toxicol 92:8–16

Nuñez-Sánchez MA, González-Sarrías A, García-Villalba R, Monedero-Saiza T, García-Talavera NV, Gómez-Sánchez MB et al (2017) Gene expression changes in colon tissues from colorectal cancer patients following the intake of an ellagitannin-containing pomegranate extract: a randomized clinical trial. J Nutr Biochem 42:126–133

Orgil O, Schwartz E, Baruch L, Matityahu I, Mahajna J, Amir R (2014) The antioxidative and anti-proliferative potential of non-edible organs of the pomegranate fruit and tree. LWT-Food Sci Technol 58:571–577

Pacheco-Palencia LA, Noratto G, Hingorani L, Talcott ST, Mertens-Talcott SU (2008) Protective effects of standardized pomegranate (*Punica granatum* L.) polyphenolic extract in ultraviolet-irradiated human skin fibroblasts. J Agricul Food Chem 56:8434–8441

Paller CJ, Ye X, Wozniak PJ, Gillespie BK, Sieber PR, Greengold RH et al (2013a) A randomized phase II study of pomegranate extract for men with rising PSA following initial therapy for localized prostate cancer. Prostate Cancer Prostatic Dis 16:50–55

Paller CJ, Olatoye D, Xie S, Zhou X, Denmeade SR, Eisenberger MA et al (2013b) The effect of the frequency and duration of PSA measurement on PSA doubling time calculations in men with biochemically recurrent prostate cancer. Prostate Cancer Prostatic Dis 17:28–33

Paller JC, Pantuck A, Carducci MA (2017) A review of pomegranate in prostate cancer. Prostate Cancer Prostatic Dis 20:265–270. https://doi.org/10.1038/pcan.2017.19

Pantuck AJ, Leppert JT, Zomorodian N, Aronson W, Hong J, Barnard RJ et al (2006) Phase II study of pomegranate juice for men with rising prostate-specific antigen following surgery or radiation for prostate cancer. Clin Cancer Res 12:4018–4026

Pantuck AJ, Pettaway CA, Dreicer R, Corman J, Katz A, Ho A et al (2015) A randomized, double-blind, placebo-controlled study of the effects of pomegranate extract on rising PSA levels in men following primary therapy for prostate cancer. Prostate Cancer Prostatic Dis 18:242–248

Paur I, Lilleby W, Bohn SK, Hulander E, Klein W, Vlatkovic L et al (2017) Tomato-based randomized controlled trial in prostate cancer patients: effect on PSA. Clin Nutr 36:672–679

Petrelli A, Giordano S (2008) From single- to multi-target drugs in cancer therapy: when a specificity becomes an advantage. Curr Med Chem 15:422–432

Pogribny IP, Rusyn I (2013) Environmental toxicants, epigenetics, and cancer. Adv Exp Med Biol 754:215–232

Prakash CVS, Prakash I (2011) Bioactive chemical constituents from pomegranate (*Punica granatum*) juice, seed and peel-a review. Int J Res Chem Environ 1:1–18

Qasim FK, Qadir FA, Karim KJ (2013) Effects of pomegranate seed oil and tamoxifen on mastectomy breast cancer women. IOSR J Pharm 3:44–51

Rahimi HR, Arastoo M, Ostad SN (2012) A comprehensive review of *Punica granatum* (pomegranate) properties in toxicological, pharmacological, cellular and molecular biology researches. Iran J Pharm Res 11:385–400

Renneville A, Roumier C, Biggio V, Nibourel O, Boissel N, Fenaux P et al (2008) Cooperating gene mutations in acutemyeloid leukemia: a review of the literature. Leukemia 22:915–931

Rettig MB, Heber D, An J, Seeram NP, Rao JY, Liu H et al (2008) Pomegranate extract inhibits androgen-independent prostate cancer growth through a nuclear factor-κB-dependent mechanism. Mol Cancer Ther 7:2662–2671

Richmond E, Viner JL (2003) Chemoprevention of skin cancer. Semin Oncol Nurs 19:62–69

Rocha A, Wang L, Penichet M, Martins-Green M (2012) Pomegranate juice and specific components inhibit cell and molecular processes critical for metastasis of breast cancer. Breast Cancer Res Treat 136:647–658

Roig JT (1974) Plantas medicinales, aromáticas o venenosas de Cuba. Ciencia y Técnica:401–402

Sadik NA, Shaker OG (2013) Inhibitory effect of a standardized pomegranate fruit extract on Wnt signalling in 1, 2-dimethylhydrazine induced rat colon carcinogenesis. Dig Dis Sci 58:2507–2517

Saltz LB (ed) (2007) Colorectal cancer: evidence-based chemotherapy strategies. Current Clinical Oncology™, Markman M, MD (Series ed). Humana, Totowa. ISBN: 1-58829-751-9, E-ISBN: 1-59745-215-7

Sanna V, Pala N, Sechi M (2014) Targeted therapy using nanotechnology: focus on cancer. Int J Nanomedicine 9:467–483

Sartippour MR, Seeram NP, Rao YJ, Moro A, Harris DM, Henning SM et al (2008) Ellagitannin-rich pomegranate extract inhibits angiogenesis in prostate cancer in vitro and in vivo. Int J Oncol 32:475–480

Scher HI, Helabi S, Tannock I, Morris M, Sternberg CN, Carducci MA et al (2008) Design and end points of clinical trials for patients with progressive prostate cancer and castrate levels of testosterone: recommendations of the prostate cancer clinical trials working group. J Clin Oncol 26:1148–1159

Seeram NP, Lee R, Heber D (2004) Bioavailability of ellagic acid in human plasma after consumption of ellagitannins from pomegranate (*Punica granatum* L.) juice. Clin Chim Acta 348:63–68

Seeram NP, Adams LS, Henning SM, Niu Y, Zhang Y, Nair MG et al (2005) In vitro antiproliferative, apoptotic and antioxidant activities of punicalagin, ellagic acid and a total pomegranate tannin extract are enhanced in combination with other polyphenols as found in pomegranate juice. J Nutr Biochem 16:360–367

Seeram NP, Henning SM, Zhang Y, Suchard M, Li Z, Heber D (2006) Pomegranate juice ellagitannin metabolites are present in human plasma and some persist in urine for up to 48 hours. J Nutr 136:2481–2485

Seeram NP, Aronson WJ, Zhang Y, Henning SM, Moro A, Lee RP et al (2007) Pomegranate ellagitannin-derived metabolites inhibit prostate cancer growth and localize to the mouse prostate gland. J Agric Food Chem 55:7732–7737

Seeram NP, Zhang Y, McKeever R, Henning SM, Lee RP, Suchard MA et al (2008) Pomegranate juice and extracts provide similar levels of plasma and urinary ellagitannin metabolites in human subjects. J Med Food 11:390–394

Seidi K, Jahanban-Esfahlan R, Abasi M, Abbasi MM (2016) Antitumoral properties of *Punica granatum* (pomegranate) seed extract in different human cancer cells. Asian Pac J Cancer Prev 17:1119–1122

Selma MV, Espín JC, Tomás-Barberán FA (2009) Interaction between phenolics and gut microbiota: role in human health. J Agricu Food Chem 57:6485–6501

Sen V, Bozkurt M, Söker S, Ece A, Güneş A, Uluca Ü et al (2014) The effects of pomegranate and carvacrol on methotrexate-induced bone marrow toxicity in rats. Clin Invest Med 37:E93–E101

Seoane J (1984) El folklor médico de Cuba. Provincia de Camagüey. Ciencias Sociales, Habana, pp 29, 256, 285, 311, 412, 454, 629, 642

Sepehr KS, Baradaran B, Mazandarani M, Yousefi B, Alitappeh MA, Khori V (2014) Growth-inhibitory and apoptosis-inducing effects of *Punica granatum L. var. spinosa* (Apple Punice) on fibrosarcoma cell lines. Adv Pharm Bull 4(Suppl 2):583–590

Shaoul R, Moati D, Schwartz B, Pollak Y, Sukhotnik I (2018) Effect of pomegranate juice on intestinal recovery following methotrexate-induced intestinal damage in a rat model. J Am Coll Nutr 37:406–414. https://doi.org/10.1080/07315724.2017.1413961

Sharma M, Li L, Celver J, Killian C, Kovoor A, Seeram NP (2010) Effects of fruit ellagitannin extracts, ellagic acid, and their colonic metabolite, urolithin A, on Wnt signaling. J Agric Food Chem 58:3965–3969

Shaygannia E, Bahmani M, Zamanzad B, Rafieian-Kopaei M (2016) A review study on *Punica granatum* L. J Evid Based Complement Altern Med 21:221–227

Shirode AB, Kovvuru P, Chittur SV, Henning SM, Heber D, Reliene R (2014) Antiproliferative effects of pomegranate extract in MCF-7 breast cancer cells are associated with reduced DNA repair gene expression and induction of double strand breaks. Mol Carcinog 53:458–470

Shirode AB, Bharali DJ, Nallanthighal S, Coon JK, Mousa SA, Reliene R (2015) Nanoencapsulation of pomegranate bioactive compounds for breast cancer chemoprevention. Int J Nanomedicine 10:475–484

Siegel R, Ward E, Brawley O, Jemal A (2011) Cancer statistics, 2011: the impact of eliminating socioeconomic and racial disparities on premature cancer deaths. CA Cancer J Clin 61:212–236

Siegel R, Ma J, Zou Z, Jemal A (2014) Cancer statistics, 2014. CA Cancer J Clin 64:9–29

Siegel RL, Miller KD, Jemal A (2016) Cancer statistics, 2016. CA Cancer J Clin 66:7–30
Sreeja S, Santhosh Kumar TR, Lakshmi BS, Sreeja S (2012) Pomegranate extract demonstrate a selective estrogen receptor modulator profile in human tumor cell lines and in vivo models of estrogen deprivation. J Nutr Biochem 23:725–732
Sreekumar S, Sithul H, Muraleedharan P, Azeez JM, Sreeharshan S (2014) Pomegranate fruit as a rich source of biologically active compounds. Biomed Res Int 686921. https://doi.org/10.1155/2014/686921
Srinivas NR (2013) Is pomegranate juice a potential perpetrator of clinical drug-drug interactions? Review of the in vitro, preclinical and clinical evidence. Eur J Drug Metab Pharmacokinet 38:223–229
Stenner-Liewen F, Liewen H, Cathomas R, Renner C, Petrausch U, Sulser T et al (2013) Daily pomegranate intake has no impact on PSA levels in patients with advanced prostate cancer – results of a phase IIb randomized controlled trial. J Cancer 4:597–605
Sturgeon SR, Ronnenberg AG (2010) Pomegranate and breast cancer: possible mechanisms of prevention. Nutr Rev 68:122–128
Suzuki R, Noguchi R, Ota T, Abe M, Miyashita K, Kawada T (2001) Cytotoxic effect of conjugated trienoic fatty acids on mouse tumor and human monocytic leukemia cells. Lipids 36:477–482
Syed DN, Malik A, Hadi N, Sarfaraz S, Afaq F, Mukhtar H (2006) Photochemopreventive effect of pomegranate fruit extract on UVA-mediated activation of cellular pathways in normal human epidermal keratinocytes. Photochem Photobiol 82:398–405
Syed DN, Chamcheu J-C, Adhami VM, Mukhtar H (2013) Pomegranate extracts and cancer prevention: molecular and cellular activities. Anti Cancer Agents Med Chem 13:1149–1161
Takigawa Y, Brown AMC (2008) Wnt signaling in liver cancer. Curr Drug Targets 9:1013–1024
Tang JM, Min J, Li BS, Hong SS, Liu C, Hu M et al (2016) Therapeutic effects of punicalagin against ovarian carcinoma cells in association with β-Catenin signaling inhibition. Int J Gynecol Cancer 26:1557–1563
Tezcan F, Gültekin- Özgüven M, Diken T, Özcelik B, Erim FB (2009) Antioxidant activity and total phenolic, organic acid and sugar content in commercial pomegranate juices. Food Chem 115:873–877
Thomas R, Williams M, Sharma H, Chaudry A, Bellamy P (2014) A double-blind, placebo controlled randomised trial evaluating the effect of a polyphenol-rich whole food supplement on PSA progression in men with prostate cancer—the U.K. NCRN Pomi-T study. Prostate Cancer Prostatic Dis 17:180–186
Tibullo D, Caporarello N, Giallongo C, Anfuso CD, Genovese C, Arlotta C et al (2016) Antiproliferative and antiangiogenic effects of *Punica granatum* juice (PGJ) in Multiple Myeloma (MM). Nutrients 8(10):E611
Toi M, Bando H, Ramachandran C, Melnick SJ, Imai A, Fife RS et al (2003) Preliminary studies on the anti-angiogenic potential of pomegranate fractions in vitro and in vivo. Angiogenesis 6:121–128
Tomás-Barberán FA, Seeram NP, Espín JC (2006) Bioavailability of pomegranate polyphenols. In: Seeram NP, Schulman RN, Heber D (eds) Pomegranates. Ancient roots to modern medicine. CRC, Boca Raton, pp 45–60
Tomás-Barberán FA, Espín JC, García-Conesa MT (2009) Bioavailability and metabolism of ellagic acid and ellagitannins. In: Quideau S (ed) Chemistry and biology of ellagitannins. World Scientific, Hackensack, pp 293–297
Torre LA, Bray F, Siegel RL, Ferlay J, Lortet-Tieulent J, Jemal A (2015) Global cancer statistics, 2012. CA Cancer J Clin 65:87–108
Tran HNA, Bae S-Y, Song B-H, Lee B-H, Bae Y-S, Kim Y-H et al (2010) Pomegranate (*Punica granatum*) seed linolenic acid isomers: concentration-dependent modulation of estrogen receptor activity. Endocr Res 35:1–16
Turk G, Ateshahin A, Sonmez M, Cheribashi AO, Yuce A (2008) Improvement of cisplatin-induced injuries to sperm quality, the oxidant-antioxidant system, and the histologic structure of the rat testis by ellagic acid. Fertil Steril 89:1474–1481

Turrini E, Ferruzzi L, Fimognari C (2015) Potential effects of pomegranate polyphenols in cancer. Prevention and therapy. Oxid Med Cell Longev 938475, 19 p. https://doi.org/10.1155/2015/938475

Valadares MC, Pereira ERT, Benfica PL, Paula JR (2010) Assessment of mutagenic and antimutagenic effects of *Punica granatumin* mice. Braz J Pharm Sci 46:121–127

Valko M, Rhodes CJ, Moncol J, Izakovic MM, Mazur M (2006) Free radicals, metals and antioxidants in oxidative stress-induced cancer. Chem Biol Interact 160:1–40

van Die MD, Bone KM, Emery J, Williams SG, Pirotta MV, Paller CJ (2016) Phytotherapeutic interventions in the management of biochemically recurrent prostate cancer: a systematic review of randomised trials. BJU Int 117(Suppl 4):17–34

Van Elswijk DA, Schobel UP, Lansky EP, Irth H, Van Der Greef J (2004) Rapid dereplication of estrogenic compounds in pomegranate (*Punica granatum*) using on-line biochemical detection coupled to mass spectrometry. Phytochemistry 65:233–241

Van Ryswyk K, Villeneuve PJ, Johnson KC (2016) Dietary patterns and the risk of female breast cancer among participants of the Canadian National Enhanced Cancer Surveillance System. Can J Public Health 107:49–55

Vanella L, Barbagallo I, Acquaviva R, di Giacomo C, Cardile V, Abraham NG et al (2013a) Ellagic acid: cytodifferentiating and antiproliferative effects in human prostatic cancer cell lines. Curr Pharm Design 19:2728–2736

Vanella L, di Giacomo C, Acquaviva R, Barbagallo I, Li Volti G, Cardile V et al (2013b) Effects of ellagic acid on angiogenic factors in prostate cancer cells. Cancers 5:726–738

Vargas AJ, Thompson PA (2012) Diet and nutrient factors in colorectal cancer risk. Nutr Clin Pract 27:613–623

Vasudev SS, Ahmad FJ, Khar RK, Bhatnagar A, Kamal YT, Talegaonkar S et al (2012) Validated HPLC method for the simultaneous determination of taxol and ellagic acid in a *Punica granatum* fruit extract containing combination formulation. Pharmazie 67:834–838

Vini R, Sreeja S (2015) *Punica granatum* and its therapeutic implications on breast carcinogenesis: a review. Biofactors 41:78–89

Vini R, Juberiya AM, Sreeja S (2016) Evidence of pomegranate methanolic extract in antagonizing the endogenous SERM, 27-hydroxycholesterol. IUBMB Life 68:116–121

Vinod BS, Maliekal TT, Anto RJ (2013) Phytochemicals as chemosensitizers: from molecular mechanism to clinical significance. Antioxid Redox Signal 18:1307–1348

Viuda-Martos M, Fernandez-Lopez J, Perez–Alvarez JA (2010) Pomegranate and its many functional components as related to human health: a review. Compr Rev Food Sci Food Saf 9:635–654

Vlachojannis C, Zimmermann BF, Chrubasik-Hausmann S (2015) Efficacy and safety of pomegranate medicinal products for cancer. Evid Based Complement Altern Med 2015:258598, 15 p. https://doi.org/10.1155/2015/258598

von Holtz RL, Fink CS, Awad AB (1998) beta-Sitosterol activates the sphingomyelin cycle and induces apoptosis in LNCaP human prostate cancer cells. Nutr Cancer 32:8–12. https://doi.org/10.1080/01635589809514709

Waly MI, Ali A, Guizani N, Al-Rawahi AS, Farooq SA, Rahman MS (2012) Pomegranate (*Punica granatum*) peel extract efficacy as a dietary antioxidant against azoxymethane-induced colon cancer in rat. Asian Pac J Cancer Prev 13:4051–4055

Waly MI, Al-Rawahi AS, Al-Riyami M, Al-Kindi MA, Al-Issaei HK, Farooq SA, Al-Alawi A, Rahman MS (2014) Amelioration of azoxymethane induced-carcinogenesis by reducing oxidative stress in rat colon by natural extracts. BMC Comp Alter Med 14:60–69

Wang L, Martins-Green M (2014) Pomegranate and its components as alternative treatment for prostate cancer. Int J Mol Sci 15:14949–14966

Wang SG, Huang MH, Li JH, Lai FI, Lee HM, Hsu YN (2013) Punicalagin induces apoptotic and autophagic cell death in human 87MG glioma cells. Acta Pharmacol Sin 34:1411–1419

Wang Y, Zhang S, Iqbal S, Chen Z, Wang X, Wang YA et al (2014) Pomegranate extract inhibits the bone metastatic growth of human prostate cancer cells and enhances the in vivo efficacy of docetaxel chemotherapy. Prostate 74:497–508

Weinberg HD, Robert A (2011) Hallmarks of cancer: the next generation. Cell 144:646–674

Wu TF, Hsu LT, Tsang BX, Huang LC, Shih WY, Chen LY (2016) Clarification of the molecular pathway of Taiwan local pomegranate fruit juice underlying the inhibition of urinary bladder urothelial carcinoma cell by proteomics strategy. BMC Complement Altern Med 16:96. https://doi.org/10.1186/s12906-016-1071-7

Xu X, Ho W, Zhang X, Bertrand N, Farokhzad O (2015) Cancer nanomedicine: from targeted delivery to combination therapy. Trends Mol Med 21:223–232

Yaseen NJ, Mustafa Al-Attar MS (2014) Protective effects of *Punica granatum* seed extract against ifosfamide induced sperm abnormalities in male albino mice. Zanco J Pure Appl Sci 26:97–104

Yazici ZM, Meric A, Midi A, ArInc YV, Kahya V, HafIz G (2012) Reduction of cisplatin ototoxicity in rats by oral administration of pomegranate extract. Eur Arch Otorhinolaryngol 269:45–52

Yildirim NC, Kandemir FM, Ceribasi S, Ozkaraca M, Benzer F (2013) Pomegranate seed extract attenuates chemotherapy-induced liver damage in an experimental model of rabbits. Cell Mol Biol (Noisy-le-Grand) 59(Suppl):OL1842–OL1847

Yoshimura M, Watanabe Y, Kasai K, Yamakoshi J, Koga T (2005) Inhibitory effect of an ellagic acid-rich pomegranate extract on tyrosinase activity and ultraviolet-induced pigmentation. Biosci Biotechnol Biochem 69:2368–2373

Zahin M, Ahmad I, Gupta RC, Aqil F (2014) Punicalagin and ellagic acid demonstrate antimutagenic activity and inhibition of benzo[a]pyrene induced DNA adducts. BioMed Res Intern 467465, 10 p. https://doi.org/10.1155/2014/467465

Zaid MA, Afaq F, Khan N, Mukhtar H (2007) Protective effects of pomegranate derived products on UVB-induced DNA damage, PCNA expression and MMPs in human reconstituted skin. J Invest Dermatol 127:143–153

Zhou B, Yi H, Tan J, Wu Y, Liu G, Qiu Z (2015) Anti-proliferative effects of polyphenols from pomegranate rind (*Punica granatum* L.) on EJ bladder cancer cells via regulation of p53/miR-34a axis. Phytother Res 29:415–422

Zhou Y, Li Y, Zhou T, Zheng J, Li S, Li HB (2016) Dietary natural products for prevention and treatment of liver cancer. Nutrients 8:156. https://doi.org/10.3390/nu8030156

Chapter 14
Cancer Chemopreventive Potential of Epidermal Growth Factor Receptor Inhibitors from Natural Products

Duc-Hiep Bach, Donghwa Kim, and Sang Kook Lee

Abstract Receptor tyrosine kinases (RTKs) are cell membrane-anchored receptors that bind to growth factors, cytokines, and hormones for signal transduction and regulate various signaling cascades. Among the diverse RTKs, epidermal growth factor receptor (EGFR) has been suggested to be upstream of major signaling pathways and regarded as a therapeutic target in cancer metastasis, tumorigenesis or drug resistance. The EGFR belongs to the ErbB RTK family and is significantly overexpressed or mutated in various epithelial malignancies. Many anticancer drugs are used to target EGFR (EGFR tyrosine kinase inhibitors, EGFR TKIs) in the clinic, but critical limitations of those drugs persist. Targeted therapies have improved the prognosis and survival of cancer patients. However, large numbers of patients treated with EFGR TKIs acquire drug resistance, for which multiple mechanisms have been suggested. Therefore, there remains an important need to develop antitumor agents targeting EGFR through the use of natural products with high efficacy. A variety of natural products have been investigated to identify novel antitumor agents that could regulate EGFR via different mechanisms. In addition, combination approaches employing natural products and molecular target therapies have been widely discussed. In the present review, we will summarize the critical roles of EGFR in tumor progression and provide a list of natural products that regulate the EGFR signaling pathway. Targeting EGFR signaling using natural products with different mechanisms may effectively overcome EFGR TKI acquired drug resistance and provide an additional strategy in the treatment of cancer.

D.-H. Bach · D. Kim · S. K. Lee (✉)
Natural Products Research Institute, College of Pharmacy, Seoul National University, Seoul, South Korea
e-mail: sklee61@snu.ac.kr

J. M. Pezzuto, O. Vang (eds.), *Natural Products for Cancer Chemoprevention*,
https://doi.org/10.1007/978-3-030-39855-2_14

14.1 Introduction

Epidermal growth factor receptor (EGFR), a member of the ErbB receptor tyrosine kinase (TKI) family, is typically expressed at high levels in various cancer types and commonly elicited to correspond to a poor prognosis (Bach et al. 2018a, b). It is known that EGFR functions upstream of several major signaling pathways, including PI3K or vascular endothelial growth factor (VEGF), and it can bind to several ligands including epidermal growth factor (EGF). Subsequently, the critical role of EGFR is significantly correlated with various diseases, typically tumorigenesis. Increased expression of EGFR is critically related to a poor prognosis, aggressive tumors, and resistance to treatment with cytotoxic agents, including chemotherapy.

Alternatively, for more than 50 years, natural products have been suggested to be the most significant sources for the development of anticancer agents (Demain and Vaishnav 2011; Duc-Hiep and Sang Kook 2018). There is still an urgent need to develop new anti-EGFR agents with potential therapeutic activity (Xiaoyu et al. 2018). It is also important to develop the principles of combining molecular target therapeutics and chemotherapy to target EGFR and overcome drug resistance in cancer treatment.

Herein, we will provide an overview of EGFR in cancer progression and suggest EGFR as a predictive and potentially therapeutic target in cancer treatment. In addition, natural product-derived compounds for targeting EGFR signaling will be suggested as potential cancer chemotherapeutic or chemopreventive agents in the treatment of EGFR-activated cancers.

14.2 EGFR Overview

14.2.1 Landscape of EGFR in Cancer

The critical role of epidermal growth factor receptor (EGFR), one of the most well-investigated signaling pathways in cancer development, has been indicated to contribute to various human tumors, such as lung, breast and colorectal cancers, by stimulating tumor growth, metastasis and invasion (Bach et al. 2018a, b; Sigismund et al. 2018). EGFR has been suggested to be a member of the erbB family of tyrosine kinase receptors (TKRs), which comprise EGFR/HER1/erbB1, HER2/erbB2, HER3/erbB3, and HER4/erbB4, and this erbB family significantly contributes to the ability to transmit a growth-accelerating signal to cells stimulated by an EGFR ligand (e.g., EGF and TGFα) (Sasaki et al. 2013). In normal tissues, the function of EGFR ligands is tightly modulated to assure the kinetics of cell growth precisely match tissue requirements for homeostasis (Sasaki et al. 2013). However, in tumor tissues, EGFR is commonly observed to be perpetually accelerated due to the sustained production of EGFR ligands in the evolution of cancer (Sasaki et al. 2013). Additionally, alteration of the expression of EGFR or TGFα by tumors typically correlates with a more aggressive phenotype and, hence, is commonly employed for the prediction of poor prognosis in cancer patients (Sasaki et al. 2013). Consequently, due to a multidimensional function in cancer development, the EGFR and its family members have been considered attractive targets for therapeutic intervention.

14.2.2 EGF-Like Ligands and EGFR

EGFR has been indicated to be activated by various ligands and belong to a family of TKRs (Sibilia et al. 2007). There are several known ligands for EGFR, including epidermal growth factor (EGF), amphiregulin (AR), epiregulin (EREG), transforming growth factor-α (TGF-α), β-cellulin (BTC) and heparin-binding EGF (HB-EGF) (Sibilia et al. 2007). EGFR binding to its ligands can lead to phosphorylation and dimerization of the receptor, recruitment of proteins containing the domains of phosphotyrosine-binding (PTB) and Src homology 2 (SH2), and stimulation of various downstream signaling pathways, such as the phospholipase C-γ (PLC-γ), phosphatidylinositol 3-kinase (PI3K) or the mitogen-activated protein kinase (MAPK) pathway (Oldrini et al. 2017).

14.2.3 EGFR and Cancer Biomarkers

Various studies have suggested that the expression of EGFR is significantly associated with a poor prognosis of cancer patients, and the EGFR mutational status in particular can serve as a potential biomarker of current value. To illustrate this feature, in evaluating 3026 lung adenocarcinomas, it was found that the probability of EGFR mutation was much higher in male non-smokers than smokers (Dogan et al. 2012). However, potential biomarkers of EGFR can also have indirect value as predictors of sensitivity to radiotherapy or molecularly targeted agents, to the drug pemetrexed specifically, or to chemotherapy in general (Vincent et al. 2012). A recent study indicated that the combination of EGFR with other receptors, such as HER2 and AR, could provide useful prognostic and diagnostic biomarkers for molecular apocrine breast cancer (MABC), and they further suggested that this combination would serve as potential therapeutic targets for MABC in improving the life quality of cancer patients with MABC (Liu et al. 2018). In glioblastoma, mTOR and Akt signaling can act as predictive biomarkers for the EGFR antibody nimotuzumab (Ronellenfitsch et al. 2018).

14.3 EGFR in the Hallmarks of Cancer

Recent studies have demonstrated a critical role of EGFR, with important correlations with ten properties in the next generation of hallmarks of cancer, including tumor-promoted inflammation, proliferative signaling, avoidance of immune destruction, evasion of growth suppressors, induction of angiogenesis, resistance to cell death, enabling of replicative immortality, genome instability and mutation, evasion of growth suppressors, activation of invasion and metastasis (Bach and Lee 2018).

14.3.1 Sustaining Proliferative Signaling

The degradation and internalization of EGFR after ligand binding can limit the intensity of proliferative signaling, consequently supporting the maintenance of cell integrity, especially in tumors; the deregulation of EGFR trafficking has various effects on tumor development (Al-Akhrass et al. 2017). For instance, a recent study has shown that HER2/EGFR-Akt signaling can switch TGF-β from suppressing cell proliferation to stimulating cell migration in breast cancer (Huang et al. 2018a). In detail, Huang et al. observed that suppression of HER2/EGFR activity may induce the anti-proliferative activity of TGF-β while attenuating its pro-migratory role (Huang et al. 2018a). Alternatively, they suggested that stimulation of HER2/EGFR could stimulate SMAD3 phosphorylation at Ser208 of the linker region through Akt, which could stimulate the nuclear accumulation of SMAD3 and subsequent expression of genes correlated to EMT and cell migration (Huang et al. 2018a). Hyperactivation of EGFR/PI3K/Akt is also considered to be a prominent characteristic of various cancer patients. To illustrate this association, a recent report has shown that an imbalance in the reciprocal inhibitory loop between EGFR/PI3K/Akt and the ubiquitin-specific protease USP43 could significantly drive breast carcinogenesis (He et al. 2018). Cross-talk between EphA2 and EGFR though the Akt-PIKyve axis has been suggested to contribute to cellular sensitivity to EGF (Shi and Wang 2018). Alternatively, the long noncoding RNA EGFR-AS1 stimulates cell growth by stimulating the stability of EGFR mRNA in gastric cancer (Hu et al. 2018).

14.3.2 Evasion of Growth Suppressors/Impairment of Differentiation Signals

In human cancers, tumor suppressors will commonly lose their functional role as a result of binding or genomic alterations by inactivation factors. The EGFR may therefore also act as a tumor promoter by modulating a variety of targets. To illustrate, in colorectal cancer, PEAK1 is suggested to act as a tumor promoter and is modulated by EGFR/KRAS signaling (Huang et al. 2018b), and HOXA4 may induce tumor progression to act as a promoter by stimulating the EGFR/MAPK signaling pathway (Zhang et al. 2018c). Loss of MED12 can stimulate tumor dormancy via downregulation of EGFR in human epithelial ovarian cancer (Luo et al. 2018). In detail, MED12 knockout decreases EGFR expression, while restoration of the expression of EGFR in MED12 KO cells might restore proliferation (Luo et al. 2018). Alternatively, miR-452-3p can act as a potential tumor promoter to target the CPEB3/EGFR axis in human hepatocellular carcinoma (Tang et al. 2017).

14.3.3 Avoiding Immune Destruction

Various recent investigations have indicated the critical role of EGFR in modulating immune destruction of cancer cells, and many treatments for tumors bearing EGFR include anti-EGFR monoclonal antibodies, which are also commonly employed in conjunction with the standard radiation therapy, chemotherapy. There are FDA-approved EGFR antibodies, including panitumumab, cetuximab, and necitumumab, which are clinically available for use in different types of cancer patients (Rosner et al. 2018). In head and neck cancer, EGFR overexpression can lead to the activation of multiple downstream signaling pathways that act simultaneously to inhibit type 1 cytokine-stimulated production of chemokines to amplify the attraction of T cells (Ma et al. 2018). Koopmans et al. constructed a bispecific antibody (bsAb), designated PD-L1xEGFR, to direct PD-L1-blockade to EGFR-expressing cancer cells by more selective reactivation of anticancer T cells (Koopmans et al. 2018). A recent study employed a high-throughput immune-oncology screen to identify inhibitors of EGFR as potent enhancers of antigen-specific cytotoxic T-lymphocyte tumor cell killing and suggested that the combination of an EGFR inhibitor and PD-1 blockade should be continuously conducted (Lizotte et al. 2018).

14.3.4 Enabling Replicative Immortality

It is well-known that normal cells have limited replicative potential, while tumor cells have been suggested to have seemingly unlimited replicative potential. Beck et al. observed that the telomerase activity-independent function of telomerase reverse transcriptase (TERT) can allow glioma cells to attain cancer stem cell features by stimulating the expression of EGFR (Beck et al. 2011). In bladder cancer cells, suppression of hTERT expression may downregulate EGFR (Kraemer et al. 2006).

14.3.5 Tumor-Promoted Inflammation

It has been suggested that EGFR signaling in keratinocytes can modulate significant factors included in the innate host defense, the barrier role and skin inflammation (Lichtenberger et al. 2013), and the expression of EGFR is frequently correlated with inflammatory bowel disease (IBD)-associated intestinal cancer (Svrcek et al. 2007). A recent study has shown that cross-talk between EGFR and IL-6 may drive oncogenic signaling and therefore offer therapeutic possibilities in cancer treatment (Ray et al. 2018). Alternatively, HIF-1α may stimulate the inflammatory response in chronic obstructive pulmonary disease through stimulating the EGFR/PI3K/Akt pathway (Zhang et al. 2018b). Consistently, Wang et al. also found that amphiregulin could potentiate mucus hypersecretion and airway inflammation stimulated by urban particulate matter through the EGFR/PI3K/Akt pathway (Wang et al. 2018a).

14.3.6 Activation of Invasion and Metastasis

Activation of EGFR signaling pathway has been indicated to lead to significant cancer metastasis and invasion through the binding of ligands such as TGF-α or EREG (Ferguson et al. 2003). For instance, loss of EGFR signaling-modulated miR-203 has been observed to stimulate tyrosine kinase inhibitors resistance and prostate cancer bone metastasis (Siu et al. 2014). Chang et al. observed that CCN2 could suppress lung cancer metastasis by stimulating EGFR degradation and further suggested a potential therapeutic synergy between the anti-EGFR-antibody and CCN2 for lung cancer treatment (Chang et al. 2013). Targeting EGFR with chemotherapy can also suppress metastasis and invasion. Kang et al. recently showed salidroside (*p*-hydroxyphenethyl-β-D-glucoside) may suppress angiogenesis and migration through modulating EGFR/STAT3 signaling in breast cancer cells (Kang et al. 2018). Alternatively, upregulation of long noncoding RNA UCA1 can stimulate the migration of hypoxia-resistant gastric cancer cells through the EGFR/miR-7-5p axis (Yang et al. 2018).

14.3.7 Induction of Angiogenesis

A significant association between EGFR and angiogenesis has been observed in various cancer patients (Skirnisdottir et al. 2018) and further supports the significant treatment of various patients carrying a subtype of the EGFR mutation with anti-angiogenesis therapy (Yuan et al. 2018). For instance, Keller et al. suggested that EGFR and EGFRvIII stimulate angiogenesis and cell invasion in glioblastoma and further described potential combination therapies for effective treatment (Keller and

Schmidt 2017). Ju et al. found that the use of an EGFR inhibitor, AG1478, may suppress angiogenesis and inflammatory infiltration in mice with diabetic retinopathy (Ju et al. 2018). Consistently, leucine-rich repeats and immunoglobulin-like domain 2 downregulation can suppress angiogenesis of glioma and inhibit HUVEC migration and tube formation by modulating the EGFR/VEGF-A pathway (Yang et al. 2017a).

14.3.8 *Resisting Cell Death*

The survival of cancer cells may be maintained by EGFR independent of its kinase activity by preventing cells from undergoing autophagic death (Weihua et al. 2008). Hence, this critical role of EGFR could endow tumor cells with an enhanced survival capacity even in the presence of TKIs or chemotherapeutic agents (Weihua et al. 2008). Alternatively, Fung et al. found that suppression of EGFR tyrosine kinase can stimulate LC3 lipidation, while induction of autophagy in EGFR-TKI resistant cells may sensitize them to erlotinib (Fung et al. 2012). Chen et al. demonstrated the switch in cancer cells between cell survival and cell death stimulated by autophagy in hypoxia can be modulated by the tyrosine kinase receptor EGFR (Chen et al. 2016). Importantly, Wei et al. suggested that EGFR mediates the phosphorylation of Beclin 1 in autophagy suppression, tumor chemo-resistance and tumor development (Wei et al. 2013).

14.3.9 *Deregulating Cellular Energetics*

EGFR plays a significant role in cancer energy metabolism, and hence, understanding the critical function of EGFR in tumor cell metabolism is important to enhance novel treatment strategies for cancer. A recent study demonstrated that targeting the suppression of EGFR and glutaminase can stimulate metabolic crisis in EGFR mutant lung cancer patients (Momcilovic et al. 2017). In triple-negative breast cancer cells, EGFR signaling can promote aerobic glycolysis to enhance tumor progression and the immune escape program (Lim et al. 2016). Alternatively, Serizawa et al. suggested that enhanced glutamine metabolism can serve as a surrogate marker, which may be employed to predict the likelihood of patients to respond to EGFR-TKIs (Serizawa et al. 2014).

14.4 Therapeutic Approaches to Target EGFR in Cancer

Cytotoxic chemotherapy lacks specificity and has limited efficacy in many types of solid tumors because of their biological diversity (Savage et al. 2009). To enhance the effect, epidermal growth factor receptor tyrosine kinase inhibitors (EGFR-TKIs) such as erlotinib (Tarceva) and gefitinib (Iressa) were developed for non-small-cell lung cancer (NSCLC) patients (Comis 2005). The clinical data suggest that EGFR-TKIs improve progression-free survival but not overall survival, and the efficacy is greater in the East Asian, female, non-smoking, adenocarcinoma pathological type 3,4 and mutant EGFR patient group (Yang et al. 2017b). The first-generation drugs, gefitinib and erlotinib, are reversible EGFR-TKIs, and the second-generation drug, afatinib, is an irreversible ErbB-family inhibitor. However, treatment failure occurs when patients become resistant to EGFR-TKIs (Culy and Faulds 2002). In efforts to overcome resistance, a third-generation EGFR-TKI was developed, osimertinib (Tagrisso), which is an irreversible inhibitor of both mutant EGFR and T790M but not wild-type EGFR (Cross et al. 2014). Although initially developed as a second or third-line therapy, first-line osimertinib clinically improved progression-free survival relative to standard-of-care EGFR-TKIs (Cho et al. 2017). The structures of gefitinib, erlotinib, afatatinib, and osimertinib are shown in Fig. 14.1. Cetuximab (Erbitux) is a chimeric EGFR monoclonal antibody, which was approved by the US Food and Drug Administration in 2004 for use in metastatic colorectal cancer patients (Wong 2005). Although EGFR genes are overexpressed in 60–80% of colorectal cancer, the presence of the KRAS gene mutation would cause resistance to cetuximab (Gomez et al. 2013). Therefore, it is important to determine the genetic background of patients to choose the correct EGFR inhibitor for treatment.

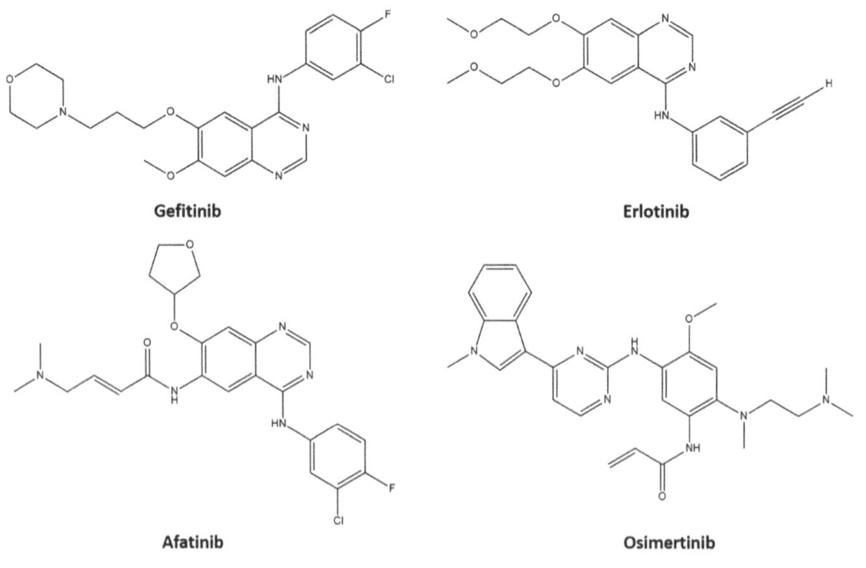

Fig. 14.1 Structures of EGFR-TKIs

14.5 Limitations of Current EGFR Inhibitors

Tyrosine kinase inhibitors compete with the ATP binding site of tyrosine kinases, which play a crucial role in growth factor signaling (Arora and Scholar 2005). However, the acquisition of resistance is the major problem in cancer therapy using kinase inhibitors (Engelman and Settleman 2008). For example, NSCLC, which harbors an EGFR mutation, is very sensitive to EGFR-TKI treatment, but a secondary mutation in exon 20 of EGFR often occurs. Other resistance mechanisms have been identified in clinical or preclinical research, which mostly consist of alternative pathway activation such as MET amplification, AXL overexpression, and EMT (Bean et al. 2007; Postel-Vinay and Ashworth 2012; Yue et al. 2018). To overcome resistance, second and third-generation EGFR-TKIs have been developed, yet they also cause resistance with limited efficacy for similar resistance mechanisms of first-generation EGFR-TKIs (Wu and Shih 2018). Cetuximab is mostly used for colorectal cancer patients, and there are multiple acquired resistance mechanisms such as KRAS/NRAS mutations or amplification, HER2 amplification, and VEGF signaling alterations (Van Emburgh et al. 2014).

14.6 Natural Products Targeting EGFR

Although there are several approaches to target EGFR for cancer treatment, they normally cause drug resistance and a limited time of progression-free survival. At present, oncoprotein degradation by ubiquitination is regarded as a superior therapeutic approach for cancer therapy (Welcker and Clurman 2014). Many natural products have been reported to target either total EGFR, phosphorylated EGFR or both, in cancer cells. EGFR degradation is reported to mediated by ubiquitin like USP22 or caspase-3 (Zhang et al. 2018a; Zhuang et al. 2003). Therefore, the precise mechanism of each natural product still needs to be investigated to identify advanced drug candidates from natural products. Moreover, some natural products can enhance the efficacy of EGFR-TKIs that are currently used in the clinic. The list of natural products based on a literature search is summarized in Table 14.1, followed by brief information about each natural product compound.

Artesunate is a semisynthetic derivative of artemisinin extracted from *Artemisia annua*, which has been reported to exhibit a variety of pharmacological activities such as anti-inflammatory, anti-anigiogenesis, and anti-malarial effects (Yang et al. 2012; Chen et al. 2004; Li and Weina 2010). Artesunate inhibits the growth of A549 cells, which are non-small cell lung cancer (NSCLC) cells, by targeting EGFR and ABCG2 (Ma et al. 2011). Both phosphorylated EGFR and total EGFR are reduced by artesunate treatment. In the same paper, artesunate inhibited tumor growth in the xenograft model when administered at 60 and 120 mg/kg, without a change in the body weight. In addition, artesunate showed a synergistic effect with OSI-774, the EGFR-TKI, in glioblastoma multiforme cell lines (Efferth et al. 2004).

Table 14.1 EGFR targeting of natural product-derived compounds

No	Compound	Source	Mechanism	References
1	Artesunate	*Artemisia annua*	Suppresses EGFR expression in non-small cell lung cancer cells and exhibits synergistic effects with EGFR tyrosine kinase inhibitor OSI-774 in glioblastoma multiforme cells	Ma et al. (2011), Efferth et al. (2004)
2	Berberine	*Berberis aquifolium*, *Berberis aristata*, *Berberis vulgaris*	Inhibits IL-8 expression via the EGFR/MEK/ERK pathway in triple-negative breast cancer cells	Kim et al. (2018)
3	Cardiotoxin III	*Naja naja atra*	Inhibits phosphorylated EGFR in oral squamous cell carcinoma cells	Chien et al. (2009)
4	Curcumin	*Curcuma longa*	Induces EGFR degradation and potentiates the effects of gefitinib in human lung adenocarcinoma cells	Lee et al. (2011)
5	Deguelin	*Mundulea sericea*	Has a significant therapeutic effect on triple-negative breast cancer cells and a combination effect with AG1478 in head and neck squamous carcinoma cells	Mehta et al. (2013), Baba et al. (2017)
6	Fucoxanthin	*Laminaria japonica*, *Undaria pinnatifida*, *Hijikia fusiformis*	Targets STAT3/EGFR signaling in sarcoma 180 xenograft-bearing mice	Wang et al. (2012)
7	Gossypol	*Gossypium herbaceum*	Inhibits the kinase activity of EGFR(L858R/T790M) in non-small cell lung cancer cells	Wang et al. (2018b)
8	Honokiol	*Magnolia obovata*, *Magnolia officinalis*	Downregulates EGFR in breast, head and neck squamous cell carcinoma, and in lung adenocarcinoma cells	Park et al. (2009), Singh et al. (2015), Dai et al. (2018)
9	Magnolol	*Magnolia obovata*, *Magnolia officinalis*	Inhibits EGFR/PI3K/AKT signaling in a wide range of cancer cells, e.g., gastric adenocarcinoma, breast, prostate cancer cells	Lee et al. (2009), Liu et al. (2013), Rasul et al. (2012)
10	Morusin	*Morus alba* L.	Downregulates EGFR and sensitizes glioblastoma cells to TRAIL inhibition	Park et al. (2016)
11	Physakengose G	*Physalis alkekengi* var. *Franchetii*	Exhibits anti-proliferative activity against human osteosarcoma cells by inhibiting EGFR/mTOR signaling	Lin et al. (2018)
12	Resveratrol	*Cassia quinquangulata*	Overcomes resistance in gefitinib-resistant non-small cell lung cancer cells treated with a combination of gefitinib or erlotinib and resveratrol	Zhu et al. (2015), Nie et al. (2015)

(continued)

Table 14.1 (continued)

No	Compound	Source	Mechanism	References
13	Shikonin	*Lithospermum erythrorhizon*	Inhibits EGFR signaling and synergistically suppress cell viability with erlotinib in glioblastoma cells, and induces EGFR degradation in gefitinib-resistant non-small cell lung cancer cells	Zhao et al. (2015), Li et al. (2017)
14	Silibinin	*Silybum marianum*	Reduces the activity of EGFR, can overcome T790M-mediated drug resistance in combination with erlotinib, and reverses EMT-driven erlotinib resistance	Rho et al. (2010), Cufi et al. (2013)
15	Yuanhuadine	*Daphne genkwa*	EGFR pathway suppression in non-small cell lung cancer cells and synergistic with EGFR-TKIs	Hong et al. (2011), Bae et al. (2015)

Berberine is a benzylisoquinoline alkaloid found in many plants, such as *Hydrastis canadensis*, *Berberis aquifolium*, *Berberis aristata*, and *Berberis vulgaris*, and it has been examined for various pharmacological activities for almost 3000 years (Kumar et al. 2015). Berberine has been reported to have anti-tumor activities in many cancer cells. In triple-negative breast cancer cells, berberine inhibits IL-8 expression via the EGFR/MEK/ERK pathway (Kim et al. 2018). Total expression of EGFR is decreased, but p-EGFR could not be detected.

Cardiotoxin III is a natural product isolated from the snake venom of Formosan cobra *Naja naja atra*, and it has been reported to induce apoptosis in various cancer cells (Yen et al. 2013). Cardiotoxin III can decrease phosphorylated EGFR, STAT5, STAT3, Akt, and ERK without affecting the total forms in oral squamous cell carcinoma Ca9-22 cells (Chien et al. 2009).

Curcumin is a bioactive compound found in dietary spice turmeric and herbal remedy that has been used as a traditional medicine with a long history (Noorafshan and Ashkani-Esfahani 2013). Based on the screening of 598 different herbal and natural compounds, curcumin was selected as a potential agent in gefitinib-resistant NSCLC cell lines by screening (Lee et al. 2011). Curcumin can induce EGFR degradation in both wild type EGFR and mutant EGFR NSCLC cell lines. Moreover, the combination treatment of gefitinib and curcumin has shown synergistic effects in both in vitro and in vivo models.

Deguelin is a plant-derived rotenoid and has been studied in cancer research for decades (Gerhauser et al. 1997). A recent study has shown that deguelin inhibits the proliferation of triple-negative breast cancer cells via targeting total EGFR and c-MET (Mehta et al. 2013). In addition, combinational treatment of EGFR-TKI AG1478 and deguelin enhances anti-tumor activity in head and neck squamous cell carcinoma (HNSCC) cells carrying the PI3KCA mutation (Baba et al. 2017). High doses of deguelin monotherapy can also inhibit HNSCC cells by targeting phosphorylated AKT and ERK.

Fucoxanthin is a marine carotenoid isolated from sargassum that has been studied in many cancer cells for antiproliferative activity (Wang et al. 2012). In S180 xenograft-bearing mice, fucoxanthin has demonstrated anti-tumor activity via inhibiting total EGFR and STAT3 expression.

Gossypol is a phenolic compound that is produced by the pigment glands of several parts of *Gossipium* spp. and is known to have toxic effects on human health (Gadelha et al. 2014). Nonetheless, gossypol inhibits the cell proliferation of gefitinib-resistant NSCLC with potent kinase inhibitory activity of $EGFR^{L858R/T790M}$ (EC_{50}: 150.1 nM) (Wang et al. 2018b). Moreover, the molecular docking model showed that gossypol binds to $EGFR^{L858R/T790M}$. Gossypol also dose-dependently suppresses phosphorylated EGFR, AKT, and ERK without affecting their total forms.

Honokiol is a phytochemical in *Magnolia obocata* and *Magnolia officinalis*, the extracts of which have been used as traditional medicines for thousands of years (Sarrica et al. 2018). In breast cancer cells, honokiol effectively modulates the cell cycle and apoptosis by suppressing c-SRC/EGFR-mediated downstream signaling (Park et al. 2009). In PC9 human lung adenocarcinoma cells, honokiol downregulates the EGFR signaling pathway by targeting Lyn kinase (Dai et al. 2018). Honokiol also inhibits the cell viability of different subsites of HNSCC cell lines (SCC-1, SCC-5, OSC-19, and FaDu) by inducing apoptosis through EGFR downregulation (Singh et al. 2015).

Magnolol is found in the same plants as honokiol. Treatment of magnolol in prostate cancer cells induces apoptosis and inhibits phosphorylated EGFR and its downstream pathway (Lee et al. 2009).

Morusin is isolated from the root bark of *Morus alba* L., which is reported to have many biological activities, such as anti-inflammatory, antimicrobial, and scavenging activities (Park et al. 2016). In glioblastoma cells, morusin regulates both phosphorylated and total EGFR protein expression, and it synergistically increases cytotoxicity when combined with TRAIL treatment. In NSCLC, morusin suppresses cell growth, which is related to the induction of apoptosis via EGFR/STAT3 inhibition (Park et al. 2018).

Physakengose G is isolated from *Physalis alkekengi* var. *franchetii*, which has been used as anti-carcinogenic traditional Chinese medicine (Lin et al. 2018). Physakengose G shows effective anti-proliferative effects in human osteosarcoma cells by targeting phosphorylated EGFR without affecting total EGFR expression.

Resveratol is a stilbenoid that is commonly found in grapes and has been widely studied for its chemopreventive activity (Jang et al. 1997). Resveratrol is found to be synergistic with both erlotinib and gefitinib in NSCLC cells (Nie et al. 2015; Zhu et al. 2015). Nie et al. showed that resveratrol exhibits synergistic antineoplastic effects with erlotinib in both erlotinib-sensitive and resistant NSCLC cells by increasing the number of apoptotic cells. Zhu et al. demonstrated that autophagy inhibition induces apoptosis when resveratrol and gefitinib are applied together to gefitinib-resistant PC9 cells.

Shikonin is a natural naphthoquinone that is isolated from the roots of the Chinese herb *Lithospermum erythrorhizon* (Zhao et al. 2015). Zhao et al. tested the binding activity and synergistic ability of shikonin and its derivatives in glioblastoma cells. Shikonin inhibited phosphorylated EGFR as well as the PI3K/Akt/mTOR signaling cascade. The drug combination of shikonin and erlotinib shows additive effects in a dose-dependent manner. Moreover, shikonin inhibits the cell proliferation of gefitinib-resistant NSCLC cells by inducing EGFR degradation (Li et al. 2017).

Silibinin is a flavonolignan extracted from milk thistle seeds and has been shown to enhance the efficacy of EGFR-TKIs in hepatocellular carcinoma and NSCLC cells (Rho et al. 2010; Cufi et al. 2013; Gu et al. 2015). Rho et al. tested effects of silibinin in various NSCLC cells and found it decreases phosphorylated EGFR only in cells harboring EGFR mutations. Moreover, the addition of silibinin to EGFR-TKIs could overcome drug resistance caused by the EGFR T790M mutation. Gu et al. found that treatment with silibinin and gefitinib inhibits cell proliferation of hepatocellular carcinoma cells mainly through Akt signaling. Although silibinin alone cannot reduce the phosphorylated EGFR expression, the combined treatment can suppress phosphorylated EGFR more than the single treatment. Cufi et al. investigated the precise role of silibinin in overcoming erlotinib resistance in NSCLC cells and tumors. They found that silibinin could overcome drug resistance and reverse EMT via targeting miR-21 and miR-200c.

Yuanhuadine is a daphnane-type diterpene ester isolated from the flowers of *Daphne genkwa* (Thymelaeaceae) (Hong et al. 2010). Yuanhuadine inhibits both gefitinib-sensitive and resistant NSCLC cells with nanomolar IC_{50} values without showing cytotoxic effects in normal lung cancer cells (Hong et al. 2011). The anti-proliferative activities occurred via cell-cycle arrest and suppression of the EGFR, Akt/mTOR, and cMet signaling pathways. Moreover, yuanhuadine showed synergistic effects with gefitinib in gefitinib-resistant NSCLC cells by targeting AXL degradation (Bae et al. 2015). Recently, yuanhuadine has been shown to delay the emergence of gefitinib resistance and can overcome acquired resistance when co-administered with gefitinib or osimertinib (Kim et al. 2019). The chemical structures of natural products targeting EGFR discussed in this chapter are depicted in Fig. 14.2.

14.7 Conclusions

In summary, there are abundant compounds in nature that target EGFR signaling and show pharmacologically effective cytotoxicity. Despite the large amount of research data obtained in vitro and in vivo, clinical data for active natural products targeting EGFR are still lacking. Therefore, further studies on the precise mechanism of each natural product are needed to expand our knowledge in this area.

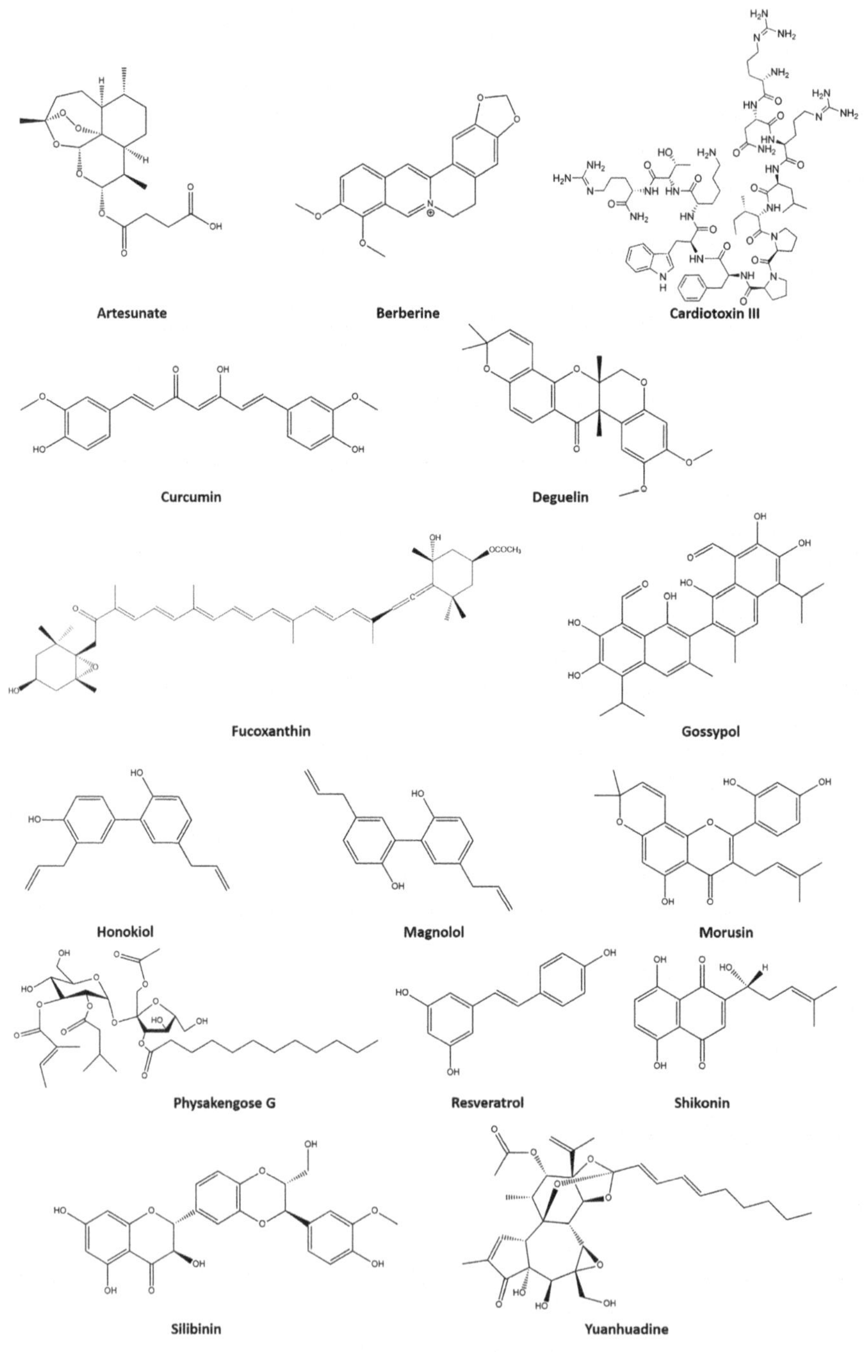

Fig. 14.2 Natural products targeting EGFR

References

Al-Akhrass H, Naves T, Vincent F, Magnaudeix A, Durand K, Bertin F, Melloni B, Jauberteau MO, Lalloue F (2017) Sortilin limits EGFR signaling by promoting its internalization in lung cancer. Nat Commun 8:1182

Arora A, Scholar EM (2005) Role of tyrosine kinase inhibitors in cancer therapy. J Pharm Exp Ther 315:971–979

Baba Y, Maeda T, Suzuki A, Takada S, Fujii M, Kato Y (2017) Deguelin potentiates apoptotic activity of an EGFR tyrosine kinase inhibitor (AG1478) in PIK3CA-mutated head and neck squamous cell carcinoma. Int J Mol Sci 18:E262

Bach D-H, Lee SK (2018) Long noncoding RNAs in cancer cells. Cancer Lett 419:152–166

Bach D-H, Kim D, Bae SY, Kim WK, Hong J-Y, Lee H-J, Rajasekaran N, Kwon S, Fan Y, Luu T-T-T, Shin YK, Lee J, Lee SK (2018a) Targeting nicotinamide N-methyltransferase and miR-449a in EGFR-TKI-resistant non-small-cell lung cancer cells. Mol Ther – Nucleic Acids 11:455–467

Bach D-H, Luu T-T-T, Kim D, An YJ, Park HJ, Park S, Lee SK (2018b) BMP4 upregulation is associated with acquired drug resistance and fatty acid metabolism in EGFR-mutant non-small cell lung cancer cells. Mol Ther – Nucleic Acids 12:817–828

Bae SY, Hong JY, Lee HJ, Park HJ, Lee SK (2015) Targeting the degradation of AXL receptor tyrosine kinase to overcome resistance in gefitinib-resistant non-small cell lung cancer. Oncotarget 6:10146–10160

Bean J, Brennan C, Shih JY, Riely G, Viale A, Wang L, Chitale D, Motoi N, Szoke J, Broderick S, Balak M, Chang WC, Yu CJ, Gazdar A, Pass H, Rusch V, Gerald W, Huang SF, Yang PC, Miller V, Ladanyi M, Yang CH, Pao W (2007) MET amplification occurs with or without T790M mutations in EGFR mutant lung tumors with acquired resistance to gefitinib or erlotinib. Proc Natl Acad Sci USA 104:20932–20937

Beck S, Jin X, Sohn YW, Kim JK, Kim SH, Yin J, Pian X, Kim SC, Nam DH, Choi YJ, Kim H (2011) Telomerase activity-independent function of TERT allows glioma cells to attain cancer stem cell characteristics by inducing EGFR expression. Mol Cells 31:9–15

Chang CC, Yang MH, Lin BR, Chen ST, Pan SH, Hsiao M, Lai TC, Lin SK, Jeng YM, Chu CY, Chen RH, Yang PC, Chin YE, Kuo ML (2013) CCN2 inhibits lung cancer metastasis through promoting DAPK-dependent anoikis and inducing EGFR degradation. Cell Death Differ 20:443–455

Chen HH, Zhou HJ, Wu GD, Lou XE (2004) Inhibitory effects of artesunate on angiogenesis and on expressions of vascular endothelial growth factor and VEGF receptor KDR/flk-1. Pharmacology 71:1–9

Chen Y, Henson ES, Xiao W, Huang D, Mcmillan-Ward EM, Israels SJ, Gibson SB (2016) Tyrosine kinase receptor EGFR regulates the switch in cancer cells between cell survival and cell death induced by autophagy in hypoxia. Autophagy 12:1029–1046

Chien CM, Lin KL, Su JC, Chang LS, Lin SR (2009) Inactivation of epidermal growth factor receptor and downstream pathways in oral squamous cell carcinoma Ca9-22 cells by cardiotoxin III from Naja naja atra. J Nat Prod 72:1735–1740

Cho BC, Chewaskulyong B, Lee KH, Dechaphunkul A, Sriuranpong V, Imamura F, Ohe Y, Nogami N, Kurata T, Okamoto I, Zhou C, Cheng Y, Cho EK, Jye VP, Lee JS, Mann H, Saggese M, Reungwetwattana T (2017) Osimertinib vs standard of care (SoC) EGFR-TKI as first-line treatment in patients with EGFR-TKI sensitising mutation (EGFRm) positive advanced non-small cell lung cancer (NSCLC): FLAURA Asian subset. Ann Oncol 28:190–190

Comis RL (2005) The current situation: Erlotinib (Tarceva (R)) and gefitinib (Iressa (R)) in non-small cell lung cancer. Oncologist 10:467–470

Cross DA, Ashton SE, Ghiorghiu S, Eberlein C, Nebhan CA, Spitzler PJ, Orme JP, Finlay MR, Ward RA, Mellor MJ, Hughes G, Rahi A, Jacobs VN, Red Brewer M, Ichihara E, Sun J, Jin H, Ballard P, Al-Kadhimi K, Rowlinson R, Klinowska T, Richmond GH, Cantarini M, Kim DW, Ranson MR, Pao W (2014) AZD9291, an irreversible EGFR TKI, overcomes T790M-mediated resistance to EGFR inhibitors in lung cancer. Cancer Discov 4:1046–1061

Cufi S, Bonavia R, Vazquez-Martin A, Oliveras-Ferraros C, Corominas-Faja B, Cuyas E, Martin-Castillo B, Barrajon-Catalan E, Visa J, Segura-Carretero A, Joven J, Bosch-Barrera J, Micol V, Menendez JA (2013) Silibinin suppresses EMT-driven erlotinib resistance by reversing the high miR-21/low miR-200c signature in vivo. Sci Rep 3:2459

Culy CR, Faulds D (2002) Gefitinib. Drugs 62:2237–2248. discussion 2249-50

Dai X, Li RZ, Jiang ZB, Wei CL, Luo LX, Yao XJ, Li GP, Leung ELH (2018) Honokiol inhibits proliferation, invasion and induces apoptosis through targeting Lyn kinase in human lung adenocarcinoma cells. Front Pharmacol 9:558

Demain AL, Vaishnav P (2011) Natural products for cancer chemotherapy. Microbial Biotechnol 4:687–699

Dogan S, Shen R, Ang DC, Johnson ML, D'angelo SP, Paik PK, Brzostowski EB, Riely GJ, Kris MG, Zakowski MF, Ladanyi M (2012) Molecular epidemiology of EGFR and KRAS mutations in 3,026 lung adenocarcinomas: higher susceptibility of women to smoking-related KRAS-mutant cancers. Clin Cancer Res 18:6169–6177

Duc-Hiep B, Sang Kook L (2018) The potential impacts of tylophora alkaloids and their derivatives in modulating inflammation, viral infections, and cancer. Curr Med Chem 25:1–16

Efferth T, Ramirez T, Gebhart E, Halatsch ME (2004) Combination-treatment of glioblastoma multiforme cell lines with the anti-malarial artesunate and the epidermal growth factor receptor tyrosine kinase inhibitor OSI-774. Biochem Pharmacol 67:1689–1700

Engelman JA, Settleman J (2008) Acquired resistance to tyrosine kinase inhibitors during cancer therapy. Curr Opin Genet Dev 18:73–79

Ferguson KM, Berger MB, Mendrola JM, Cho HS, Leahy DJ, Lemmon MA (2003) EGF activates its receptor by removing interactions that autoinhibit ectodomain dimerization. Mol Cell 11:507–517

Fung C, Chen X, Grandis JR, Duvvuri U (2012) EGFR tyrosine kinase inhibition induces autophagy in cancer cells. Cancer Biol Ther 13:1417–1424

Gadelha IC, Fonseca NB, Oloris SC, Melo MM, Soto-Blanco B (2014) Gossypol toxicity from cottonseed products. ScientificWorldJournal 2014:231635

Gerhauser C, Lee SK, Kosmeder JW, Moriarty RM, Hamel E, Mehta RG, Moon RC, Pezzuto JM (1997) Regulation of ornithine decarboxylase induction by deguelin, a natural product cancer chemopreventive agent. Cancer Res 57:3429–3435

Gomez D, de Rosa A, Addison A, Brooks A, Malik HZ, Cameron IC (2013) Cetuximab therapy in the treatment of metastatic colorectal cancer: the future frontier? Int J Surg 11:507–513

Gu HR, Park SC, Choi SJ, Lee JC, Kim YC, Han CJ, Kim J, Yang KY, Kim YJ, Noh GY, No SH, Jeong JH (2015) Combined treatment with silibinin and either sorafenib or gefitinib enhances their growth-inhibiting effects in hepatocellular carcinoma cells. Clin Mol Hepatol 21:49–59

He L, Liu X, Yang J, Li W, Liu S, Liu X, Yang Z, Ren J, Wang Y, Shan L, Guan C, Pei F, Lei L, Zhang Y, Yi X, Yang X, Liang J, Liu R, Sun L, Shang Y (2018) Imbalance of the reciprocally inhibitory loop between the ubiquitin-specific protease USP43 and EGFR/PI3K/AKT drives breast carcinogenesis. Cell Res 28:934–951

Hong JY, Nam JW, Seo EK, Lee SK (2010) Daphnane diterpene esters with anti-proliferative activities against human lung cancer cells from Daphne genkwa. Chem Pharm Bull (Tokyo) 58:234–237

Hong JY, Chung HJ, Lee HJ, Park HJ, Lee SK (2011) Growth inhibition of human lung cancer cells via down-regulation of epidermal growth factor receptor signaling by yuanhuadine, a daphnane diterpene from Daphne genkwa. J Nat Prod 74:2102–2108

Hu J, Qian Y, Peng L, Ma L, Qiu T, Liu Y, Li X, Chen X (2018) Long noncoding RNA EGFR-AS1 promotes cell proliferation by increasing EGFR mRNA stability in gastric cancer. Cell Physiol Biochem 49:322–334

Huang F, Shi Q, Li Y, Xu L, Xu C, Chen F, Wang H, Liao H, Chang Z, Liu F, Zhang XH, Feng XH, Han JJ, Luo S, Chen YG (2018a) HER2/EGFR-AKT signaling switches TGF-beta from inhibiting cell proliferation to promoting cell migration in breast cancer. Cancer Res 78:6073–6085

Huang L, Wen C, Yang X, Lou Q, Wang X, Che J, Chen J, Yang Z, Wu X, Huang M, Lan P, Wang L, Iwamoto A, Wang J, Liu H (2018b) PEAK1, acting as a tumor promoter in colorectal cancer, is regulated by the EGFR/KRas signaling axis and miR-181d. Cell Death Dis 9:271

Jang M, Cai L, Udeani GO, Slowing KV, Thomas CF, Beecher CW, Fong HH, Farnsworth NR, Kinghorn AD, Mehta RG, Moon RC, Pezzuto JM (1997) Cancer chemopreventive activity of resveratrol, a natural product derived from grapes. Science 275:218–220

Ju X, Yang X, Yan T, Chen H, Song Z, Zhang Z, Wu W, Wang Y (2018) EGFR inhibitor, AG1478, inhibits inflammatory infiltration and angiogenesis in mice with diabetic retinopathy. Clin Exp Pharmacol Physiol

Kang DY, Sp N, Kim DH, Joung YH, Lee HG, Park YM, Yang YM (2018) Salidroside inhibits migration, invasion and angiogenesis of MDAMB 231 TNBC cells by regulating EGFR/Jak2/ STAT3 signaling via MMP2. Int J Oncol 53:877–885

Keller S, Schmidt MHH (2017) EGFR and EGFRvIII promote angiogenesis and cell invasion in Glioblastoma: combination therapies for an effective treatment. Int J Mol Sci 18

Kim S, You D, Jeong Y, Yu J, Kim SW, Nam SJ, Lee JE (2018) Berberine down-regulates IL-8 expression through inhibition of the EGFR/MEK/ERK pathway in triple-negative breast cancer cells. Phytomedicine 50:43–49

Kim D, Bach DH, Fan Y, Luu TTT, Hong JY, Park HJ, Lee SK (2019) AXL degradation in combination with EGFR-TKI can delay and overcome acquired resistance in human non-small cell lung cancer cells. Cell Death Dis 10:361

Koopmans I, Hendriks D, Samplonius DF, van Ginkel RJ, Heskamp S, Wierstra PJ, Bremer E, Helfrich W (2018) A novel bispecific antibody for EGFR-directed blockade of the PD-1/PD-L1 immune checkpoint. Oncoimmunology 7:e1466016

Kraemer K, Schmidt U, Fuessel S, Herr A, Wirth MP, Meye A (2006) Microarray analyses in bladder cancer cells: inhibition of hTERT expression down-regulates EGFR. Int J Cancer 119:1276–1284

Kumar A, Ekavali, Chopra K, Mukherjee M, Pottabathini R, Dhull DK (2015) Current knowledge and pharmacological profile of berberine: an update. Eur J Pharmacol 761:288–297

Lee DH, Szczepanski MJ, Lee YJ (2009) Magnolol induces apoptosis via inhibiting the EGFR/ PI3K/Akt signaling pathway in human prostate cancer cells. J Cell Biochem 106:1113–1122

Lee JY, Lee YM, Chang GC, Yu SL, Hsieh WY, Chen JJ, Chen HW, Yang PC (2011) Curcumin induces EGFR degradation in lung adenocarcinoma and modulates p38 activation in intestine: the versatile adjuvant for gefitinib therapy. PLoS One 6:e23756

Li Q, Weina P (2010) Artesunate: the best drug in the treatment of severe and complicated malaria. Pharmaceutic (Basel) 3:2322–2332

Li X, Fan XX, Jiang ZB, Loo WT, Yao XJ, Leung EL, Chow LW, Liu L (2017) Shikonin inhibits gefitinib-resistant non-small cell lung cancer by inhibiting TrxR and activating the EGFR proteasomal degradation pathway. Pharmacol Res 115:45–55

Lichtenberger BM, Gerber PA, Holcmann M, Buhren BA, Amberg N, Smolle V, Schrumpf H, Boelke E, Ansari P, Mackenzie C, Wollenberg A, Kislat A, Fischer JW, Rock K, Harder J, Schroder JM, Homey B, Sibilia M (2013) Epidermal EGFR controls cutaneous host defense and prevents inflammation. Sci Transl Med 5:199ra111

Lim S-O, Li C-W, Xia W, Lee H-H, Chang S-S, Shen J, Hsu JL, Raftery D, Djukovic D, Gu H, Chang W-C, Wang H-L, Chen M-L, Huo L, Chen C-H, Wu Y, Sahin A, Hanash SM, Hortobagyi GN, Hung M-C (2016) EGFR signaling enhances aerobic glycolysis in triple-negative breast cancer cells to promote tumor growth and immune escape. Cancer Res 76:1284–1296

Lin H, Zhang C, Zhang H, Xia YZ, Zhang CY, Luo J, Yang L, Kong LY (2018) Physakengose G induces apoptosis via EGFR/mTOR signaling and inhibits autophagic flux in human osteosarcoma cells. Phytomedicine 42:190–198

Liu Y, Cao W, Zhang B, Liu YQ, Wang ZY, Wu YP, Yu XJ, Zhang XD, Ming PH, Zhou GB, Huang L (2013) The natural compound magnolol inhibits invasion and exhibits potential in human breast cancer therapy. Sci Rep 3:3098

Liu X, Feng C, Liu J, Liu J, Li C, Xu C, Niu Y (2018) The importance of EGFR as a biomarker in molecular apocrine breast cancer. Hum Pathol 77:1–10

Lizotte PH, Hong RL, Luster TA, Cavanaugh ME, Taus LJ, Wang S, Dhaneshwar A, Mayman N, Yang A, Kulkarni M, Badalucco L, Fitzpatrick E, Kao HF, Kuraguchi M, Bittinger M, Kirschmeier PT, Gray NS, Barbie DA, Janne PA (2018) A high-throughput immune-oncology screen identifies EGFR inhibitors as potent enhancers of antigen-specific cytotoxic T-lymphocyte tumor cell killing. Cancer Immunol Res 6:1511–1523

Luo XL, Deng CC, Su XD, Wang F, Chen Z, Wu XP, Liang SB, Liu JH, Fu LW (2018) Loss of MED12 induces tumor dormancy in human epithelial ovarian cancer via downregulation of EGFR. Cancer Res 78:3532–3543

Ma H, Yao Q, Zhang AM, Lin S, Wang XX, Wu L, Sun JG, Chen ZT (2011) The effects of artesunate on the expression of EGFR and ABCG2 in A549 human lung cancer cells and a xenograft model. Molecules 16:10556–10569

Ma W, Concha-Benavente F, Santegoets S, Welters MJP, Ehsan I, Ferris RL, van der Burg SH (2018) EGFR signaling suppresses type 1 cytokine-induced T-cell attracting chemokine secretion in head and neck cancer. PLoS One 13:e0203402

Mehta R, Katta H, Alimirah F, Patel R, Murillo G, Peng X, Muzzio M, Mehta RG (2013) Deguelin action involves c-met and EGFR signaling pathways in triple negative breast cancer cells. PLoS One 8:e65113

Momcilovic M, Bailey ST, Lee JT, Fishbein MC, Magyar C, Braas D, Graeber T, Jackson NJ, Czernin J, Emberley E, Gross M, Janes J, Mackinnon A, Pan A, Rodriguez M, Works M, Zhang W, Parlati F, Demo S, Garon E, Krysan K, Walser TC, Dubinett SM, Sadeghi S, Christofk HR, Shackelford DB (2017) Targeted inhibition of EGFR and glutaminase induces metabolic crisis in EGFR mutant lung cancer. Cell Rep 18:601–610

Nie P, Hu W, Zhang T, Yang Y, Hou B, Zou Z (2015) Synergistic induction of erlotinib-mediated apoptosis by resveratrol in human non-small-cell lung cancer cells by down-regulating survivin and up-regulating PUMA. Cell Physiol Biochem 35:2255–2271

Noorafshan A, Ashkani-Esfahani S (2013) A review of therapeutic effects of curcumin. Curr Pharm Des 19:2032–2046

Oldrini B, Hsieh WY, Erdjument-Bromage H, Codega P, Carro MS, Curiel-Garcia A, Campos C, Pourmaleki M, Grommes C, Vivanco I, Rohle D, Bielski CM, Taylor BS, Hollmann TJ, Rosenblum M, Tempst P, Blenis J, Squatrito M, Mellinghoff IK (2017) EGFR feedback-inhibition by ran-binding protein 6 is disrupted in cancer. Nat Commun 8:2035

Park EJ, Min HY, Chung HJ, Hong JY, Kang YJ, Hung TM, Youn UJ, Kim YS, Bae K, Kang SS, Lee SK (2009) Down-regulation of c-Src/EGFR-mediated signaling activation is involved in the honokiol-induced cell cycle arrest and apoptosis in MDA-MB-231 human breast cancer cells. Cancer Lett 277:133–140

Park D, Ha IJ, Park SY, Choi M, Lim SL, Kim SH, Lee JH, Ahn KS, Yun M, Lee SG (2016) Morusin induces TRAIL sensitization by regulating EGFR and DR5 in human glioblastoma cells. J Nat Prod 79:317–323

Park HJ, Min TR, Chi GY, Choi YH, Park SH (2018) Induction of apoptosis by morusin in human non-small cell lung cancer cells by suppression of EGFR/STAT3 activation. Biochem Biophys Res Comm 505:194–200

Postel-Vinay S, Ashworth A (2012) AXL and acquired resistance to EGFR inhibitors. Nat Genet 44:835–836

Rasul A, Yu B, Khan M, Zhang K, Iqbal F, Ma T, Yang H (2012) Magnolol, a natural compound, induces apoptosis of SGC-7901 human gastric adenocarcinoma cells via the mitochondrial and PI3K/Akt signaling pathways. Int J Oncol 40:1153–1161

Ray K, Ujvari B, Ramana V, Donald J (2018) Cross-talk between EGFR and IL-6 drives oncogenic signaling and offers therapeutic opportunities in cancer. Cytokine Growth Factor Rev 41:18–27

Rho JK, Choi YJ, Jeon BS, Choi SJ, Cheon GJ, Woo SK, Kim HR, Kim CH, Choi CM, Lee JC (2010) Combined treatment with silibinin and epidermal growth factor receptor tyrosine kinase inhibitors overcomes drug resistance caused by T790M mutation. Mol Cancer Ther 9:3233–3243

Ronellenfitsch MW, Zeiner PS, Mittelbronn M, Urban H, Pietsch T, Reuter D, Senft C, Steinbach JP, Westphal M, Harter PN (2018) Akt and mTORC1 signaling as predictive biomarkers for the EGFR antibody nimotuzumab in glioblastoma. Acta Neuropathol Comm 6:81

Rosner T, Kahle S, Montenegro F, Matlung HL, Jansen JHM, Evers M, Beurskens F, Leusen JHW, Van Den Berg TK, Valerius T (2018) Immune effector functions of human IgG2 antibodies against EGFR. Mol Cancer Ther 18:75–88

Sarrica A, Kirika N, Romeo M, Salmona M, Diomede L (2018) Safety and toxicology of magnolol and honokiol. Planta Med 84:1151–1164

Sasaki T, Hiroki K, Yamashita Y (2013) The role of epidermal growth factor receptor in cancer metastasis and microenvironment. Biomed Res Int 2013:546318

Savage P, Stebbing J, Bower M, Crook T (2009) Why does cytotoxic chemotherapy cure only some cancers? Nat Clinic Pract Oncol 6:43–52

Serizawa M, Kusuhara M, Zangiacomi V, Urakami K, Watanabe M, Takahashi T, Yamaguchi K, Yamamoto N, Koh Y (2014) Identification of metabolic signatures associated with erlotinib resistance of non-small cell lung cancer cells. Anticancer Res 34:2779–2787

Shi X, Wang B (2018) Caught in the "Akt": cross-talk between EphA2 and EGFR through the Akt-PIKfyve axis maintains cellular sensitivity to EGF. Sci Signal 11:eaau1207

Sibilia M, Kroismayr R, Lichtenberger BM, Natarajan A, Hecking M, Holcmann M (2007) The epidermal growth factor receptor: from development to tumorigenesis. Differentiation 75:770–787

Sigismund S, Avanzato D, Lanzetti L (2018) Emerging functions of the EGFR in cancer. Mol Oncol 12:3–20

Singh T, Gupta NA, Xu S, Prasad R, Velu SE, Katiyar SK (2015) Honokiol inhibits the growth of head and neck squamous cell carcinoma by targeting epidermal growth factor receptor. Oncotarget 6:21268–21282

Siu MK, Abou-Kheir W, Yin JJ, Chang Y-S, Barrett B, Suau F, Casey O, Chen W-Y, Fang L, Hynes P, Hsieh Y-Y, Liu Y-N, Huang J, Kelly K (2014) Loss of EGFR signaling-regulated miR-203 promotes prostate cancer bone metastasis and tyrosine kinase inhibitors resistance. Oncotarget 5:3770–3784

Skirnisdottir I, Akerud H, Seidal T (2018) Clinical significance of growth factor receptor EGFR and angiogenesis regulator VEGFR2 in patients with ovarian cancer at FIGO stages I-II. Int J Oncol 53:1633–1642

Svrcek M, Cosnes J, Tiret E, Bennis M, Parc Y, Flejou JF (2007) Expression of epidermal growth factor receptor (EGFR) is frequent in inflammatory bowel disease (IBD)-associated intestinal cancer. Virchows Arch 450:243–244

Tang H, Zhang J, Yu Z, Ye L, Li K, Ding F, Feng X, Meng W (2017) Mir-452-3p: a potential tumor promoter that targets the CPEB3/EGFR axis in human hepatocellular carcinoma. Technol Cancer Res Treat 16:1136–1149

Van Emburgh BO, Sartore-Bianchi A, DI Nicolantonio F, Siena S, Bardelli A (2014) Acquired resistance to EGFR-targeted therapies in colorectal cancer. Mol Oncol 8:1084–1094

Vincent MD, Kuruvilla MS, Leighl NB, Kamel-Reid S (2012) Biomarkers that currently affect clinical practice: EGFR, ALK, MET, KRAS. Curr Oncol 19:S33–S44

Wang J, Chen S, Xu S, Yu X, Ma D, Hu X, Cao X (2012) In vivo induction of apoptosis by fucoxanthin, a marine carotenoid, associated with down-regulating STAT3/EGFR signaling in sarcoma 180 (S180) xenografts-bearing mice. Mar Drugs 10:2055–2068

Wang J, Zhu M, Wang L, Chen C, Song Y (2018a) Amphiregulin potentiates airway inflammation and mucus hypersecretion induced by urban particulate matter via the EGFR-PI3Kalpha-AKT/ERK pathway. Cell Signal 53:122–131

Wang Y, Lai H, Fan X, Luo L, Duan F, Jiang Z, Wang Q, Leung ELH, Liu L, Yao X (2018b) Gossypol inhibits non-small cell lung cancer cells proliferation by targeting EGFR(L858R/T790M). Front Pharmacol 9:728

Wei Y, Zou Z, Becker N, Anderson M, Sumpter R, Xiao G, Kinch L, Koduru P, Christudass CS, Veltri RW, Grishin NV, Peyton M, Minna J, Bhagat G, Levine B (2013) EGFR-mediated Beclin 1 phosphorylation in autophagy suppression, tumor progression, and tumor chemoresistance. Cell 154:1269–1284

Weihua Z, Tsan R, Huang W-C, Wu Q, Chiu C-H, Fidler IJ, Hung M-C (2008) Survival of cancer cells is maintained by EGFR independent of its kinase activity. Cancer Cell 13:385–393

Welcker M, Clurman BE (2014) Oncoprotein ubiquitylation: dimers, degrons, and degradation. Cell Cycle 13:1829–1830

Wong SF (2005) Cetuximab: an epidermal growth factor receptor monoclonal antibody for the treatment of colorectal cancer. Clin Therap 27:684–694

Wu SG, Shih JY (2018) Management of acquired resistance to EGFR TKI-targeted therapy in advanced non-small cell lung cancer. Mol Cancer 17:38

Xiaoyu W, Linfeng X, Yuanzhi L, Hongmei Z, Hongxi X (2018) Natural products targeting EGFR signaling pathways as potential anticancer drugs. Curr Protein Pept Sci 19:380–388

Yang Z, Ding J, Yang C, Gao Y, Li X, Chen X, Peng Y, Fang J, Xiao S (2012) Immunomodulatory and anti-inflammatory properties of artesunate in experimental colitis. Curr Med Chem 19:4541–4551

Yang HK, Chen H, Mao F, Xiao QG, Xie RF, Lei T (2017a) Downregulation of LRIG2 expression inhibits angiogenesis of glioma via EGFR/VEGF-A pathway. Oncol Lett 14:4021–4028

Yang Z, Hackshaw A, Feng Q, Fu X, Zhang Y, Mao C, Tang J (2017b) Comparison of gefitinib, erlotinib and afatinib in non-small cell lung cancer: a meta-analysis. Int J Cancer 140:2805–2819

Yang Z, Shi X, Li C, Wang X, Hou K, Li Z, Zhang X, Fan Y, Qu X, Che X, Liu Y (2018) Long non-coding RNA UCA1 upregulation promotes the migration of hypoxia-resistant gastric cancer cells through the miR-7-5p/EGFR axis. Exp Cell Res 368:194–201

Yen CY, Liang SS, Han LY, Chou HL, Chou CK, Lin SR, Chiu CC (2013) Cardiotoxin III inhibits proliferation and migration of oral cancer cells through MAPK and MMP signaling. Sci World J 2013:1–5

Yuan XH, Yang J, Wang XY, Zhang XL, Qin TT, Li K (2018) Association between EGFR/KRAS mutation and expression of VEGFA, VEGFR and VEGFR2 in lung adenocarcinoma. Oncol Lett 16:2105–2112

Yue J, Lv D, Wang C, Li L, Zhao Q, Chen H, Xu L (2018) Epigenetic silencing of miR-483-3p promotes acquired gefitinib resistance and EMT in EGFR-mutant NSCLC by targeting integrin beta3. Oncogene 37:4300–4312

Zhang H, Han B, Lu H, Zhao Y, Chen X, Meng Q, Cao M, Cai L, Hu J (2018a) USP22 promotes resistance to EGFR-TKIs by preventing ubiquitination-mediated EGFR degradation in EGFR-mutant lung adenocarcinoma. Cancer Lett 433:186–198

Zhang HX, Yang JJ, Zhang SA, Zhang SM, Wang JX, Xu ZY, Lin RY (2018b) HIF-1alpha promotes inflammatory response of chronic obstructive pulmonary disease by activating EGFR/PI3K/AKT pathway. Eur Rev Med Pharmacol Sci 22:6077–6084

Zhang X, Liu G, Ding L, Jiang T, Shao S, Gao Y, Lu Y (2018c) HOXA3 promotes tumor growth of human colon cancer through activating EGFR/Ras/Raf/MEK/ERK signaling pathway. J Cell Biochem 119:2864–2874

Zhao Q, Kretschmer N, Bauer R, Efferth T (2015) Shikonin and its derivatives inhibit the epidermal growth factor receptor signaling and synergistically kill glioblastoma cells in combination with erlotinib. Int J Cancer 137:1446–1456

Zhu Y, He W, Gao X, Li B, Mei C, Xu R, Chen H (2015) Resveratrol overcomes gefitinib resistance by increasing the intracellular gefitinib concentration and triggering apoptosis, autophagy and senescence in PC9/G NSCLC cells. Sci Rep 5:17730

Zhuang S, Ouedraogo GD, Kochevar IE (2003) Downregulation of epidermal growth factor receptor signaling by singlet oxygen through activation of caspase-3 and protein phosphatases. Oncogene 22:4413–4424

Chapter 15
Anti-cancer Dynamics of Natural Phytochemical Inhibitors of Cyclin-Dependent Kinases

Shyam N. Sundar and Gary L. Firestone

Abstract Cyclin dependent kinases (CDK), classically thought of as cell cycle regulatory enzymes, have been emerging as multifaceted proteins in normal and transformed cells. This class of multi-functional kinases have thus become promising targets for clinical cancer management, from not only an anti-proliferative perspective, but also to be efficacious in altering the cancer biology of the neoplasm. Anti-cancer phytochemicals have, in the recent decades, have been shown to trigger a plethora of effects on the growth, differentiation, and metastasis of many cancer cell types. These phytochemicals have been shown to disrupt cell cycle dynamics, and stimulate apoptosis in different cancers, both in cell culture as well as in animal models. Several promising classes of these phytochemicals exert their anti-proliferative effects by altering the expression, stability, localization, protein-protein interactions and other critical processes that control the cellular utilization and function of specific CDKs. This chapter aims to discuss the molecular and cellular mechanisms by which natural CDK inhibitors mediate their anti-cancer responses, and to compare the effects of natural compounds to pharmacologically designed drugs that inhibit CDK activity. These natural agents potentially can also synergize with the designer inhibitors, enhancing their efficacy, and decreasing the required individual dosage in cancer management.

15.1 Cyclin Dependent Kinases Structure and Function

The human Cyclin Dependent Kinase (CDK) gene family is comprised of 21 distinct serine/threonine protein kinases. CDK function requires the formation of a heterodimer protein complex with individual CDKs binding to their respective

---

S. N. Sundar
Department of Biology, Ohlone College, Fremont, CA, USA
e-mail: ssundar@ohlone.edu

G. L. Firestone (✉)
Department of Molecular and Cell Biology, University of California at Berkeley, Berkeley, CA, USA
e-mail: glfire@berkeley.edu

J. M. Pezzuto, O. Vang (eds.), *Natural Products for Cancer Chemoprevention*,
https://doi.org/10.1007/978-3-030-39855-2_15

cyclin(s) activators and CDK inhibitor (CDKI) proteins to control the selective phosphorylation of target proteins such as the retinoblastoma gene product (pRb). Similar to most protein kinases, CDKs have an active site located between two structural lobes, the carboxy terminus rich in alpha helices and the amino terminus containing numerous beta-pleated sheets. CDK activation usually requires the orchestrated function of several domains that make up the catalytic region, namely the cyclin binding domain, the conserved ATP binding pocket, and the activating T loop. In the cyclin-free form, the T loop inhibits the catalytic domain, and for most CDKs, cyclin binding triggers the displacement of the T loop, which causes a conformational change in the active site of the enzyme that primes the enzyme for activation. The T loop of certain CDKs contain phosphorylation sites that can serve as activation sites and influence substrate binding. In CDK7 null mouse fibroblasts, T loop phosphorylation of other CDK proteins is reduced, suggesting that CDK7 is a CDK activating kinase, or CAK, and represents an intriguing therapeutic target. Other regulatory sites in CDKs include a P loop, which upon activation by phosphorylation, can disrupt ATP binding. The amino terminus has a glycine-rich region called the G loop that is positioned opposite the T-loop and contains the critical inhibitory sites, such as Threonine-14 and Tyrosine-15 in CDK2. Phosphorylation of Threonine-15 (or of both sites) by the Wee1 and/or Myt1 protein kinases inhibits CDK activity by causing the misalignment of ATP and conformational changes within the G Loop, which in turn reduces substrate affinity (Cheng et al. 2019; Kalra et al. 2017).

One of the critical functions of CDKs in eukaryotic cell cycle is to control the cell cycle, which consists of the following four general phases: G1, S (DNA synthesis), G2, and M (mitosis). Daughter cells from mitosis undergo a growth phase called G1 characterized by increased production of proteins and other macromolecules accompanied by an increase in cell size. The cell then initiates the duplication of DNA in the S phase after a G1/S check point. Post S phase, the cell goes through another gap phase called G2 and after passing through another checkpoint, namely, G2/M, the cell undergoes mitosis. Transition of cells through this cycle of events is orchestrated by a complex set of signaling events that are highly regulated and converge on activation and inactivation of specific CDKs that function at distinct steps in cell cycle, through the regulated interactions with specific sets of cyclins and CDK Inhibitor proteins to control the selective phosphorylation of target proteins. The regulated expression and stability of individual cyclins and CDK Inhibitor proteins play important roles in controlling CDK activity and cell cycle progression, and these processes represent potential therapeutic targets.

The classical model of progression through the G1 phase of the cell cycle and the G1-S transition requires the hyperphosphorylation of pRb by CDK4 and CDK6 that are bound to Cyclin D, and the maintenance of hyperphosphorylated pRb by active CDK2 bound to Cyclin E (Poon 2016; Swaffer et al. 2016). Aspects of this classical model has been challenged by findings from transgenic mouse models. CDK4 null mice and CDK6 null mice were viable and showed some disrupted endocrine function and lowered blood cell counts, respectively, indicating that CDK4 and CDK6 may potentially compensate for each other. The double knockout mouse model lacking both CDK4 and CDK6 did not survive due to anemia, but a number of other tissues displayed normal rates of proliferation. Embryonic fibroblasts from the double knockout mice showed a slower entry into S phase suggesting that CDK2 could interact with D type cyclins that normally bind to and activate CDK4 and CDK6. It is also interesting to note that the phenotype observed in the double CD4/CDK6 knockout bears some similarity to toxicity observed in patients treated with first generation inhibitors selective for CDK4 and CDK6 (Thill and Schmidt 2018; Malumbres et al. 2004). CDK2 null mice were also viable, although the loss of CDK2 resulted in marked effects in gametogenesis (Ray et al. 2011). In tissues such as the colon, inhibition of CDK2 does not inhibit cell proliferation, however, in other cell types such as liver and fibroblasts, loss of CDK2 caused senescence and delayed tumorigenesis. Ablation of both CDK2 and CDK4 was well tolerated and highly mitotic tissues such as the digestive tract epithelium remained unaffected (Barriere et al. 2007).

The most significant CDK involved in procession of mitosis is CDK1, whose rapid activation is ensured by positive feedback. CDK1 protein levels are constant throughout the cell cycle, but the key event for entry into mitosis is activation of CDK1 by cyclin binding as well as by phosphorylation (Kataria and Yamano 2019). CDK1 null mice are not viable and did not even yield early stage embryos indicating that CDK1 is essential for cell cycle progression (Risal et al. 2016). One explanation is that CDK1 can interact with either cyclin D or cyclin E in the absence of the other CDKs. These observations establishing the essentiality of CDK1 limits its potential as a therapeutic target.

15.2 Cyclin and CDK Inhibitor Protein Control of CDK Enzymatic Activity

Cyclin-CDK Interactions As reviewed in detailed (Satyanarayana and Kaldis 2009), individual cyclin proteins bind to and activate specific CDKs in a cell cycle-dependent context. For example, Cyclin D1 binds CDK4 and CDK6 causing the phosphorylation of retinoblastoma gene product pRb at Ser 807 and Ser 811. Cyclin D1 expression rises at the early part of G1 due to increased transcription initiated by a variety of signaling pathways including estrogen receptor-alpha, as well as the RAS-RAF-MAPK and AKT/PKB-β-Catenin pathways. The rise in cyclin D levels can also be attributed to stabilization of cyclin D1 protein due to GSK3β inactivation which prevents proteasomal degradation of cyclin D1 protein (Liu et al. 2017).

The hyperphosphorylation of pRb releases E2F leading to increased transcription of and increased cyclin E protein levels. Cyclin E then binds to and activates CDK2, resulting in maintaining the hyperphosphorylated state of pRb, allowing E2F to transcribe a large number of genes involved in S phase progression, including cyclin E and cyclin A. CDK2 bound to cyclin E or cyclin A then activates a helicase leading to the initiation of replication (Moiseeva and Bakkenist 2018). Cyclin E is degraded during S phase and Cyclin A-CDK2 phosphorylates the helicase, which signals the exclusion of the helicase from the nucleus, resulting in an inhibition of re-replication. CyclinA-CDK2 complex also causes phosphorylation of E2F1 and E2F3 decreasing their DNA binding and subsequent transcription of S phase genes (Blais 2012). As such, CDK2 and Cyclin E represents intriguing therapeutic targets.

Cyclin B and cyclin A gene families are the cyclins involved in mitosis progression (Kalaszczynska et al. 2009; Strauss et al. 2018). Cyclin B1 is the predominant CDK1 partner in most mammalian cells, and formation of and nuclear localization of the cyclin B1-CDK1 protein complex is highly regulated by critical phosphorylation events. For example, phosphorylation by the protein kinase PLK1 triggers translocation of cyclin B1 into the nucleus, and another protein kinase, MASTL, inhibits the PP2A-B55 phosphatase that normally dephosphorylates CDK1-Cyclin B1 complex (Serra and Chetty 2018). MASTL is activated by the active CDK1 protein complex and functions to maintain the activated status of CDK1 via CDC25-mediated mechanisms during mitosis, preventing retro entry into G2. Cyclin A is rapidly degraded during mitosis and cyclin B1 transcription is orchestrated by many transcription factors in a way that ensures its accumulation at the end of G2 and decline post mitotically.

Inhibitors of CDK Activity Inhibition of CDK activity is achieved in the cell by the actions of specific CDK Inhibitor proteins that bind to their complementary CDKs at distinct stages of the cell cycle (Serra and Chetty 2018; Drexler 1998; Abbastabar et al. 2018; Zohny et al. 2019). Members of the INK4 (CDK4 inhibitor) and CIP/KIP (cyclin dependent kinase inhibitor/kinase inhibitory protein) gene families are inherent modulators of CDK activity. The INK4 family consists of $p16^{INK4A}$, $p15^{INK4B}$, $p18^{INK4C}$, and $p19^{INK4D}$. Of these, p16 is the most well studied, and is induced by a variety of signals such as Transforming Growth Factor-beta, and contact inhibition. The p16 protein has been shown to directly inhibit CDK4 activity and indirectly by interfering with Heat Shock Protein-90 induced folding of CDK4 in the cytoplasm. In contrast, the members of the CIP/KIP family are ubiquitously expressed with the exception of $p57^{KIP2}$. The other members of this family are $p21^{CIP1}$ and $p27^{KIP1}$. Also, the CIP/KIP family members have demonstrated binding to all CDK and can have positive or negative effects in regulating CDK activity. The members of CIP/KIP family can bind CDK4-Cyclin D complex, sequester this complex and favor the activation of CDK2.

15.3 Non-cell Cycle Functions of CDK

CDK are very versatile and their functional repertoire far exceeds regulation of cell cycle progression. For example, individual CDKs have been shown to modulate critical cell signaling pathways that regulate cell division, affect transcription in general, as well as cell differentiation, and even embryonic development (Bendris et al. 2015). As such, these non-cell cycle functions could potentially account for unanticipated side effects of the therapeutic use of natural CDK regulators.

The atypical CDK with the most diverse functions is CDK5, which binds cyclin Y, can localize to the membrane, and is expressed in terminally differentiated tissues such as neurons (Bhonsule et al. 2017). CDK5 has been shown to influence the beta-catenin Wnt signaling pathway and plays a role in neuronal migration and neurite outgrowth as well as synapse formation. Ablation of cyclin Y produced a phenotype similar to loss of Wnt function in Xenopus embryo model. CDK5 through Wnt activation facilitates organization of the mitotic spindle as well as chromosome segregation, and CDK5 has also been shown to be involved with insulin secretion and glycogen synthesis.

Some members of the CDK gene family play critical roles in transcription, and hence can influence both cell cycle and non-cell cycle effects such as differentiation, and apoptosis. The transcriptional CDKs include CDK7, CDK8, CDK9, CDK10, CDK11 and CDK12. Several of the typical CDKs, such as CDK1, CDK2 and CDK6, have been shown to have "atypical" cellular functions in addition to their "typical" role in cell cycle progression. For instance, CDK6 unbound to cyclin D, can associate with a number of transcription factors such as the Jun-Fos complex on the EGR1 promoter, and with c-Jun on the VEGF-A promoter (Schmitz and Kracht 2016). The CDK6-cyclinD1 complex can also bind STAT3 on the p16 promoter. CDK1, CDK2 and several of the transcriptional CDKs have been shown to phosphorylate the C-terminal repeat domain (CTD) of the largest subunit of RNA polymerase II, which typically serves as a binding scaffold for nuclear factors that bind depending in the phosphorylation pattern of the CTD, and which regulates the processive elongation of the enzyme. CDK7 bound with cyclin H is a major activator of the RNA polymerase II CTD and is critical for initiation of transcription. Interestingly, CDK7 is overexpressed in majority of ER-positive breast cancer and loss of CDK7 resulted in lower levels of phosphorylated ERα (Ser 118) (Chen et al. 2000). CDK7 has also been shown to associate with androgen receptor and causes phosphorylation of the AR at S515 leading to its proteasomal degradation CDK9 (bound to cyclin T1 or cyclin T2) and CDK12 (bound to cyclin K) have been shown to release the RNA polymerase II from a pause and continue elongation.

CDK8 and CDK19 are very similar and bind cyclin C, but these complexes are repressors of transcription and have been shown to play a role in gene transcription by p53, Wnt, Smad, and thyroid hormone receptors. CDK11 binds L type cyclins and plays a role in alternate splicing of genes. CDK11 has also been shown to increase transcription of the AR gene in osteosarcoma cells. CDK11 is associated with proper formation of mitotic spindles and sister chromatid cohesion. CDK10 binds cyclin M and this CDK protein complex is responsible for proteasomal degradation of the transcription factor Ets2, causing decreased levels of Raf and dampening of the MAPK pathway. CDK10 has also been shown to dampen steroid receptor signaling by increasing receptor association with heat shock proteins. CDK20 has been shown to have CAK activity for CDK2, and shares similarity with CDK7 functionally, and can function as an activator of the Wnt signaling pathway, as well as promote beta-catenin dependent cell cycle progression (Bacon and D'Orso 2019; Guen et al. 2017; Zhou et al. 2016; Malumbres 2014).

15.4 CDK and Cancer

CDK activity is regulated by many signaling pathways and, in turn, CDKs can influence a number of important intracellular signaling cascades. CDK activity is influenced by gene mutations, expression levels, protein stability, protein-protein interactions, and by cellular compartmentalization. Depending on the cancer cell type, the dysregulation of CDK activity can be influenced by any of these processes. Excessive activity of individual CDKs can influence the promotion of tumorigenesis that result from several distinct mechanisms that include, but not limited to, point mutations in the CDK that cause its constitutive activation and prevent inhibitor binding, gene amplification, delocalization and nonsense mutations leading to truncated cyclins that can trigger higher levels of CDK activity.

Even though mouse knockout studies suggest that CDK1 is the essential CDK to drive cell cycle progression, current studies suggest that each CDK has a distinct role in tumorigenesis. This concept fits well with the consensus that tumorigenesis is not only cell cycle dependent, but rather it is also dependent on processes such as angiogenesis, differentiation, apoptosis and DNA damage. Studies from various models of human cancer suggest a role for many CDKs, both positive and negative, in tumorigenesis. Thus, CDKs are potentially effective therapeutic targets because the modulation of each CDK activity may affect several processes involved with tumorigenesis, including the cell cycle. This is a double-edged sword because of the potential for toxic side effects in normal cells. An ideal therapeutic molecule should selectively effect tumor cells with little or no side effects in normal cells. Many natural compounds, discussed later, have this property. The following discusses each of the individual CDKs in the context of human cancers.

CDK1 appears to be the most essential CDK for cell cycle progression, and not surprisingly it has been reported to be the least mutated kinases in human cancers. Some ovarian cancers display a missense mutation (73 Asp→His). Overexpression of CDK1 has been reported in a few cancers such as melanoma, lymphoma and lung cancer. The low levels of cytoplasmic CDK1 has been correlated to resistance to chemotherapy and poor overall survival (Malumbres 2014; Brown et al. 2015).

CDK2 is reported to be overexpressed in some melanoma, breast cancers and laryngeal squamous cell cancers. Even though mutations in CDK2 have been reported in many cancers, elevated activity of CDK2 has been primarily due to elevated expression of wild type and mutated cyclins E and A (Malumbres 2014; Chohan et al. 2015).

CDK3 is a transcriptional CDK that has been shown to be overexpressed in tamoxifen resistant breast cancer. CDK3 phosphorylates at Ser 104/116 and promotes antiestrogen resistance. Inhibition of CDK3 expression and activity caused a reversal to tamoxifen sensitivity in these cells (Zheng et al. 2018). In skin cancer models, CDK3 activates NFAT3 and together they promote in vitro and in vivo transformation including elevated proliferation and anchorage independent growth (Xiao et al. 2017). In the nervous system, elevated CDK3 expression was elevated in cancer cell lines and tumors compared to normal tissue, and with higher activity of transcription factor ATF1 (Zheng et al. 2008).

The CDK4-Cyclin D-p16-pRb signaling pathway represents the lion share of mutations associated with human cancer. Almost 50% of all human cancers display an aberration in one of these components. Gene amplification of CDK4 has been reported in osteosarcoma, melanoma, breast cancer, glioblastoma, neuroblastoma, and liposarcoma. The most reported mutation in CDK4 is the R24C mutation that occurs in melanoma, lymphoma and some lung cancers, and which prevents p16 from binding CDK4 complex, and leading to CDK4 hyperactivity. The most common aberration from this complex is from the cyclin D family, with reports of gene amplification, overexpression, inappropriate localization and alternative splicing. It is worth noting that the CDK4 pathway (CDK4-Cyclin D-p16-pRb) is dysregulated in over 90% of melanoma, and in a significant number of lung cancers. Mouse models of non-small cell lung carcinoma show a clear dependence of tumorigenesis on CDK4 hyperactivity. Selective inhibition of CDK4 is a promising anti-cancer strategy for melanoma and lung cancer management (Malumbres 2014; O'Leary et al. 2016).

CDK5 hyperactivity is significantly associated with neurodegenerative diseases such as Alzheimer's and Parkinson's disease. Upregulation of CDK5 has been detected in a variety of cancers such as glioblastoma, neuroblastoma, colorectal, head-neck, breast, lung, ovarian, prostate, myeloma, bladder cancers and lymphoma. Lung cancers expressing CDK5/p35 are associated with poorer prognosis. Single Nucleotide Polymorphisms (SNP) in the promoter region of CDK5 are associated with increased risk for lung cancer. In prostate cancer cells, CDK5 has been associated with increased metastasis. In mantle cell lymphoma, decreased methylation of the CDK5 promoter results in its elevated expression. CDK5's role in pancreatic cancer is very multifaceted. CDK5 and its partners are expressed at very low levels in normal pancreatic ductal epithelium; however, 60% of pancreatic adenocarcinomas display overexpressed CDK5 due to gene amplification. Additionally, CDK5 has also been implicated in progression as well as migration of pancreatic cancer cells. In breast cancer, TGF-β causes an increased expression of CDK5 as well as p35 and mediates Epithelial-Mesenchymal Transition. Such a transition causes increased migration of cells and an enrichment of cancer stem cells. It is becoming clear that CDK5 plays an important role in cell motility, and this CDK is potentially an important target in the management of metastasis (Malumbres 2014; Pozo and Bibb 2016).

CDK6 mutations are not a frequent event correlating with human cancer development. However, CDK6 overexpression is known to be a characteristic of many leukemias and lymphomas. Chromosomal translocation of CDK6 has been known to be causative for B lymphoid malignancy and amplification of the CDK6 locus has been reported in glioblastoma as well as in pancreatic cancer. CDK6 has been implicated in acute myeloid leukemia and in the progression of mixed lineage leukemia in mice where CDK6 hyperactivity causes cell to remain undifferentiated (Malumbres 2014; VanArsdale et al. 2015).

CDK7 exerts two major classes of effects in cells. CDK7 acts as a CAK to phosphorylate other CDKs, and CDK7 forms a transcription module that activates RNA polymerase. CDK7 is associated with increased expression of oncogenes such as BCL2, hTERT, and c-Myc in cervical cancer cells. Also, in a xenograft transplant model of these cervical cancer cells, inhibition of CDK7 by THZ1 showed marked inhibition of tumor growth (Malumbres 2014; Fisher 2019).

CDK8 overexpression is most commonly observed in cancers of the gastrointestinal tract, melanoma and breast cancer. It is also a transcriptional CDK and is required as a functional connection between transcription factors and RNA polymerase II. CDK8 is closely related to β-catenin function, especially in colorectal cancer cells. 47% of colorectal cancer appears to have elevated levels of CDK8 and is associated with poor prognosis. Expression of CDK8 becomes elevated in cancer cells compared to preneoplastic lesions and normal mammary tissue. In breast cancer, CDK8 expression is also correlated with estrogen receptor-alpha expression and with levels of the phosphorylated receptor. In breast cancer cells, CDK8 appears to be downstream of estrogen receptor-alpha in that CDK8 kinase activity is required for transcription by the steroid receptor (McDermott et al. 2017). CDK8 is also implicated in Epithelial-Mesenchymal Transition in pancreatic and ovarian cancer, which is attributable to its regulation of β-catenin (Xu et al. 2015). In prostate, colorectal, pancreatic and hepatic cancer models, CDK8 is associated with increased β-catenin expression leading to increased matrix metalloproteinase and decreased tissue inhibitor of matrix metalloproteinase expression, and in these cell types, knockdown of CDK8 does not affect proliferation significantly (Chi et al. 2014).

CDK9 overexpression has been reported in two major classes of human cancer, namely cancers of the immune system and neural cancers. CDK9 overexpression has been found in a majority of lymphoma and leukemia such as Burkitts lymphoma, Hodgkins lymphoma, myeloid leukemia, and other B and T cell precursor derived lymphomas (Morales and Giordano 2016; Franco et al. 2018).

CDK10 has negative effects on the cell cycle in hepatocellular carcinoma. Expression of CDK10 is found to be reduced in hepatic cancers compared to normal cells and restoration of CDK10 expression caused a G1 cell cycle arrest as well as increased sensitivity to chemotherapy and apoptotic agents. CDK10 levels are suppressed in almost half of breast cancer samples, and the lowered expression is associated with a poor prognosis. Silencing of CDK10 expression causes an increase in ETS2 driven transcription of RAF, enhanced MAPK signaling and reduced dependence on estrogen for growth as well as with increased tamoxifen resistance. The silencing of CDK10 expression is due to an increased promoter methylation (Malumbres 2014; Iorns et al. 2008).

CDK11's significance in cancer still needs much more investigation. The p110 isoform of CDK11 is very highly expressed in cancers, and CDK11 expression is associated with poor prognosis. In breast cancer as well as in osteosarcoma models where expression of CDK11 is marked, CDK11 is associated with high levels of cell cycle progression, growth, migration, and resistance to apoptosis. In liposarcoma, elevated CDK11 levels have the same effects as observed in breast cancer and osteosarcoma, additionally, CDK11 expression also induces chemotherapy resistance. In multiple myeloma, CDK11 increases cell proliferation as well as cell survival. In colon cancer cells, CDK11 is a positive modulator of the Wnt–βcatenin pathway. Interestingly, the p58 isoform of CDK11 is expressed at lower levels in prostate cancer compared to normal tissues. Elevated expression of p58 in prostate cancer cells led to decreased levels of androgen receptors, and lowered metastasis rates by lowering expression of MMP2 and Integrin β3. These effects were observed in androgen receptor expressing cell lines but not in androgen receptor deficient cell lines. Loss of CDK11 in melanoma cells has been shown to be result in G1 cell cycle arrest (Malumbres 2014; Chi et al. 2014).

CDK12, CDK13, CDK14, CDK15 and CDK16 have all been shown to positively influence the cell cycle. CDK12 and CDK13 are involved in transcription elongation and promote cancer cell cycle progression. CDK14 causes increased cell proliferation in addition to increased migration and modulation of Wnt pathways. CDK15 and CDK16 enhancer of cell cycle progression and increased cell proliferation (Malumbres 2014; Greenleaf 2019).

15.5 Therapeutic Targeting of CDK in Cancer

One of the initial strategies employed to target inhibition of CDK activity was to develop small molecule inhibitors that act at the ATP binding site. These compounds are also called competitive or type I inhibitors. They are typically flavonoid, purine, indenopyrazole, arylcarbazole, indolinone, oxindole, pyrimidine, thiazole, indirubin, hymenialdisine or paullone derivatives. The first set of CDK inhibitors resulted in non-selective or pan inhibition of CDK family of kinases. Since then, more selective inhibitors have surfaced utilizing a variety of strategies.

Peptidomimetics Inhibition of cyclin binding to CDK would be an ideal strategy to dampen most CDK activities and as a targeted strategy for anticancer therapy. However, the binding of CDK to its cyclins is so tight that no designed molecule to date has come close to inhibiting this binding interaction. The activities of CDK/cyclin complexes require protein-protein interactions and small peptides have been designed that disrupt this protein-protein interaction with high specificity. These peptide molecules are limited by their poor tumor penetrating properties as well as their short half-life. One chimeric peptides designed to target CDK4 was successful in inducing a cell cycle arrest and apoptosis in cancer cell lines as well as inhibit the growth of tumors in xenograft models. MM-D37K, derived from p16INK4a peptide and penetratin (cell penetrating peptide) acts as a surrogate of endogenous p16INK4a inhibition targets CDK4 and CDK6. This peptide induced a G1 cell cycle arrest, inhibited growth in colorectal and lung cancer tumor xenograft models, and synergized with 5′-fluorouracil, a chemotherapy agent. Another strategy involved inhibiting an allosteric site close to the ATP binding pocket, which worked to inhibit CDK2 and cause G1 cell cycle arrest in the micromolar range. Another example of a non-competitive inhibitor is THZ1, a compound that exhibits specificity towards CDK7. THZ1 has shown efficacy at inhibiting cell proliferation in acute T cell lymphoblastic leukemia both in culture and in xenografts with no observable side effects. ATP competitive drugs (type I) such as flavopiridol and roscovitine failed to show specificity and act as pan CDK inhibitors, resulting in excessive cytotoxicity (McInnes et al. 2003; Heptinstall et al. 2018; Malínková et al. 2015).

Small molecule CDK inhibitors

Drug	Targets	Effects	Side effects/efficacy
Alvocidib	CDK 1, 2, 4, 6, 7, 9	G1 and G2 arrest	Hepatotoxicity, Nausea, Cytopenia
Seliciclib	CDK 1, 2, 5, 7, 9	G1 and G2 arrest	Short Half Life
Dinaciclib	CDK 1, 2, 5, 9	Growth inhibition	Cytopenia
AT 7519	CDK 1, 2, 4, 5, 6, 9	G1 and G2 arrest	Cardiac problems
Palbociclib	CDK4 and CDK6	G1 arrest	Rb needed, synergy with tamoxifen and letrozole. Decreases tamoxifen resistance
Ademaciclib	CDK4 and CDK6	G1 arrest	Synergy with tamoxifen/Trastuzumab
Ribociclib	CDK4 and CDK6	G1 arrest	Rb needed /cytopenia

Alvocidib (Flavopiridol) is one of the earliest CDK inhibitors that was developed, which depending on the cancer cell type induced either G1 or G2 cell cycle arrests as well as an apoptotic response. Initially, alvocidib was thought to inhibit the G1-acting CDK2 and CDK4; however, recent reports have suggested that the apoptotic and growth arrest effects of alvocidib are due to inhibition of transcriptional CDKs such as CDK7 and CDK9. Alvocidib stabilize the disease in approximately 35% of tested cancer (breast, ovarian and pancreatic) patients, although the side effects are significant (Zeidner and Karp 2015; Dai and Grant 2003).

Dinaciclib was developed as a more selective inhibitor of CDK activity, but in clinical trials involving breast and lung cancer, dinaciclib caused a hastened progression and the study was terminated (Blachly and Byrd 2013). In studies that employed dinaciclib with other anticancer drugs, a 50% enhanced efficacy was reported but severe cytopenia was a side effect that forced the studies to terminate early. Another promising pan CDK inhibitor is AT7519 developed using fragment based medicinal chemistry techniques linked to X ray crystallography. This drug showed high efficacy against multiple myeloma and B cell lymphoma cell lines by strongly inhibiting CTD phosphorylation of the RNA polymerase and subsequent global transcriptional inhibition. Interestingly, recent reports have also shown a marked activation of GSK3β (dephosphorylation at Ser 9) (Glycogen Synthase Kinase) in addition to RNA polymerase II inhibition. These two effects have been shown to be independent of each other. GSK3β is a key enzyme that regulates β catenin, NFκB, and Akt pathways all linked to cell survival. Initial clinical trials showed cardiac abnormalities such as prolonged QT values and the trials had to be discontinued. In another study involving non Hodgkins lymphoma, these cardiac effects were not observed. AT7519, similar to other pan CDK inhibitors, showed neutropenia, with marked inhibition of CDK9 even at lower concentrations. In a different tumor xenograft model of neuroblastoma, AT7519 showed almost complete inhibition of tumor growth, although the report did not address CDK9 activity and reported a marked inhibition of CDK2. It is interesting to note that the pan CDK inhibitors show significant growth inhibition in mice tumor xenografts; however, in humans, the best effect appears to be stabilization of disease. Many other inhibitors that target multiple CDKs have been developed but have not progressed beyond early clinical studies for a variety of reasons, but hematological complications have been reported in almost all of them. Induction of apoptosis in leukocytes due to inhibition of kinases that are related to CDK such as GSK3β and Akt might be the primary reason for cytopenia (Roskoski Jr 2016; Santo et al. 2010).

Palbociclib has been reported to be a much more selective inhibitor than the ones described above. This drug primarily inhibits CDK4 and CDK6, and as expected is efficacious in Rb positive cell lines. Palbociclib treatment resulted in G1 induced cytostasis and a near ablation of Rb phosphorylation. In cancer models that depend on cyclin D1 driven cell cycle progression, palbociclib was reported to particularly effective. These models include estrogen receptor-positive/ HER2 amplified breast cancers, mantle cell lymphoma, multiple myeloma, and colorectal cancers where expression of cyclin D and Rb is high. In estrogen receptor-positive breast cancer cells, treatment with palbociclib caused cyclin D to bind CDK2 and amplification of cyclin E, which in turn resulted in lowered dependence on CDK 4 and CDK6 for G1/S transition, resulting in a palbociclib-resistant state. Palbociclib has shown most promise in management of Estrogen Receptor-positive/HER2-negative breast cancer. The combination of palbociclib and letrozole doubled disease-free survival. Treatment with letrozole can lead to endocrine resistance and palbociclib along with fulvestrant also showed improved survival (Turner et al. 2015; Herrera-Abreu et al. 2016).

Abemaciclib is another selective inhibitor of CDK4 and CDK6 and shows much reduced activity against other CDKs. Similar to Palbociclib, abemaciclib shows dependence on the MAPK and the Cyclin D/Rb pathways. In melanoma, abemaciclib resulted in reversal of BRAF resistance and in apoptosis. This drug has been tested in various cancer models including NSCLC, Estrogen Receptor-positive/HER2-negative breast cancer, colorectal, ovarian, melanoma and glioblastoma, and has shown much higher efficacy than other CDK4 and CDK6 inhibitors. It is interesting to note that 88% of the patients experienced neutropenia, with diarrhea, fatigue and nausea being other frequent side effects. Abemaciclib has been shown to exhibit low toxicity with fulvestrant and is currently being tested in metastatic breast cancer. These effects are also exhibited by Ribociclib, another CDK4 and CDK6 selective inhibitor. Trials are underway to explore the synergism between tamoxifen and ribociclib as well as letrozole and ribociclib in human breast cancer. Ribociclib has been effective in curbing growth in a mouse xenograft model of neuroblastoma, primary liposarcoma, and lymphoma. Ribociclib, similar to palbociclib and abemaciclib, is efficacious in cells that depend on CDK4/CDK6/CyclinD/Rb for cell cycle progression. Ribociclib treatment has shown the reduction of FOXM1 transcription factor activity (a known target of CDK4 and CDK6). Ribociclib has been in clinical testing in various cancer models since 2016, and like the other CDK4 and CDK6 inhibitors, side effects include neutropenia and thrombocytopenia, with QT prolongation at higher doses (Tripathy et al. 2017; Bilgin et al. 2017).

15.6 Targeting of Transcriptional CDKs

The inhibition of transcriptional CDKs such as CDK7 and CDK9 have shown to be selective to cancer cells and not as much toward non-transformed cells, presenting these inhibitors as drugs that might produce reduced side effects. CDK7 has a cysteine near its catalytic domain that is not found in other CDKs and makes this an excellent therapeutic target. THZ1 and the improved version of THZ1, THZ2 are phenylaminopyramidine derivatives that display a selective inhibition of CDK7, and both compounds inhibit tumor growth of neuroblastoma, triple negative breast cancer as well as small cell lung cancer. These cancer cells all have amplification of at least one family member of the Myc family. It is also interesting to note that these cancers are "addicted" to CDK7 based transcription for survival. One area of concern is that CDK7 inhibition might eradicate pluripotent cells in the body, as observed in CDK7 null mice (Ganuza et al. 2012).

Inhibition of CDK9 also shows a similar profile as CDK7 inhibitors, but needs more investigation, especially in clinical studies. Effects are more pronounced in cancer cells than in non-cancer cells. Inhibitors that have been developed to target CDK9 have been either non-selective [Flavopiridol, DRB (5,6-dichloro-1-β-D-ribofuranosylbenzimidazole), LDC067] or need more characterization (iCDK9) or has poor pharmacology (Atuveciclib). Inhibition of CDK9 has been shown to decrease tumor growth in xenograft models (HeLa, NSCLC, leukemia cell lines), and as expected, decreased transcript levels of cell survival genes such as Myc.

CDK8, another transcriptional CDK modulates activity of transcription factors such as NFκB, and STATs. Most CDK8/CDK19 inhibitors have been projected to face challenges as therapeutics due to possibly high levels of cytotoxicity. Both type I and type II inhibitors have been developed for CDK8/CDK19 and some are even specific for one versus the other. Cortistatin is a naturally derived compound known to cause anti-angiogenic effects. Even though cortistatin has high affinity for both CDK8 and CDK19, it has only been tested in cell lines (leukemia) and in some mouse models. Cortistatin appears to de-repress genes responsible for differentiation, and inhibiting phosphorylation of transcription factors such as SMAD, STAT and CTD. Senexin A and its improved version Senexin B are still being investigated. In NSCLC, Senexin A has been shown to inhibit β-catenin transcriptional activity, and in Estrogen receptor-positive breast cancer, suppress Estrogen receptor-alpha transcription as well as cell proliferation. Another type I inhibitor derived from 6-azabenzothio-phene and a type II inhibitor derived from sorafenib showed high affinity for CDK8/CDK19 but had low efficacy in controlling proliferative rates. Pyridine based inhibitors for CDK8/CDK19 proved toxic in dogs and rats (Whittaker et al. 2017).

15.7 Modulation of CDK Function and Expression by Natural Phytochemicals

The following describes several well characterized examples of natural plant products that can alter CDK function, cellular localization, and expression through distinct cellular pathways in human cancer cells. These examples are illustrative of the various ways by which individual CDKs can be targeted by phytochemicals, and the mechanistic concepts are applicable to understanding the responses of a much larger number of bioactive plant products.

15.7.1 Indole-3-Carbinol (I3C)

This phytochemical is found enriched as the glucobrassicin precursor in cruciferous vegetables from plants belonging to the *Brassica* genus such as broccoli, cabbage, cauliflower and Brussels sprouts. I3C is derived from hydrolysis of glucobrassicin, as is the natural I3C dimer 3,3′-diindolylmethane discussed below. Early studies in mice bearing mammary tumors showed a marked inhibition of tumor growth when fed diets rich in I3C (Grubbs et al. 1995), and this phytochemical was effective in curbing the carcinogenic potential of dimethyl benzanthracene, a potent indirect acting chemical carcinogen in several organs such as mammary gland, endometrium, pituitary gland, skin and lung (Brignall 2001). A number of cellular studies demonstrated that the anti-tumor effects of I3C can be accounted for, in part, by the marked cell cycle arrest in various human cancers such as breast, prostate, melanoma, leukemic as well as colorectal to name a few (Dandawate et al. 2016). As detailed below, the mechanism by which I3C targets the cell cycle can differ depending on the tissue origin, phenotypes, expressed genes and hormone-responsive properties of the cancer cells.

In both hormone responsive and hormone unresponsive breast cancer cell lines, I3C has been shown to exert a strong G1 cell cycle arrest. One study demonstrated that I3C almost ablated CDK6 gene expression at the transcriptional level by disruption of the interactions of the transcription factors Sp1 and Ets1 with the CDK6 promoter (Cram et al. 2001). Interestingly, in estrogen responsive breast cancer cells, I3C was shown to inhibit Estrogen receptor-alpha/Sp1 interactions at the telomerase promoter (Marconett et al. 2011), suggesting that the ability of I3C to disrupt transcription factor-promoter interactions occurs at several distinct target genes that ultimately contribute to the G1 cell cycle arrest. I3C treatment also caused a significant decrease in CDK2 kinase activity, an important G1-acting CDK, along with a predominant cytoplasmic localization of the CDK2/Cyclin E complex (Garcia et al. 2005). One mechanism that explains some of these results is the ability of I3C to directly bind to and inhibit cellular elastase activity (Nguyen et al. 2008). One consequence of the I3C inhibition of elastase activity is the disruption of cyclin E protein cleavage, which is a substrate of elastase, with the larger cyclin E protein now accessible to bind to CDK2, causing reduced CDK activity and translocation to the cytoplasm. In this regard, the lower molecular weight cyclin E isoform that is formed in the presence of active elastase, is associated with worse prognosis and increased cancer cell proliferation.

In prostate cancer cell lines such as androgen responsive LNCaP cells, I3C has been shown to cause a G1 cell cycle arrest that is characterized by transcriptional downregulation of CDK6, increased levels of the p16, p21 and p27 CDK inhibitors (Zhang et al. 2003). The increase in p21 was shown to be due to I3C-mediated increase in activated p53 tumor suppressor protein, although in some cancer cell lines, I3C induction of p21 was p53 independent (Hsu et al. 2006). Expression of CDK2 and CDK4 was not altered by I3C in these cells, although the kinase activity of both CDKs were inhibited by I3C treatment. The mechanism of these effects is yet to be determined and was reported in two independent studies employing different prostate cancer cell lines. Many of the I3C effects on expression and activity of CDKs were observed in human cancer cells treated with highly potent I3C derivatives, such a 1-benzyl-I3C (Nguyen et al. 2010).

I3C has also been shown to cause a G1 cell cycle arrest in a myeloid leukemia cell line by upregulation of the p21 and p27 CDK inhibitors, and downregulation of CDK2 (Mohammadi et al. 2017). The mechanism of these effects is yet to be clearly established. In a nasopharyngeal carcinoma cell line model, treatment with I3C caused a marked G1 cell cycle arrest accompanied by downregulation of CDK4, CDK6, cyclin D1 and phospho-Rb. The report did not detail the mechanisms of how I3C brought about these changes, but did report that there was significant reduction in phosphorylation of p38-Mitogen Activated Protein Kinase (MAPK), NFκB and their downstream target proteins in the cell lines as well as in the cancer cell-derived tumor xenografts in mice (Chen et al. 2013). It is important to note that the I3C effects on p38MAPK and NFκB were also reported in prostate cancer cell lines (Sarkar and Li 2004).

15.7.2 3,3′-Diindolylmethane (DIM)

DIM is a natural acid condensation product of I3C and has also displayed cytostatic and anti-cancer effects in many model systems. It is of particular interest to note that I3C and DIM appear to exert similar growth inhibitory effects by distinct mechanisms. For instance, DIM treated breast cancer cells displayed a marked G1 cell cycle arrest to an extent similar to that of I3C, however, DIM treatment only showed a decrease in CDK2 activity due to a transcriptional increase in the p21 CDK inhibitor. Also, DIM increased Sp1 activity at the p21 promoter in these cells. No other effects on other cell cycle regulators were observed in breast cancer cells (Hong et al. 2002).

In human esophageal squamous cell carcinoma cell lines, DIM has been shown to cause a G1 cell cycle arrest accompanied by a drastic reduction in kinase activities of CDK4 and CDK6 due to increased expression of the p15 and p27 CDK inhibitors, and because of lowered levels of cyclin D1 and cyclin E2 (Kim et al. 2012). DIM-arrested gastric cancer cells displayed an increase in the apoptotic protein caspase 9, which likely accounts for the apoptotic response of DIM in these cells. In gastric cancer cells, DIM increased paclitaxel's ability to downregulate CDK4 and cyclin D1 in a FOXM1-dependent manner (Jin et al. 2015). These effects are observed in gastric cancer cells exposed to a higher dose of DIM (40 μM), whereas at lower doses, DIM has been reported to enhance beta-catenin activity associated with increased tumorigenicity (Zhu et al. 2016). A similar study employing athymic mouse xenografts of the SGC7901 human gastric cancer cell line reported that DIM triggered an apoptotic effect that was accompanied by a proportional decrease in expression of the Aryl hydrocarbon receptor (AhR), although potential effects on CDK were not examined (Su et al. 2017). This study also reported that DIM did not cause any gastric, hepatic or renal toxicity, and all other toxicity parameters showed DIM at this dosage to be very safe. It is interesting to note that a modulation of AhR function was also reported with I3C in breast cancer cells as well as in human colorectal cell lines under conditions in which this phytochemical triggers a G1 cell cycle arrest. In cell lines of T cell acute lymphoblastic leukemia (T-ALL), DIM caused a G1 cell cycle arrest, but in these cells, DIM treatment led to decreased levels of CDK4 and CDK6 as well as of cyclin D3 proteins. Interestingly, the study reports that concomitant with the G1 cell cycle arrest, I3C downregulated CDK4, CDK6 and cyclin D3 levels (Shorey et al. 2012). This study is one of the very few examples where I3C and DIM showed an identical profile of cellular changes both in vitro and in vivo.

DIM was shown to induce a marked G1 and G2 cell cycle arrest in HT29 human colon cancer cell line that is accompanied by decreases in CDK4, cyclin A, cyclin B1 and cyclin D1 levels (Choi et al. 2009). Whether this effect was at the transcriptional level remains unclear. However, there was a significant increase in mRNA and protein levels of the p21 and p27 CDK inhibitors, which likely plays an important role in the cell cycle arrest. Another intriguing mechanistic feature not addressed in the study was that even though total CDK2 protein levels included a significant portion of the 34 kDa isoform of CDK2, the level of this CDK2 isoform was nearly ablated in DIM treated cells. In human ovarian cancer cell lines, DIM treatment causes a G2/M cell cycle arrest brought about by activation of the checkpoint kinase chk2, elevation of chk2 kinase protein levels and a downregulation of cyclin B1 as well as CDK1. Studies have shown that the chk2 is integral to DIM induced G2/M arrest in these cells and that downregulation of CDK1 and cyclin B1 appears to be downstream of DIM induced protein degradation of CDC25C phosphatase (Kandala and Srivatsava 2010). In bladder cancer cell lines, DIM induced a G1 or G2 cell cycle arrest depending on the phenotype of the cell line employed. The radioresistant bladder cancer cells were resistant to DIM; whereas, a radiosensitive cancer cell line (RT112) treated with DIM exhibited a G1 cell cycle arrest with decreased protein levels of CDK6 and cyclin D1. Interestingly, DIM treatment of bladder cancer cells with intermediate radiosensitivity induced a G2 cell arrest concomitant with decreased CDK1 and cyclin B1 levels (Sun et al. 2013).

DIM treatment caused a very different profile of cell cycle regulation in breast, lung and glial cancer cells that expressed mutated Epidermal Growth Factors receptors (EGFR). The EGFR mutant in estrogen responsive MCF7 breast cancer cells employed is this study was delE746-A750, which exerts a tamoxifen resistant state. In glioma cells this mutation causes resistance to chemotherapy and radiation, whereas in lung cancer cells (L858R+T790M) this mutant EGFR confers resistance to tyrosine kinase inhibitors. In breast cancer cells expression the mutant EGF receptor, DIM treatment caused an ablation of CDK6, CDK4 and cyclin D1 levels, concomitant with a G1 cell cycle arrest. In contrast, in breast cancer cells expressing wild-type EGFR, DIM did not have a the same cell cycle effect and instead there was no alteration in cyclin D1 or CDK4 or CDK6 levels (Rahimi et al. 2010). Similarly, in lung cancer cells, DIM strongly downregulated CDK4, CDK6 and cyclin D1 protein levels in cells expression mutant EGFR (L858R+T790M), and in all glioma cell lines DIM downregulated the expression of CDK6, although the extent of the downregulation was much greater in cells expressing a mutant form of EGFR (delE746-A750) compared to cells expressing wild type EGFR. The mechanistic connection between EGFR signaling and this profile of cell cycle regulation is not well understood but provides an intriguing platform to test the effects of DIM in cancer cells expressing mutated forms of EGF receptors. This observation is also consistent with a report utilizing Ishikawa endometrial cancer cells in which the DIM stimulation of TGF-alpha levels, a growth factor that binds to EGFR and is normally associated with proliferation, was required for the DIM-mediated G1 cell cycle arrest, and was shown to be highly estrogen receptor dependent (Leong et al. 2001).

15.7.3 Artemisinin (ART)

ART is a phytochemical derived from the sweet wormwood leaves and has been used for centuries in China as a cure for fever and other maladies (Klayman 1985). ART is FDA approved for use in humans as an antimalarial agent, and in the past three decades, there has been many studies that have characterized the potent anti-cancer activities of ART in a variety of human cancer types (Zhang et al. 2018). A number of these studies have established that ART acts, in part, by inducing a cell cycle arrest through the disrupted function and expression of specific CDKs.

ART has been shown to cause a potent G1 cell cycle arrest in breast cancer cell lines, such as estrogen responsive MCF cells, by the transcriptional downregulation of CDK2, CDK4, Cyclin E, Cyclin D1 and E2F1. The transcriptional effects of ART on CDK2 and cyclin E can be attributed to the ablation of E2F1 transcription factor expression (Tin et al. 2012). Similarly, in LNCaP prostate cancer cells, ART treatment caused a G1 cell cycle arrest concomitant with the downregulation of CDK2 and CDK4 expression. The mechanism by which ART downregulated CDK4 expression in the prostate cancer cells involved a different transcription factor, namely Sp1. Overexpression of Sp1 partially reversed the ART induced G1 cell cycle arrest of LNCaP cells, which functionally establishes the role of Sp1 in the ART mediated cell cycle arrest (Willoughby Sr et al. 2009).

In endometrial cancer cells (Ishikawa cells), ART treatment induced a strong G1 cell cycle arrest along with the transcriptional downregulation of both CDK2 and CDK4. However, in contrast to the breast cancer and prostate cancer cells, in the endometrial cancer cells, ART disrupted NFκB localization leading to the loss of CDK4 expression. Importantly, overexpression of NFκB in the Ishikawa endometrial cancer cells partially reversed the G1 cell cycle arrest induced by ART in Ishikawa cells. A very similar effect has been reported in pancreatic cancer cells exposed to dihydroartemisinin, wherein the disruption of NFκB expression and localization led to marked decrease in CDK2, CDK4, and cyclin E expression and a G1 cell cycle arrest in all cell lines tested (Tran et al. 2014). This profile of CDK2, CDK4, cyclin D1 and cyclin E downregulation was also observed in ART treated hepatoma cells, in neuroblastoma cells and in esophageal squamous cell cancer cells (Hou et al. 2008; Du et al. 2013; Zhu et al. 2014). In a human skin cancer cell line (A431), ART treatment caused a G1 cell cycle arrest by downregulating the expression of the G1-acting CDKs, namely CDK6, CDK4 and CDK2 as well as of cyclin D1, and upregulation of the p21 and p27 CDK inhibitors. In the skin cancer model, the authors highlighted the dependency of ART on iron levels and that normal human keratinocyte cells were not affected by ART (Jia et al. 2016).

In gall bladder cancer cell lines, ART treatment caused a G1 cell cycle arrest that led to massive apoptosis and exhibited a mechanism quite similar to its anti-malarial effects in that ART treatment led to an increase in reactive oxygen species in these cells. The G1 cell cycle arrest was accompanied by a decrease in CDK4 and cyclin D1 and an increase in the levels of the p16 CDK inhibitor (Luo et al. 2013). A contrasting effect of ART on the cell cycle progression of cancer cells was reported in HeLa cervical cancer cell line, where ART reversed the radiation induced G2 cell cycle arrest (Gong et al. 2012). ART treatment of irradiated HeLa cells led to undetectable levels of the Wee1 kinase, causing the cells to progress into mitosis and eventual cell death due to severe DNA damage by irradiation. ART was able to significantly enhance growth inhibition of these irradiated cells in xenograft models (Gong et al. 2012).

In the majority of human cancer cells examined, the cell cycle effects of ART can be accounted for by the disruption of cellular cascades required for the activity and expression of specific transcription factors are required for expression of G1-acting cell cycle components, such as CDK2 and CDK4. ART exerts a plethora of other cell cycle effects through different signaling pathways. ART's ability to influence many different pathways that control the cell cycle of human cancer cells makes it a very promising candidate as an anticancer agent.

15.7.4 Resveratrol (RES)

RES is a polyphenol with a stilbene structure that has been shown to exert antiproliferative effects in a variety of cancer cells such as prostate, liver, breast, lung and skin.

RES is found enriched in grapes, red wine and peanuts as well as some berries.

In A549 lung cancer cells, RES treatment caused a strong G1 cell cycle arrest that was associated with an increase in the levels of the functional p53 tumor suppressor protein as evidenced by an increase expression of the p21 CDK inhibitor protein. In these cells, RES strongly inhibited the protein levels of the G1-acting CDK4, CDK6 and cyclin D1 (Yuan et al. 2015). The precise mechanism of this effect has not been established. In this regard, inhibition of p53 did not reverse the RES-mediated cell cycle effects suggesting that this phytochemical may trigger a p53-independent mechanism that leads to the disrupted expression of G1-acting CDKs. Similarly, in human colon cancer cells, RES elicited a G1 cell cycle arrest, along with the downregulation of CDK2, CDK4 and cyclin D1. It is interesting to note that RES treatment also downregulated expression of the p21 CDK inhibitor; however, the Caco2 colon cancer cells used for the study expresses a mutated p53, suggesting that the effects on p21 are independent of the p53 status (Fouad et al. 2013).

Several studies indicate that RES inhibits CDK activity through effects on the corresponding CDK inhibitors and cyclin binding partners. In the T-ALL T cell acute lymphoblastic leukemia cell line, RES treatment induced a G1 cell cycle arrest followed by an apoptotic response. In these cells, RES did not alter levels of CDKs, but showed an increase in the levels of the p21 and p27 CDK inhibitors and decrease in the level of cyclin D1 and cyclin A (Ge et al. 2013). In another leukemia cell line (HL60 cells), treatment with the RES derivative (digalloyl RES) caused an increase in Chk2 kinase and a simultaneous downregulation of Cdc25A and a rapid downregulation of cyclin D1 (Madlener et al. 2010). It is interesting to note that RES synergized with roscovitine, a selective CDK2 inhibitor in arresting HL60 cells in the G1 phase (Komina and Wesierska-Gadek 2008), which implicates a potential therapeutic use of this phytochemical in several different cancer types because the RES-roscovitine synergy was also reported in MCF7 breast cancer cells (Wesierska-Gadek et al. 2008).

RES treatment can disrupt CDK expression in certain cancer cell types. For example, similar to the effects of other anti-cancer phytochemicals described earlier, in MCF7 breast cancer cells, RES induced a G1 cell cycle arrest through the downregulation of all three G1-acting CDKs (CDK2, CDK4 and CDK6) as well as of cyclin D1, cyclin D3 and cyclin E. Additionally, RES also caused an increase in CDK inhibitors such as p15, p16, p21 and p27 (Pan et al. 2010). The profile of cell cycle effects of RES in prostate cancer cells was somewhat different. In androgen responsive LNCaP prostate cancer cells, RES treatment induced a G1 cell cycle arrest concomitant with the downregulation of CDK4, cyclin D1 and cyclin E as well as a modest induction of the p21 CDK inhibitor. RES also decreased cyclin B1 and CDK1 levels (Pan et al. 2010). RES was less effective in causing a G1 cell cycle arrest in androgen insensitive PC3 prostate cancer cells, but this phytochemical did downregulate the levels of cyclins E and cyclin B1, and CDK1 (Benitez et al. 2007). Another report describing cell cycle effects of RES in DU145 androgen insensitive prostate cancer cells reported a downregulation of CDK4 and cyclin D with a reduction in CDK2 kinase activity, which was likely due to an increase in the levels of the p21 CDK inhibitor (Singh et al. 2017).

Generally, similar to reproductive cancer cells, in human A431 skin cancer cells, RES treatment caused a significant loss of CDK2, CDK4 and CDK6 levels along with the rapid disappearance of cyclin D1 and cyclin D2. There was also a sharp rise in the levels of the p21 and p27 CDK inhibitors in these cells, with the subsequent increased association of these inhibitors with the residual CDK complexes. The authors reported a massive dampening of signaling from key transcription factors such as the AP1 heterodimer and disruption of p42/44 MAPK activity that likely accounts for some of the observed effects on CDK gene expression (Kim et al. 2006). In vascular smooth muscle cells, RES was able to reverse the proliferation induced by TNF-alpha, which acts through the EGF receptor. It is very interesting to note that RES treatment reversed the TNF-alpha induced levels of the G1-acting CDK2, CDK4, cyclin D and cyclin E, as well as increase the levels and CDK2 association of the p21 CDK inhibitor (Lee and Moon 2005), thereby accounting for the cell cycle effects of this phytochemical. It is of interest to note is that the TNF-alpha-mediated decrease in level of the p27 CDK inhibitor was not reversed with RES. In SH-SY5Y neuroblastoma cells, RES caused an S phase arrest by elevating the levels of cyclin A and cyclin E (Rigolio et al. 2005).

Taken together, current evidence shows that RES has strong anti-proliferative properties by stimulating a G1 cell cycle arrest and apoptosis in most cancer cell types, which in a large number of cancer cell types is associated with the loss of specific G1-acting CDKs and cyclins and an increase in the level of the p21 CDK inhibitor. RES also generated apoptosis upon prolonged exposure in almost all the cell types examined, implicating this phytochemical as a promising adjuvant in anti-cancer therapeutic strategies.

15.7.5 Curcumin (CUR)

Curcumin is a polyphenolic derived from the *Curcuma longa* or the turmeric rhizome. Curcumin has emerged as a very promising phytochemical that exerts antiproliferative effects in many cancer types. The major obstacle in the translation of bench to bedside appears to be its low bioavailability in vivo.

In a urothelial cancer cell line, curcumin showed very poor efficacy in curbing cell growth in the absence of irradiation. However, exposure to visible light appeared to significantly enhance CUR's ability to halt cell division as early as 24 h. In all three cancer cell lines employed (RT112, UMUC3, TCCSUP), curcumin and radiation caused protein levels of CDK1, CDK2 and cyclin D1 to decrease by approximately 50% compared to untreated controls (Roos et al. 2019). Similarly, in renal cancer cell lines (A498, Caki1, and KTCTL-26), light exposure was required for CUR to be effective. In these cells, CUR treatment resulted in lower levels of CDK1, CDK2 and CDK4 (Zhang et al. 2015), and in an earlier study CUR treatment was shown to decrease the levels of cyclin A and cyclin B1 (Rutz et al. 2019).

In a number of studies, the CUR G1 cell cycle arrest was shown to be mediated by the downregulation of CDKs, and their associated cyclins as well as with the upregulation of specific sets of the corresponding CDK inhibitors. In RB Y79 retinoblastoma cells, the CUR-mediated cell cycle arrest was associated with the decreased protein levels of CDK2, CDK6 and cyclin D3 and with a sharp increase in levels of the p21 and p27 CDK inhibitors (Li et al. 2018). In several breast cancer cell lines (BT483 or MDA-MB-468 cells), CUR treatment triggered a downregulation of CDK4 and cyclin D1 and an increase in the p21 CDK inhibitor (Hu et al. 2018). In this study the authors reported a marked inhibition of NFκB activity, which is an important transcription factor that directly targets CDK4 expression.

Several studies show that CUR treatment alters the protein stabilization of specific cell cycle components. In MDA-MB 231 breast cancer cells that overexpress the HER2 form of the EGF receptor, CUR exposure inhibited the ubiquitination and disrupted degradation of the p27 protein, resulting in the stabilization of this CDK inhibitor and decreased CDK2 kinase activity (Sun et al. 2012). CUR treatment of these cells also decreased cyclin E levels, although the mechanism of this response is not known. Similarly, in LNCaP and PC3 prostate cancer cells, CUR induced a G1 cell cycle arrest as early as 24 h and modest apoptosis by 48 h. In both cell lines, CUR treatment downregulated the levels of the G1-acting cyclin D1 and cyclin E, which was shown to be due to their increased proteasomal degradation (Guo et al. 2013). Interestingly, the authors also established that p21-mediated cell cycle arrest was required for CUR to produce apoptosis in both these cell lines. In contrast to these G1 cell cycle arrest effects, CUR produced a marked G2 cell cycle arrest in T24 bladder cancer cell line (Park et al. 2006). This arrest was attributed to an increase in p21, which appeared to be at the transcriptional level, and a decrease in cyclin A, which appeared to be a post transcriptional regulatory mechanism. It is also interesting to note that the upregulation of the p21 CDK inhibitor was p53 independent in this cell line.

15.7.6 (−)-Epigallocatechin-3-Gallate (EGCG)

EGCG is a polyphenol derived from green tea that has been shown to have anti-proliferative, anti-angiogenic, anti-inflammatory and antioxidant effects in cancer cells. EGCG has also been shown to retard tumorigenesis and tumor progression in many models.

In A431 and SCC13 human skin cancer cells, EGCG exposure led to a decrease in cell viability and caused a sharp decrease in the levels of the G1-acting CDK2, CDK4, cyclin D1 and cyclin D2. These effects were shown to be mediated by inhibition of cyclooxygenase COX-2 by EGCG (Singh and Katiyar 2013). The study also reported that COX2 inhibition led to beta-catenin inactivation which could explain the decrease in cyclin D levels. Similar results were reported in SGC7901 gastric cancer cells, DLD1 and SW480 colon cancer stem cell line, A549 and H1299 lung cancer cells exposed to EGCG (Fu et al. 2019; Chen et al. 2017; Zhu et al. 2017). The cell cycle effects of EGCG varied in cell type- and phenotype-dependent manner in breast cancer cell lines. In estrogen unresponsive MDA-MB-231 breast cancer cells exposed to EGCG initially underwent a G1 cell cycle arrest before apoptosis, concomitant with the EGCG-mediated downregulation of CDK1, CDK4, cyclin D1 and cyclin E (Thangapazham et al. 2007). In contrast, estrogen responsive T47D breast cancer cells treated with EGCG displayed G2 cell cycle arrest due to a downregulation of cyclin B1 and cdc2 (Deguchi et al. 2002). However, in MCF7 estrogen responsive breast cancer cells, EGCG caused a G1 cell cycle arrest, which was attributed to diminished CDK kinase activity due to p21 induction by rising p53 levels (Liang et al. 1999). The underlying mechanisms of these responses are generally poorly understood.

In oral carcinoma cells and in Hs294T melanoma cells, EGCG treatment resulted in marked increases in the levels of the p16, p21, and p27 CDK inhibitors, and a downregulation of CDK2 and cyclin D1 (Singh and Katiyar 2011). Large increases in p21 and p27 CDK inhibitors and decreases of cyclin D1 and cyclin E were reported in LNCaP and DU145 prostate cancer cells arrested in the G1 phase of the cell cycle after treatment with EGCG. All three G1-acting CDKs were found to be downregulated with EGCG in both cell lines. The study also found that the residual cyclin E bound less to CDK2 in the presence of EGCG, although the underlying mechanism remains unknown (Gupta et al. 2003). In A431 keratinocyte cancer model cell line, the EGCG induced G1 cell cycle arrest was attributed to downregulation of CDK4 and CDK6 but not CDK2 (Ahmad et al. 2000). However, the kinase activities of all three G1 CDKs were markedly reduced, probably due to rising levels of the p16, and p21 CDK inhibitors (Ahmad et al. 2000). A very similar effect has been described for the EGCG G1 cell cycle arrest in in pancreatic cancer cells (Shankar et al. 2007). Exposure to EGCG triggered the downregulation of CDK4, CDK6, and cyclin D1 and the upregulation of the p21 and p27 CDK inhibitors. In HNSCC head and neck squamous carcinoma cells EGCG treatment abolished CDK kinase activity by the inducing the levels of the p21 and p27 CDK inhibitors, with little effect on expression of the G1-acting CDKs (Masuda et al. 2001).

Several studies have shown that the EGCG G1 cell cycle arrest and increased levels of specific CDK inhibitors is due to the selective phytochemical-mediated stabilization of CDK inhibitor proteins and of regulators of transcription factors that target G1 cell cycle genes. For example, in Jurkat and prostate cancer cells, EGCG has been shown to increase the protein levels of p27 and of IκB, an inhibitor of the transcription factor NFκB, through the stabilization of each protein by inhibition of proteasomal activity (Lu et al. 2006). CDKs are well known target genes for NFκB, and the inhibition of NκFB by a stabilized IκB protein accounts, in part, for the G1 cell cycle arrest. It is important to note that normal fibroblasts were resistant to EGCG's proteasomal inhibitory effects, and the efficacy of the EGCG response correlated with the transformation state of the cells (Park et al. 2008).

15.8 Perspectives and Future Directions

A number of natural plant products have potent anti-cancer activities, although, for the most part the mechanisms of action are poorly understood. An in depth understanding of how individual phytochemicals target CDK function, stability, expression, accessibility that leads to the arrest of cell cycle progression will be important for the development of new therapeutic strategies using the phytochemicals alone or in synergistic combinations with other anti-cancer agents. The natural plant compounds discussed in this chapter represent the best characterized and promising anti-cancer agents, which generally target the CDKs as well as their critical cyclin and CDK inhibitor binding partners. Most of the natural phytochemicals regulate a number of cellular pathways, such as Mitogen Activated Protein Kinase (MAPK) activated stress cascades and of the protein kinase Akt, which interface with and regulate the actions of the transcriptional CDKs. Therefore, an important future direction will be to understand how the transcriptional CDKs are targeted by natural phytochemicals and how these effects contribute to the anti-cancer activities of these plant compounds. An important eventual goal will be to develop personalized medicines with enhanced efficacies for cancer management that is based on the actions of natural phytochemicals.

References

Abbastabar M, Kheyrollah M, Azizian K, Bagherlou N, Tehrani SS, Maniati M, Karimian A (2018) Multiple functions of p27 in cell cycle, apoptosis, epigenetic modification and transcriptional regulation for the control of cell growth: a double-edged sword protein. DNA Repair (Amst) 69:63–72

Ahmad N, Cheng P, Mukhtar H (2000) Cell cycle dysregulation by green tea polyphenol epigallocatechin-3-gallate. Biochem Biophys Res Commun 275(2):328–334

Bacon CW, D'Orso I (2019) CDK9: a signaling hub for transcriptional control. Transcription 10(2):57–75

Barriere C, Santamaria D, Cerqueira A, Galan J, Martin A, Ortega S, Malumbres M, Dubus P, Barbacid M (2007) Mice thrive without Cdk4 and Cdk2. Mol Oncol 1(1):72–83

Bendris N, Lemmers B, Blanchard JM (2015) Cell cycle, cytoskeleton dynamics and beyond: the many functions of cyclins and CDK inhibitors. Cell Cycle 14(12):1786–1798

Benitez DA, Pozo-Guisado E, Alvarez-Barrientos A, Fernandez-Salquero PM, Castellion EA (2007) Mechanisms involved in resveratrol-induced apoptosis and cell cycle arrest in prostate cancer-derived cell lines. J Andol 28(2):282–293

Bhonsule AS, Bhatt LK, Prabhavalkar KS, Oza M (2017) Cyclin dependent kinase 5: a novel avenue for Alzheimer's disease. Brian Res Bull 132(28-38)

Bilgin B, Sendur MAN, Şener Dede D, Akıncı MB, Yalçın B (2017) A current and comprehensive review of cyclin-dependent kinase inhibitors for the treatment of metastatic breast cancer. Curr Med Res Opin 33(9):1559–1569

Blachly JS, Byrd JC (2013) Emerging drug profile: cyclin dependent kinase inhibitors. Leuk Lymphoma 54(10):2133–2143

Blais A (2012) A new mode of cell cycle stimulation: cyclin E and CDK2-mediated cytoplasmic retention of repressive E2F complexes. Cell Cycle 11(16):2978

Brignall MS (2001) Prevention and treatment of cancer with indole-3-carbinol. Altern Med Rev 6(6):580–589

Brown NR, Korolchuk S, Martin MP, Stanley WA, Moukhametzianov R, Noble MEM, Endicott JA (2015) CDK1 structures reveal conserved and unique features of the essential cell cycle CDK. Nat Commun 6:6769

Chen D, Riedl T, Washbrook E, Pace PE, Coombes RC, Egly JM, Ali S (2000) Activation of estrogen receptor alpha by S118 phosphorylation involves a ligand-dependent interaction with TFIIH and participation of CDK7. Mol Cell 6(1):127–137

Chen Z, Tao ZZ, Chen SM, Chen C, Li F, Xiao BK (2013) Indole-3-carbinol inhibits nasopharyngeal carcinoma growth through cell cycle arrest in vivo and in vitro. PLoS One 8(12):e82288

Chen Y, Wang XQ, Zhang Q, Zhu JY, Li Y, Xie CF, Li XT, Wu JS, Geng SS, Zhong CY, Han HY (2017) (-)-Epigallocatechin-3-gallate inhibits colorectal cancer stem cells by suppressing Wnt/β-catenin pathway. Nutrients 9(6):E572

Cheng W, Yang Z, Wang S, Li Y, Wei H, Tian X, Kan Q (2019) Recent development of CDK inhibitors: an overview of CDK/inhibitor co-crystal structures. Eur J Med Chem 164:615–639

Chi Y, Wang L, Xiao X, Wei P, Wang Y, Zhou X (2014) Abnormal expression of CDK11p58 in prostate cancer. Cancer Cell Int 14(1):2–12

Chohan TA, Qian H, Pan Y, Chen JZ (2015) Cyclin-dependent kinase-2 as a target for cancer therapy: progress in the development of CDK2 inhibitors as anti-cancer agents. Curr Med Chem 22(2):237–263

Choi HJ, Lim DY, Park JH (2009) Induction of G1 and G2/M cell cycle arrests by the dietary compound 3,3′-diindolylmethane in HT-29 human colon cancer cells. BMC Gastroenterol 9:39

Cram EJ, Liu BD, Bjeldanes LF, Firestone GL (2001) Indole-3-carbinol inhibits CDK6 expression in human MCF-7 breast cancer cells by disrupting Sp1 transcription factor interactions with a composite element in the CDK6 gene promoter. J Biol Chem 276(25):22332–22340

Dai Y, Grant S (2003) Cyclin dependent kinase inhibitors. Curr Opin Pharmacol 3(4):362–370

Dandawate PR, Subramaniam D, Jensen RA, Anant S (2016) Targeting cancer stem cells and signaling pathways by phytochemicals: novel approach for breast cancer therapy. Semin Cancer Biol 40–41:192–208

Deguchi H, Fujii T, Nakagawa S, Koga T, Shirouzu K (2002) Analysis of cell growth inhibitory effects of catechin through MAPK in human breast cancer cell line T47D. Int J Oncol 21(6):1301–1305

Drexler HG (1998) Review of alterations of the cyclin-dependent kinase inhibitor INK4 family genes p15, p16, p18 and p19 in human leukemia-lymphoma cells. Leukemia 12(60): 845–859

Du XX, Li YJ, Wu CL, Zhou JH, Han Y, Sui H, Wei XL, Liu L, Huang P, Yuan HH, Zhang TT, Zhang WJ, Xie R, Lang XH, Jia DX, Bai YX (2013) Initiation of apoptosis, cell cycle arrest and autophagy of esophageal cancer cells by dihydroartemisinin. Biomed Pharmacother 67(5):417–424

Fisher RP (2019) Cdk7: a kinase at the core of transcription and in the crosshairs of cancer drug discovery. Transcription 10(2):47–56

Fouad MA, Agha AM, Merzabani MM, Shouman SA (2013) Resveratrol inhibits proliferation, angiogenesis and induces apoptosis in colon cancer cells: calorie restriction is the force to the cytotoxicity. Hum Exp Toxicol 32(10):1067–1080

Franco LC, Morales F, Boffo S, Giordano A (2018) CDK9: a key player in cancer and other diseases. J Cell Biochem 119(2):1273–1284

Fu JD, Yao JJ, Wang H, Cui WG, Leng L, Ding LY, Fan KY (2019) Effects of EGCG on proliferation and apoptosis of gastric cancer SGC7901 cells via down-regulation of HIF-1α and VEGF under a hypoxic state. Eur Rev Med Pharmacol Sci 23(1):155–161

Ganuza M, Sáiz-Ladera C, Cañamero M, Gómez G, Schneider R, Blasco MA, Pisano D, Paramio JM, Santamaría D, Barbacid M (2012) Genetic inactivation of Cdk7 leads to cell cycle arrest and induces premature aging due to adult stem cell exhaustion. EMBO J 21(11):2498–2510

Garcia HH, Brar GA, Nguyen DH, Bjeldanes LF, Firestone GL (2005) Indole-3-carbinol (I3C) inhibits cyclin-dependent kinase-2 function in human breast cancer cells by regulating the size distribution, associated cyclin E forms, and subcellular localization of the CDK2 protein complex. J Biol Chem 280(10):8756–8764

Ge J, Liu Y, Li Q, Guo X, Gu L, Ma ZG, Zhu YP (2013) Resveratrol induces apoptosis and autophagy in T-cell acute lymphoblastic leukemia cells by inhibiting Akt/mTOR and activating p38-MAPK. 26(11):902–911

Gong XM, Zhnag Q, Torossian A, Cao JP, Fu S (2012) Selective radiosensitization of human cervical cancer cells and normal cells by artemisinin through the abrogation of radiation-induced G2 block. Int J Gynecol Cancer 22(5):718–724
Greenleaf AL (2019) Human CDK12 and CDK13: multitasking CTD kinases for the new millennium. Transcription 10(2):91–110
Grubbs CJ, Steele VE, Casebolt T, Juliana MM, Eto I, Whitaker LM, Dragnev KH, Kelloff GJ, Lubet RL (1995) Chemoprevention of chemically-induced mammary carcinogenesis by indole-3-carbinol. Anticancer Res 15(3):709–716
Guen VJ, Gamble C, Lees JA, Colas P (2017) The awakening of the CDK10/Cyclin M protein kinase. Oncotarget 8(30):50714–50186
Guo H, Xu YM, Ye ZQ, Yu JH, Hu XY (2013) Curcumin induces cell cycle arrest and apoptosis of prostate cancer cells by regulating the expression of IkappaBalpha, c-Jun and androgen receptor. Pharmazie 68(6):431–434
Gupta S, Hussain T, Mukhtar H (2003) Molecular pathway for (-)-epigallocatechin-3-gallate-induced cell cycle arrest and apoptosis of human prostate carcinoma cells. Arch Biochem Biophys 410(1):177–185
Heptinstall AB, Adiyasa I, Cano C, Hardcastle IR (2018) Recent advances in CDK inhibitors for cancer therapy. Future Med Chem 10(11):1369–1388
Herrera-Abreu MT, Palafox M, Asghar U, Rivas MA, Cutts RJ, Garcia-Murillas I, Pearson A, Guzman M, Rodriguez O, Grueso J, Bellet M, Cortés J, Elliott R, Pancholi S, Baselga J, Dowsett M, Martin LA, Turner NC, Serra V (2016) Early adaptation and acquired resistance to CDK4/6 inhibition in estrogen receptor-positive breast cancer. Cancer Res 76(8):2301–2313
Hong C, Kim HA, Firestone GL, Bjeldanes LF (2002) 3,3′-Diindolylmethane (DIM) induces a G (1) cell cycle arrest in human breast cancer cells that is accompanied by Sp1-mediated activation of p21(WAF1/CIP1) expression. Carcinogenesis 23(8):1297–1305
Hou J, Wang D, Zhang R, Wang H (2008) Experimental therapy of hepatoma with artemisinin and its derivatives: in vitro and in vivo activity, chemosensitization, and mechanisms of action. Clin Cancer Res 14(7):5519–5530
Hsu JC, Dev A, Wing A, Brew CT, Bjeldanes LF, Firestone GL (2006) Indole-3-carbinol mediated cell cycle arrest of LNCaP human prostate cancer cells requires the induced production of activated p53 tumor suppressor protein. Biochem Pharmacol 72(12):1714–1723
Hu S, Xu Y, Meng L, Huang L, Sun H (2018) Curcumin inhibits proliferation and promotes apoptosis of breast cancer cells. Exp Ther Med 16(2):1266–1272
Iorns E, Turner NC, Elliott R, Syed N, Garrone O, Gasco M, Tutt AN, Crook T, Lord CJ, Ashworth A (2008) Identification of CDK10 as an important determinant of resistance to endocrine therapy for breast cancer. Cancer Cell 13(2):91–104
Jia J, Qin Y, Zhang L, Guo C, Wang Y, Yue X, Qian J (2016) Artemisinin inhibits gallbladder cancer cell lines through triggering cell cycle arrest and apoptosis. Mol Med Rep 13(5):4461–4468
Jin H, Park MH, Kim SM (2015) 3,3′-Diindolylmethane potentiates paclitaxel-induced antitumor effects on gastric cancer cells through the Akt/FOXM1 signaling cascade. Oncol Rep 33(4):2031–2036
Kalaszczynska I, Geng Y, Iino T, Mizuno S, Choi Y, Kondrartiuk I, Silver DP, Wolgemuth DJ, Akashi K, Sicinki P (2009) Cyclin A—redundant in fibroblasts, essential in hematopoietic and embryonal stem cells. Cell 138(2):352–365
Kalra S, Joshi G, Munshi A, Kumar R (2017) Structural insights of cyclin dependent kinases: implications in design of selective inhibitors. Eur J Med Chem 142:424–458
Kandala PK, Srivatsava SK (2010) Activation of checkpoint kinase 2 by 3,3′-diindolylmethane is required for causing G2/M cell cycle arrest in human ovarian cancer cells. Mol Pharmacol 78(2):297–309
Kataria M, Yamano H (2019) Interplay between phosphatases and the anaphase-promoting complex/cyclosome in mitosis. Cells 8(8):2–33

Kim AL, Zhu Y, Zhu H, Han L, Kopelovich L, Bickers DR, Athar M (2006) Resveratrol inhibits proliferation of human epidermoid carcinoma A431 cells by modulating MEK1 and AP-1 signaling pathways. Exp Dermatol 15(7):538–546

Kim SJ, Lee JS, Kim SM (2012) 3,3′-Diindolylmethane suppresses growth of human esophageal squamous cancer cells by G1 cell cycle arrest. Oncol Rep 27(5):1669–1673

Klayman DL (1985) Qinghaosu (artemisinin): an antimalarial drug from China. Science 228:1049–1055

Komina O, Wesierska-Gadek J (2008) Action of resveratrol alone or in combination with roscovitine, a CDK inhibitor, on cell cycle progression in human HL-60 leukemia cells. Biochem Pharmacol 76(11):1554–1562

Lee B, Moon SK (2005) Resveratrol inhibits TNF-alpha-induced proliferation and matrix metalloproteinase expression in human vascular smooth muscle cells. J Nutr 135(12):2767–2773

Leong H, Firestone GL, Bjeldanes LF (2001) Cytostatic effects of 3,3′-diindolylmethane in human endometrial cancer cells result from an estrogen receptor-mediated increase in transforming growth factor-α expression. Carcinogenesis 22(11):1809–1817

Li Y, Sun W, Han N, Zou Y, Yin D (2018) Curcumin inhibits proliferation, migration, invasion and promotes apoptosis of retinoblastoma cell lines through modulation of miR-99a and JAK/STAT pathway. BMC Cancer 18(1):1230

Liang YC, Lin-Shiau SY, Chen CF, Lin JK (1999) Inhibition of cyclin-dependent kinases 2 and 4 activities as well as induction of Cdk inhibitors p21 and p27 during growth arrest of human breast carcinoma cells by (-)-epigallocatechin-3-gallate. J Cell Biochem 75(1):1–12

Liu SL, Liu Z, Zhang LD, Zhu HQ, Guo JH, Zhao M, Wu YL, Liu F, Gao FH (2017) GSK3-β-dependent cyclin D1 and cyclin E1 degradation is indispensable for NVP-BEZ235 induced G0/G1 arrest in neuroblastoma cells. Cell Cycle 16(24):2386–2395

Lu M, Dou QP, Kitson RP, Smith DM, Goldfarb RH (2006) Differential effects of proteasome inhibitors on cell cycle and apoptotic pathways in human YT and Jurkat cells. J Cell Biochem 97(1):122–134

Luo J, Chen X, Chen G, Zhou X, Lu X, Ling Y, Zhang S, Zhu W, Cao J (2013) Dihydroartemisinin induces radiosensitivity in cervical cancer cells by modulating cell cycle progression. Saudi Med J 34(3):254–260

Madlener S, Saiko P, Vonach C, Viola K, Huttary N, Stark N, Popescu R, Gridling M, Vo NT, Herbacek I, Davidovits A, Giessrigl B, Venkateswarlu S, Geleff S, Jäger W, Grusch M, Kerjaschki D, Mikulits W, Golakoti T, Fritzer-Szekeres M, Szekeres T, Krupitza G (2010) Multifactorial anticancer effects of digalloyl-resveratrol encompass apoptosis, cell-cycle arrest, and inhibition of lymphendothelial gap formation in vitro. Br J Cancer 102(9):1361–1370

Malínková V, Vylíčil J, Kryštof V (2015) Cyclin dependent kinase inhibitors for cancer therapy: a patent review. Expert Opin Ther Pat 25(9):953–970

Malumbres M (2014) Cyclin-dependent kinases. Genome Biol 15(6):122–132

Malumbres M, Sotillo R, Santamaria D, Galan J, Cerezo A, Ortega S, Dubus P, Barbacid M (2004) Mammalian cells cycle without the D-type cyclin-dependent kinases Cdk4 and Cdk6. Cell 118(4):493–504

Marconett CN, Sundar SN, Tseng M, Tin AS, Tran KQ, Mahuron KM, Bjeldanes LF, Firestone GL (2011) Indole-3-carbinol downregulation of telomerase gene expression requires the inhibition of estrogen receptor-alpha and Sp1 transcription factor interactions within the hTERT promoter and mediates the G1 cell cycle arrest of human breast cancer cells. Carcinogenesis 32(9):1315–1323

Masuda M, Suzui M, Weinstein B (2001) Effects of epigallocatechin-3-gallate on growth, epidermal growth factor receptor signaling pathways, gene expression, and chemosensitivity in human head and neck squamous cell carcinoma cell lines. Clin Cancer Res 7(12):4220–4229

McDermott MS, Chumanevich AA, Lim CU, Liang J, Chen M, Altilia S, Oliver D, Rae JM, Shtutman M, Kiaris H, Győrffy B, Roninson IB, Broude EV (2017) Inhibition of CDK8 mediator kinase suppresses estrogen dependent transcription and the growth of estrogen receptor positive breast cancer. Oncotarget 8(8):12558–12575

McInnes C, Andrews MJ, Zheleva DI, Lane DP, Fischer PM (2003) Peptidomimetic design of CDK inhibitors targeting the recruitment site of the cyclin subunit. Curr Med Chem Anticancer Agents 3(1):57–69
Mohammadi S, Seyedhosseini FS, Behnampour N, Yazdani Y (2017) Indole-3-carbinol induces G1 cell cycle arrest and apoptosis through aryl hydrocarbon receptor in THP-1 monocytic cell line. J Recept Signal Transduct Res 37(5):506–514
Moiseeva TN, Bakkenist CJ (2018) Regulation of the initiation of DNA replication in human cells. DNA Repair (Amst) 72:99–106
Morales F, Giordano A (2016) Overview of CDK9 as a target in cancer research. Cell Cycle 15(4):519–527
Nguyen HH, Aronchik I, Brar GA, Nguyen DH, Bjeldanes LF, Firestone GL (2008) The dietary phytochemical indole-3-carbinol is a natural elastase enzymatic inhibitor that disrupts cyclin E protein processing. Proc Natl Acad Sci USA 105(50):19750–19755
Nguyen HH, Lavrenov SN, Sundar SN, Nguyen DH, Tseng M, Marconett CN, Kung J, Staub RE, Preobrazhenskaya MN, Bjeldanes LF, Firestone GL (2010) 1-Benzyl-indole-3-carbinol is a novel indole-3-carbinol derivative with significantly enhanced potency of anti-proliferative and anti-estrogenic properties in human breast cancer cells. Chem Biol Interact 186(3):255–266
O'Leary B, Finn RS, Turner NC (2016) Treating cancer with selective CDK4/6 inhibitors. Nat Rev Clin Oncol 13(7):417–430
Pan MH, Lin CL, Tsai JH, Ho CT, Chen WJ (2010) 3,5,3′,4′,5′-pentamethoxystilbene (MR-5), a synthetically methoxylated analogue of resveratrol, inhibits growth and induces G1 cell cycle arrest of human breast carcinoma MCF-7 cells. J Agric Food Chem 58(1):226–234
Park C, Kim GY, Kim GD, Choi BT, Park YM, Choi YH (2006) Induction of G2/M arrest and inhibition of cyclooxygenase-2 activity by curcumin in human bladder cancer T24 cells. Oncol Rep 15(5):1225–1231
Park G, Yoon BS, Moon JH, Kim B, Jun EK, Oh S, Kim H, Song HJ, Noh JY, Oh C, You S (2008) Green tea polyphenol epigallocatechin-3-gallate suppresses collagen production and proliferation in keloid fibroblasts via inhibition of the STAT3-signaling pathway. J Invest Dermatol 128(10):2429–2441
Poon RY (2016) Cell cycle control: a system of interlinking oscillators. Methods Mol Biol 1342:3–19
Pozo K, Bibb JA (2016) The emerging role of Cdk5 in cancer. Trends Cancer 2(10):606–618
Rahimi M, Huang KL, Tang CK (2010) 3,3′-Diindolylmethane (DIM) inhibits the growth and invasion of drug-resistant human cancer cells expressing EGFR mutants. Cancer Lett 295(1):59–68
Ray D, Terao Y, Christov K, Kaldis P, Kiyokawa H (2011) Cdk2-null mice are resistant to ErbB-2-induced mammary tumorigenesis. Neoplasia 13(5):439–444
Rigolio R, Miloso M, Nicolini G, Villa D, Scuteri A, Simone M, Tredici G (2005) Resveratrol interference with the cell cycle protects human neuroblastoma SH-SY5Y cell from paclitaxel-induced apoptosis. Neurochem Int 46(3):205–211
Risal S, Adhikari D, Liu K (2016) Animal models for studying the in vivo functions of cell cycle CDKs. Methods Mol Biol 1336:155–166
Roos F, Binder K, Rutz J, Maxeiner S, Bernd A, Kippenberger S, Zöller N, Chun FK, E J, Blaheta RA (2019) The antitumor effect of curcumin in urothelial cancer cells is enhanced by light exposure in vitro. Evid Based Complement Alternat Med 2019:6374940
Roskoski R Jr (2016) Cyclin-dependent protein kinase inhibitors including palbociclib as anticancer drugs. Pharmacol Res 107:249–275
Rutz J, Maxeiner S, Juengel E, Bernd A, Kippenberger S, Zöller N, Chun FK, Blaheta RA (2019) Growth and proliferation of renal cell carcinoma cells is blocked by low curcumin concentrations combined with visible light irradiation. Int J Mol Sci 20(6):E1464
Santo L, Vallet S, Hideshima T, Cirstea D, Ikeda H, Pozzi S, Patel K, Okawa Y, Gorgun G, Perrone G, Calabrese E, Yule M, Squires M, Ladetto M, Boccadoro M, Richardson PG, Munshi NC, Anderson KC, Raje N (2010) AT7519, A novel small molecule multi-cyclin-dependent kinase inhibitor, induces apoptosis in multiple myeloma via GSK-3beta activation and RNA polymerase II inhibition. Oncogene 29(16):2325–2336

Sarkar FH, Li Y (2004) Indole-3-carbinol and prostate cancer. J Nutr 134(12 Suppl):3493S–3498S

Satyanarayana A, Kaldis P (2009) Mammalian cell-cycle regulation: several Cdks, numerous cyclins and diverse compensatory mechanisms. Oncogene 28(33):2925–2939

Schmitz ML, Kracht M (2016) Cyclin-dependent kinases as coregulators of inflammatory gene expression. Trends Pharmacol Sci 37(2):101–113

Serra S, Chetty R (2018) P16. J Clin Pathol 71(10):853–858

Shankar S, Suthakar G, Srivastava RK (2007) Epigallocatechin-3-gallate inhibits cell cycle and induces apoptosis in pancreatic cancer. Front Biosci 12:5039–5051

Shorey LE, Hagman AM, Williams DE, Ho E, Dashwood RH, Benninghoff AD (2012) 3,3-′-Diindolylmethane induces G1 arrest and apoptosis in human acute T-cell lymphoblastic leukemia cells. PLoS One 7(4):e34975

Singh T, Katiyar SK (2011) Green tea catechins reduce invasive potential of human melanoma cells by targeting COX-2, PGE2 receptors and epithelial-to-mesenchymal transition. PLoS One 6(10):e25224

Singh T, Katiyar SK (2013) Green tea polyphenol, (-)-epigallocatechin-3-gallate, induces toxicity in human skin cancer cells by targeting β-catenin signaling. Toxicol Appl Pharmacol 272(2):418–424

Singh SK, Banerjee S, Acosta EP, Lillard JW, Singh R (2017) Resveratrol induces cell cycle arrest and apoptosis with docetaxel in prostate cancer cells via a p53/ p21WAF1/CIP1 and p27KIP1 pathway. Oncotarget 8(10):17216–17228

Strauss B, Harrison A, Coelho PA, Yata K, Zernicka-Goetz M, Pines J (2018) Cyclin B1 is essential for mitosis in mouse embryos, and its nuclear export sets the time for mitosis. J Cell Biol 217(1):179–193

Su M, Qian C, Hu Y, Lu W, Huang R, Chen M, Chen J (2017) Inhibitory effect of the low-toxic exogenous aryl hydrocarbon receptor modulator 3′3-diindolylmethane on gastric cancer in mice. Oncol Lett 14(6):8100–8105

Sun SH, Huang HC, Huang C, Lin JK (2012) Cycle arrest and apoptosis in MDA-MB-231/Her2 cells induced by curcumin. Eur J Pharmacol 690(1–30): 22–30

Sun Y, Cheng MK, Griffiths TR, Mellon JK, Kai B, Kriajevska M, Manson MM (2013) Inhibition of STAT signalling in bladder cancer by diindolylmethane: relevance to cell adhesion, migration and proliferation. Curr Cancer Drug Targets 13(1):57–68

Swaffer MP, Jones AW, Flynn HR, Snijders AP, Nurse P (2016) CDK substrate phosphorylation and ordering the cell cycle. Cell 167(7):1750–1761

Thangapazham RL, Singh AK, Sharma A, Warren J, Gaddipati JP, Maheshwari RK (2007) Green tea polyphenols and its constituent epigallocatechin gallate inhibits proliferation of human breast cancer cells in vitro and in vivo. Cancer Lett 245(1–2):232–241

Thill M, Schmidt M (2018) Management of adverse events during cyclin-dependent kinase 4/6 (CDK4/6) inhibitor-based treatment in breast cancer. Ther Adv Med Oncol 10:1–12

Tin AS, Sundar SN, Tran KQ, Park AH, Poindexter KM, Firestone GL (2012) Antiproliferative effects of artemisinin on human breast cancer cells requires the downregulated expression of the E2F1 transcription factor and loss of E2F1-target cell cycle genes. Anticancer Drugs 23(4):370–379

Tran KQ, Tin AS, Firestone GL (2014) Artemisinin triggers a G1 cell cycle arrest of human Ishikawa endometrial cancer cells and inhibits cyclin-dependent kinase-4 promoter activity and expression by disrupting nuclear factor-κB transcriptional signaling. Anticancer Drugs 25(3):270–281

Tripathy D, Bardia A, Sellers WR (2017) Ribociclib (LEE011): mechanism of action and clinical impact of this selective cyclin-dependent kinase 4/6 inhibitor in various solid tumors. Clin Cancer Res 23(13):3251–3262

Turner NC, Ro J, André F, Loi S, Verma S, Iwata H, Harbeck N, Loibl S, Huang Bartlett C, Zhang K, Giorgetti C, Randolph S, Koehler M, Cristofanilli M (2015) Palbociclib in hormone-receptor-positive advanced breast cancer. N Engl J Med 373(3):209–219

VanArsdale T, Boshoff C, Arndt KT, Abraham RT (2015) Molecular pathways: targeting the cyclin D-CDK4/6 axis for cancer treatment. Clin Cancer Res 21(13):2905–2910

Wesierska-Gadek J, Kramer MP, Maurer M (2008) Resveratrol modulates roscovitine-mediated cell cycle arrest of human MCF-7 breast cancer cells. Food Chem Toxicol 46(4):1327–1333

Whittaker SR, Mallinger A, Workman P, Clarke PA (2017) Inhibitors of cyclin dependent kinases as cancer therapeutics. Pharmacol Ther 173:83–105

Willoughby JA Sr, Sundar SN, Cheung M, Tin AS, Modiano J, Firestone GL (2009) Artemisinin blocks prostate cancer growth and cell cycle progression by disrupting Sp1 interactions with the cyclin-dependent kinase-4 (CDK4) promoter and inhibiting CDK4 gene expression. J Biol Chem 284(4):2203–2213

Xiao T, Zhu JJ, Huang S, Peng C, He S, Du J, Hong R, Chen X, Bode AM, Jiang W, Dong Z, Zheng D (2017) Phosphorylation of NFAT3 by CDK3 induces cell transformation and promotes tumor growth in skin cancer. Onocgene 36(20):2835–2845

Xu W, Wang Z, Zhang W, Qian K, Li H, Kong D, Li Y, Tang Y (2015) Mutated K-ras activates CDK8 to stimulate the epithelial-to-mesenchymal transition in pancreatic cancer in part via the Wnt/β-catenin signaling pathway. Cancer Lett 356(2PtB):613–627

Yuan L, Zhang Y, Xia J, Liu B, Zhang Q, Liu J, Luo L, Peng Z, Song Z, Zhu R (2015) Resveratrol induces cell cycle arrest via a p53-independent pathway in A549 cells. Mol Med Rep 11(4):2459–2464

Zeidner JF, Karp JE (2015) Clinical activity of alvocidib (flavopiridol) in acute myeloid leukemia. Leuk Res 39(12):1312–1318

Zhang J, Hsu BAJC, Kinseth BAMA, Bjeldanes LF, Firestone GL (2003) Indole-3-carbinol induces a G1 cell cycle arrest and inhibits prostate-specific antigen production in human LNCaP prostate carcinoma cells. Cancer 98(11):2511–2520

Zhang H, Xu W, Li B, Zhang K, Wu Y, Xu H, Wang J, Zhang J, Fan R, Wei J (2015) Curcumin promotes cell cycle arrest and inhibits survival of human renal cancer cells by negative modulation of the PI3K/AKT signaling pathway. Cell Biochem Biophys 73(3):681–686

Zhang Y, Xu G, Zhang S, Wang D, Saravana Prabha P, Zuo Z (2018) Antitumor research on artemisinin and its bioactive derivatives. Nat Prod Bioprospect 8(4):303–319

Zheng D, Cho YY, Lau AT, Zhang J, Ma WY, Bode AM, Dong Z (2008) Cyclin-dependent kinase 3-mediated activating transcription factor 1 phosphorylation enhances cell transformation. Cancer Res 68(18):7650–7660

Zheng L, Meng X, Li X, Zhang Y, Li C, Xiang C, Xing Y, Xia Y, Xi T (2018) miR-125a-3p inhibits ERα transactivation and overrides tamoxifen resistance by targeting CDK3 in estrogen receptor-positive breast cancer. FASEB J 32(2):588–600

Zhou Y, Shen JK, Hornicek FJ, Kan Q, Duan Z (2016) The emerging roles and therapeutic potential of cyclin dependent kinase 11 in human cancer. Oncotarget 7(26):40486–40859

Zhu S, Liu W, Ke X, Li J, Hu R, Cui H, Song G (2014) Artemisinin reduces cell proliferation and induces apoptosis in neuroblastoma. Oncol Rep 32(3):1094–1100

Zhu Y, Zhang B, Gong A, Fu H, Zhang X, Shi H, Sun Y, Wu L, Pan Z, Mao F, Zhu W, Qian H, Xu W (2016) Anti-cancer drug 3,3′-diindolylmethane activates Wnt4 signaling to enhance gastric cancer cell stemness and tumorigenesis. Oncotarget 7(13):16311–16324

Zhu J, Jiang Y, Yang X, Wang S, Xie C, Li X, Li Y, Chen Y, Wang X, Meng Y, Zhu M, Wu R, Huang C, Ma X, Geng S, Wu J, Zhong C (2017) Wnt/β-catenin pathway mediates (-)-Epigallocatechin-3-gallate (EGCG) inhibition of lung cancer stem cells. Biochem Biophys Res Commun 482(1):15–21

Zohny SF, Al-Malki AL, Zamzami MA, Choudhry H (2019) $p21^{Waf1/Cip1}$: its paradoxical effect in the regulation of breast cancer. Breast Cancer 26(2):131–137

Chapter 16
Pro-apoptotic Properties of Chemopreventive Agents

Christiana M. Neophytou, Yiota Gregoriou, and Andreas I. Constantinou

Abstract Natural chemopreventive agents have long been validated to induce apoptosis in cancer cells. Extensive research is being conducted to elucidate the molecular pathways activated by natural agents and cause cellular death. They can act by directly suppressing molecules that inhibit apoptosis, activating pro-apoptotic proteins or by inhibiting pathways that promote survival. Understanding the mode of action of these natural compounds is of great value as this can lead to the development of targeted anti-cancer therapies. The use of natural agents as leads to develop chemotherapeutic drugs is preferred because of diminished side effects. This chapter focuses on natural compounds that have been established, by numerous studies, to be effective as anti-cancer agents. We describe the major apoptotic mechanisms of action of selected natural chemopreventive agents, including vitamin E, curcumin EGCG, quercetin, resveratrol and genistein. We also investigate the effects of these compounds in combination with natural or synthetic drugs. Finally, we take a detailed look at the efforts being made to incorporate these agents in nanoparticle formulations.

C. M. Neophytou (✉)
Laboratory of Cancer Biology and Chemoprevention, Department of Biological Sciences, Faculty of Pure and Applied Sciences, University of Cyprus, Nicosia, Cyprus

European University Research Center, Nicosia, Cyprus
e-mail: cneoph01@ucy.ac.cy

Y. Gregoriou
Laboratory of Cancer Biology and Chemoprevention, Department of Biological Sciences, Faculty of Pure and Applied Sciences, University of Cyprus, Nicosia, Cyprus

A. I. Constantinou
Laboratory of Cancer Biology and Chemoprevention, Department of Biological Sciences, Faculty of Pure and Applied Sciences, University of Cyprus, Nicosia, Cyprus

University of Nicosia Medical School, Nicosia, Cyprus

J. M. Pezzuto, O. Vang (eds.), *Natural Products for Cancer Chemoprevention*,
https://doi.org/10.1007/978-3-030-39855-2_16

16.1 Apoptosis

Programmed cell death (PCD) or apoptosis is a tightly regulated physiological process that plays a critical role in various processes, including normal embryonic development, the maintenance of tissue homeostasis and proper functioning of the immune system (Elmore 2007). Apoptosis also occurs as a defense mechanism by eliminating damaged or harmful cells. Proper apoptotic signaling is very important in maintaining the integrity of the genome, and the evasion of apoptosis has been established as a prominent hallmark of cancer (Hanahan and Weinberg 2011). In addition to tumorigenesis, deregulation of apoptosis can lead to autoimmune and degenerative diseases (Plati et al. 2011); potent apoptosis-inducing compounds can prevent tumor promotion, progression, and the occurrence of inflammation.

Apoptosis is morphologically distinct from necrosis, another form of cell death. The form of cell death being activated depends on the developmental stage of the organism, the physiological environment of tissues and the type and/or the degree of the initiating death signal. Generally, low doses of stimuli such as radiation, heat, hypoxia or cytotoxic anticancer drugs induce apoptosis. However, higher doses of these same stimuli could result in necrosis (Lennon et al. 1991). The two processes may occur independently, in sequence or simultaneously, in cells (Hirsch et al. 1997; Zeiss 2003). Characteristics of apoptosis include cell shrinkage, cytoplasmic membrane blebbing, chromatin condensation, DNA fragmentation, cytoplasmic condensation, nuclear fragmentation and formation of apoptotic bodies. Necrosis is morphologically distinct from apoptosis and involves loss of membrane integrity, swollen endoplasmic reticulum, cell swelling, formation of cytoplasmic vacuoles, ruptured mitochondria and release of the contents of the cytoplasm into the surrounding tissue leading to an inflammatory reaction (Majno and Joris 1995; Trump et al. 1997; Kurosaka et al. 2003). Apoptosis is a highly regulated process that does not induce an inflammatory reaction. In contrast to necrotic cells, apoptotic cells do not release their cellular contents into the surrounding tissues but are quickly phagocytosed by surrounding cells (Kurosaka et al. 2003; Savill and Fadok 2000). Initially, necrotic cell death was thought to not involve gene expression and to be a passive process. In any case, evidence in the literature suggests that necrosis may also be a highly regulated cell death process and may occur in a controlled fashion (Moubarak et al. 2007; Vanden Berghe et al. 2004; Saelens et al. 2005).

Apoptosis is divided into two major pathways: (1) the death receptor or extrinsic pathway, activated by binding of pro-apoptotic ligands to cell surface death receptors, and (2) the mitochondrial or intrinsic pathway, activated by internal signals such as genotoxic stress, and involves the disruption of mitochondrial membrane integrity (Elmore 2007). Caspases are cysteinyl, aspartate-specific proteases that play a central role in both the extrinsic and intrinsic pathway of apoptosis (Li and Yuan 2008). There are 14 caspases that have been identified, 11 of which are present in mammals. Depending on their activity, caspases are divided into pro-inflammatory (caspases 1, 4, 5, 11, 12, 13 and 14) and pro-apoptotic caspases (caspases 2, 3, 6, 7, 8, 9 and 10). The function of pro-inflammatory caspases has not been entirely characterized.

Caspase-11 has been reported to take part during septic shock in order to regulate apoptosis and cytokine maturation (Kang et al. 2002) while caspase-12 can mediate endoplasmic-specific apoptosis in mice and rats. Caspase-13 has been found to be expressed only in cattle while caspase-14 is highly expressed in embryonic tissues (Burz et al. 2009).

Caspases are widely expressed in an inactive pro-enzyme form in most cells with an N-terminal pro-domain and a C-terminal catalytic domain that is comprised by a p20 large subunit and a p10 small subunit (Pop and Salvesen 2009). Based on which stage they are activated during apoptosis, caspases are generally categorized into initiators (caspase-2,-8,-9,-10) or executioners (caspase-3,-6,-7) (Cohen 1997). Initiator caspases possess a longer pro-domain than the effector caspases, whose pro-domain is very small. The pro-domain of the initiator caspases contain either a caspase-recruitment domain (CARD) (e.g., caspases-2 and -9) or a death effector domain (DED) (caspases-8 and -10) that is responsible for the interaction of caspases with molecules that regulate their activity. Following a pro-apoptotic signal, the initiator caspases are clustered and activated automatically by dimerization (Pop and Salvesen 2009). Active initiator caspases proceed to activate effector caspases by cleavage at aspartate residues; the large and small subunits are separated and then the N-terminal domain is removed (Degterev et al. 2003). This leads to the execution of a proteolytic cascade that amplifies the apoptotic signaling pathway.

Based on the implication of caspases in the apoptotic cascade, programmed cell death can also be characterized as caspase-dependent (CD-PCD) or caspase-independent (CI-PCD) (Constantinou et al. 2009).

16.1.1 Caspase-Dependent Programmed Cell Death (CD-PCD)

Caspases play a central role in both the extrinsic and intrinsic pathway of apoptosis. The extrinsic pathway is initiated by binding of death ligands to the extracellular domains of transmembrane cell surface death receptors. These receptors belong to the tumor necrosis factor (TNF) receptor superfamily. The best-characterized death receptors and their corresponding ligands include TNFR1/TNF-α, FasR/FasL, DR3/Apo3L, DR4/Apo2L and DR5/Apo2L (Suliman et al. 2001; Ashkenazi and Dixit 1998; Chicheportiche et al. 1997; Peter and Krammer 1998; Rubio-Moscardo et al. 2005). Following ligand binding, death receptors assemble into active homotrimers which leads to the aggregation of their intracellular cytoplasmic domain of about 80 amino acids called the death domain (DD) (Guicciardi and Gores 2009; Boldin et al. 1995). FAS-associated death domain protein (FADD) or TNFR1-associated death domain protein (TRADD), are adaptor proteins that are recruited to the intracellular domain of the FAS or TNF receptor, respectively (Wajant 2002; Hsu et al. 1995). These adaptor proteins include the DED protein interaction module, that sequesters the inactive initiator caspase-8 with a DED in its

Table 16.1 Members of the Bcl-2 protein family are categorized as anti-apoptotic, pro-apoptotic and BH3-only, according to their function and their composition in BH3 domains

Anti-apoptotic	Pro-apoptotic	Pro-apoptotic, BH3-only
Bcl-2, Bcl-xL, Bcl-w, A1, Mcl-1, Boo	Bax, Bok/Mtd, Bcl-xs, Bak, Bcl-GL,	Bad, Bik/Nbk/Blk, Bid, Hrk/DP5, Bim/Bod, Bmf, Noxa, Puma/Bbc3, BNIP3, BNIP3L

prodomain, to form the Death Inducing Signaling Complex (DISC) (Jin and El-Deiry 2005). DISC formation mediates the oligomerization and consequent auto-catalytic activation of caspase-8 (Kischkel et al. 1995). Subsequently, active caspase-8 can activate downstream effector caspase-3 (Fig. 16.2).

The intrinsic pathway of apoptosis is activated by a range of stress signals, including growth factor, hormone, cytokine or growth-factor deprivation, UV radiation, gamma irradiation, heat, viral virulence factors, DNA-damaging agents such as toxins or free radicals, hypoxia and the activation of some oncogenic factors. Mitochondria play a central role in the execution of the intrinsic pathway. Apoptotic signals cause changes in the mitochondrial membrane that induce the opening of the mitochondrial permeability transition (MPT) pore and loss of the mitochondrial transmembrane potential. This leads to mitochondrial outer membrane permeabilization (MOMP) and release of pro-apoptotic proteins from the inter-membrane space (IMS) into the cytosol (Saelens et al. 2004).

The members of the Bcl-2 protein family are responsible for controlling the MOMP and subsequently the induction of apoptosis. Bcl-2 proteins are broadly classified into three subgroups, one anti-apoptotic and two pro-apoptotic, based on their function and the number of BH domains present (Table 16.1). Anti-apoptotic multidomain members, contain three to four BH domains, pro-apoptotic multidomain members, contain BH1, BH2, and BH3 domains, and the third class is a subset of pro-apoptotic proteins that contain only the BH3 domain (Giam et al. 2008; Danial 2007). The BH1, BH2, and BH3 domains of multidomain Bcl-2 proteins form a hydrophobic groove at the surface of the protein that can bind BH3 domains of BH3-only proteins (Youle and Strasser 2008; Hinds and Day 2005). This heterodimerization plays a key role in the mechanisms by which Bcl-2 proteins regulate apoptosis; BH3-only proteins promote apoptosis by inhibiting anti-apoptotic Bcl-2 proteins and/or by binding to and activating pro-apoptotic Bax and Bak (Ghiotto et al. 2010). Anti-apoptotic Bcl-2 family members, including Bcl-2 itself, decrease apoptosis mainly by neutralizing the activity of pro-apoptotic members (BH3 only protein and multidomain members) and preventing MOMP (Youle and Strasser 2008). Overexpression of Bcl-2 has been reported in various cancers and has been associated with aggressive disease and/or chemoresistance (Campana et al. 1993; Mason et al. 2008). A decrease in the Bcl-2/Bax ratio is considered a prominent indicator during the induction of apoptosis. Furthermore, the subcellular localization of certain Bcl-2 family members changes during apoptotic stimuli; Bax localizes from the cytosol to the mitochondria in apoptotic cells while Bcl-2 is constitutively membrane-bound at the mitochondria. The C-terminal tail of Bcl-2 is anchored in the membrane while the remaining residues reside in the cytosol (Youle and Strasser 2008).

One example of the "cross-talk" between the extrinsic pathway and the intrinsic pathway is by caspase-8 mediated cleavage of Bid (Vancompernolle et al. 1998). This generates the activated Bid fragment (tBid) which then translocates to the mitochondria and induces the release of pro-apoptotic factors (Esposti 2002).

Following MOMP, pro-apoptotic proteins are released from the intermembrane space of the mitohondria into the cytosol. These proteins include cytochrome c, Smac/DIABLO, and the serine protease HtrA2/Omi (Du et al. 2000; van Loo et al. 2002; Garrido et al. 2006). Cytochrome c binds and activates Apaf-1 and recruits procaspase-9 that is also activated following aggregation. Cytochrome c, Apaf-1 and active caspase-9 form the apoptosome which subsequently activates effector caspases (Chinnaiyan 1999; Hill et al. 2004). Smac/DIABLO and HtrA2/Omi induce apoptosis by hindering the activity of Inhibitors of Apoptosis Proteins (IAPs) (van Loo et al. 2002; Schimmer 2004). At later stages of apoptosis, the caspase-activated DNase (CAD) is also released from the mitochondria. CAD is normally associated with the Inhibitor of Caspase-Activated DNase (ICAD) which is cleaved by caspase-3 during apoptosis. Upon activation, CAD translocates to the nucleus and induces oligonucleosomal DNA fragmentation at ~180-bp intervals (Enari et al. 1998).

16.1.2 Mediators of Caspase Independent Programmed Cell Death (CI-PCD)

In addition to caspase-dependent death, cells undergo apoptosis without the involvement of caspase activation. The CI-PCD pathway may be induced by the same signals that induce CD-PCD and the two pathways may be activated simultaneously and are interlinked (Constantinou et al. 2009).

Apoptosis inducing factor (AIF) and endonuclease G (Endo G) are well known mediators of caspase-independent death that are released from the mitochondria at a later stage of apoptosis, when the cell has committed to die. In the absence of apoptotic stimuli, AIF co-localizes with Hsp60 in the IMS. During apoptosis, AIF is cleaved by proteases calpains (calcium activated neutral proteases) and cathepsins and following MOMP, it is slowly released from mitochondria and translocates to the nucleus (Lorenzo and Susin 2007). AIF fragments DNA into ~50–300 kb pieces and induces condensation of peripheral nuclear chromatin (Joza et al. 2001). It has also been suggested that AIF promotes cell death by contributing to loss of mitochondrial function; cells that do not express AIF are defective in electron transport chain complex I/III activity (Klein et al. 2002; Vahsen et al. 2004). Endo G is an endonuclease located in the mitochondrial IMS and is thought to be involved in DNA synthesis and repair and in the regulation of mitochondrial biogenesis. Endo G also translocates to the nucleus following MOMP in a caspase-independent manner and cleaves nuclear chromatin to produce high molecular weight DNA fragments (approximately 50 kb) (Bahi et al. 2006; Li et al. 2001).

The proteases calpains and cathepsins that are regulated by the ER and lysosomes respectively are mediators of CI-PCD in addition to AIF and Endo G. Cathepsins are lysosomal proteins that take part in apoptotic signaling by inducing translocation of Bax to the mitochondria and cleavage and translocation of Bid thereby inducing MOMP (Bidere et al. 2003; Cirman et al. 2004). In addition, as previously mentioned, cathepsins can directly cleave AIF leading to its release from the mitochondria (Lorenzo and Susin 2007). Furthermore, cathepsins may also activate several caspases, thereby contributing to CD-PCD (Vancompernolle et al. 1998). In the absence of apoptotic signals, calpains normally reside in the cytosol as inactive zymogens. Following ER stress, calpains are activated by intracellular calcium influx subsequently activating Bax and Bid and releasing lysosomal cathepsins (reviewed by Constantinou et al. 2009). Calpains can also induce AIF cleavage and release from the mitochondria contributing to the induction of CI-PCD (Lorenzo and Susin 2007).

16.1.3 Execution Phase of Apoptosis

The extrinsic and intrinsic pathways are linked and converge to the execution pathway which is initiated by the cleavage of effector or executioner caspases-3, -6 and -7 (Igney and Krammer 2002). Caspase-3 can be activated by both caspase-9 and -8, while caspase-7 is directly activated by caspase-9. Effector caspase-6 is a downstream substrate of caspase-3 (Cullen and Martin 2009). Active effector caspases are responsible for the activation of endonucleases that cleave DNA, as well as proteases that degrade nuclear and cytoskeletal proteins. Other substrates of effector caspases include cytokeratins, PARP-1, alpha-fodrin and the nuclear protein NuMA that ultimately lead to the morphological and biochemical changes seen in apoptotic cells (Slee et al. 2001). Caspase-3, the most important effector caspase, also induces cytoskeletal reorganization by cleavage of gelsolin, an actin binding protein. Gelsolin is a cytoplasmic, calcium-regulated protein; it binds to the ends of actin filaments, preventing monomer exchange (Weeds et al. 1986). Caspase-3 cleaves gelsolin and leads to cleavage of actin filaments in a calcium independent manner, resulting in cytoskeletal disorganization (Kothakota et al. 1997).

The caspase substrates PARP-1 and alpha-fodrin are cleaved with equal efficiency by caspases-3 and -7. PARP-1 is an abundant nuclear protein, involved in the DNA-base-excision-repair system. It is a 116 kDa protein that contains three main functional domains: The amino-terminal DNA-binding domain (42 kDa) which contains a nuclear localization signal; the central automodification domain (16 kDa) which contains specific glutamate and lysine residues that serve as acceptors of ADP-ribose units that allow the enzyme to poly(ADP-ribosyl)ate itself, as well as a BRCA1 carboxy-terminal (BRCT) protein–protein interaction domain that is found in other proteins of the DNA damage response pathway; finally, the C-terminal, catalytic domain (55 kDa) sequentially transfers ADP-ribose subunits from NAD^+ to protein acceptors, thereby forming ADP-ribose polymers (pADPr) (reviewed by Rouleau et al. 2010). On average, there is approximately one molecule of PARP-1 present per 1000 bp of DNA. In response to DNA damage, including nicks and DNA double strand brakes, PARP-1 is quickly recruited to the modified DNA site and its catalytic activity is rapidly increased 10–500-fold. Activation of PARP-1 results in the synthesis of protein-conjugated long branched pADPr chains 15–30 s after damage (Rouleau et al. 2010). PARP-1 transfers 50–200 residues of PAR to itself and to acceptor proteins such as histones, DNA polymerases, topoisomerases, DNA ligase-2, high-mobility-group proteins and transcription factors (Hong et al. 2004). Through (ADP-ribosyl)ation of these substrates, PARP-1 regulates cellular repair, transcription and replication of DNA, protein degradation, cytoskeletal organization and other cellular activities (Hong et al. 2004). The intensity of PARP-1 activation determines whether cells die or survive following DNA damage. Cleavage of PARP-1 by caspases is considered to be a hallmark of apoptosis. During the execution phase of apoptosis, PARP-1 is inactivated by caspases-3 and -7 by cleavage into a ~25-kDa N-terminal and a ~89-kDa C-terminal fragment (Soldani and Scovassi 2002; Kaufmann et al. 1993). Cleavage of PARP-1 eliminates its activation in response to DNA fragmentation during apoptosis and helps commit cells to the apoptotic pathway.

Alpha-fodrin is an abundant and highly conserved plasma membrane cytoskeletal protein thought to be responsible for coupling a variety of membrane-spanning cell surface proteins to cytoplasmic elements (Vanags et al. 1996). alpha-Fodrin is a known substrate of caspases-3 and -7, as well as of calpain I that cleave the 240 kDa protein into 150 and 120 kDa fragments (Elmore 2007). Fodrin cleavage is thought to result in a reduced ability to cross-link actin filaments leading to plasma membrane blebbing and cellular fragmentation (Vanags et al. 1996).

In addition to caspases, other proteases can cleave PARP-1 and alpha-fodrin. As previously mentioned, calpains play a crucial role in mediating apoptotic cell death but are also known to take part in necrotic cell death. m-Calpain and μ-calpain are the best understood of all the calpain isoforms. μ-Calpain, isolated from calf thymus, has been found to generate ~40–70 kDa N-terminal PARP-1 fragments (Buki et al. 1997). However, it is not yet established whether the 40–70 kDa PARP-1 fragment appears only during necrotic conditions or also during calpain-mediated caspase independent apoptosis. α-Fodrin is also cleaved by calpains to calpain-specific 150 and 140 kDa fragments (Reimertz et al. 2001). During necrosis, cathepsin isoforms B and D produce 55 and 42 kDa PARP-1 fragments. The 89 kDa PARP-1 fragment, which appears during apoptotic cell death, may also be produced by these isoforms (Gobeil et al. 2001).

Characteristic alterations of apoptotic cells also include chromatin condensation, exposure of phosphatidylserine at the external surface of the cell membrane and shrinkage of the cytoplasm (Luthi and Martin 2007; Khosravi-Far and Esposti 2004).

At the final stages of apoptosis, apoptotic bodies are formed and ligands for phagocytic cell receptors are expressed leading to uptake by phagocytic cells (Elmore 2007).

16.2 Survival Pathways Targeted by Natural Chemopreventive Agents

Chemopreventive agents induce apoptosis by targeting specific survival pathways that are often upregulated in cancer cells, including the PI3K/AKT and NFκB pathways. NFκB is a transcription factor that regulates the expression of several proteins involved in survival, proliferation, invasion and angiogenesis. The natural vitamin E isoform γ-TT inhibits the transcriptional activity of NFκB, thereby leading to the downregulation of anti-apoptotic proteins such as Bcl-2, Bcl-xL, c-IAP-1, c-IAP-2 and XIAP and the activation of caspases that induce CD-PCD.

Protein kinase B (PKB), also known as AKT, is a serine/threonine kinase that plays a central role in the regulation of apoptosis, metabolism, transcription and cell cycle progression. Binding of ligands, such as growth factors or insulin, to receptor tyrosine kinases (RTKs), stimulate PI3K which becomes active by autophosphorylation, allowing for the translocation of AKT from the cytoplasm to the plasma membrane where it is also activated by phosphorylation. The tumor suppressor phosphatase and tensin homology deleted on chromosome ten (PTEN) inhibits AKT activity (Stambolic et al. 1998). PTEN stability is achieved via phosphorylation (Vazquez et al. 2000). AKT is phosphorylated on Thr308 and Ser473 by phosphoinositide-dependent kinase-1 and -2 (PDK1 and PDK2) respectively (Stephens et al. 1998; Sarbassov et al. 2005; Jacinto et al. 2006). Phosphorylation of Thr308 partially activates AKT, while phosphorylation of both sites is required for full activation (Alessi et al. 1996). Once activated at the plasma membrane, phosphorylated AKT translocates to the cytosol or the nucleus.

Activated AKT promotes cell survival by phosphorylating an array of downstream proteins that are known to regulate apoptosis such as Bad, glycogen synthase kinase-3 (GSK-3), pro-caspase 9, IκB kinase (IKK), forkhead transcription factors (FOXO1, FOXO2, FOXO3a and FOXO4) and yes-associated protein (YAP) (Sale and Sale 2008). Phosphorylation and activation of the transcription factor cyclic AMP response element-binding protein (CREB) IKK, a positive regulator of NFκB, by AKT leads to the activation of important anti-apoptotic proteins including Bcl-2, IAPs such as survivin, Mcl-1, Bfl-1 and Bcl-xL (Asanuma et al. 2005; Crawford and Nahta 2011; Du and Montminy 1998; Song et al. 2005). Furthermore, AKT can phosphorylate pro-apoptotic protein Bad at S136, preventing in this manner Bad interaction with Bcl-xL and restoring its anti-apoptotic function. AKT regulates cRAF activity by phosphorylation at multiple sites leading to activation of the MEK-MAP kinase pathway which contributes to the survival and proliferation of cancer cells (Somanath et al. 2009). AKT can also block the caspase cascade by

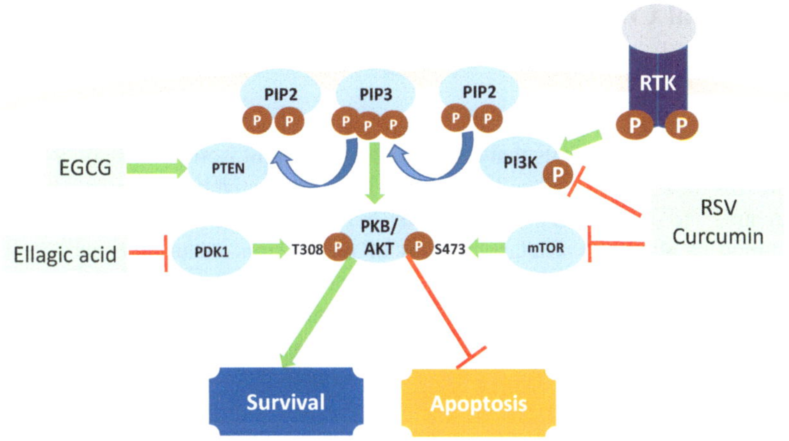

Fig. 16.1 Effects of natural chemopreventive agents on the PI3K/mTOR/AKT pathway. Resveratrol (RSV) and curcumin suppress the phosphorylation of PI3K and AKT. EGCG increases the mRNA and protein levels of PTEN while ellagic acid downregulates PDK1, thereby reducing phosphorylation of AKT at T308

directly phosphorylating and inhibiting pro-caspase 9 on S196 (Manning and Cantley 2007). AKT phosphorylation of FOXO transcription factors leads to their cytoplasmic sequestration and promotes cell survival since FOXOs regulate the transcription of pro-apoptotic proteins such as death receptor ligands TRAIL and Fas and of BH3-only proteins Bim and BNIP3 (Zhang et al. 2011).

Several natural compounds have been reported to inhibit the PI3K/AKT pathway and induce apoptosis (Fig. 16.1). For example curcumin has been reported to inhibit the activation of PI3K/AKT/mTOR pathway and to suppress epithelial-mesenchymal transition (EMT) and angiogenesis in lung cancer cells; Curcumin was also effective in reducing tumor growth in animal models (Jiao et al. 2016). Resveratrol is another natural compound that can suppress the PI3K/AKT/mTOR pathway. In breast cancer cells, resveratrol caused a time-dependent reduction in PI3K/AKT and reduced tumor volume in vivo (She et al. 2001); Resveratrol also inhibits the phosphorylation of PI3K, PKB/AKT and reduced cyclin D1 levels in prostate cancer cells (Frojdo et al. 2007; Benitez et al. 2007). EGCG was reported to upregulate mRNA and protein levels of PTEN, to downregulate the expression of p-mTOR and p-AKT, leading to the inhibition of proliferation and the induction of apoptosis in PANC-1 pancreatic cancer cells (Liu et al. 2013). Ellagic acid also suppresses this pathway by downregulating PDK1 and inhibiting HIF-1a-induced VEGF/VEGFR2 (Kowshik et al. 2014). A more detailed approach on the effects of selective chemopreventive agents on the pathways leading to apoptosis is provided below.

16.3 Natural Compounds That Induce Apoptosis

16.3.1 Vitamin E

Vitamin E is a family of agents that exists in nature in eight isoforms: α-, β-, γ-, and δ-tocopherols (α-TOC, β-TOC, γ-TOC, and δ-TOC, respectively) and α-, β-, γ-, and δ-tocotrienols (α-TT, β-TT, γ-TT, and δ-TT, respectively) (reviewed by Constantinou et al. 2008). Dietary sources of tocopherols include vegetable oils and nuts, while tocotrienols can be found in rice bran, palm oil, wheat germ, rye, oat, and barley. The chemopreventive properties of vitamin E have been well established since the mid-1980s. Initially, their anti-cancer effects were attributed to their anti-oxidant effect and studies were mostly centered on α-TOC, the isoform with the strongest anti-oxidant effects. However, over the last few years, it has become increasingly evident that vitamin E natural isoforms and synthetic derivatives have pro-apoptotic, anti-inflammatory, anti-angiogenic and anti-proliferative activity against cancer cells.

Their structure is comprised by a chroman head containing one heterocyclic ring and one phenolic acid ring, and a phytyl tail. Tocopherols have a saturated phytyl tail while tocotrienols have an unsaturated phytyl tail. The chroman head of the two groups also has a different number of methyl groups (Kamal-Eldin and Appelqvist 1996). The apoptotic properties of the vitamin E isoforms are mainly attributed to their functional domain, composed by the redox-active hydroxyl group which is responsible for their antioxidant activity, as well as to the structure of their aliphatic chain that may modify membrane docking and lipid solubility (Neuzil 2003).

The pro-apoptotic, anticancer effects of vitamin E natural isoforms are now well established (reviewed in Sylvester 2007). Tocotrienols have been reported to induce both the intrinsic and the extrinsic apoptotic pathways in several cancer cell lines. γ-TT regulates the translocation of Bax to the mitochondria, causes cleavage and activation of Bid and translocation of the latter to the mitochondria. Translocation of both Bax and cleaved Bid cause MMOP and allow the release of cytochrome c, the formation of apoptosome and the activation of caspase-9. This leads to the activation of the execution pathway which is initiated by the activation of caspase-3. In addition to CD-PCD, evidence in the literature suggests that vitamin E isoforms can induce caspase-independent pathways of apoptosis.

In addition to the natural isoforms of vitamin E, several synthetic molecules have been developed. Most notably, alpha-tocopherol polyethylene glycol succinate (TPGS), a synthetic derivative prepared form the esterification of alpha-TOC, has been widely used as a platform for the development of novel drug delivery systems (DDS) and is extensively studied for its own anti-cancer properties. TPGS inhibits the p-AKT pathway, reduces the levels of Bcl-2 and survivin and induces G1 cell cycle arrest and apoptosis in breast cancer cells (Neophytou et al. 2014). TPGS has been evaluated in different systems, including in vitro and in vivo models. Importantly, based on its use as a therapeutic adjuvant its safety limits in humans have been determined. In addition to increasing the bioavailability and distribution of other drugs, synergistic effects of TPGS with other compounds have been described due to its own anticancer properties. TPGS has been found to induce apoptosis in lung cancer cells in combination with DOX (Hou et al. 2016), to decrease MDR by inhibiting the P-Gp efflux pump, facilitating the effect of PTX in epidermal carcinoma cells (Ma et al. 2014) and to facilitate the delivery of drugs that act synergistically by multi-drug loading in lung cancer cells (Gu et al. 2016). The apoptotic pathways induced by natural isoforms and synthetic derivatives of vitamin E have been extensively described (Constantinou et al. 2008; Choudhury et al. 2017).

16.3.2 Curcumin

Curcumin (diferulolylmethane), is a diarylheptanoid isolated from turmeric (*Curcuma longa*), a member of the ginger family. It was first isolated in 1815 but was used traditionally in Ayurvedic medicine, a system developed in the Indian subcontinent. Curcumin has been used to treat many systemic diseases including dermatological, pulmonary, and gastrointestinal disorders. Even though studies have shown that curcumin has antioxidant, antifungal, antibacterial, antiviral, anti-inflammatory and anti-cancer properties, its medicinal uses when taken orally have not been substantiated.

Curcumin is comprised of three chemical entities in its structure: two phenolic groups connected by a diketone moiety. Its biological activity has been attributed to its ability to act as a ROS scavenger, mainly through its phenol-OH group. The first anticancer effects of curcumin were reported by Aggarwal et al. in the 1990s, who discovered that curcumin could suppress the activation of NFκB in human myeloid ML-1a cells treated with tumor necrosis factor (TNF) (Singh and Aggarwal 1995).

Turmeric has been found to induce apoptosis in prostate cancer cells by modulating the EGFR pathway (Dorai et al. 2000). Interestingly, curcumin can induce apoptosis in PC3 cells via caspase-independent pathways, by affecting proteins of the Bcl-2 family, producing ROS and prompting the release of AIF (Hilchie et al. 2010). The mode of action of curcumin in prostate cancer cells seems to be androgen receptor-independent; Curcumin induced apoptosis in both DU145 (AR-independent) and LNCaP (AR-dependent) cells by inhibiting the NFκB and AP-1 survival pathways, downregulation of the expression of Bcl-2 and Bcl-xL and activation of procaspase-3 and procaspase-8 (Mukhopadhyay et al. 2001). In vivo studies also showed that curcumin can reduce tumor growth and metastasis of prostate cancer cells (Hong et al. 2006). The mitochondrial pathway of apoptosis was also induced by curcumin in colon cancer cells HT-29. Curcumin decreased the levels of Bcl-2, Bcl-xL and survivin at concentrations ranging from 10 to 80 μmol/L curcumin. The levels of pro-apoptotic Bax and Bad increased in the presence of curcumin which also induced release of cytochrome *c*, activation of caspase-3, and cleavage of PARP (Wang et al. 2009). Curcumin has exhibited apoptotic potency in osteosarcomas (OS). High concentration of curcumin caused apoptosis in OS by inducing ROS production, prompting the release of cytochrome c from the mitochondria and causing cleavage of caspase-3 (Chang et al. 2014). By inhibiting the Notch pathway, curcumin effectively arrested proliferation, activated apoptosis, induced G2/M phase cell cycle arrest (by downregulating cyclin D1), and reduced the ability of OS cells to invade and metastasize (Li et al. 2012).

Curcumin has been shown to synergize with both natural and synthetic compounds in cancer cells. In combination with α-tomatine, a glycoalkaloid found in tomatoes, curcumin inhibited the growth and induced apoptosis in prostate cancer PC-3 cells. Their synergistic action involved inhibition of NF-κB activity and reduction in its downstream target, Bcl-2. In addition, the phosphorylation of Akt and ERK1/2 was reduced in the presence of both compounds. Their effect was also measured in vivo where they potently inhibited the growth of PC-3 tumors compared to either agent alone (Huang et al. 2015). Curcumin has also displayed synergistic action with conventional drug 5-fluorouracil (5-Fu) in colon cancer cells, both in vitro and in vivo (Zhang et al. 2017).

16.3.3 EGCG

Epigallocatechin-3-gallate (EGCG), the ester of epigallocatechin and gallic acid, is the most abundant catechin in tea, comprising of 65% of the total catechin content. EGCG has been found by many studies to act therapeutically against cancer, heart disease, diabetes, and obesity. The chemopreventive properties of EGCG have been attributed to its ability to act as an anti-oxidant, to inhibit inflammatory processes, to enhance gap junctional communication between cells protecting from tumor development, to bind to certain carcinogens and to inhibit angiogenesis and metastasis. However, recently it has been reported that excessive intake of EGCG may cause liver damage. This prompted the EFSA and the FDA to issue warnings on the daily intake of EGCG that should not exceed 800 mg.

Structurally, its chemopreventive properties are attributed to the presence of di-hydroxyl groups on the B-ring and the meta-5,7-dihydroxyl groups on the A ring. The phenolic groups contained in EGCG are sensitive to oxidation and can generate quinone. Its antioxidative activity is further enhanced by the presence of the trihydroxyl structure in its D ring. EGCG has been extensively studied in the laboratory and its mode of action against cancer involves several pathways including inhibition of proliferation, MAP kinases, activator protein-1 (AP-1), NFκB, EGFR- or insulin-like growth factor (IGF)-1 mediated pathways, metalloproteinases, proteosome or urokinase-plasminogen activator activities, and induction of apoptosis. EGCG has been found to induce apoptosis and cell cycle arrest at the G1 phase in prostate cancer cells. In LNCaP cells, apoptosis involved modulation of the NFκB pathway and of p53; EGCG affected the Bax/Bcl-2 ratio, activated caspases 3, 8 and 9 and caused cleavage of PARP (Hastak et al. 2003). In cervical cancer cells, EGCG was able to increase p53 levels and inhibit the EGFR pathway, ultimately leading to apoptosis (Sah et al. 2004). EGCG has been shown to induce apoptosis in cancer cells by binding to surface receptors. Zeta-chain-associated protein kinase 70 (ZAP

70), a protein that is part of the T cell receptor, is highly expressed in leukemia. EGCG induced caspase-dependent apoptosis in ZAP70-expressing leukemia cells in a dose-dependent manner, while ZAP70-deficient cells were resistant to EGCG treatment (Shim et al. 2008). The extrinsic pathway of apoptosis is also induced by EGCG in leukemic cells, where treatment with the compound activated caspase-8; DNA fragmentation in this instance was abolished in the presence of a caspase-8 inhibitor. It is therefore plausible that EGCG may activate death receptors on the surface of cells (Hayakawa et al. 2001).

EGCG has also shown synergistic affects with other natural compounds and therapeutic drugs. EGCG enhanced the effect of curcumin in inducing apoptosis in resistant breast cancer cells; specifically, the combination of these compounds inhibited the p-glycoprotein efflux pump and activated the caspase-dependent apoptotic pathway (Wang et al. 2014). In addition, the synergistic action of curcumin and EGCG, potentiated the effect of DOX and increased its accumulation in the cell. Combination of erlotinib and EGCG induced apoptosis in head and neck cancers. Even though the agents did not affect the mRNA levels of Bim, p21, p27 or Bcl-2, these proteins were regulated posttranscriptionally by the combination of erlotinib and EGCG (Haque et al. 2015).

16.3.4 Quercetin

Quercetin [5,7-dihydroxy-2-(4-hydroxyphenyl)chromen-4-one] is a flavonoid (plant pigment) found in many plants and foods, such as green tea, apples, red wine, onions, berries, *Ginkgo biloba*, St. John's wort, and others. The name is derived from quercetum (oak forest), after Quercus. Uses of quercetin, reported since 1857, include treatment of hay fever, peptic ulcer, diabetes, cataracts, asthma, gout inflammation and viral infections. The chemopreventive activity of quercetin has been attributed to its structure since it enables it to act as an anti-oxidant and reduce free radicals. It contains five hydroxyl groups and a carbonyl group in the four position. Quercetin has direct antioxidant properties that protect against DNA damage, but can also target multiple signaling pathways associated with carcinogenesis and tumor progression. Pathways affected by quercetin include DNA damage and inflammation-related pathways.

The apoptotic pathways activated by quercetin have been described in many types of cancer. In human hepatoma cells (HepG2), treatment with quercetin induced the mitochondrial pathway of apoptosis. The Bcl-xL/Bcl-xS ratio was increased, Bax was translocated to the mitochondria apoptosis and by the activation of caspases-3 and -9 were activated in HepG2 cells. The survival pathway Akt and the extracellular regulated kinase (ERK) were inhibited in quercetin-treated cells (Granado-Serrano et al. 2006). In HL-60 leukemic cells, a caspase-3 dependent mitochondrial pathway was also induced and this was accompanied by cycloocygenase-2 (Cox-2) mRNA and Cox-2 protein inhibition (Niu et al. 2011). The levels of anti-apoptotic protein survivin were also reduced by quercetin in human glioma cells, where ERK and AKT were also inhibited and apoptosis was induced via caspases (Kim et al. 2008). The extrinsic pathway of apoptosis has also been implicated in the mode of action of this compound. In human oral cancer cells, quercetin increased Fas, Fas-Ligand, FADD and caspase-8, all of which associated with the death receptor pathway (Ma et al. 2018).

Combination studies with quercetin have been applied to evaluate whether resistant cells can become sensitive to treatment. Quercetin was able to increase tumor radiosensitivity both in vitro in DLD1, HeLa and MCF-7 tumor cell lines and in vivo in the DLD-1 human colorectal cancer xenograft model in nude mice. Mechanistically, it was shown that quercetin induced radio-sensitization by inhibiting the ATM kinase, which is one of the critical DNA damage response proteins. It is therefore possible that quercetin supplementation may benefit patients undergoing radiotherapy (Lin et al. 2012). The effect of quercetin in triple negative breast cancers (TNBC) is enhanced by combination with other natural compounds. One study reported that even though quercetin was able to induce apoptosis in MCF-7 cells through suppression of Twist via the p38MAPK pathway, it had no cytotoxic effects on the TNBC cell line MDA-MB-231, even at 100 μM concentration (Ranganathan et al. 2015). However, when combined with curcumin, they induced breast cancer type 1 susceptibility protein (BRCA1) promoter histone acetylation, enhanced BRCA1 expression and inhibited cell survival and migration of TNBC cells (Kundur et al. 2019).

16.3.5 Resveratrol

Resveratrol (3,5,4′-trihydroxy-*trans*-stilbene) (RSV), a naturally occurring phenol and phytoalexin, is produced by many plants in response to injury or pathogens. RSV has been shown to possess cancer preventive and therapeutic activities in many types of cancer. RSV was initially isolated from the roots of the *Veratrum grandiflorum* O. Loes and is also found in berries, grapes, and peanuts. In Japan and China, knotweed, which contains significant amount of RSV, has been traditionally used as a herbal remedy. Even though the chemopreventive ability of RSV has been reported by in vivo studies (Tessitore et al. 2000), the effective in vitro concentrations of the compound required for anti-cancer activity cannot be reached in the plasma. Specifically, the consumption of 1 g of RSV results to about 0.62 μM maximal plasma concentrations in humans (Brown et al. 2010). After digestion, RSV is rapidly metabolized in the liver and intestinal epithelial cells. It has been therefore suggested that the observed benefits in vivo may be attributed to metabolites of RSV or that conjugates of RSV revert back to the parent compound following hydrolysis.

Numerous in vitro studies have identified the molecular pathways of apoptosis induced by RSV. As previously described in the above sections, RSV can inhibit the PI3K/AKT pathway. Even though there have been reports that RSV can induce apoptosis in p53-mutant tumor cells, there is a consensus among the literature that RSV induces apoptosis in most cancer types via p53-dependent mechanisms.

Interestingly, RSV has been found to induce apoptosis independently of caspases. In MCF-7 cells, RSV decreased Bcl-2 levels but this did not involve cytochrome c release or cleavage of caspases, it rather implicated the inhibition of NFκB and calpain activity (Pozo-Guisado et al. 2005). Treatment of prostate cancer cells with RSV caused apoptosis via inhibition of the PI3K/AKT and induction of the mitochondrial pathway. RSV causes loss of mitochondrial membrane potential, reduction of the anti-apoptotic Bcl-2 protein and increase in pro-apoptotic Bax, Bak, Bid, and Bad (Aziz et al. 2006). RSV was also found to be effective against DMBA-induced skin tumors in Wistar rats through the induction of apoptosis (Hu et al. 2016).

RSV has also displayed enhanced apoptotic properties when combined with chemotherapeutic drugs. In prostate cancer cells RSV in combination with docetaxel (DTX) upregulated pro-apoptotic genes including Bax, Bid and Bak, caused cleavage of PARP and downregulated anti-apoptotic Mcl-1, Bcl-2 and Bcl-xL, promoting apoptosis (Singh et al. 2017). When combined with conventional chemotherapeutic agent 5-fluorouracil, RSV simultaneously inhibited the STAT3 and Akt signaling pathways, induced S-phase specific cell cycle arrest, and increased apoptosis in colorectal cancer cells (Chung et al. 2018). Resveratrol also synergizes with other natural compounds and produces enhanced anti-cancer effects. Combination of RSV with curcumin inhibited the growth of colon cancer HCT-116 cells, regardless of p53 status in in vitro and in vivo mouse models, more potently than either agent alone. Their mode of action included both inhibition of proliferation and induction of apoptosis by suppressing NFκB activity, which was possibly modulated via the inhibition of EGFR and IGF-1R (Majumdar et al. 2009).

16.3.6 Genistein

Genistein, one of the major functional constituents of soy, first isolated in 1899 from *Genista tinctoria* (dyer's broom). Genistein is a known chemopreventive and chemotherapeutic agent that has shown efficacy against various types of cancer. Genistein is a multi-functional bioactive molecule that exhibits anti-cancer action by inducing apoptosis, inhibiting cell cycle progression, angiogenesis and metastasis. Genistein has been reported to bind to estrogen receptors (ER), to topoisomerase and to receptor tyrosine kinases (RTK) and inhibit their function. In addition, genistein modulates a number of key signalling pathways implicated in cell survival such as the PI3K/AKT signaling pathway and the NFκB pathway; by affecting these pathways, genistein induces growth arrest and apoptosis in cancer cells (Fig. 16.2).

The mechanism of genistein's cytotoxicity against a wide range of cancer cells is considered to comprise an inhibitory effect on topoisomerase II (Topo II). Topo II is a nuclear protein catalyzing the reaction of breakage and relinking of DNA, which plays an important part in preservation of DNA topology required for DNA replication, transcription, and recombination of cellular genes. It is believed that genistein binds to and stabilizes the topoisomerase-DNA complex, causing DNA strand breakage and induction of apoptosis (Salti et al. 2000). Alternatively, by binding

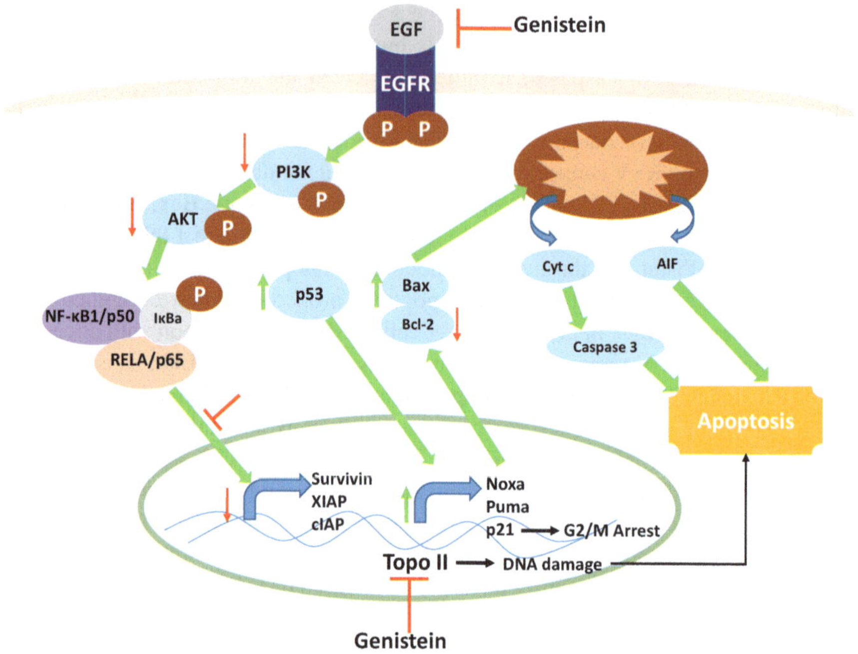

Fig. 16.2 Apoptotic mechanism of action of genistein. Genistein inhibits the activity of the EGF receptor leading to the inhibition of the PI3K/AKT pathway and subsequently of the translocation of the NFκB transcription factor to the nucleus. Target genes of NFκB, including the anti-apoptotic survivin, XIAP and cIAP are downregulated. In addition, genistein induces upregulation and stabilization of p53 which promotes the transcription of p21 leading to G2/M arrest. Noxa and Puma, which are also p53 target genes, are upregulated and induce an increase in the Bax/Bcl-2 ratio. Due to MOMP, cytochrome c is released from the mitochondria, inducing the cleavage of caspase-3 and apoptosis. Caspase-independent apoptosis is also induced following release of AIF from the mitochondria. Genistein also inhibits topoisomerase II resulting in DNA strand breakage and induction of apoptosis. AIF, apoptosis inducing factor; Cyt c, cytochrome c; EGFR, epidermal growth factor receptor, MOMP, mitochondrial outer membrane permeabilization; Topo II, topoisomerase II

to the estrogen receptors (ERs), genistein displays both estrogenic and anti-estrogenic actions depending on its concentration. At low concentrations, genistein has a stimulatory (estrogenic) effect on tumor growth, while at higher concentrations, over 60 μM, it displays inhibitory (anti-estrogenic) effects and it induces apoptotic cell death in cancer cells (El Touny and Banerjee 2009; Constantinou et al. 1998a). Genistein is also known to inhibit the tyrosine-specific protein kinase activity of epidermal growth factor (EGF) receptor (Akiyama et al. 1987). The dual role of genistein as a Topo II and tyrosine kinase inhibitor, are essential for inducing apoptosis. In MCF-7 breast cancer cells, genistein induced the phosphorylation of p21 and stabilized the tumor suppressor p53, resulting in cell cycle arrest at the G2/M phase and the induction of apoptosis (Constantinou et al. 1998b).

The arrest of the cell cycle at the G2/M phase by genistein, as well as the dependency of apoptosis induction on the activation of p53 (Zhang et al. 2013), has been reported in many cell lines; in ovarian cancer cells, genistein downregulated p-FAK, p-PI3K, p-AKT, p-GSK3β, and upregulated p21, leading to G2/M arrest (Chan et al. 2018). In lung and colon cancer cells, genistein induced the intrinsic pathway of apoptosis by allowing the release of cytochrome c from the mitochondria, promoting Bax/Bcl-2 expression and cleaving caspase-3 (Liu et al. 2016; Zhou et al. 2017). In addition, genistein has been found to induce the extrinsic pathway of apoptosis by upregulating the levels of the FAS receptor and causing cleavage of initiator caspase-8 (Seo et al. 2011). Across several cell lines, genistein has been shown to induce apoptosis by inhibiting the NFκB pathway, by decreasing nuclear p65 translocation and IκBα phosphorylation and downregulating IAPs including XIAP, survivin and cIAP (Prietsch et al. 2014); its potential use as a SMAC inhibitor remains to be evaluated. Interestingly, genistein was found to induce caspase-independent apoptotic pathways, releasing AIF from the mitochondria to the cytosol (Yamasaki et al. 2013).

Moreover, genistein shows synergistic behavior with well-known anticancer drugs, such as adriamycin, docetaxel, and tamoxifen, suggesting a potential role in combination therapy. Combination therapy with several chemotherapeutic drugs or targeted therapies with genistein led to synergistic effects in vivo, by targeting the same pathways as in vitro. Low concentrations of cisplatin in combination with genistein, induced significantly greater growth inhibition in a xenograft model of the A549 non-small-cell lung cancer (NSCLC) cells compared with either agent alone, and increased apoptosis by targeting the PI3K/AKT pathway (Liu et al. 2014). In human malignant neuroblastoma SH-SY5Y xenografts, combination of a synthetic retinoid and genistein, led to mitochondrial apoptosis by increasing the Bax/Bcl-2 ratio, allowing the release of Smac/Diablo to the cytosol and cleavage of caspase-3. Caspase-independent apoptosis was also induced via activation of calpains and release of AIF while endoplasmic reticulum (ER) stress was also involved via the cleavage of caspase-4 (Karmakar et al. 2011). In xenografts bearing human osteosarcoma tumors, combination of genistein and gemcitabine augmented tumor growth inhibition through the down-regulation of NFκB activity and Akt activation (Liang et al. 2012). Overall, these results suggest that the anti-cancer effects of genistein observed in pre-clinical studies are transferable in in vivo models and, importantly, that genistein improves the efficacy of numerous therapeutic agents.

To date, growing evidence suggests that genistein can regulate biological molecules, such as the androgen or estrogen receptor, protein-tyrosine kinase, NFκB, MAPK and AKT pathways, leading to inhibition of cancer cell proliferation and induction of cancer cell apoptosis. Genistein can induce cell apoptosis and cell cycle G2/M arrest in many kinds of human cancer cells including breast, neuroblastoma, lung and colon cancer cells. Recent anti-cancer studies have proven that cell apoptosis induced by genistein correlates with the expression of several genes including those encoding p53, p21WAF1, caspases, Bax, Cdc25C, cyclin B1, and Bcl-2. Furthermore, it was found that genistein inhibits cancer cell proliferation by controlling the expression of certain transcription factors, such as STAT-3, Nrf1, Nrf2, AP-1 and CREB.

The inhibition of topo II by genistein is of special interest to us, as it can find applications in cancer chemotherapy. We have shown that genistein is a topo II poison, stabilizing the topo II protein-DNA cleavable complex, which is similar to the mechanism of action of several anticancer agents commonly used in chemotherapy and collectively known as topo II poisons. These drugs block the ligation step of enzymatic reaction of topo II, generating double stranded breaks that harm the integrity of the genome. Constantinou et al. (1990) were the first to report that genistein inhibited specifically the enzymatic activity of purified topo II without affecting the activity of topo I. Furthermore, they demonstrated that genistein enhanced the topo II-DNA reaction intermediate (the cleavable complex) and in this capacity genistein functioned as a topo II poison (Constantinou et al. 1990). Several of these topo II poisons, including etoposide, doxorubicin, mitoxantone and amsacrine, are effective antitumor drugs being used in conventional chemotherapy. The induction of DNA-cleavage, as determined by alkaline elution technique, was evident in the extracts of clonal variants of human promyelocytic (HL-60) and erythroid leukemia (K-562) cells that had been treated with 10-30 μg/ml concentrations of genistein for as little as 1 h (Constantinou et al. 1990). Following this report, subsequent studies confirmed the topo II inhibitory effects of genistein (Markovits et al. 1995; Bandele and Osheroff 2007; Michael McClain et al. 2006; Kaufmann 1998). It was also established that two isoforms of topo II (topo II alpha and topo II beta) are expressed in many cell lines. Resistance to genistein in leukemic T cell line (CCRF-CEM) was demonstrated to be associated with reduced levels of topo II beta isoform (Markovits et al. 1995), suggesting that genistein-induced DNA breakage requires topo II. Drug-induced topo II-mediated strand breakage can be due to either increased DNA cleavage or blocked religation. It was determined that genistein (similarly to amsacrine, ellipticine and azatoxin) acted by enhancing topo II-mediated DNA cleavage, whereas etoposide and its derivatives blocked DNA relegation, downstream of the DNA cleavage step (van Hille et al. 1999).

It is well established that if the DNA damage is beyond repair, cellular mechanisms leading to apoptosis are being activated. Following treatment of HT-29, SW-620 or SW-1116 colon cancer cells or MCF-7 cells with genistein concentrations sufficient to form the topo II cleavable complex (over 60 μM), the apoptotic pathway of cell death was initiated (Salti et al. 2000; Constantinou et al. 1998b). The molecular events underlying genistein-induced apoptosis in MCF-7 cells included Bcl-2 phosphorylation (leading to its inactivation as an antiapoptotic protein) p53 protein stabilization and Bcl-2 downregulation. These molecular events delayed cell cycle progression in the G2/M phase, a characteristic of topo II poisons (Constantinou et al. 1998b). The ability of genistein to bind to the topo II-DNA complex, resulting in topo II-mediated double strand DNA breakage and leading to apoptosis, is now well established in a variety of in vitro systems (Salti et al. 2000; Constantinou et al. 1998b; Bandele and Osheroff 2007; Michael McClain et al. 2006; Kaufmann 1998; van Hille et al. 1999).

Importantly, recently it has been demonstrated to occur in vivo. Specifically, juvenile male Wistar rats that received a single dose of genistein subcutaneously (10 mg/kg of body weight) showed a significant increase in the amount of covalent topo II-alpha and topo II-beta -DNA complexes in their gut and colon. Interestingly, rats receiving isoflavone-rich diet as glycosides (25–50 mg/kg BW) either from in utero or the lactation phase, did not significantly increase such topo II complexes (Baechler et al. 2016). These results suggest that subcutaneously administrated genistein targets topo II in vivo, whereas the isoflavone-rich diet may not reach the required concentrations to form topo II poisons (Zhou et al. 2009). In a more recent article it was reported that topo II of the African Swine Fever Virus (ASFV) was inhibited by genistein and formed topo II cleavable complex, hindering the transcription of late viral genes and the synthesis of late viral proteins. It seems that genistein interacts with four residues of the ATP-binding site of ASFV-topo II (Asn-144, Val-146, Gly-147 and Leu-148) with a higher affinity than ATP. In this manner, genistein reduced viral progeny. ASFV causes a highly-contagious and fatal disease of domestic pigs. Therefore, the ability of genistein to stabilize the topo II-mediated cleavable complex has been confirmed in vivo and this information is being applied to eradicate a fatal animal disease (Arabyan et al. 2018).

The requirement of pharmacological doses of genistein for the induction of apoptosis in cancer cells justifies current efforts to use nanoparticles for targeting, and introducing high doses of this isoflavone, specifically to cancer cells, as detailed in the next section of this chapter.

16.4 Nanochemoprevention: The Future of Apoptosis-Inducing Natural Agents

Nanotechnology refers to the branch of science, engineering, and technology conducted at the nanoscale (10^9 nm), and involves developing materials or devices on that scale. Although definitions vary, nanocarriers, also known as nanoparticles (NPs) or drug delivery systems (DDS) can be composed of almost any material and will have at least one dimension of between 1 and 500 nm (Clancy et al. 2010). NPs are of special interest because they display unique optical, electronic, magnetic, and structural properties, at the nanoscale, that are not observed at bulk or atomic scales (Clancy et al. 2010). These unique properties that NPs possess have been evaluated and employed in various areas of cancer diagnosis and therapy, a field of science generally referred to as nanotheranostics, with hopeful developments. Cancer nanotheranostics is a strategy that combines targeting, drug release, and diagnostic imaging into a single platform, the NP. A schematic of a multifunctional nanotheranostic agent can be seen in Fig. 16.3. Typically, theranostic NPs are built upon four basic components: signal emitter, therapeutic payload, payload carrier, and targeting ligand (Men et al. 2014). The signal emitter is an entity that is either encapsulated within the payload carrier or conjugated to its outer surface.

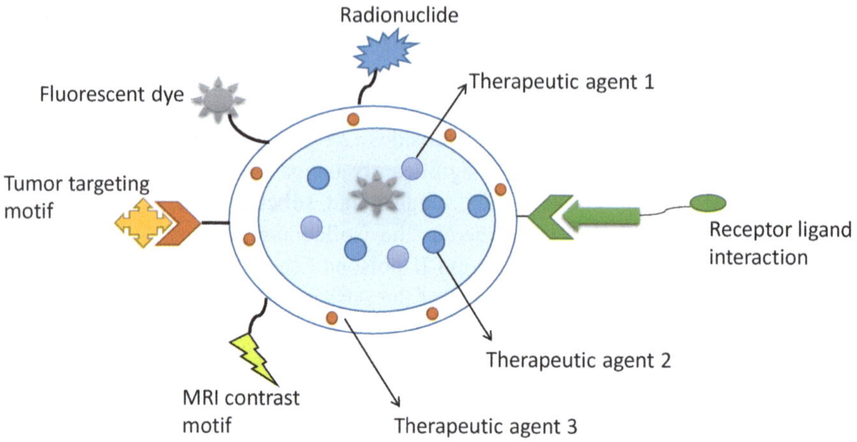

Fig. 16.3 Multifunctional nanomaterial in action for diverse applications simultaneously. Modified from Kumar et al. (2012)

Signal emitters are entities with unique physical properties (optical, magnetic, or radioactive) and emit a signal upon excitation by an external source. In cancer therapeutics the payload is a chemotherapeutic drug. Generally, the chemotherapeutic drug is either hydrophobic and is encapsulated within the inner core of the NP or hydrophilic which is loaded in the outer layer. Typically, the chemotherapeutic drug is delivered to the cancer tissue via the enhanced permeability and retention effect (EPR). Passive tissue targeting is achieved by extravasation of NPs through increased permeability of the tumor vasculature and ineffective lymphatic drainage. When the EPR effect is not suitable or inefficient, a targeting ligand is added to guide the NP to specific pathogenic sites. The targeting ligand aids selective delivery of the NPs to diseased tissues and is always covalently attached to the surface of the carrier.

The engineering of nanomaterials that interact with cancer cells at the molecular level is a novel approach that significantly improves the effectiveness and specificity of anticancer agents including natural products that have shown great promise in cancer chemoprevention. Nanomaterial-based therapy is often referred as the new generation of cancer treatment because it is capable of facilitating site-selective drug delivery with reduced side effects. In addition, NPs demonstrate the competence to overcome many of the characteristic problems associated with bioactive natural products (stability, solubility and toxicity) by offering protection from degradation, enabling controlled release and biodistribution and increasing bioavailability through specific targeting (Nguyen et al. 2014). This novel concept of using nanotechnology to improve the outcome of chemopreventive intervention was coined 'nanochemoprevention' (Siddiqui et al. 2009) which was used to refer to the merging of progressive nanotechnology and natural products. Depending on the material of the delivery payload carrier, NPs are divided into the following three main groups: (1) Polymer-based NPs including nanospheres, nanocapsules and polymersomes,

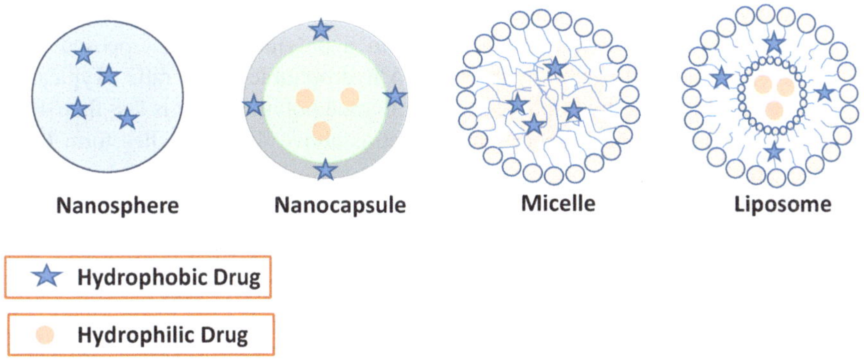

Fig. 16.4 Versatile drug delivery systems include, nanospheres, nanocapsules, micelles and liposomes (modified from Neophytou and Constantinou, 2015). Stars illustrate hydrophobic drugs whereas hydrophilic drugs are illustrated by a circle

(2) polymeric and lipid micelles, and (3) lipid-based NPs and lipid-polymer hybrid NPs (Fig. 16.4).

We briefly describe below the main characteristics of each group of nanoparticles:

1. **Polymer-based nanoparticles** are submicron-sized polymeric, colloidal particles that are extensively studied as carriers of natural products. Polymers are widely used for developing NP-based carriers and reports exploiting polymers for NP facilitated drug delivery trace back to 1979 (Couvreur et al. 1979; Men et al. 2014). Polymeric NPs are composed of a wide variability of biodegradable and biocompatible polymers of either natural origin, such as chitosan, alginate, gelatin, or synthetic ones, such as polylactic acid (PLA), polylactide-*co*-glycolic acid (PLGA), poly(ε-caprolactone) (PCL), polymethyl methacrylate (PMMA), and polyglycolic acid (PGA), to name a few (Kumari et al. 2010). The drugs confined within the polymeric structure can be released controllably via various mechanisms such as surface erosion, diffusion through the polymer matrix, or in response to the local environment (Peer et al. 2007). FDA approved polymeric NP formulations for clinical use include methoxy-PEG-poly (D, L-lactide) taxol (Genexol-PM®) from Samyang biopharmaceuticals, L-Glutamic acid, L-alanine, L-lysine, and L-tyrosine copolymer (Copaxone®) from TEVA Pharmaceuticals, and many more are currently under clinical trials (Men et al. 2014). Depending on the method of fabrication polymeric NPs can be nanocapsules or nanospheres. When the drug is contained within the core, the particles are termed "nanocapsules," and when the drug is adsorbed on the surface or entrapped in the matrix structure of the system, the nanoparticles are termed "nanospheres" (Macagnan et al. 2016; Labhasetwar et al. 1997). The polymeric nanocapsule structure is especially interesting because it allows for encapsulation of both hydrophilic drugs in its central aqueous reservoir and hydrophobic drugs in its thick hydrophobic lamellar membrane. Polymersomes are a distinct type of nanocapsule that is very similar to a liposome which is formed by the self-

assembly of amphiphilic diblock or triblock copolymers (Levine et al. 2008). Amphiphilic copolymers self-assemble into a polymersome as opposed to a micelle, by controlling the hydrophilic to hydrophobic block ratio. Typically, when the ratio of the hydrophilic segment to total polymer mass is less than 45% polymersomes can be formed, while at ratios above 45%, micelles form (Zhu et al. 2014).

2. **Polymeric and lipid micelles** are nanoscopic core/shell structures formed from the self-assembly of amphiphilic block copolymers (Xu et al. 2013). Polymeric NPs are attractive candidates for use in biomedical applications due to the fact that they are biocompatible and biodegradable. Additionally, the degradation of polymeric NPs can be tuned enabling the controlled release of the drug they carry at the pathogenic site of interest (Alotaibi et al. 2013; Granja et al. 2016; Elsabahy and Wooley 2012). Micellization or aggregation of unimers takes place around the Critical Micelle Concentration (CMC) of the polymer used. The CMC is defined as the concentration of surfactants above which micelles start to form spontaneously. Typically the sizes of amphiphilic block copolymer micelles are 5–100 nm. The resulting core/shell structures have the ability to increase the solubility of hydrophobic molecules. This is attributed to their unique structural composition comprised by a hydrophobic core sterically stabilized by a hydrophilic shell. Drug molecules can be incorporated in the hydrophobic core by means of chemical, electrostatic or physical interactions, depending on the drug's physicochemical properties. The type of polymer used to form the core of a micelle is the major factor for the most important properties polymeric micelles possess such as stability, drug loading capacity, and drug release profile (Carstens et al. 2008). The most common constituents of polymeric micelles include poly (propylene oxide) (PPO) (Rapoport 2004) which belongs to Pluronics, poly (esters) such as poly(lactic acid) (PLA) (Ruan and Feng 2003), hydrophobic poly(amino acids) (Bae and Kataoka 2009) copolymers of lactic acid and glycolic acids (Kim et al. 2009), and poly(caprolactone) (PCL) (Meier et al. 2005). Additionally, the chemical nature and the molecular weight of the hydrophilic block polymer used, greatly affects the nanoparticle's stealth properties and determines its kinetics in vivo. Poly(ethylene glycol) (PEG) is the most frequently used hydrophilic block copolymer. PEG is an ideal choice as it is a nontoxic polymer that is FDA approved. The act of adding PEG to a nanoparticle is known as PEGylation and benefits include, but are not limited to, prolonged circulation in the blood which promotes enhanced tumor accumulation.
3. **Lipid-based nanoparticles**, commonly known as liposomes (50 nm to several micrometers), are the most common and well-investigated nanocarriers for targeted drug delivery. Liposomes are defined as phospholipid vesicles consisting of one or more lipid bilayers enclosing an interior aqueous space (Sercombe et al. 2015). Liposomes are of great importance owing to the fact that they are biodegradable and non-toxic (Granja et al. 2016; Fang et al. 2006). They are made up of a lipid bilayer that can be composed of cationic, anionic, or neutral phospholipids and cholesterol, surrounding an aqueous core. PEGylation is often used to improve liposome stability and to enhance circulation times in vivo (Sercombe

et al. 2015). Liposomal systems have the unique ability to entrap both lipophilic and hydrophilic drugs which allows for a diverse array of applications. Hydrophobic drugs are entrapped into the bilayer membrane, and hydrophilic molecules can be encapsulated in the aqueous center (Koning and Storm 2003). Additionally, the outer surface can be modified by the addition of a peptide or an antibody against a specific receptor overexpressed in cancer cells, to enable enhanced targeted delivery to the tumor site. FDA has approved some liposomal products for clinical use including Doxil® in 1995 which was the first liposomal drug formulation approved by the FDA for the treatment of patients with HIV-associated Kaposi's sarcoma (Zhang et al. 2008; Northfelt et al. 1998). Encapsulation of chemopreventive natural agents by liposomes is a desired method for developing novel nanoformulations for cancer prevention. A special class of lipid nanoparticles include the solid lipid nanoparticle (SLN). An SLN is an alternative carrier system made of lipids that remains solid at room temperature and also at human body temperature and is stabilized by a suitable surfactant. These lipidic materials usually contain purified triglycerides, complex glyceride mixtures, or waxes. SLNs are of special interest as they are characterized by improved stability and longer circulation times in vivo but suffer from low drug loading capacity (Wissing and Muller 2003).

16.4.1 Vitamin E-TPGS Nanoformulations

Vitamin E TPGS or TPGS is a synthetic derivative of alpha-tocopherol that has been widely studied in the development of drug delivery systems (DDS) and has also shown promising anti-cancer effects as a single agent (Neophytou et al. 2014; Neophytou and Constantinou 2015). TPGS is prepared from the esterification of α-TOS and polyethylene glycol (PEG) 1000. As such, it possesses the advantages of PEG and vitamin E in applications of various nanocarriers for drug delivery, including the ability to extend the half-life of the drug in the plasma. TPGS having hydrophilic liphophilic balance (HLB) value of 13.2 and a relatively low critical micelle concentration (CMC) of 0.02% w/w makes it ideal for applications in developing various DDS. TPGS is thus used as an absorption enhancer, emulsifier, solubilizer, additive, permeation enhancer and stabilizer. TPGS has been used as an effective emulsifier, enhancing the performance of NPs, increasing cellular uptake of the drug and improving in vivo pharmacokinetics (Feng 2006; Win and Feng 2006; Parhi et al. 2011). The co-administration of TPGS has been shown to enhance drug solubility, to inhibit P-glycoprotein (P-gp) mediated multi-drug resistance (MDR) and increase the oral bioavailability of anti-cancer drugs (Mu and Feng 2002; Pan et al. 2008; Dintaman and Silverman 1999; Mu et al. 2005).

Polymeric nanoparticles incorporating vitamin E TPGS have been reported. Specifically, garcinol was loaded into PLGA NPs using vitamin E TPGS as an emulsifier (Gaonkar et al. 2017). The nanoparticles caused a high amount of cytotoxicity in B16F10, HepG2 and KB cells. A considerable amount of cell apoptosis was observed in B16f10 melanoma and KB cell lines exhibiting pronounced nuclear condensation of both cell lines. Interestingly, free garcinol exhibited a lower effect on cellular apoptosis than the nanoformulation. Additionally, in a different study by Wang et al. (Wang et al. 2018), polymeric polylactide-TPGS (PLA-TPGS) NPs for targeting gastric cancer cells were fabricated. These NPs were surface modified with polydopamine (pD) and conjugated with galactosamine (Gal) (Gal-pD-PLA-TPGS/NPs). Results showed enhanced apoptosis in Gal-pD-PLA-TPGS/NPs-treated cancer cells, accompanied with the up-regulation of apoptosis-related protein expression as compared to the blank NPs. In vivo, Gal-pD-PLA-TPGS/NPs were targeted to the tumor site and exhibited higher anti-tumor effects resulting in reduced tumor volume and reduced tumor weight.

Micellar formulations made from vitamin E TPGS have a relatively high critical micelle concentration (CMC) value of 0.2 mg/mL (Zhang et al. 2012) making them unstable and easily dissociated in plasma after intravenous injection. Consequently, TPGS is often used together with other polymers to form mixed micelles. In a study by Zhang et al. (2014), a mixed micelle system was developed from vitamin E TPGS-graft-PLGA (TPGS-g-PLGA) copolymer and Pluronic F68. The mixed micelle was used as a carrier of Tanshinone IIA (TAN). TAN-loaded mixed micelles compared with free TAN, had higher cytotoxicity and pro-apoptotic effects against human hepatocellular carcinoma HepG2 cells. The significant enhancement on pro-apoptosis by TAN micelles was evidenced by increased chromosome condensation, mitochondria membrane potential loss, and cleavage of caspase-3 and PARP. Moreover, in a study by Wang et al. (2015) a mixed micelle system made of methoxy poly (ethylene glycol)-b-polycaprolactone (mPEG-PCL) and TPGS was prepared for the encapsulation of resveratrol (Res) to form Res-loaded mixed micelles. The uptake of Res by Dox-resistant breast cancer MCF-7/ADR cells and the apoptotic cell death was highly increased in the mixed micellar formulation. This was assessed by the accumulation of Sub G1 phases of cell cycle, nuclear staining and Annexin-FITC/propidium iodide assay. Additionally, Res-loaded mixed micelles increased Dox-induced cytotoxicity and moreover increased drug accumulation by down-regulating P-glycoprotein (P-gp). In a more recent study, mixed micelles were developed from two biocompatible copolymers of polyvinyl caprolactam–polyvinyl acetate–polyethylene glycol (Soluplus®) and TPGS (Bernabeu et al. 2016). The NP formulation aimed to improve the in vitro anti-tumor activity of paclitaxel (PTX) on both breast and ovarian cancer cell lines. Cells treated with TPGS and blank mixed micelles exhibited considerable cleavage of PARP compared with blank Soluplus® micelles, indicating the superior antitumor efficacy of the formulation made with TPGS.

Liposomal TPGS formulations have also shown great promise in improving cellular uptake of anticancer drugs and offering enhanced apoptosis. For example, TPGS coated liposomes were developed to improve the accumulation of luteolin in lung cancer (Li et al. 2016). Coating luteolin loaded liposomes with TPGS increased their cellular uptake by A549 cells and as a result the cytotoxicity was grealtly enhanced. Additionally, liposomes coated with TPGS showed increased accumulation in tumor tissue and inhibited tumor growth. TPGS coated liposomes loaded with resveratrol have also been developed and were tested in vitro for their anticancer potential against C6 glioma cell lines (Vijayakumar et al. 2016). RSV-TPGS-Liposomes showed significantly higher cytotoxicity than RSV-Liposomes (uncoated liposomes) and RSV alone. The higher cytotoxic potential of RSV-TPGS-liposomes was attributed to the presence of TPGS which is known for its cytotoxic potential. Additionally, apigenin and TPGS liposomes improved the delivery of apigenin to tumor cells, both in vitro and in vivo (Jin et al. 2017). The combination of apigenin TPGS liposomes and tyroservatide was cytotoxic in A549 cells, induced G2 arrest, and suppressed cell invasion more effectively than either agent alone. More importantly, the combination of apigenin TPGS liposomes and tyroservatide inhibited tumor-growth in A549 cell-bearing mice.

16.4.2 Curcumin Nanoformulations

A variety of curcumin nanoformulations have been reported in the literature in an effort to overcome its low aqueous solubility and poor bioavailability. The limitations associated with free curcumin were addressed in a study by Azandeh et al. (Azandeh et al. 2017). Polymeric nanospheres were utilized to investigate their cytotoxic activity on PC3 human cancer prostate cells. Specifically, curcumin encapsulated in PLGA nanospheres (NCur) had a considerable cytotoxic activity on PC3 cell lines, which was facilitated by induction of both apoptotic and autophagic processes. In a different study, curcumin NPs were fabricated by using PLGA as a carrier and hexadecyltrimethylammonium bromide (CTAB) as a surfactant/surface charge modifier and their anticancer potential in human triple negative breast cancer (TNBC) MDA-MB-231 cells were investigated (Arya et al. 2018). In an in vitro drug release assay, curcumin NPs showed a higher cellular incorporation than free curcumin and resulted in higher cytotoxicity. Curcumin induces the reactive oxygen species production which in turn causes DNA damage and results in p38-MAPK activation. It also reduced the expression of DNA repair genes (such as BRCA1, BRCA2, Rad51, Rad50, Mre11 and NBS1) resulting in persistent DNA damage and apoptosis. Similarly, curcumin-loaded PLGA NPs and surface-coated with chitosan and PEG (CNPs) were formulated aiming to accomplish optimum therapeutic effect in pancreatic cancer (Arya et al. 2018). Cellular studies revealed superior cytotoxicity, enhanced anti-migratory, anti-invasive and apoptosis-inducing ability of CNPs in metastatic pancreatic cancer in comparison to a free equivalent. The mode of cell death induced in pancreatic cancer cells by CNPs was due to augmented apoptosis as compared to free curcumin. Mechanistically, there was an enhanced down-regulation of anti-apoptotic protein Bcl2, enhanced expression of pro-apoptotic proteins Bax and cleavage of PARP and caspase-3 in cells treated with CNPs in comparison to the free counterpart.

Micellar systems incorporating curcumin have also been reported in the literature. For example, curcumin micelles were fabricated from modified 2000 monomethoxy-PEG (mPEG) and their cytotoxicity was tested in vitro against four cancer cell lines

(HeLa, S-65, BGC-823 and C-26 cell) (Li et al. 2014). Results indicated that the curcumin micelles were more effective than free curcumin against most cancer cell lines resulting in apoptosis of cancer cells. This effect was investigated by western blotting which revealed that the induction of apoptosis of S-65 cancer cells by curcumin micelles was due to the down-regulation of p-Rb, Blc-2, p-AKT expression and caspase-9 activation. Moreover, anti-tumor testing in nude BALB/c mouse bearing S-65 xenografts indicated that the intraperitoneal injection of curcumin micelles could significantly inhibit tumor growth as compared to the free curcumin treatment. This was accompanied by significantly increased apoptosis of tumor cells and diminished vascular endothelial growth factor expression in tumor tissue.

Curcumin was encapsulated into monomethyl poly (ethylene glycol)-poly (ε-caprolactone)-poly (trimethylene carbonate) (MPEG-P(CL-co-TMC)) micelles (Yang et al. 2015). The results of the in vitro anticancer studies confirmed that apoptosis induction and cellular uptake of colon CT26 carcinoma cells was significantly higher in curcumin micelles compared with free curcumin. Additionally, curcumin micelles were effective in suppressing the growth of carcinoma cells in vivo, by inhibiting tumor cell proliferation and angiogenesis and increased apoptosis of tumor cells. Moreover, fabricated curcumin-loaded methoxy polyethylene glycol–polylactide (CUR/mPEG–PLA) polymeric micelles have also been reported in the literature (Zhu et al. 2017). CUR/mPEG–PLA micelles inhibited A549 cell proliferation, increased cell cytotoxicity, induced G2/M stage arrest and promoted apoptosis. Curcumin encapsulated in a diblock copolymer micelle was also potent in inducing apoptosis against mouse mammary tumors by decreasing the Bcl-2/Bax ratio (Alizadeh et al. 2015).

Liposomal nanoparticles of curcumin were also formulated in a delivery system that allowed intravenous administration (Li et al. 2005). The in vitro and in vivo effects of this formulation were evaluated on pancreatic carcinoma cells. Liposomal curcumin consistently suppressed NF-kappaB transcriptional activity and consequently decreased the expression of NF-kappaB-regulated proteins, including cyclooxygenase-2 and interleukin-8, both of which have been implicated in tumor growth and tumor invasiveness. These in vitro changes were associated with concentration and time-dependent antiproliferative activity and proapoptotic effects. The preclinical anticancer activity of a liposomal curcumin formulation was also examined in colorectal cancer (Anand et al. 2007). Specifically, liposomal curcumin was compared to oxaliplatin, a standard chemotherapeutic agent for colorectal cancer. Results from in vitro studies showed a synergistic effect between liposomal curcumin and oxaliplatin in LoVo cells. Furthermore, in animal studies, significant tumor growth inhibition was observed in Colo205 and LoVo xenografts in mice, with the liposomal curcumin showing greater tumor inhibition than oxaliplatin in Colo205 cells. In a different study, curcumin liposomes modified with *p*-aminophenyl-α-D-mannopyranoside, which facilitates the transport of liposomes across the blood–brain barrier, demonstrated anti-tumor effects in glioma cells. In particular, the targeted liposomes induced apoptosis and endocytosis in C6 glioma cells and glioma stem cells (Wang et al. 2017a). Furthermore, the targeted liposomes increased the survival period of brain glioma-bearing mice and inhibited the growth of gliomas. The anticancer activity of curcumin-loaded cationic liposomes has also been investigated against Hela and SiHa cervical cancer cells where it was found to cause apoptosis (Saengkrit et al. 2014). Additionally, the effects of curcumin-loaded liposomes on breast cancer were examined and showed that liposomes composed of salmon's lecithin improved curcumin bioavailability compared to those constituted of rapeseed and soya lecithins and induced cell cycle arrest and apoptosis in vitro (Hasan et al. 2014).

16.4.3 EGCG Nanoformulations

EGCG is one of few hydrophilic anticancer natural compounds with poor cellular absorption and compromised in vivo bioefficiency. Polymeric and liposomal nanoformulations that incorporate hydrophilic components are used to enhance the lipophilicity of EGCG nanoformulations and to improve its cellular absorption and bioavailability in vivo. The efficiency of polymeric PLA-PEG encapsulated EGCG NPs against human prostate cancer was determined in both in vitro and in vivo studies (Siddiqui et al. 2009). EGCG NPs induced a 15-fold increase in apoptosis of PC3 cells compared with free EGCG by increasing the Bax/Bcl-2 ratio. Moreover, EGCG-loaded NPs were able to efficiently inhibit angiogenesis. Athymic nude mice injected with androgen-responsive 22Rν1 cells were treated with EGCG NPs or unecapsulated EGCG. Tumor growth inhibition was achieved with a tenfold lower dose of nano-EGCG compared to the unecapsulated form. Additionally, PLGA-casein nanocapsules were also synthesized (Narayanan et al. 2014) consisting of an EGCG shell and entrapping paclitaxel in the core. The idea was that an early release of EGCG would substantially increase the sensitivity of cancer cells to paclitaxel, thereby providing improved therapeutics at lower concentrations, with less toxicity. NPs revealed a longer circulatory lifespan and increased biocompatibility both in vitro and in vivo. EGCG-paclitaxel nanocapsules were also effective against MDA-MB-231 breast cancer cells and patient-derived tumor cells (Narayanan et al. 2015). Moreover, some of the NPs were functionalized with antibodies specific for the cell surface receptors anti-EGFR and anti-HER2. The results indicated an enhanced cellular uptake by MDA-MB-231 cells and a higher rate of apoptosis compared to encapsulated paclitaxel and EGCG. As expected, results were additionally improved when NPs were functionalized with anti-EGFR. Likewise, in a different study the antitumor efficacy of chitosan nano EGCG was evaluated in subcutaneously implanted 22Rν1 tumor xenografts in athymic nude mice (Khan et al. 2014). Chitosan nano EGCG caused significant inhibition of tumor growth and secreted prostate-specific antigen levels compared with EGCG and control groups. In tumor tissues of mice treated with Chitosan nano EGCG, compared with groups treated with EGCG and controls, there was significant induction of PARP cleavage, increased Bax/Bcl-2 ratio, activation of caspases and reduction in Ki-67 proliferation index.

Uncommonly, ECGC has been applied in the form of micelles. Methoxy poly (ethylene glycol)-b-poly[5-methyl-5-(3, 4, 5-trimethoxybenzoyol)-1, 3-dioxan-2-one-co-lactide copolymeric micelles were synthesized for the delivery of EGCG and cyclopamine to pancreatic cancer cells (Sun et al. 2014). The combination of EGCG and cyclopamine (CyA) inhibited the growth of Mia PaCa-2 pancreatic cancer cells and induced apoptosis. The expression level of Gli-1 was greatly downregulated by cyclopamine treatment, but treatment with EGCG provided an additional inhibition of the phosphorylation of EGFR in Mia PaCa-2 cells.

There is a plethora of studies utilizing liposomes for delivery of EGCG to cancer cells (Granja et al. 2016). For example, a liposomal co-delivery system comprising EGCG and paclitaxel was fabricated for addressing breast cancer in vitro utilizing an MDA-MB-231 breast cancer cell line (Ramadass et al. 2015). The results showed a synergistic effect in inducing cancer cell apoptosis and inhibiting cell invasion as demonstrated by an increase in caspase-3 activity and a decrease in matrix metalloproteinase expression (MMP) expression. Most importantly, these effects were augmented in comparison to the individual drug-loaded liposomes. Furthermore, in a different study, EGCG was encapsulated in the hydrophilic core of liposomes formed by cholesterol and phosphatidylcholine and coated with chitosan (de Pace et al. 2013). In vitro studies demonstrated chitosan-coated liposomes showed significant anti-proliferative and pro-apoptotic effects with a significant decrease of MCF7 cells proliferation compared with free EGCG and induction of apoptosis. Additionally, the use of liposomal formulations for basal cell carcinoma in vivo after intra-tumoral administration has also been reported in the literature (Fang et al. 2006). The synthesized liposomes enabled higher EGCG accumulation in tumor tissues and induced higher levels of BCC cell death and higher apoptosis induction compared to free EGCG.

16.4.4 Quercetin Nanoformulations

Quercetin's low aqueous solubility, poor cellular permeability and instability in physiological media have limited its widespread application in the pharmaceutical field. Herein, we present various nanocarriers that have been reported in the literature and designed to overcome these limitations.

Quercetin loaded polymeric chitosan nanoparticles (QCT-CS NPs) were developed and tested both in vitro and in vivo (Baksi et al. 2018). In vitro cytotoxicity assay on A549 and MDA MB 468 cell lines showed significantly reduced IC_{50} value for QCT-CS treated cells compared to free QCT. Additionally, intra venous treatment of QCT-CS NPs in tumor xenograft mice with A549 and MDA MB 468 cells caused a substantial reduction in tumour volume compared to control groups. In a different study, gold-quercetin was loaded into poly (DL-lactide-co-glycolide) NPs (NQ) and the biological activity on HepG2 hepatocarcinoma cells was tested (Bishayee et al. 2015). A cytotoxicity assay indicated that NQ preferentially killed cancer cells, compared to normal cells and induced apoptosis in HepG2 cells by activating p53-ROS crosstalk. Moreover, methoxy poly(ethylene glycol)-poly (lactide) NPs encapsulating quercetin have been reported in the literature and shown to act as an effective anticancer agent by inducing apoptosis in breast cancer (Sharma et al. 2015).

An effective drug delivery system consisting of polymeric micelles has been reported for quercetin (Xu et al. 2015). In this drug delivery system, quercetin was encapsulated into an amphiphilic block copolymer of monomethoxy poly(ethylene glycol)-poly(ε-caprolactone) (MPEG-PCL). The quercetin-loaded MPEG-PCL micelles exhibited improved apoptosis induction and cell growth inhibition effects in CT26 cells in vitro compared with free quercetin. Moreover, in a mouse subcutaneous CT26 colon cancer model quercetin-loaded MPEG-PCL micelles were more effective in inhibiting the growth of colon tumor compared to free quercetin. Additionally, quercetin-loaded MPEG-PCL micelles were superior in inducing cell apoptosis, inhibiting tumor angiogenesis, and restraining cell proliferation. In a different study, quercetin-loaded mixed micelles were fabricated for the treatment of lung cancer (Zhao et al. 2017). The mixed micelles comprised TPGS and a 1,2-distearoyl-*sn*-glycero-3-phosphatidylethanolamine derivative of polyethylene glycol. Interestingly, the prepared micelles exhibited a pH-responsive and controlled release of quercetin that could be advantageous in cancer therapy. MTT assay showed that the anticancer effect of quercetin-loaded mixed micelles in A549 cancer cells is enhanced compared to free quercetin. Additionally, confocal microscopy of A549 cells treated with QUR-M showed severe chromatin condensation and apoptotic body formation of the nuclei. Another micellar preparation was shown by Gao et al. (Gao et al. 2012) who encapsulated quercetin into monomethoxy poly(ethylene glycol)-poly(ε-caprolactone) (MPEG-PCL) micelles for the treatment of ovarian cancer. In vivo, quercetin MPEG-PCL micelles significantly suppressed the growth of established xenograft A2780S ovarian tumors by cell apoptosis and inhibition of angiogenesis.

To overcome quercetin's poor water solubility, Yuan et al. (2006) developed liposomal quercetin and investigated its antitumor efficacy both in vivo and in vitro. PEGylated liposomal quercetin induced apoptosis in vitro and significantly inhibited tumor growth in vivo in a dose-dependent manner. Liposomal quercetin down-regulated the expression of heat shock protein 70 (Hsp70) in tumor tissues, inhibited tumor angiogenesis as assessed by CD31 staining and induced tumor cell apoptosis as assessed by DNA fragmentation in tumor tissue. Additionally, PEGylated liposomal quercetin was shown to induce apoptosis and to inhibit angiogenesis in both cisplatin-sensitive (A2780s) and cisplatin-resistant (A2780cp) ovarian cancers (Long et al. 2013). In vitro, experiments suggested that PEGylated liposomal quercetin inhibited cell proliferation, induced apoptosis, and induced cell cycle arrest in both cisplatin-sensitive and cisplatin-resistant human ovarian tumor xenograft models in nude mice. PEGylated liposomal quercetin significantly suppressed tumor growth in both models compared to free quercetin, blank liposomes, or saline. In a mouse model, liposomal quercetin was found to enhance the sensitivity of colon carcinoma to thermotherapy and thermochemotherapy by inhibiting the expression of Hsp70 (He et al. 2013).

16.4.5 Resveratrol Nanoformulations

Despite the aforementioned therapeutic possibilities of resveratrol, its efficacy is limited by its poor bioavailability (less than 1%) due to its poor aqueous solubility (0.03 g/L). Additionally, resveratrol suffers from extensive metabolism in the intestine and liver called enterohepatic recirculation. To overcome these limitations, various nanonoformulations have been developed.

For example polymeric NPs made from PLGA for the encapsulation of resveratrol have been developed (Nassir et al. 2018). The NPs' cytotoxic and mode of apoptotic cell death was tested against a prostate cancer cell line (LNCaP). Resveratrol loaded PLGA NPs caused a decrease in cell viability in LNCaP cells, caused cell cycle arrest at G1/S transition phase and induced apoptosis as confirmed by externalization of phosphatidylserine, DNA cleavage, loss of mitochondrial membrane potential and ROS generation. Furthermore, significantly greater cytotoxicity to LNCaP cells was observed with NPs as compared to that of free resveratrol. When resveratrol loaded human serum albumin (HSA), NPs conjugating RGD (arginine–glycine–aspartate) were used to target pancreatic tumors (Geng et al. 2017) and apoptotic cell death was evident. Moreover, Jung et al. (2015) prepared resveratrol (RSV)-loaded PEG-PLA polymer NPs and investigated its anti-tumor effect in vitro and in vivo. The apoptotic effect of RSV-NP was demonstrated by increased annexin V staining and by capspase-3 and PARP cleavage. When resveratrol NP was intravenously administered to CT26 tumor bearing mice, there was a reduction of radiopharmaceutical ^{18}F FDG uptake. Longer treatment led to retardation of tumor growth accompanied by an improvement in survival compared to injected controls of empty NPs.

Resveratrol NPs were also efficient in overcoming chemoresistance in breast cancer. To overcome issues associated with poor absorption and rapid metabolism, Wang et al. (2015) designed a mixed micelle system made of methoxy poly (ethylene glycol)-b-polycaprolactone (mPEG-PCL) and TPGS. The mixed micellar formulation increased drug uptake efficiency of resveratrol by doxorubicin-resistant breast cancer MCF-7/ADR cells and induced higher rates of apoptotic cell death (compared to free resveratrol) as assessed by the accumulation of Sub G1 phases of cell cycle, nuclear staining and annexin V/propidium iodide assay. As previously mentioned, Res-loaded mixed micelles enhanced Dox-induced cytotoxicity in MCF-7/ADR cells by increasing accumulation of Dox and by downregulating the expression of P-glycoprotein (P-gp). Polymer micelles have also been employed for the successive delivery of Resveratrol (RES) and paclitaxel (PTX) (Hu et al. 2014). PTX and RES co-encapsulated micelles were prepared from mPEG-*b*-PLA block copolymers. In vitro cytotoxicity tests showed that the time-dependent sequential release of the two drugs increased the sensitivity of PTX-resistant human lung adenocarcinoma epithelial (A549/T) and mice sarcoma 180 (S180) cells to PTX, possibly due to the enhanced PTX-induced apoptosis in the presence of RES. The combination therapy caused tumor regression and achieved the best antitumor effect in all treatment groups in S180 bearing mice. In a different study redox-sensitive pluronic F127-SS-α-tocopherol (TOC) micelles loaded with resveratrol (F127-SS-TOC/RES) were prepared and their cytotoxicity in human breast cancer cells was tested (Liu et al. 2017). Redox-sensitive F127-SS-TOC/RES micelles induced apoptosis and elevated the intracellular reactive oxygen species (ROS) level against human breast cancer cells MCF-7 and MDA-MB-231 in relation to free RES and non-redox-responsive F127-TOC/RES micelles.

Moreover, Wang et al. (2011) developed a strategy using liposomes modified with a dequalinium polyethylene glycol-distearoylphosphatidyl ethanolamine conjugate to target mitochondria and induce apoptosis in cisplatin-resistant lung cancer cells. Results indicated that mitochondrial targeting resveratrol liposomes provide a potential strategy to treat the inherent resistant lung cancers by inducing apoptosis via the mitochondria signaling pathway. In a different study, the anti-cancer effect of resveratrol solid lipid NPs (SLNs) was found to be superior compared to that of free RSV (Wang et al. 2017b). The Res-SLNs inhibited the proliferation, invasion and migration of MDA-MB-231 cells, increased the Bax/Bcl-2 ratio and decreased the expression of cyclin D1 and c-Myc. These results indicate that the Res-SLN may could potentially be used for the treatment of breast cancer.

16.4.6 Genistein Nanoformulations

Genistein also suffers from poor bioavailability because of its low aqueous solubility and absorption. Polymeric NPs of genistein have been reported in the literature and include a novel polymeric folic acid-conjugated chitosan NP (FGCN) that was used for specific delivery of genistein to cervical cancer (Cai et al. 2017). Results from this study showed that FGCN nanoformulations exhibited a superior cytotoxic effect compared to that of non-targeted formulations. Additionally, apoptosis studies indicated that the FGCN NPs exhibited a remarkable apoptosis of cancer cells compared to that of non-targeted formulations.

Additionally, micellar formulations of genistein have been utilized. Genistein loaded into lipidic micelles made from vitamin E TPGS and PEG2000-PE produced significant cytotoxicity in hepatic and colon carcinomas, compared to free genistein and drug-free lipidic micelles (Pham et al. 2013). This cytotoxicity was due to the mitochondria-specific accumulation of genistein NPs and consequently the activation of intrinsic apoptotic pathway markers such as cytosolic cytochrome c and caspase-9.

Liposomes loaded with genistein have been similarly used to aid genistein's clinical use. For example effective liposomal delivery of genistein to cancer cells resulted in marked enhancement in the overall in vitro cytotoxicity against breast, ovarian and prostate carcinomas (Phan et al. 2013). Genistein-loaded liposomes produced P53-independent apoptosis including mitochondrial polarization and caspase-3/7 cleavage.

16.5 Conclusions and Recommendations

Vitamin E isoforms, gurcumin, EGCG, quercetin, resveratrol and genistein have all been extensively studied and shown to possess pro-apoptotic properties by activating the extrinsic and intrinsic pathway of programmed cell death, including caspase-dependent and independent mechanisms. The effects of these compounds have been investigated as single agents as well as in combination studies both in vitro and in vivo. Natural compounds have been combined either amongst them or with established anti-cancer drugs, as in the case of curcumin or resveratrol and 5-FU, respectively. The ultimate aim, and especially when administered with chemotherapeutics, is to create a synergistic, enhanced effect, lower the drug dosage and protect normal cells from damage.

The mechanism of action shows similarity across natural compounds and across different types of cancers. Resveratrol, curcumin, ellagic acid and EGCG inhibit the PI3K/AKT survival pathway, either by blocking the activation of the main proteins involved or by positively regulating tumor suppressor genes, such as PTEN, that suppress signal transduction. Many natural compounds block the transcription of anti-apoptotic genes including survivin and XIAP while others increase the levels of pro-apoptotic molecules such as Noxa and Puma. Members of the Bcl-2 superfamily are also affected by natural agents, so that pro-apoptotic members are upregulated and induce the release of cytochrome c and AIF from the mitochondria that catalyze both caspase-dependent and independent programmed cell death. Figure 16.5 shows how some of the major apoptotic pathways are affected by natural agents.

Clinical trials involving natural agents have not shown great promise, mostly because of the limited bioavailability of these compounds and their effective biodistribution. The advancement of nanoformulation technology can provide solutions to these limitations. Nanoshperes, nanocapsules, liposomes and micelles have all been extensively applied for the encapsulation of natural agents and have shown enhanced effects across a range of different malignancies. NPs loaded with natural compounds induce similar apoptotic pathways as described above, however, they display many advantages, including prolonged circulation time in the blood, enhanced tumor accumulation, encapsulation of hydrophobic compounds that would otherwise have been unavailable in vivo, targeted delivery to the tumor site due to the addition of a molecule against a specific receptor overexpressed in cancer cells, excellent cellular uptake, improved stability and many more. The same properties that make nanoparticles unique and their allotropic physicochemical behaviour could result in many potential clinical implications. Limitations associated with nanodelivery systems include, but are not limited to, low drug loading capacity, low bioavailability due to immature degradation, insufficient tumor uptake via the EPR effect, unforeseen toxic activity and over and/or under activation of the innate immune system.

The development of the nanochemoprevention field may be the future for unlocking the anti-cancer potential of natural compounds.

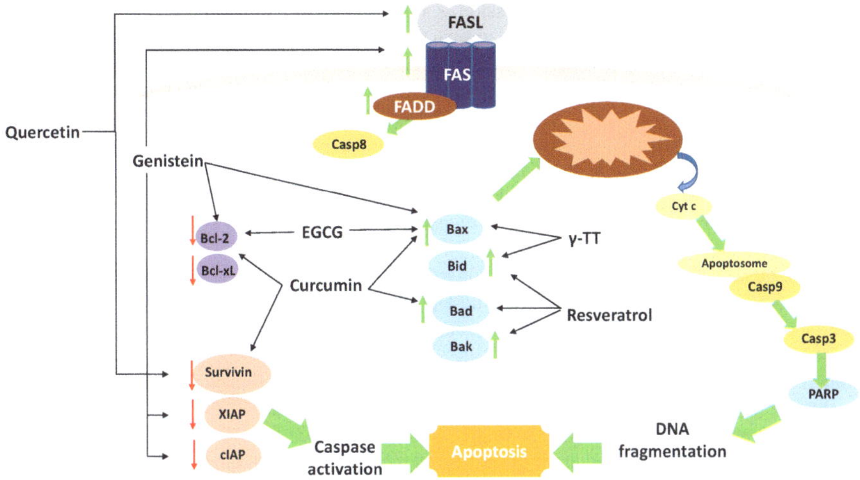

Fig. 16.5 Main apoptotic pathways affected by natural compounds. The Bcl-2 superfamily plays a central role in the apoptosis induced by natural agents. Pro-apoptotic members Bax, Bid, Bad and Bak are upregulated while anti-apoptotic Bcl-2 and Bcl-xL are downregulated. This leads to MOMP and release of cyt c from the mitochondria to form the apoptosome and activate caspase-9. Caspase-3 activation and PARP cleavage ultimately lead to DNA fragmentation and apoptosis. Other natural compounds lower the levels of IAPs such as survivin, XIAP and cIAP further enhancing caspase activation. Finally, the extrinsic pathway of apoptosis may be initiated by increasing the levels of FASL, FAS and FADD. Cyt c, cytochrome c; MOMP, mitochondrial outer membrane permeabilization

Acknowledgments This work was supported by funding from the University of Cyprus and was co-funded by the European Regional Development Fund and the Republic of Cyprus through the Research and Innovation Foundation (Project: INTERNATIONAL/OTHER/0118/0017).

References

Akiyama T et al (1987) Genistein, a specific inhibitor of tyrosine-specific protein kinases. J Biol Chem 262(12):5592–5595

Alessi DR et al (1996) Mechanism of activation of protein kinase B by insulin and IGF-1. EMBO J 15(23):6541–6551

Alizadeh AM et al (2015) Encapsulation of curcumin in diblock copolymer micelles for cancer therapy. Biomed Res Int 2015:824746

Alotaibi A et al (2013) Tea phenols in bulk and nanoparticle form modify DNA damage in human lymphocytes from colon cancer patients and healthy individuals treated in vitro with platinum-based chemotherapeutic drugs. Nanomedicine (Lond) 8(3):389–401

Anand P et al (2007) Bioavailability of curcumin: problems and promises. Mol Pharm 4 (6):807–818

Arabyan E et al (2018) Genistein inhibits African swine fever virus replication in vitro by disrupting viral DNA synthesis. Antiviral Res 156:128–137

Arya G, Das M, Sahoo SK (2018) Evaluation of curcumin loaded chitosan/PEG blended PLGA nanoparticles for effective treatment of pancreatic cancer. Biomed Pharmacother 102:555–566

Asanuma H et al (2005) Survivin expression is regulated by coexpression of human epidermal growth factor receptor 2 and epidermal growth factor receptor via phosphatidylinositol 3-kinase/AKT signaling pathway in breast cancer cells. Cancer Res 65(23):11018–11025

Ashkenazi A, Dixit VM (1998) Death receptors: signaling and modulation. Science 281 (5381):1305–1308

Azandeh SS et al (2017) Anticancer activity of curcumin-loaded PLGA nanoparticles on PC3 prostate cancer cells. Iran J Pharm Res 16(3):868–879

Aziz MH et al (2006) Resveratrol-caused apoptosis of human prostate carcinoma LNCaP cells is mediated via modulation of phosphatidylinositol 3′-kinase/Akt pathway and Bcl-2 family proteins. Mol Cancer Ther 5(5):1335–1341

Bae Y, Kataoka K (2009) Intelligent polymeric micelles from functional poly(ethylene glycol)-poly (amino acid) block copolymers. Adv Drug Deliv Rev 61(10):768–784

Baechler SA et al (2016) Topoisomerase poisoning by genistein in the intestine of rats. Toxicol Lett 243:88–97

Bahi N et al (2006) Switch from caspase-dependent to caspase-independent death during heart development: essential role of endonuclease G in ischemia-induced DNA processing of differentiated cardiomyocytes. J Biol Chem 281(32):22943–22952

Baksi R et al (2018) In vitro and in vivo anticancer efficacy potential of quercetin loaded polymeric nanoparticles. Biomed Pharmacother 106:1513–1526

Bandele OJ, Osheroff N (2007) Bioflavonoids as poisons of human topoisomerase II alpha and II beta. Biochemistry 46(20):6097–6108

Benitez DA et al (2007) Non-genomic action of resveratrol on androgen and oestrogen receptors in prostate cancer: modulation of the phosphoinositide 3-kinase pathway. Br J Cancer 96 (10):1595–1604

Bernabeu E et al (2016) Novel Soluplus((R))-TPGS mixed micelles for encapsulation of paclitaxel with enhanced in vitro cytotoxicity on breast and ovarian cancer cell lines. Colloids Surf B Biointerfaces 140:403–411

Bidere N et al (2003) Cathepsin D triggers Bax activation, resulting in selective apoptosis-inducing factor (AIF) relocation in T lymphocytes entering the early commitment phase to apoptosis. J Biol Chem 278(33):31401–31411

Bishayee K, Khuda-Bukhsh AR, Huh SO (2015) PLGA-loaded gold-nanoparticles precipitated with quercetin downregulate HDAC-Akt activities controlling proliferation and activate p53-ROS crosstalk to induce apoptosis in hepatocarcinoma cells. Mol Cells 38(6):518–527

Boldin MP et al (1995) Self-association of the "death domains" of the p55 tumor necrosis factor (TNF) receptor and Fas/APO1 prompts signaling for TNF and Fas/APO1 effects. J Biol Chem 270(1):387–391

Brown VA et al (2010) Repeat dose study of the cancer chemopreventive agent resveratrol in healthy volunteers: safety, pharmacokinetics, and effect on the insulin-like growth factor axis. Cancer Res 70(22):9003–9011

Buki KG, Bauer PI, Kun E (1997) Isolation and identification of a proteinase from calf thymus that cleaves poly(ADP-ribose) polymerase and histone H1. Biochim Biophys Acta 1338(1):100–106

Burz C et al (2009) Apoptosis in cancer: key molecular signaling pathways and therapy targets. Acta Oncol 48(6):811–821

Cai L et al (2017) Folate receptor-targeted bioflavonoid genistein-loaded chitosan nanoparticles for enhanced anticancer effect in cervical cancers. Nanoscale Res Lett 12(1):509

Campana D et al (1993) Prolonged survival of B-lineage acute lymphoblastic leukemia cells is accompanied by overexpression of bcl-2 protein. Blood 81(4):1025–1031

Carstens MG, Rijcken CJ, Nostrum CF, Hennink WE (2008) Pharmaceutical micelles: combining longevity, stability, and stimuli sensitivity. In: Multifunctional pharmaceutical nanocarriers. Springer, New York, pp 263–308

Chan KKL et al (2018) Estrogen receptor modulators genistein, daidzein and ERB-041 inhibit cell migration, invasion, proliferation and sphere formation via modulation of FAK and PI3K/AKT signaling in ovarian cancer. Cancer Cell Int 18:65

Chang Z, Xing J, Yu X (2014) Curcumin induces osteosarcoma MG63 cells apoptosis via ROS/Cyto-C/Caspase-3 pathway. Tumour Biol 35(1):753–758

Chicheportiche Y et al (1997) TWEAK, a new secreted ligand in the tumor necrosis factor family that weakly induces apoptosis. J Biol Chem 272(51):32401–32410

Chinnaiyan AM (1999) The apoptosome: heart and soul of the cell death machine. Neoplasia 1 (1):5–15

Choudhury H et al (2017) Recent advances in TPGS-based nanoparticles of docetaxel for improved chemotherapy. Int J Pharm 529(1–2):506–522

Chung SS et al (2018) Combination of resveratrol and 5-flurouracil enhanced anti-telomerase activity and apoptosis by inhibiting STAT3 and Akt signaling pathways in human colorectal cancer cells. Oncotarget 9(68):32943–32957

Cirman T et al (2004) Selective disruption of lysosomes in HeLa cells triggers apoptosis mediated by cleavage of Bid by multiple papain-like lysosomal cathepsins. J Biol Chem 279 (5):3578–3587

Clancy AA et al (2010) Measuring properties of nanoparticles in embryonic blood vessels: towards a physicochemical basis for nanotoxicity. Chem Phys Lett 488(4-6):99–111

Cohen GM (1997) Caspases: the executioners of apoptosis. Biochem J 326(Pt 1):1–16

Constantinou A, Kiguchi K, Huberman E (1990) Induction of differentiation and DNA strand breakage in human HL-60 and K-562 leukemia cells by genistein. Cancer Res 50(9):2618–2624

Constantinou AI, Krygier AE, Mehta RR (1998a) Genistein induces maturation of cultured human breast cancer cells and prevents tumor growth in nude mice. Am J Clin Nutr 68 (6 Suppl):1426S–1430S

Constantinou AI, Kamath N, Murley JS (1998b) Genistein inactivates bcl-2, delays the G2/M phase of the cell cycle, and induces apoptosis of human breast adenocarcinoma MCF-7 cells. Eur J Cancer 34(12):1927–1934

Constantinou C, Papas A, Constantinou AI (2008) Vitamin E and cancer: an insight into the anticancer activities of vitamin E isomers and analogs. Int J Cancer 123(4):739–752

Constantinou C, Papas KA, Constantinou AI (2009) Caspase-independent pathways of programmed cell death: the unraveling of new targets of cancer therapy? Curr Cancer Drug Targets 9(6):717–728

Couvreur P et al (1979) Adsorption of antineoplastic drugs to polyalkylcyanoacrylate nanoparticles and their release in calf serum. J Pharm Sci 68(12):1521–1524

Crawford A, Nahta R (2011) Targeting Bcl-2 in herceptin-resistant breast cancer cell lines. Curr Pharmacogenomics Person Med 9(3):184–190

Cullen SP, Martin SJ (2009) Caspase activation pathways: some recent progress. Cell Death Differ 16(7):935–938

Danial NN (2007) BCL-2 family proteins: critical checkpoints of apoptotic cell death. Clin Cancer Res 13(24):7254–7263

Degterev A, Boyce M, Yuan J (2003) A decade of caspases. Oncogene 22(53):8543–8567

de Pace RC et al (2013) Anticancer activities of (-)-epigallocatechin-3-gallate encapsulated nanoliposomes in MCF7 breast cancer cells. J Liposome Res 23(3):187–196

Dintaman JM, Silverman JA (1999) Inhibition of P-glycoprotein by D-alpha-tocopheryl polyethylene glycol 1000 succinate (TPGS). Pharm Res 16(10):1550–1556

Dorai T, Gehani N, Katz A (2000) Therapeutic potential of curcumin in human prostate cancer. II. Curcumin inhibits tyrosine kinase activity of epidermal growth factor receptor and depletes the protein. Mol Urol 4(1):1–6

Du K, Montminy M (1998) CREB is a regulatory target for the protein kinase Akt/PKB. J Biol Chem 273(49):32377–32379

Du C et al (2000) Smac, a mitochondrial protein that promotes cytochrome c-dependent caspase activation by eliminating IAP inhibition. Cell 102(1):33–42

Elmore S (2007) Apoptosis: a review of programmed cell death. Toxicol Pathol 35(4):495–516

Elsabahy M, Wooley KL (2012) Design of polymeric nanoparticles for biomedical delivery applications. Chem Soc Rev 41(7):2545–2561

El Touny LH, Banerjee PP (2009) Identification of a biphasic role for genistein in the regulation of prostate cancer growth and metastasis. Cancer Res 69(8):3695–3703

Enari M et al (1998) A caspase-activated DNase that degrades DNA during apoptosis, and its inhibitor ICAD. Nature 391(6662):43–50

Esposti MD (2002) The roles of Bid. Apoptosis 7(5):433–440

Fang JY et al (2006) Effect of liposome encapsulation of tea catechins on their accumulation in basal cell carcinomas. J Dermatol Sci 42(2):101–109

Feng SS (2006) New-concept chemotherapy by nanoparticles of biodegradable polymers: where are we now? Nanomedicine (Lond) 1(3):297–309

Frojdo S et al (2007) Resveratrol is a class IA phosphoinositide 3-kinase inhibitor. Biochem J 406 (3):511–518

Gao X et al (2012) Anticancer effect and mechanism of polymer micelle-encapsulated quercetin on ovarian cancer. Nanoscale 4(22):7021–7030

Gaonkar RH et al (2017) Garcinol loaded vitamin E TPGS emulsified PLGA nanoparticles: preparation, physicochemical characterization, in vitro and in vivo studies. Sci Rep 7(1)

Garrido C et al (2006) Mechanisms of cytochrome c release from mitochondria. Cell Death Differ 13(9):1423–1433

Geng T et al (2017) Resveratrol-loaded albumin nanoparticles with prolonged blood circulation and improved biocompatibility for highly effective targeted pancreatic tumor therapy. Nanoscale Res Lett 12(1):437

Ghiotto F, Fais F, Bruno S (2010) BH3-only proteins: the death-puppeteer's wires. Cytometry A 77 (1):11–21

Giam M, Huang DC, Bouillet P (2008) BH3-only proteins and their roles in programmed cell death. Oncogene 27(Suppl 1):S128–S136

Gobeil S et al (2001) Characterization of the necrotic cleavage of poly(ADP-ribose) polymerase (PARP-1): implication of lysosomal proteases. Cell Death Differ 8(6):588–594

Granado-Serrano AB et al (2006) Quercetin induces apoptosis via caspase activation, regulation of Bcl-2, and inhibition of PI-3-kinase/Akt and ERK pathways in a human hepatoma cell line (HepG2). J Nutr 136(11):2715–2721

Granja A, Pinheiro M, Reis S (2016) Epigallocatechin gallate nanodelivery systems for cancer therapy. Nutrients 8(5)

Gu Y et al (2016) Nanomicelles loaded with doxorubicin and curcumin for alleviating multidrug resistance in lung cancer. Int J Nanomedicine 11:5757–5770

Guicciardi ME, Gores GJ (2009) Life and death by death receptors. FASEB J 23(6):1625–1637

Hanahan D, Weinberg RA (2011) Hallmarks of cancer: the next generation. Cell 144(5):646–674

Haque A et al (2015) Combination of erlotinib and EGCG induces apoptosis of head and neck cancers through posttranscriptional regulation of Bim and Bcl-2. Apoptosis 20(7):986–995

Hasan M et al (2014) Liposome encapsulation of curcumin: physico-chemical characterizations and effects on MCF7 cancer cell proliferation. Int J Pharm 461(1-2):519–528

Hastak K et al (2003) Role of p53 and NF-kappaB in epigallocatechin-3-gallate-induced apoptosis of LNCaP cells. Oncogene 22(31):4851–4859

Hayakawa S et al (2001) Apoptosis induction by epigallocatechin gallate involves its binding to Fas. Biochem Biophys Res Commun 285(5):1102–1106

He B et al (2013) Quercetin liposome sensitizes colon carcinoma to thermotherapy and thermochemotherapy in mice models. Integr Cancer Ther 12(3):264–270

Hilchie AL et al (2010) Curcumin-induced apoptosis in PC3 prostate carcinoma cells is caspase-independent and involves cellular ceramide accumulation and damage to mitochondria. Nutr Cancer 62(3):379–389

Hill MM et al (2004) Analysis of the composition, assembly kinetics and activity of native Apaf-1 apoptosomes. EMBO J 23(10):2134–2145

Hinds MG, Day CL (2005) Regulation of apoptosis: uncovering the binding determinants. Curr Opin Struct Biol 15(6):690–699

Hirsch T et al (1997) The apoptosis-necrosis paradox. Apoptogenic proteases activated after mitochondrial permeability transition determine the mode of cell death. Oncogene 15 (13):1573–1581

Hong SJ, Dawson TM, Dawson VL (2004) Nuclear and mitochondrial conversations in cell death: PARP-1 and AIF signaling. Trends Pharmacol Sci 25(5):259–264
Hong JH et al (2006) The effects of curcumin on the invasiveness of prostate cancer in vitro and in vivo. Prostate Cancer Prostatic Dis 9(2):147–152
Hou W et al (2016) pH-Sensitive self-assembling nanoparticles for tumor near-infrared fluorescence imaging and chemo-photodynamic combination therapy. Nanoscale 8(1):104–116
Hsu H, Xiong J, Goeddel DV (1995) The TNF receptor 1-associated protein TRADD signals cell death and NF-kappa B activation. Cell 81(4):495–504
Hu M, Zhu J, Qiu L (2014) Polymer micelle-based combination therapy of paclitaxel and resveratrol with enhanced and selective antitumor activity. RSC Adv 4:64151–64161
Hu YQ, Wang J, Wu JH (2016) Administration of resveratrol enhances cell-cycle arrest followed by apoptosis in DMBA-induced skin carcinogenesis in male Wistar rats. Eur Rev Med Pharmacol Sci 20(13):2935–2946
Huang H et al (2015) Combination of alpha-tomatine and curcumin inhibits growth and induces apoptosis in human prostate cancer cells. PLoS One 10(12):e0144293
Igney FH, Krammer PH (2002) Death and anti-death: tumour resistance to apoptosis. Nat Rev Cancer 2(4):277–288
Jacinto E et al (2006) SIN1/MIP1 maintains rictor-mTOR complex integrity and regulates Akt phosphorylation and substrate specificity. Cell 127(1):125–137
Jiao D et al (2016) Curcumin inhibited HGF-induced EMT and angiogenesis through regulating c-Met dependent PI3K/Akt/mTOR signaling pathways in lung cancer. Mol Ther Oncolytics 3:16018
Jin Z, El-Deiry WS (2005) Overview of cell death signaling pathways. Cancer Biol Ther 4 (2):139–163
Jin X, Yang Q, Zhang Y (2017) Synergistic apoptotic effects of apigenin TPGS liposomes and tyroservatide: implications for effective treatment of lung cancer. Int J Nanomed 12:5109–5118
Joza N et al (2001) Essential role of the mitochondrial apoptosis-inducing factor in programmed cell death. Nature 410(6828):549–554
Jung KH et al (2015) Resveratrol-loaded polymeric nanoparticles suppress glucose metabolism and tumor growth in vitro and in vivo. Int J Pharm 478(1):251–257
Kamal-Eldin A, Appelqvist LA (1996) The chemistry and antioxidant properties of tocopherols and tocotrienols. Lipids 31(7):671–701
Kang SJ et al (2002) Distinct downstream pathways of caspase-11 in regulating apoptosis and cytokine maturation during septic shock response. Cell Death Differ 9(10):1115–1125
Karmakar S et al (2011) Induction of mitochondrial pathways and endoplasmic reticulum stress for increasing apoptosis in ectopic and orthotopic neuroblastoma xenografts. J Cancer Ther 2 (2):77–90
Kaufmann SH (1998) Cell death induced by topoisomerase-targeted drugs: more questions than answers. Biochim Biophys Acta 1400(1-3):195–211
Kaufmann SH et al (1993) Specific proteolytic cleavage of poly(ADP-ribose) polymerase: an early marker of chemotherapy-induced apoptosis. Cancer Res 53(17):3976–3985
Khan N et al (2014) Oral administration of naturally occurring chitosan-based nanoformulated green tea polyphenol EGCG effectively inhibits prostate cancer cell growth in a xenograft model. Carcinogenesis 35(2):415–423
Khosravi-Far R, Esposti MD (2004) Death receptor signals to mitochondria. Cancer Biol Ther 3 (11):1051–1057
Kim EJ et al (2008) Underlying mechanism of quercetin-induced cell death in human glioma cells. Neurochem Res 33(6):971–979
Kim TG et al (2009) Controlled release of paclitaxel from heparinized metal stent fabricated by layer-by-layer assembly of polylysine and hyaluronic acid-g-poly(lactic-co-glycolic acid) micelles encapsulating paclitaxel. Biomacromolecules 10(6):1532–1539
Kischkel FC et al (1995) Cytotoxicity-dependent APO-1 (Fas/CD95)-associated proteins form a death-inducing signaling complex (DISC) with the receptor. EMBO J 14(22):5579–5588

Klein JA et al (2002) The harlequin mouse mutation downregulates apoptosis-inducing factor. Nature 419(6905):367–374

Koning GA, Storm G (2003) Targeted drug delivery systems for the intracellular delivery of macromolecular drugs. Drug Discov Today 8(11):482–483

Kothakota S et al (1997) Caspase-3-generated fragment of gelsolin: effector of morphological change in apoptosis. Science 278(5336):294–298

Kowshik J et al (2014) Ellagic acid inhibits VEGF/VEGFR2, PI3K/Akt and MAPK signaling cascades in the hamster cheek pouch carcinogenesis model. Anticancer Agents Med Chem 14 (9):1249–1260

Kumar S et al (2012) Nanotechnology as emerging tool for enhancing solubility of poorly water-soluble drugs. BioNanoScience 2(4):227–250. https://doi.org/10.1007/s12668-012-0060-7

Kumari A, Yadav SK, Yadav SC (2010) Biodegradable polymeric nanoparticles based drug delivery systems. Colloids Surf B Biointerfaces 75(1):1–18

Kundur S et al (2019) Synergistic anticancer action of quercetin and curcumin against triple-negative breast cancer cell lines. J Cell Physiol 234(7):11103–11118

Kurosaka K et al (2003) Silent cleanup of very early apoptotic cells by macrophages. J Immunol 171(9):4672–4679

Labhasetwar V, Song CX, Levy RJ (1997) Nanoparticle drug delivery system for restenosis. Adv Drug Deliv Rev 24(1):63–85

Lennon SV, Martin SJ, Cotter TG (1991) Dose-dependent induction of apoptosis in human tumour cell lines by widely diverging stimuli. Cell Prolif 24(2):203–214

Levine DH et al (2008) Polymersomes: a new multi-functional tool for cancer diagnosis and therapy. Methods 46(1):25–32

Li J, Yuan J (2008) Caspases in apoptosis and beyond. Oncogene 27(48):6194–6206

Li LY, Luo X, Wang X (2001) Endonuclease G is an apoptotic DNase when released from mitochondria. Nature 412(6842):95–99

Li L, Braiteh FS, Kurzrock R (2005) Liposome-encapsulated curcumin: in vitro and in vivo effects on proliferation, apoptosis, signaling, and angiogenesis. Cancer 104(6):1322–1331

Li Y et al (2012) Curcumin inhibits proliferation and invasion of osteosarcoma cells through inactivation of Notch-1 signaling. FEBS J 279(12):2247–2259

Li X et al (2014) Preparation of curcumin micelles and the in vitro and in vivo evaluation for cancer therapy. J Biomed Nanotechnol 10(8):1458–1468

Li J et al (2016) Vitamin E TPGS modified liposomes enhance cellular uptake and targeted delivery of luteolin: an in vivo/in vitro evaluation. Int J Pharm 512(1):262–272

Liang C et al (2012) Genistein potentiates the anti-cancer effects of gemcitabine in human osteosarcoma via the downregulation of Akt and nuclear factor-kappaB pathway. Anticancer Agents Med Chem 12(5):554–563

Lin C et al (2012) Combination of quercetin with radiotherapy enhances tumor radiosensitivity in vitro and in vivo. Radiother Oncol 104(3):395–400

Liu S et al (2013) PI3K/AKT/mTOR signaling is involved in (-)-epigallocatechin-3-gallate-induced apoptosis of human pancreatic carcinoma cells. Am J Chin Med 41(3):629–642

Liu D et al (2014) Genistein enhances the effect of cisplatin on the inhibition of non-small cell lung cancer A549 cell growth in vitro and in vivo. Oncol Lett 8(6):2806–2810

Liu XX et al (2016) Genistein mediates the selective radiosensitizing effect in NSCLC A549 cells via inhibiting methylation of the keap1 gene promoter region. Oncotarget 7(19):27267–27279

Liu Y, Lin L, Song J, Zhao Y, Chao Z, Li H (2017) Preparation, characterization and anticanceractivities of resveratrol loaded redox-sensitive F127-SS-TOC micelles. RSC Adv 7:47091–47098

Long Q et al (2013) Induction of apoptosis and inhibition of angiogenesis by PEGylated liposomal quercetin in both cisplatin-sensitive and cisplatin-resistant ovarian cancers. J Biomed Nanotechnol 9(6):965–975

Lorenzo HK, Susin SA (2007) Therapeutic potential of AIF-mediated caspase-independent programmed cell death. Drug Resist Updat 10(6):235–255

Luthi AU, Martin SJ (2007) The CASBAH: a searchable database of caspase substrates. Cell Death Differ 14(4):641–650

Ma Y et al (2014) Combinational delivery of hydrophobic and hydrophilic anticancer drugs in single nanoemulsions to treat MDR in cancer. Mol Pharm 11(8):2623–2630

Ma YS et al (2018) Quercetin induced apoptosis of human oral cancer SAS cells through mitochondria and endoplasmic reticulum mediated signaling pathways. Oncol Lett 15(6):9663–9672

Macagnan FT, da Silva LP, Hecktheuer LH (2016) Dietary fibre: the scientific search for an ideal definition and methodology of analysis, and its physiological importance as a carrier of bioactive compounds. Food Res Int 85:144–154

Majno G, Joris I (1995) Apoptosis, oncosis, and necrosis. An overview of cell death. Am J Pathol 146(1):3–15

Majumdar AP et al (2009) Curcumin synergizes with resveratrol to inhibit colon cancer. Nutr Cancer 61(4):544–553

Manning BD, Cantley LC (2007) AKT/PKB signaling: navigating downstream. Cell 129 (7):1261–1274

Markovits J et al (1995) Genistein resistance in human leukaemic CCRF-CEM cells: selection of a diploid cell line with reduced DNA topoisomerase II beta isoform. Biochem Pharmacol 50 (2):177–186

Mason KD et al (2008) In vivo efficacy of the Bcl-2 antagonist ABT-737 against aggressive Myc-driven lymphomas. Proc Natl Acad Sci USA 105(46):17961–17966

Meier MAR, Aerts SNH, Staal BBP, Rasa M, Schubert US (2005) PEO-b-PCL block copolymers: synthesis, detailed characterization, and selected micellar drug encapsulation behavior. Macromol Rapid Comm 26:1918–1924

Men K et al (2014) Nanoparticle-delivered quercetin for cancer therapy. Anti Cancer Agents Med Chem 14(6):826–832

Michael McClain R et al (2006) Genetic toxicity studies with genistein. Food Chem Toxicol 44 (1):42–55

Moubarak RS et al (2007) Sequential activation of poly(ADP-ribose) polymerase 1, calpains, and Bax is essential in apoptosis-inducing factor-mediated programmed necrosis. Mol Cell Biol 27 (13):4844–4862

Mu L, Feng SS (2002) Vitamin E TPGS used as emulsifier in the solvent evaporation/extraction technique for fabrication of polymeric nanospheres for controlled release of paclitaxel (Taxol). J Control Release 80(1–3):129–144

Mu L, Elbayoumi TA, Torchilin VP (2005) Mixed micelles made of poly(ethylene glycol)-phosphatidylethanolamine conjugate and d-alpha-tocopheryl polyethylene glycol 1000 succinate as pharmaceutical nanocarriers for camptothecin. Int J Pharm 306(1-2):142–149

Mukhopadhyay A et al (2001) Curcumin downregulates cell survival mechanisms in human prostate cancer cell lines. Oncogene 20(52):7597–7609

Narayanan S et al (2014) Sequentially releasing dual-drug-loaded PLGA-casein core/shell nanomedicine: design, synthesis, biocompatibility and pharmacokinetics. Acta Biomater 10 (5):2112–2124

Narayanan S et al (2015) Sequential release of epigallocatechin gallate and paclitaxel from PLGA-casein core/shell nanoparticles sensitizes drug-resistant breast cancer cells. Nanomedicine 11 (6):1399–1406

Nassir AM et al (2018) Resveratrol-loaded PLGA nanoparticles mediated programmed cell death in prostate cancer cells. Saudi Pharm J 26(6):876–885

Neophytou CM, Constantinou AI (2015) Drug delivery innovations for enhancing the anticancer potential of vitamin E isoforms and their derivatives. Biomed Res Int 2015:584862

Neophytou CM et al (2014) D-alpha-tocopheryl polyethylene glycol succinate (TPGS) induces cell cycle arrest and apoptosis selectively in Survivin-overexpressing breast cancer cells. Biochem Pharmacol 89(1):31–42

Neuzil J (2003) Vitamin E succinate and cancer treatment: a vitamin E prototype for selective antitumour activity. Br J Cancer 89(10):1822–1826

Nguyen T et al (2014) Designing a better theranostic nanocarrier for cancer applications. Nanomedicine 9(15):2371–2386

Niu G et al (2011) Quercetin induces apoptosis by activating caspase-3 and regulating Bcl-2 and cyclooxygenase-2 pathways in human HL-60 cells. Acta Biochim Biophys Sin (Shanghai) 43 (1):30–37

Northfelt DW et al (1998) Pegylated-liposomal doxorubicin versus doxorubicin, bleomycin, and vincristine in the treatment of AIDS-related Kaposi's sarcoma: results of a randomized phase III clinical trial. J Clin Oncol 16(7):2445–2451

Pan J, Wang Y, Feng SS (2008) Formulation, characterization, and in vitro evaluation of quantum dots loaded in poly(lactide)-vitamin E TPGS nanoparticles for cellular and molecular imaging. Biotechnol Bioeng 101(3):622–633

Parhi P, Mohanty C, Sahoo SK (2011) Enhanced cellular uptake and in vivo pharmacokinetics of rapamycin-loaded cubic phase nanoparticles for cancer therapy. Acta Biomater 7 (10):3656–3669

Peer D et al (2007) Nanocarriers as an emerging platform for cancer therapy. Nat Nanotechnol 2 (12):751–760

Peter ME, Krammer PH (1998) Mechanisms of CD95 (APO-1/Fas)-mediated apoptosis. Curr Opin Immunol 10(5):545–551

Pham J, Brownlow B, Elbayoumi T (2013) Mitochondria-specific pro-apoptotic activity of genistein lipidic nanocarriers. Mol Pharm 10(10):3789–3800

Phan V et al (2013) Enhanced cytotoxicity of optimized liposomal genistein via specific induction of apoptosis in breast, ovarian and prostate carcinomas. J Drug Target 21(10):1001–1011

Plati J, Bucur O, Khosravi-Far R (2011) Apoptotic cell signaling in cancer progression and therapy. Integr Biol (Camb) 3(4):279–296

Pop C, Salvesen GS (2009) Human caspases: activation, specificity, and regulation. J Biol Chem 284(33):21777–21781

Pozo-Guisado E et al (2005) Resveratrol-induced apoptosis in MCF-7 human breast cancer cells involves a caspase-independent mechanism with downregulation of Bcl-2 and NF-kappa B. Int J Cancer 115(1):74–84. (Erratum in vol 116, pg 1004, 2005)

Prietsch RF et al (2014) Genistein induces apoptosis and autophagy in human breast MCF-7 cells by modulating the expression of proapoptotic factors and oxidative stress enzymes. Mol Cell Biochem 390(1-2):235–242

Ramadass SK et al (2015) Paclitaxel/epigallocatechin gallate coloaded liposome: a synergistic delivery to control the invasiveness of MDA-MB-231 breast cancer cells. Colloids Surf B Biointerfaces 125:65–72

Ranganathan S, Halagowder D, Sivasithambaram ND (2015) Quercetin suppresses twist to induce apoptosis in MCF-7 breast cancer cells. PLoS One 10(10):e0141370

Rapoport N (2004) Combined cancer therapy by micellar-encapsulated drug and ultrasound. Int J Pharm 277(1-2):155–162

Reimertz C et al (2001) Ca(2+)-induced inhibition of apoptosis in human SH-SY5Y neuroblastoma cells: degradation of apoptotic protease activating factor-1 (APAF-1). J Neurochem 78 (6):1256–1266

Rouleau M et al (2010) PARP inhibition: PARP1 and beyond. Nat Rev Cancer 10(4):293–301

Ruan G, Feng SS (2003) Preparation and characterization of poly(lactic acid)-poly(ethylene glycol)-poly(lactic acid) (PLA-PEG-PLA) microspheres for controlled release of paclitaxel. Biomaterials 24(27):5037–5044

Rubio-Moscardo F et al (2005) Characterization of 8p21.3 chromosomal deletions in B-cell lymphoma: TRAIL-R1 and TRAIL-R2 as candidate dosage-dependent tumor suppressor genes. Blood 106(9):3214–3222

Saelens X et al (2004) Toxic proteins released from mitochondria in cell death. Oncogene 23 (16):2861–2874

Saelens X et al (2005) Protein synthesis persists during necrotic cell death. J Cell Biol 168 (4):545–551

Saengkrit N et al (2014) Influence of curcumin-loaded cationic liposome on anticancer activity for cervical cancer therapy. Colloids Surf B Biointerfaces 114:349–356

Sah JF et al (2004) Epigallocatechin-3-gallate inhibits epidermal growth factor receptor signaling pathway. Evidence for direct inhibition of ERK1/2 and AKT kinases. J Biol Chem 279 (13):12755–12762

Sale EM, Sale GJ (2008) Protein kinase B: signalling roles and therapeutic targeting. Cell Mol Life Sci 65(1):113–127

Salti GI et al (2000) Genistein induces apoptosis and topoisomerase II-mediated DNA breakage in colon cancer cells. Eur J Cancer 36(6):796–802

Sarbassov DD et al (2005) Phosphorylation and regulation of Akt/PKB by the rictor-mTOR complex. Science 307(5712):1098–1101

Savill J, Fadok V (2000) Corpse clearance defines the meaning of cell death. Nature 407 (6805):784–788

Schimmer AD (2004) Inhibitor of apoptosis proteins: translating basic knowledge into clinical practice. Cancer Res 64(20):7183–7190

Seo HS et al (2011) Phytoestrogens induce apoptosis via extrinsic pathway, inhibiting nuclear factor-kappaB signaling in HER2-overexpressing breast cancer cells. Anticancer Res 31 (10):3301–3313

Sercombe L et al (2015) Advances and challenges of liposome assisted drug delivery. Front Pharmacol 6:286

Sharma G et al (2015) Methoxy poly(ethylene glycol)-poly(lactide) nanoparticles encapsulating quercetin act as an effective anticancer agent by inducing apoptosis in breast cancer. Pharm Res 32(2):723–735

She QB et al (2001) Resveratrol-induced activation of p53 and apoptosis is mediated by extracellular-signal-regulated protein kinases and p38 kinase. Cancer Res 61(4):1604–1610

Shim JH et al (2008) (-)-Epigallocatechin gallate regulates CD3-mediated T cell receptor signaling in leukemia through the inhibition of ZAP-70 kinase. J Biol Chem 283(42):28370–28379

Siddiqui IA et al (2009) Introducing nanochemoprevention as a novel approach for cancer control: proof of principle with green tea polyphenol epigallocatechin-3-gallate. Cancer Res 69 (5):1712–1716

Singh S, Aggarwal BB (1995) Activation of transcription factor Nf-kappa-B is suppressed by curcumin (diferulolylmethane). J Biol Chem 270(42):24995–25000

Singh SK et al (2017) Resveratrol induces cell cycle arrest and apoptosis with docetaxel in prostate cancer cells via a p53/p21(WAF1/CIP1) and p27(KIP1) pathway. Oncotarget 8 (10):17216–17228

Slee EA, Adrain C, Martin SJ (2001) Executioner caspase-3, -6, and -7 perform distinct, non-redundant roles during the demolition phase of apoptosis. J Biol Chem 276(10):7320–7326

Soldani C, Scovassi AI (2002) Poly(ADP-ribose) polymerase-1 cleavage during apoptosis: an update. Apoptosis 7(4):321–328

Somanath PR et al (2009) The role of PAK-1 in activation of MAP kinase cascade and oncogenic transformation by Akt. Oncogene 28(25):2365–2369

Song G, Ouyang G, Bao S (2005) The activation of Akt/PKB signaling pathway and cell survival. J Cell Mol Med 9(1):59–71

Stambolic V et al (1998) Negative regulation of PKB/Akt-dependent cell survival by the tumor suppressor PTEN. Cell 95(1):29–39

Stephens L et al (1998) Protein kinase B kinases that mediate phosphatidylinositol 3,4,5-trisphosphate-dependent activation of protein kinase B. Science 279(5351):710–714

Suliman A et al (2001) Intracellular mechanisms of TRAIL: apoptosis through mitochondrial-dependent and -independent pathways. Oncogene 20(17):2122–2133

Sun L, Zhang C, Li P (2014) Copolymeric micelles for delivery of EGCG and cyclopamine to pancreatic cancer cells. Nutr Cancer 66(5):896–903

Sylvester PW (2007) Vitamin E and apoptosis. Vitam Horm 76:329–356

Tessitore L et al (2000) Resveratrol depresses the growth of colorectal aberrant crypt foci by affecting bax and p21(CIP) expression. Carcinogenesis 21(8):1619–1622
Trump BF et al (1997) The pathways of cell death: oncosis, apoptosis, and necrosis. Toxicol Pathol 25(1):82–88
Vahsen N et al (2004) AIF deficiency compromises oxidative phosphorylation. EMBO J 23 (23):4679–4689
Vanags DM et al (1996) Protease involvement in fodrin cleavage and phosphatidylserine exposure in apoptosis. J Biol Chem 271(49):31075–31085
Vancompernolle K et al (1998) Atractyloside-induced release of cathepsin B, a protease with caspase-processing activity. FEBS Lett 438(3):150–158
Vanden Berghe T et al (2004) Differential signaling to apoptotic and necrotic cell death by Fas-associated death domain protein FADD. J Biol Chem 279(9):7925–7933
van Hille B, Perrin D, Hill BT (1999) Differential in vitro interactions of a series of clinically useful topoisomerase-interacting compounds with the cleavage/religation activity of the human topoisomerase IIalpha and IIbeta isoforms. Anticancer Drugs 10(6):551–560
van Loo G et al (2002) The serine protease Omi/HtrA2 is released from mitochondria during apoptosis. Omi interacts with caspase-inhibitor XIAP and induces enhanced caspase activity. Cell Death Differ 9(1):20–26
Vazquez F et al (2000) Phosphorylation of the PTEN tail regulates protein stability and function. Mol Cell Biol 20(14):5010–5018
Vijayakumar MR et al (2016) Pharmacokinetics, biodistribution, in vitro cytotoxicity and biocompatibility of Vitamin E TPGS coated trans resveratrol liposomes. Colloids Surf B Biointerfaces 145:479–491
Wajant H (2002) The Fas signaling pathway: more than a paradigm. Science 296(5573):1635–1636
Wang JB et al (2009) Curcumin induces apoptosis through the mitochondria-mediated apoptotic pathway in HT-29 cells. J Zhejiang Univ Sci B 10(2):93–102
Wang XX et al (2011) The use of mitochondrial targeting resveratrol liposomes modified with a dequalinium polyethylene glycol-distearoylphosphatidyl ethanolamine conjugate to induce apoptosis in resistant lung cancer cells. Biomaterials 32(24):5673–5687
Wang S et al (2014) Epigallocatechin-3-gallate potentiates the effect of curcumin in inducing growth inhibition and apoptosis of resistant breast cancer cells. Am J Chin Med 42 (5):1279–1300
Wang S et al (2015) mPEG-b-PCL/TPGS mixed micelles for delivery of resveratrol in overcoming resistant breast cancer. Expert Opin Drug Deliv 12(3):361–373
Wang Y et al (2017a) The functional curcumin liposomes induce apoptosis in C6 glioblastoma cells and C6 glioblastoma stem cells in vitro and in animals. Int J Nanomed 12:1369–1384
Wang W et al (2017b) Anticancer effects of resveratrol-loaded solid lipid nanoparticles on human breast cancer cells. Molecules 22(11)
Wang YR et al (2018) Barbaloin loaded polydopamine-polylactide-TPGS (PLA-TPGS) nanoparticles against gastric cancer as a targeted drug delivery system: studies in vitro and in vivo. Biochem Biophys Res Commun 499(1):8–16
Weeds AG et al (1986) Preparation and characterization of pig plasma and platelet gelsolins. Eur J Biochem 161(1):69–76
Win KY, Feng SS (2006) In vitro and in vivo studies on vitamin E TPGS-emulsified poly(D, L-lactic-co-glycolic acid) nanoparticles for paclitaxel formulation. Biomaterials 27 (10):2285–2291
Wissing SA, Muller RH (2003) The influence of solid lipid nanoparticles on skin hydration and viscoelasticity—in vivo study. Eur J Pharm Biopharm 56(1):67–72
Xu W, Ling P, Zhang T (2013) Polymeric micelles, a promising drug delivery system to enhance bioavailability of poorly water-soluble drugs. J Drug Deliv 2013:340315
Xu G et al (2015) Enhancing the anti-colon cancer activity of quercetin by self-assembled micelles. Int J Nanomed 10:2051–2063

Yamasaki M et al (2013) Genistein induces apoptotic cell death associated with inhibition of the NF-kappaB pathway in adult T-cell leukemia cells. Cell Biol Int 37(7):742–747
Yang X et al (2015) Curcumin-encapsulated polymeric micelles suppress the development of colon cancer in vitro and in vivo. Sci Rep 5:10322
Youle RJ, Strasser A (2008) The BCL-2 protein family: opposing activities that mediate cell death. Nat Rev Mol Cell Biol 9(1):47–59
Yuan ZP et al (2006) Liposomal quercetin efficiently suppresses growth of solid tumors in murine models. Clin Cancer Res 12(10):3193–3199
Zeiss CJ (2003) The apoptosis-necrosis continuum: insights from genetically altered mice. Vet Pathol 40(5):481–495
Zhang L et al (2008) Nanoparticles in medicine: therapeutic applications and developments. Clin Pharmacol Ther 83(5):761–769
Zhang X et al (2011) Akt, FoxO and regulation of apoptosis. Biochim Biophys Acta 1813 (11):1978–1986
Zhang Z, Tan S, Feng SS (2012) Vitamin E TPGS as a molecular biomaterial for drug delivery. Biomaterials 33(19):4889–4906
Zhang Z et al (2013) Genistein induces G2/M cell cycle arrest and apoptosis via ATM/p53-dependent pathway in human colon cancer cells. Int J Oncol 43(1):289–296
Zhang J et al (2014) TPGS-g-PLGA/Pluronic F68 mixed micelles for tanshinone IIA delivery in cancer therapy. Int J Pharm 476(1-2):185–198
Zhang P et al (2017) Curcumin synergizes with 5-fluorouracil by impairing AMPK/ULK1-dependent autophagy, AKT activity and enhancing apoptosis in colon cancer cells with tumor growth inhibition in xenograft mice. J Exp Clin Cancer Res 36(1):190
Zhao MH et al (2017) Quercetin-loaded mixed micelles exhibit enhanced cytotoxic efficacy in non-small cell lung cancer in vitro. Exp Ther Med 14(6):5503–5508
Zhou N et al (2009) Genistein inhibition of topoisomerase IIalpha expression participated by Sp1 and Sp3 in HeLa cell. Int J Mol Sci 10(7):3255–3268
Zhou P et al (2017) Genistein induces apoptosis of colon cancer cells by reversal of epithelial-to-mesenchymal via a Notch1/NF-kappaB/slug/E-cadherin pathway. BMC Cancer 17(1):813
Zhu X, Anquillare ELB, Farokhzad OC, Shi J (2014) Polymer- and protein-based nanotechnologies for cancer theranostics. In: Chen X, Wong S (eds) Cancer theranostics. Academic, Oxford pp 419–436
Zhu WT et al (2017) Delivery of curcumin by directed self-assembled micelles enhances therapeutic treatment of non-small-cell lung cancer. Int J Nanomed 12:2621–2634

Chapter 17
The Use of Anti-Inflammatory Agents for Cancer Chemoprevention

Aymeric Monteillier and Muriel Cuendet

Abstract Over 150 years have passed since the link between inflammation and cancer was first hypothesized, and this relationship is now widely accepted. Inflammation has been described as an important player in all stages in the process of carcinogenesis, and anti-inflammatory drugs have consistently demonstrated cancer chemopreventive activity in various animal models. Considering the global cancer burden and the difficulty to treat most cancers, the development of such a preventive strategy using readily available anti-inflammatory drugs is highly appealing. However, most existing anti-inflammatory drugs come with serious side effects (gastrointestinal bleeding for NSAIDs, cardiotoxicity for COX-2 inhibitors) that would hamper their long-term use in large populations at risk of cancer development. In this context, important efforts have been made by both academia and industry to discover new potent and safe anti-inflammatory compounds with cancer chemopreventive properties. Natural reservoirs are of high interest in support of this prospect, owing to their richness and the chemical diversity they offer. The present chapter recapitulates the main preclinical and clinical advances on the search for anti-inflammatory cancer chemopreventive compounds.

17.1 Inflammation and Cancer

Inflammation is a physiological immune response to infection and tissue injury that aims at delivering blood components, mainly plasma and leucocytes, to the site of injury in order to fight external agents and repair the damaged tissue (Medzhitov 2008). In the context of bacterial infection, for example, toll like receptor (TLR)-driven recognition of the microorganism by tissue macrophages results in the production of various inflammatory mediators such as chemokines, cytokines, vasoactive amines and prostaglandins. Together, these mediators are responsible

---

A. Monteillier · M. Cuendet (✉)
School of Pharmaceutical Sciences, University of Geneva, Geneva, Switzerland
e-mail: muriel.cuendet@unige.ch

J. M. Pezzuto, O. Vang (eds.), *Natural Products for Cancer Chemoprevention*,
https://doi.org/10.1007/978-3-030-39855-2_17

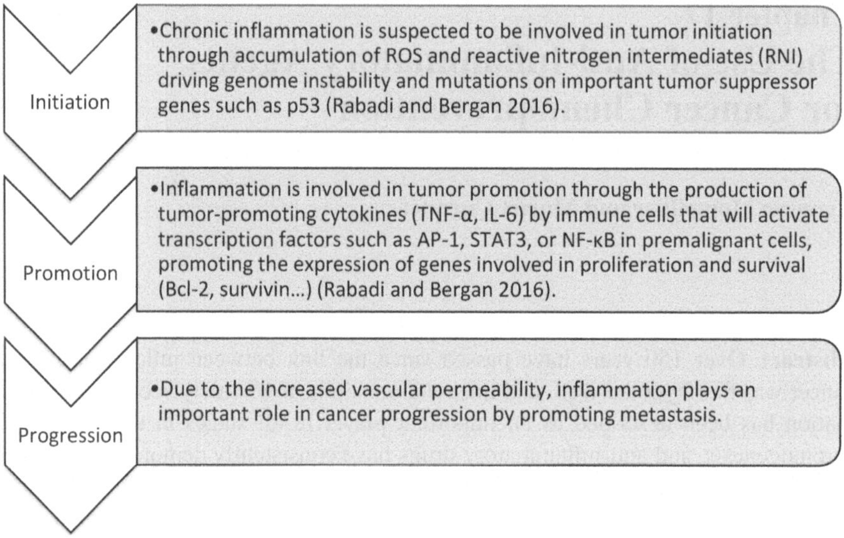

Fig. 17.1 Roles of inflammation in the carcinogenesis process

for increasing the vascular permeability, allowing plasma proteins and leukocytes (mainly neutrophils) to infiltrate the extravascular tissue and be activated. Once triggered, neutrophils release unspecific toxic molecules such as reactive oxygen species (ROS) to kill the microorganism. This process is normally well controlled and self-limited, and should be resolved by switching from production of pro-inflammatory mediators to anti-inflammatory ones such as lipoxins, resolvins, protectins, and TGF-β. This is accompanied by the recruitment of monocytes that remove the dead cells and initiate tissue remodeling.

However, dysregulation of this tightly controlled process can lead to chronic inflammation, involved in the development of several diseases, such as type 2 diabetes, cardiovascular diseases, rheumatoid arthritis and cancer (Medzhitov 2008; Ben-Neriah and Karin 2011). The link between inflammation and cancer was first hypothesized in 1863 when Rudolf Virchow observed leukocytes infiltrating tumor tissues. Since then, numerous reports confirmed and refined this hypothesis, and the implication of inflammation in all stages of the process of carcinogenesis is now widely accepted (Fig. 17.1).

17.2 NF-κB as the Driver

Among the transcription factors listed in Fig. 17.1, NF-κB was described by Ben-Neriah and Karin as the principal "matchmaker" linking inflammation and cancer (Ben-Neriah and Karin 2011). Since its discovery in 1986 in mouse B lymphocytes (Sen and Baltimore 1986), NF-κB has attracted a great deal of attention leading to a better understanding of its roles and regulatory functions. NF-κB is a family of five proteins (p50, p65 or RelA, RelB, c-Rel, and p52) ubiquitously expressed in the cytoplasm of cells of multicellular organisms, from corals to humans (Aggarwal 2004; Ben-Neriah and Karin 2011). Each protein contains a homology domain, allowing the formation of active dimers, and a nuclear localization sequence (NLS). In normal conditions, the NLS is hidden through its interaction with endogenous NF-κB inhibitors, IκB proteins, which sequestrate the dimers in the cytoplasm. When activated, NF-κB proteins can form either homo or heterodimers which are responsible for the regulation of the expression of over 500 genes involved in immune response and inflammation, but also in cell proliferation, cell survival, angiogenesis, invasion and metastasis (Barnes and Karin 1997; Aggarwal and Sung 2011).

Two main NF-κB pathways involving different dimers and resulting in various outcomes are described. The classical pathway, including p50/p65 dimers, regulates innate immunity, inflammation and cell survival, and will therefore be of particular interest in this chapter. Upon stimulation by molecules such as TNF-α or LPS, IκB proteins are phosphorylated by activated IκB kinases (IKKα/IKKβ heterodimers), ubiquitinated, and degraded by the proteasome. This releases the active dimers and allows for nuclear translocation. Once in the nucleus, p50/p65 dimers bind to DNA at the promoter region of target genes and induce expression (Fig. 17.2). An alternative pathway involves a different heterodimer, p100/RelB, and regulates lymphoid organogenesis, B-cell maturation and humoral immunity (Karin et al. 2004). In this pathway, activated IKK (IKKα/IKKα homodimers) phosphorylate p100 upon binding of cytokines from the TNF family (lymphotoxin β, RANKL). This leads to its partial proteasomal degradation into p52 and the nuclear translocation of the p52/RelB heterodimer (Karin et al. 2004). Although most research in drug discovery focuses on the classical pathway, the alternative pathway is also of importance in carcinogenesis because its activation was shown to promote the development of T-regulatory cells, and therefore allow tumors escape immunity (Lawrence 2009).

A critical aspect of both the classical and alternative pathways is nuclear import mediated by alpha members of the importin family. Importins are a group of proteins that recognize the NLS of NF-κB proteins and translocate them through the nuclear pore complexes. Nuclear translocation of p50/p65 dimers in the classical pathway involves importin α3 and α4, whereas importins α5 and α6 facilitate RelB transport (Grivennikov et al. 2010).

The classical NF-κB pathway plays a central role in both the onset and resolution of inflammation (Tang et al. 2006) and was therefore described as the conductor of inflammatory response. Consistently, it has been shown to be over-activated in many inflammatory conditions, including inflammatory bowel disease, rheumatoid arthritis, psoriasis, and cancers (Ben-Neriah and Karin 2011; Aggarwal and Sung 2011), making it a promising target for drug development (Karin et al. 2004). In the context of carcinogenesis, NF-κB is described as a "non-classical oncogene", as its activation results more often from signals produced by neighboring cells than through direct mutation (Takahashi et al. 2010).

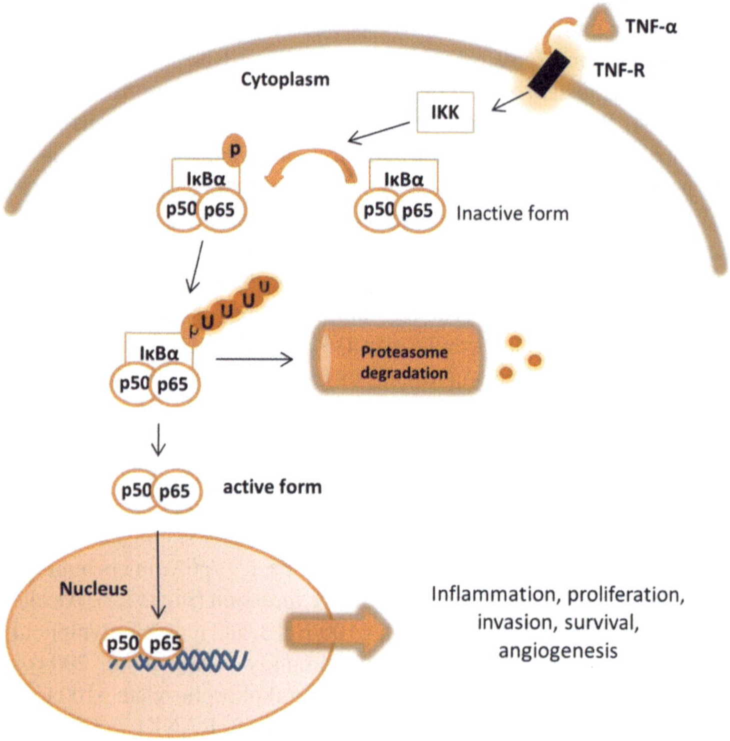

Fig. 17.2 Classical NF-κB activation pathway

17.3 Other Important Pathways

Although presented as the most important pathway because of its pivotal role in the inflammation process, NF-κB is not the only target worth investigating for inhibiting inflammation-driven carcinogenesis. At least two other proteins have been consistently shown to be involved in carcinogenesis: cyclooxygenase-2 (COX2) and inducible nitric-oxide synthase (iNOS). The first one is involved in the synthesis of prostaglandins from arachidonic acid, and the latter in the formation of nitric oxide, two crucial effectors of the inflammatory process (Dannenberg et al. 2001). Interestingly, both enzymes have been found to be overexpressed in various cancers (Dannenberg et al. 2001; Vannini et al. 2015), and their inhibition was effective for cancer chemoprevention in vivo (Oshima et al. 1996; Ramasamy et al. 2011). While the expression of both is known to be regulated by NF-κB, their specific inhibition offers theoretically the advantage of more selectivity compared to a general NF-κB inhibition that will affect all target genes.

17.4 Anti-Inflammatory Agents in Cancer Chemoprevention

Supporting the paradigm of inflammation-driven carcinogenesis, long-term use of aspirin and other non-steroidal anti-inflammatory drugs (NSAIDs) has been correlated with a reduced incidence of various cancers. Among the 12 FDA approved drugs for cancer chemoprevention, three are NSAIDs (aspirin, celecoxib, and diclofenac) (Rabadi and Bergan 2016).

17.4.1 Aspirin

The largest amount of evidence was collected for aspirin, with several clinical studies reporting a 7–10% reduction in all cancer incidence and 9–12% reduction in mortality if taken for 10 years (Cuzick 2017). The greatest extent of prevention was observed for colorectal, esophageal and gastric cancers, in which incidence was decreased by up to 30%. Therefore, and despite the risk of gastrointestinal bleeding, regular intake of aspirin is recommended by the United States Preventive Services Task Force to people aged between 50 and 59 years having a 10% risk of developing cardiovascular diseases within 10 years and no increased risk for bleeding, for prevention of cardiovascular diseases and colon cancer (The United States Preventive Services Task Force 2018). However, daily intake of aspirin for the sole prevention of colorectal cancer is not recommended because of the increased risk of severe gastrointestinal bleeding. A recent clinical trial on around 19,000 healthy persons 70 years of age or older followed for a median of 4.7 years showed that the use of low-dose aspirin did not prolong disability-free survival, but led to a higher rate of major hemorrhage than placebo (McNeil et al. 2018).

17.4.2 Celecoxib

The COX-2 selective inhibitor celecoxib was first developed for its anti-inflammatory activity and limited gastrointestinal toxicity compared to non-selective inhibitors. It was shown to reduce the number of polyps by 28% in patients with familial adenomatous polyposis (FAP) and it is now approved by the FDA in colorectal cancer chemoprevention for people with FAP (Henney 2000). Besides colorectal cancer, a double blind randomized phase II clinical trial validated the potential efficacy of celecoxib in non-small cell lung cancer (NSCLC) prevention in former smokers. In that study, treated patients exhibited reduced Ki-67 expression (a commonly used proliferation marker) and lung nodule size compared with the placebo group (Mao et al. 2011). However, its use should be restricted to people with low risk of cardiovascular disease due to the potential of cardiotoxicity, and this excludes most heavy smokers.

17.4.3 Diclofenac

Another NSAID, diclofenac, is approved for the treatment of actinic keratosis, a pre-cancerous skin lesion (Gravitz 2011). In this indication, diclofenac exhibited the same efficacy as 5-fluorouracil with less toxicity (Nelson 2011). More recently, a phase II randomized controlled clinical trial also demonstrated the efficacy of diclofenac for superficial basal cell carcinoma treatment, with a total tumor regression in 64% of treated patients (Brinkhuizen et al. 2016). Diclofenac could therefore be presented as an alternative therapy for low risk superficial basal cell carcinoma instead of the gold standard surgical excision. This effect was accompanied by a significant decrease in Ki-67 and Bcl-2 expression, highlighting the antiproliferative and proapoptotic effects of diclofenac.

17.4.4 Corticosteroids

In addition to their use for the treatment of chronic inflammatory diseases such as rheumatoid arthritis or chronic obstructive pulmonary disease (COPD), corticosteroids (e.g., dexamethasone) have been shown to exert pro-apoptotic activities in lymphoid cancers, and are used in combination with other drugs against leukemia and lymphoma (Lin and Wang 2016). The anticancer activity of corticosteroids involves complex mechanisms, among which inhibition of the NF-κB pathway. When activated through the binding of corticosteroids, the cortisol-glucocorticoid receptor complex directly interacts with NF-κB and blocks its transcriptional activity (Rhen and Cidlowski 2005). In addition to their curative properties in hematological malignancies, corticosteroids exhibited preclinical activity against lung cancer (Greenberg et al. 2002; Yao et al. 2004) and showed a lung cancer chemopreventive effect in female patients with COPD (Liu et al. 2017). However, conflicting results between prospective and retrospective studies rendered the interest in corticosteroids for lung cancer chemoprevention debatable (Greenberg et al. 2013).

17.5 Natural Anti-Inflammatory Compounds in Cancer Chemoprevention

Although some anti-inflammatory cancer chemopreventive agents are available and commonly used, their indication is limited to a few cancer types and most of them present risks when used in the long term. Therefore, finding and developing both safe and effective cancer chemopreventive drugs remains a major challenge and natural reservoirs are being actively explored for this purpose.

Natural products have been used for several thousands of years to treat numerous diseases. There is currently a resurgence of interest in natural products in all areas of drug discovery due to the low success rates of combinatorial chemistry and HTS techniques. This was emphasized by the 2015 Nobel Prizes awarded to Campbell and Omura for the development of avermectin, and by Tu for the discovery of artemisinin, generating hope towards a new Golden Age of natural products (Shen 2015). Compared to synthetic compounds, natural products are thought to be "evolutionarily optimized as drug-like molecules" (Shen 2015) and are therefore an almost inexhaustible source of bioactive compounds, some of which attracted considerable attention for their cancer chemopreventive properties. Examples of the most studied natural products with anti-inflammatory cancer chemopreventive properties are listed below.

17.5.1 Resveratrol

Resveratrol (Fig. 17.3), a phytoalexin found in various plants and food products such as grapes, peanuts and berries, is one of the most studied natural product for its cancer chemopreventive properties. In the seminal study that led to such intense interest as a chemopreventive agent (Jang et al. 1997), orally administered resveratrol was found to demonstrate a strong anti-inflammatory response in the rat paw model. More recently, even though thousands of papers have been published describing the actions of resveratrol, it has been suggested that anti-inflammatory potential is actually the greatest attribute of the compound (Pezzuto 2019). Interestingly, although resveratrol inhibits both COX-1 and -2, there is no indication that ulcer generation or gastrointestinal bleeding results from ingestion of the compound. Resveratrol has shown activity against various forms of cancers, together with a low toxicity profile (Aggarwal et al. 2004; Tome-Carneiro et al. 2013; Wahab et al. 2017; Jiang et al. 2017). The chemopreventive activity involves numerous mechanisms of action, but notably including the inhibition of NF-κB and COX (Aggarwal et al. 2004; Takahashi et al. 2010; Elshaer et al. 2018).

Nevertheless, the chemopreventive effect of resveratrol is dependent on the administration route because of its rapid and extensive liver metabolism, and in vivo efficacy was only observed in tissues exposed to high concentrations of resveratrol (Walle et al. 2004). While oral administration efficiently inhibited digestive tract carcinogenesis, only invasive intraperitoneal administration showed potential protection against more internal malignancies such as lung cancer (Hecht et al. 1999; Berge et al. 2004; Sengottuvelan and Nalini 2006; Bishayee 2009; Kurus et al. 2009; Saud et al. 2014). As such invasive parenteral administration is not feasible for the long-term daily administration of chemopreventive compounds, recent work focused on a local administration route (Monteillier et al. 2018). In one study, a cyclodextrin-based saline formulation allowed for the administration of high amounts of RES directly into the lungs through intranasal instillation in a mouse model of carcinogen-induced lung cancer. Treated mice exhibited a 45% decrease in tumor load compared to mice receiving placebo, emphasizing the efficacy of local resveratrol treatment in lung cancer chemoprevention. The relatively high number of

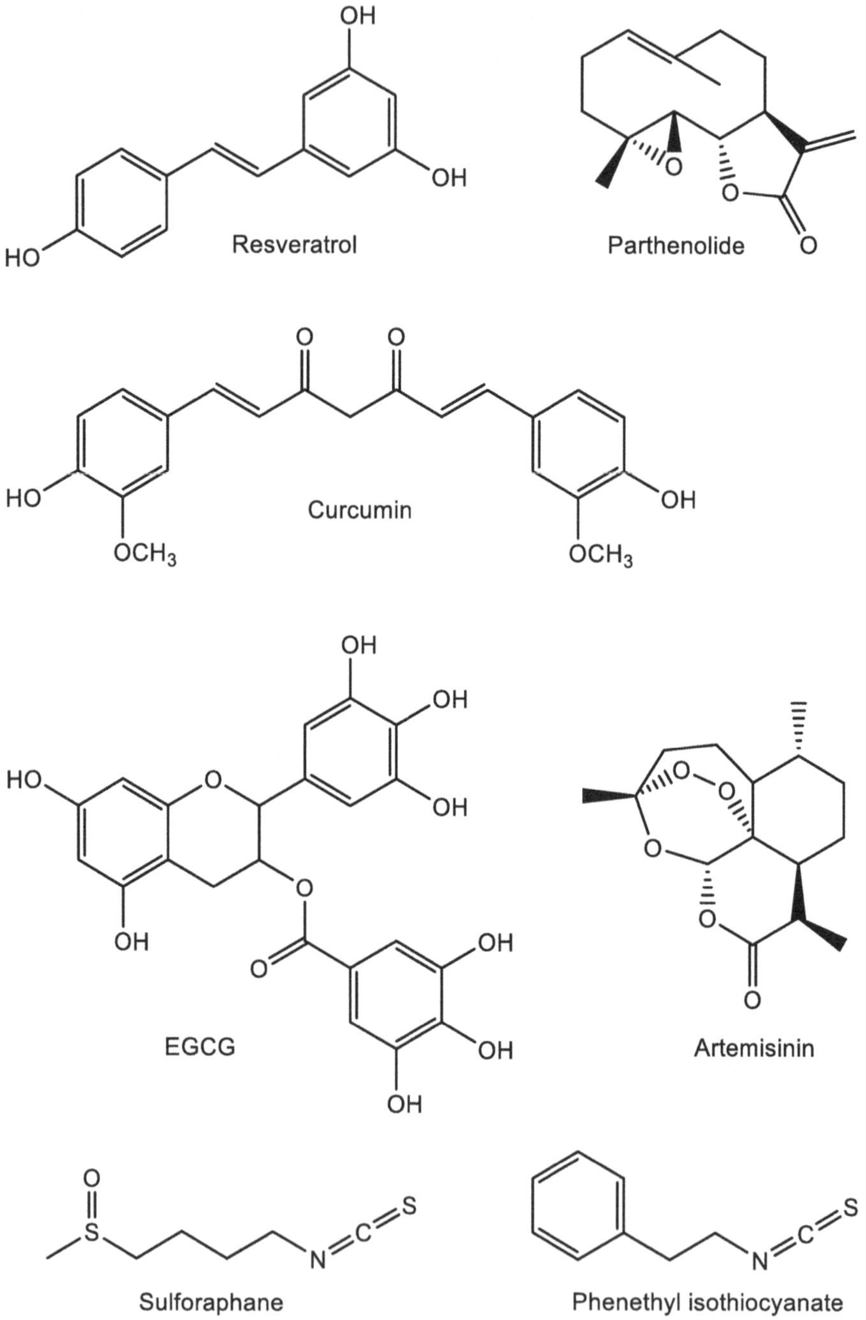

Fig. 17.3 Chemical structures of natural anti-inflammatory compounds

pathways impacted by resveratrol makes it sometimes challenging to link its in vivo activity to its anti-inflammatory properties solely. This link was however established in a study where resveratrol inhibited *N*-nitrobenzylamine-induced esophageal carcinogenesis through COX-2 downregulation, likely due to NF-κB inhibition (Li et al. 2002).

17.5.2 Curcumin

Curcumin (Fig. 17.3), a diarylheptanoid responsible for the yellow color of turmeric, is described as one of the most potent in vitro and in vivo chemopreventive natural compounds. The antiproliferative and antimetastatic properties of curcumin were partly attributed to its ability to inhibit NF-κB through IKK inhibition (Pavan et al. 2016). The clinical cancer chemopreventive properties of curcumin are being extensively studied. As an example, a phase II clinical trial reported NF-κB and COX-2 downregulation in advanced pancreatic cancer patients treated with curcumin despite bioavailability issues (Dhillon et al. 2008). More recently however, the daily administration of 3 g of curcumin for 12 weeks had no impact on number and size of polyps in patients with FAP (Cruz-Correa et al. 2018). The clinical efficacy of curcumin alone remains controversial, and several clinical trials are being conducted to assess its activity in solid tumors in combination with chemo- and radio-therapy (ClinicalTrials.gov identifiers NCT01859858, NCT03072992, NCT01490996, NCT01740323). One clinical trial investigating curcumin in breast cancer chemoprevention is also currently ongoing (ClinicalTrials.gov identifier NCT01975363).

17.5.3 Parthenolide and Derivatives

Sesquiterpene lactones are natural products mainly found in the Asteraceae family, and extensively studied for their cancer chemotherapeutic and preventive properties. Sesquiterpene lactones are known to possess strong NF-κB inhibitory properties, which have been linked to their ability to alkylate the Cys-38 residue of the p65 subunit, inhibiting its interaction with DNA and thus the transcription induction of the targeted genes (Ghantous et al. 2010). Among the sesquiterpene lactones, parthenolide (Fig. 17.3), isolated from feverfew (*Tanacetum parthenium*), has raised considerable interest in cancer chemoprevention and therapy since its discovery in the 1970s'. In vitro, parthenolide was able to inhibit NF-κB in the nanomolar range and to promote apoptosis in a wide variety of cancer cells. These results translated in vivo, where parthenolide exerted anti-proliferative and anti-metastatic effects in mice xenograft models, but its activity was again disappointing when given orally due to its poor bioavailability (Ghantous et al. 2013). This bioavailability issue was confirmed in cancer patients during a phase I study, in which parthenolide was not detectable in the plasma after the consumption of a standardized feverfew extract

(Curry et al. 2004). Therefore, dimethylamino-parthenolide (DMAPT), a more water soluble parthenolide derivative, was synthetized and exhibited improved pharmacokinetic properties, with an oral bioavailability of 70%, resulting in effective anticancer activity in vivo (Ghantous et al. 2013). However, neither parthenolide nor DMAPT were able to completely eliminate tumors when given as single agents, highlighting the potential interest of combinations with classical chemotherapeutic agents. A phase 1 clinical trial was conducted on DMAPT for the treatment of leukemia, but no results are available yet (Ghantous et al. 2013).

17.5.4 Artemisinin Derivatives

Another sesquiterpene lactone, artesunate, was the subject of many studies in the past years. Artesunate is a semi-synthetic derivative of the antimalarial drug artemisinin (Fig. 17.3), which has been reported to exert cytotoxic, antiangiogenic, antimetastatic, and anti-inflammatory activities (Ho et al. 2014). The anti-inflammatory activity of artemisinin derivatives was attributed to their ability to inhibit TLRs, PI-3K, MAPK, and the NF-κB pathway. Compared to artemisinin, artesunate has an improved in vitro cytotoxicity and induced clinical remission in patients with advanced cervical carcinoma after 28 days of oral administration during a phase I study (Jansen et al. 2011). Two other recent phase I studies concluded on the safety of both oral and intravenous artesunate administration (von Hagens et al. 2017; Deeken et al. 2018), and a phase II clinical trial is currently recruiting patients with colorectal cancers (NCT02633098).

17.5.5 Isothiocyanates

The cancer chemopreventive properties of isothiocyanates has been hypothesized since epidemiological evidence reported the link between consumption of cruciferous vegetables (plants of the Brassicaceae family) and reduced risk of developing colorectal, prostate, and lung cancers (Gründemann and Huber 2018). These compounds are produced by the hydrolysis of glucosinolates contained in the plant when the cells are broken or when they are in contact with enzymes from the gut microbiota. Among this family, sulforaphane and phenethyl isothiocyanate (Fig. 17.3) are the two most described compounds for their cancer chemopreventive properties, involving various mechanisms of action, such as an increased carcinogen detoxification (inhibition of phase I enzymes and induction of phase II enzymes) and anti-inflammatory activity. The latter has been shown to be mediated by NF-κB inhibition through direct interaction of thiol groups and p50, as well as inhibition of IκBα phosphorylation. NF-κB inhibition by sulforaphane was also shown to decrease COX-2 expression in vitro (Gründemann and Huber 2018). Animal experiments confirmed the chemopreventive activity of these compounds in models of carcinogen-induced skin, prostate, breast, and lung cancers (Gründemann and Huber 2018). Interestingly, the length of the alkyl chain seemed to affect the in vivo chemopreventive activity of phenethyl isothiocyanate derivatives, the most potent compound being the one with the longest chain [6-phenylhexyl isothiocyanate (PHITC)], allowing for a 95% decrease in lung tumor incidence in mice.

Clinical trials were performed on various isothiocyanates and led to the following results. Oral intake of 60 mg of sulforaphane for 6 months following radical prostatectomy in patients with prostate cancer significantly decreased the postoperative PSA level increase compared to placebo (Cipolla et al. 2015). In another randomized controlled clinical trial, 40 mg of phenethyl isothiocyanate/day during 1 week significantly decreased nicotine-derived nitrosamine ketone (NNK) bioactivation in smokers (Yuan et al. 2016).

Long-term studies with large sample size will be necessary to assess the effect of isothiocyanate consumption on tumor development itself. Most interestingly, a randomized controlled clinical trial is currently recruiting over 70 former smokers with bronchial dysplasia to assess the efficacy of daily intake of sulforaphane, notably looking at cell proliferation and apoptosis (NCT03232138). This study is expected to be completed in 2022 and the results will shed more light on the future development potential of isothiocyanates in cancer chemoprevention.

17.5.6 Green Tea Catechins

Green tea, the water extract of unfermented dry leaves of *Camellia sinensis*, contains many polyphenols credited with the health benefits associated with its consumption. Green tea polyphenols are mainly catechins, and the most abundant one is (−)-epigallocatechin-3-gallate (EGCG, Fig. 17.3), accounting for over 50% of all polyphenols (Guo et al. 2017). Many in vitro and in vivo studies reported the chemopreventive properties of green tea catechins and especially EGCG against prostate, lung, and digestive tract carcinogenesis (Yang and Wang 2016; Guo et al. 2017). Besides its well-described antioxidant properties, EGCG also exerts anti-inflammatory activities by inhibiting TNF-α-induced degradation of IκB in both cancer and normal cells, leading to apoptosis induction in prostate cancer cells (Nam 2006; Guo et al. 2017).

In humans, clinical trials concluded on the safety of long-term daily administration of green tea extracts containing between 200 and 843 mg of EGCG (Bettuzzi et al. 2006; Dostal et al. 2015; Kumar et al. 2016). The chemopreventive effect observed remains, however, controversial. Striking results were obtained by Bettuzzi et al. who conducted a double-blind randomized placebo-controlled trial on 60 patients with high-grade prostate intraepithelial neoplasia (PIN), a premalignant lesion of prostate cancer. Thirty patients were treated with green tea catechins, corresponding to a dose of about 300 mg of EGCG/day, during 1 year. At the 1-year follow-up, only 1 cancer was diagnosed in the treated group (3% of the patients), versus 9 in the placebo group (30% of the patients), suggesting a 90% chemopreventive efficacy (Bettuzzi et al. 2006). Subsequent follow-up 2 years after the end of the treatment confirmed a significant difference in cancer prevalence between treated and control groups ($p < 0.01$) with a 80% reduction in cancer diagnosis in the treated group (Bettuzzi et al. 2006). Conversely, a recent study using a similar protocol did not show a significant difference in prostate cancer prevalence at 1-year follow-up between patients receiving daily green tea catechins (corresponding to a dose of 400 mg of EGCG) and the control group (Kumar et al. 2015). Another recent randomized controlled trial led on postmenopausal women at increased risk of breast cancer failed to show a significant difference in mammographic density after 1-year of supplementation with green tea extracts (corresponding to a daily dose of 843 mg of EGCG) (Samavat et al. 2017). Further clinical trials are currently being conducted to investigate the interest of green tea catechins and EGCG for the prevention of liver and colorectal cancer (NCT02891538, NCT03278925), and the treatment of lung cancer (NCT01317953).

17.6 Conclusion and Future Directions

Despite over 50 years of research in cancer chemoprevention, only 12 prophylactic drugs have reached the market, covering a rather small portion of population and malignancies. Hence the need is still present, especially for the most lethal malignancies such as lung cancer (Greenberg et al. 2013; Clamon 2015). Among the various pathways involved in lung carcinogenesis, NF-κB is a promising target and its inhibition in people at high risk is predicted to provide protection against various malignancies (Tang et al. 2006; Meylan et al. 2009; Takahashi et al. 2010). The progresses made on the search for natural anti-inflammatory compounds for cancer chemoprevention have led many molecules to be tested in humans, with variable clinical outcome. Most of the natural products presented above are hampered by a poor bioavailability. Therefore, innovative modes of administration and derivatives were developed and have shown superior activity in animal models. This should now be investigated clinically.

Beside their cancer chemopreventive properties, these compounds are also of interest for chemotherapy, especially in combination with cytotoxic compounds, in an adjuvant setting. While NF-κB inhibition is not always sufficient to trigger cancer cell death (depending on their dependence for this pathway), it can be used to increase their sensitivity to conventional chemotherapy. Such combinations can allow the administration of lower doses of cytotoxic treatments, with increased efficacy and decreased side effects. For example, parthenolide was able to potentiate the efficacy of taxol in non-small cell lung cancer through NF-κB inhibition (Zhang et al. 2009). Moreover, chemotherapy-induced NF-κB is often observed in resistant cancers, and the combination of conventional chemotherapeutic drugs with NF-κB inhibitors has been shown to overcome resistance to chemotherapy. Therefore, many ongoing clinical trials are focusing on combinations between some natural products mentioned in this chapter and chemotherapies, and results will hopefully strengthen the interest in natural anti-inflammatory compounds for the management of cancer.

References

Aggarwal BB (2004) Nuclear factor-κB: the enemy within. Cancer Cell 6:203–208

Aggarwal BB, Sung B (2011) NF-κB in cancer: a matter of life and death. Cancer Discov 1:469–471

Aggarwal BB, Bhardwaj A, Aggarwal RS et al (2004) Role of resveratrol in prevention and therapy of cancer: preclinical and clinical studies. Anticancer Res 24:2783–2840

Barnes PJ, Karin M (1997) Nuclear factor-κB—a pivotal transcription factor in chronic inflammatory diseases. N Engl J Med 336:1066–1071

Ben-Neriah Y, Karin M (2011) Inflammation meets cancer, with NF-κB as the matchmaker. Nat Immunol 12:715–723

Berge G, Øvrebø S, Eilertsen E et al (2004) Analysis of resveratrol as a lung cancer chemopreventive agent in A/J mice exposed to benzo[a]pyrene. Br J Cancer 91:1380–1383

Bettuzzi S, Brausi M, Rizzi F et al (2006) Chemoprevention of human prostate cancer by oral administration of green tea catechins in volunteers with high-grade prostate intraepithelial neoplasia: a preliminary report from a one-year proof-of-principle study. Cancer Res 66:1234–1240

Bishayee A (2009) Cancer prevention and treatment with resveratrol: from rodent studies to clinical trials. Cancer Prev Res 2:409–418

Brinkhuizen T, Frencken KJA, Nelemans PJ et al (2016) The effect of topical diclofenac 3% and calcitriol 3 μg/g on superficial basal cell carcinoma (sBCC) and nodular basal cell carcinoma (nBCC): a phase II, randomized controlled trial. J Am Acad Dermatol 75:126–134

Cipolla BG, Mandron E, Lefort JM et al (2015) Effect of sulforaphane in men with biochemical recurrence after radical prostatectomy. Cancer Prev Res 8:712–719

Clamon G (2015) Chemoprevention and screening for lung cancer: changing our focus to former smokers. Clin Lung Cancer 16:1–5

Cruz-Correa M, Hylind LM, Marrero JH et al (2018) Efficacy and safety of curcumin in treatment of intestinal adenomas in patients with familial adenomatous polyposis. Gastroenterology 155:668–673

Curry EA, Murry DJ, Yoder C et al (2004) Phase I dose escalation trial of feverfew with standardized doses of parthenolide in patients with cancer. Investig New Drugs 22:299–305

Cuzick J (2017) Preventive therapy for cancer. Lancet Oncol 18:e472–e482

Dannenberg AJ, Altorki NK, Boyle JO et al (2001) Cyclo-oxygenase 2: a pharmacological target for the prevention of cancer. Lancet Oncol 2:544–551

Deeken JF, Wang H, Hartley M et al (2018) A phase I study of intravenous artesunate in patients with advanced solid tumor malignancies. Cancer Chemother Pharmacol 81:587–596

Dhillon N, Aggarwal BB, Newman RA et al (2008) Phase II trial of curcumin in patients with advanced pancreatic cancer. Clin Cancer Res 14:4491–4499

Dostal AM, Samavat H, Bedell S et al (2015) The safety of green tea extract supplementation in postmenopausal women at risk for breast cancer: results of the Minnesota Green Tea Trial. Food Chem Toxicol 83:26–35

Elshaer M, Chen Y, Wang XJ, Tang X (2018) Resveratrol: an overview of its anti-cancer mechanisms. Life Sci 207:340–349

Ghantous A, Gali-Muhtasib H, Vuorela H et al (2010) What made sesquiterpene lactones reach cancer clinical trials? Drug Discov Today 15:668–678

Ghantous A, Sinjab A, Herceg Z, Darwiche N (2013) Parthenolide: from plant shoots to cancer roots. Drug Discov Today 18:894–905

Gravitz L (2011) Chemoprevention: first line of defence. Nature 471:S5–S7

Greenberg AK, Hu J, Basu S et al (2002) Glucocorticoids inhibit lung cancer cell growth through both the extracellular signal-related kinase pathway and cell cycle regulators. Am J Respir Cell Mol Biol 27:320–328

Greenberg AK, Tsay J-C, Tchou-Wong K-M et al (2013) Chemoprevention of lung cancer: prospects and disappointments in human clinical trials. Cancers 5:131–148

Grivennikov SI, Greten FR, Karin M (2010) Immunity, inflammation, and cancer. Cell 140:883–899
Gründemann C, Huber R (2018) Chemoprevention with isothiocyanates – from bench to bedside. Cancer Lett 414:26–33
Guo Y, Zhi F, Chen P et al (2017) Green tea and the risk of prostate cancer. Medicine 96:e6426
Hecht SS, Kenney PM, Wang M et al (1999) Evaluation of butylated hydroxyanisole, myo-inositol, curcumin, esculetin, resveratrol and lycopene as inhibitors of benzo[a]pyrene plus 4-(methylnitrosamino)-1-(3-pyridyl)-1-butanone-induced lung tumorigenesis in a/J mice. Cancer Lett 137:123–130
Henney JE (2000) Celecoxib indicated for FAP. JAMA 283:1131–1131
Ho WE, Peh HY, Chan TK, Wong WSF (2014) Artemisinins: pharmacological actions beyond antimalarial. Pharmacol Ther 142:126–139
Jang M, Cai L, Udeani GO et al (1997) Cancer chemopreventive activity of resveratrol, a natural product derived from grapes. Science 275:218–220
Jansen FH, Adoubi I, Comoe JCK et al (2011) First study of oral Artenimol-R in advanced cervical cancer: clinical benefit, tolerability and tumor markers. Anticancer Res 31:4417–4422
Jiang Z, Chen K, Cheng L et al (2017) Resveratrol and cancer treatment: updates. Ann N Y Acad Sci 1403:59–69
Karin M, Yamamoto Y, Wang QM (2004) The IKK NF-κB system: a treasure trove for drug development. Nat Rev Drug Discov 3:17–26
Kumar NB, Pow-Sang J, Egan KM et al (2015) Randomized, placebo-controlled trial of green tea catechins for prostate cancer prevention. Cancer Prev Res 8:879–887
Kumar NB, Pow-Sang J, Spiess PE et al (2016) Randomized, placebo-controlled trial evaluating the safety of one-year administration of green tea catechins. Oncotarget 7:70794–70802
Kurus M, Firat Y, Cetin A et al (2009) The effect of resveratrol in tracheal tissue of rats exposed to cigarette smoke. Inhal Toxicol 21:979–984
Lawrence T (2009) The nuclear factor NF-κB pathway in inflammation. Cold Spring Harb Perspect Biol 1:a001651
Li ZG, Hong T, Shimada Y et al (2002) Suppression of N-nitrosomethylbenzylamine (NMBA)-induced esophageal tumorigenesis in F344 rats by resveratrol. Carcinogenesis 23:1531–1536
Lin K-T, Wang L-H (2016) New dimension of glucocorticoids in cancer treatment. Steroids 111:84–88
Liu S-F, Kuo H-C, Lin M-C et al (2017) Inhaled corticosteroids have a protective effect against lung cancer in female patients with chronic obstructive pulmonary disease: a nationwide population-based cohort study. Oncotarget 8:29711–29721
Mao JT, Roth MD, Fishbein MC et al (2011) Lung cancer chemoprevention with celecoxib in former smokers. Cancer Prev Res 4:984–993
McNeil JJ, Woods RL, Nelson MR et al (2018) Effect of aspirin on disability-free survival in the healthy elderly. New Engl J Med 379:1499–1508
Medzhitov R (2008) Origin and physiological roles of inflammation. Nature 454:428–435
Meylan E, Dooley AL, Feldser DM et al (2009) Requirement for NF-κB signalling in a mouse model of lung adenocarcinoma. Nature 462:104–107
Monteillier A, Voisin A, Furrer P et al (2018) Intranasal administration of resveratrol successfully prevents lung cancer in A/J mice. Sci Rep 8:14257
Nam N-H (2006) Naturally occurring NF-κB inhibitors. Mini Rev Med Chem 6:945–951
Nelson CG (2011) Diclofenac gel in the treatment of actinic keratoses. Ther Clin Risk Manag 7:207–211
Oshima M, Dinchuk JE, Kargman SL et al (1996) Suppression of intestinal polyposis in ApcΔ716 knockout mice by inhibition of cyclooxygenase 2 (COX-2). Cell 87:803–809
Pavan AR, Silva GD, Jornada DH et al (2016) Unraveling the anticancer effect of curcumin and resveratrol. Nutrients 8:628
Pezzuto JM (2019) Resveratrol: twenty years of growth, development and controversy. Biomol Ther 27:1–14

Rabadi LA, Bergan R (2016) A way forward for cancer chemoprevention: think local. Cancer Prev Res 10:14–35

Ramasamy K, Dwyer-Nield LD, Serkova NJ et al (2011) Silibinin prevents lung tumorigenesis in wild-type but not in iNOS−/− mice: potential of real-time micro-CT in lung cancer chemoprevention studies. Clin Cancer Res 17:753–761

Rhen T, Cidlowski JA (2005) Antiinflammatory action of glucocorticoids—new mechanisms for old drugs. N Engl J Med 353:1711–1723

Samavat H, Ursin G, Emory TH et al (2017) A randomized controlled trial of green tea extract supplementation and mammographic density in postmenopausal women at increased risk of breast cancer. Cancer Prev Res 10:710–718

Saud SM, Li W, Morris NL et al (2014) Resveratrol prevents tumorigenesis in mouse model of Kras activated sporadic colorectal cancer by suppressing oncogenic Kras expression. Carcinogenesis 35:2778–2786

Sen R, Baltimore D (1986) Multiple nuclear factors interact with the immunoglobulin enhancer sequences. Cell 46:705–716

Sengottuvelan M, Nalini N (2006) Dietary supplementation of resveratrol suppresses colonic tumour incidence in 1,2-dimethylhydrazine-treated rats by modulating biotransforming enzymes and aberrant crypt foci development. Br J Nutr 96:145–153

Shen B (2015) A new golden age of natural products drug discovery. Cell 163:1297–1300

Takahashi H, Ogata H, Nishigaki R et al (2010) Tobacco smoke promotes lung tumorigenesis by triggering IKKβ and JNK1 dependent inflammation. Cancer Cell 17:89–97

Tang X, Liu D, Shishodia S et al (2006) Nuclear factor-κB (NF-κB) is frequently expressed in lung cancer and preneoplastic lesions. Cancer 107:2637–2646

The United States Preventive Services Task Force (2018) Task force releases recommendations on aspirin to prevent colon cancer, heart disease. https://www.cancer.org/latest-news/task-force-releases-recommendations-on-aspirin-to-prevent-colon-cancer-heart-disease.html.

Tome-Carneiro J, Larrosa M, Gonzalez-Sarrias A et al (2013) Resveratrol and clinical trials: the crossroad from in vitro studies to human evidence. Curr Pharm Des 19:6064–6093

Vannini F, Kashfi K, Nath N (2015) The dual role of iNOS in cancer. Redox Biol 6:334–343

von Hagens C, Walter-Sack I, Goeckenjan M et al (2017) Prospective open uncontrolled phase I study to define a well-tolerated dose of oral artesunate as add-on therapy in patients with metastatic breast cancer (ARTIC M33/2). Breast Cancer Res Treat 164:359–369

Wahab A, Gao K, Jia C et al (2017) Significance of resveratrol in clinical management of chronic diseases. Molecules 22:1329

Walle T, Hsieh F, DeLegge MH et al (2004) High absorption but very low bioavailability of oral resveratrol in humans. Drug Metab Dispos 32:1377–1382

Yang CS, Wang H (2016) Cancer preventive activities of tea catechins. Molecules 21:1679

Yao R, Wang Y, Lemon WJ et al (2004) Budesonide exerts its chemopreventive efficacy during mouse lung tumorigenesis by modulating gene expressions. Oncogene 23:7746–7752

Yuan J-M, Stepanov I, Murphy SE et al (2016) Clinical trial of 2-phenethyl isothiocyanate as an inhibitor of metabolic activation of a tobacco-specific lung carcinogen in cigarette smokers. Cancer Prev Res 9:396–405

Zhang D, Qiu L, Jin X et al (2009) Nuclear factor-kappaB inhibition by parthenolide potentiates the efficacy of Taxol in non-small cell lung cancer in vitro and in vivo. Mol Cancer Res 7:1139–1149

Chapter 18
Combination Cancer Chemoprevention by Targeting the Epigenome

Clarissa Gerhauser

Abstract The past 15 years have provided a wealth of information on the influence of natural products and dietary agents on epigenetic mechanisms, including DNA methylation, histone acetylation and methylation, and miRNAs. This chapter will give an overview of studies which have investigated potential additive or synergistic effects of chemopreventive agents targeting the epigenome when used in combination. These studies have focused mainly on breast and colon cancer and investigated green tea catechins and soy isoflavones, quercetin, resveratrol and pterostilbene, withaferin A, the short chain fatty acid butyrate, sulforaphane, selenium, curcumin, synthetic triterpenoids, and docosahexaenoic acid (DHA). Up to now, investigations were limited to in vitro cell culture and animal models. The most promising finding might be the reactivation of the estrogen receptor in estrogen receptor-negative breast cancer by various combinations of DNA demethylating and histone-modifying compounds, increasing susceptibility to anti-hormonal therapy.

18.1 Introduction

The term "epigenetics" refers to modifications in gene expression caused by heritable, but potentially reversible, changes in DNA methylation and chromatin structure, without alterations in DNA sequence (Felsenfeld 2014). Major epigenetic mechanisms include DNA hyper- and hypomethylation (Jones 2012), remodeling of the chromatin, modification of histones by histone acetylation and methylation (among others) (Barnes et al. 2019), and non-coding RNAs (Guil and Esteller 2009).

C. Gerhauser (✉)
Workgroup Cancer Chemoprevention and Epigenomics, Division Cancer Epigenomics, German Cancer Research Center (DKFZ), Heidelberg, Germany
e-mail: c.gerhauser@dkfz.de

J. M. Pezzuto, O. Vang (eds.), *Natural Products for Cancer Chemoprevention*,
https://doi.org/10.1007/978-3-030-39855-2_18

18.1.1 DNA Methylation

Methylation at the C5 position of cytosines in the context of CpG dinucleotides is the most prevalent DNA-based epigenetic mark in the human genome. Considering that all cells of an organism share the same genomic information, an important feature of DNA methylation is that it regulates gene transcription in a cell-type specific manner. The DNA methyltransferase (DNMT) family of enzymes catalyzes the transfer of methyl groups from *S*-adenosyl-L-methionine (SAM) to DNA and maintains DNA methylation patterns after DNA replication. DNMT1, the maintenance methyltransferase, preferentially methylates hemimethylated DNA, whereas the methyltransferases DNMT3a and 3b are involved in methylation of fully unmethylated DNA. With few exceptions related to cell type-specific gene expression patterns, in healthy tissue, CpG-dense regions (so-called CpG islands, CGIs), located in the promoter regions of about 60% of all genes, are usually unmethylated. On the other hand, intra- and intergenic regions with lower CpG density are usually highly methylated, thus limiting accessibility of DNA and maintaining genomic stability. Also, repetitive genomic sequences are highly methylated to prevent these sites from active transcription (Stirzaker et al. 2014). Methylation at enhancer regions may protect from transcription factor binding, thus fine-tuning gene transcription. Inhibition of DNMT1 activity or downregulation of DNMT1 expression leads to passive loss of DNA methylation during cell division. Alternatively, ten-eleven translocation (TET) proteins are involved in active demethylation and can reactivate previously silenced genes (Feinberg et al. 2016).

During carcinogenesis, focal gain in methylation at CGIs in promoter regions, for example of tumor suppressor genes (TSGs), concomitant with global loss of methylation (hypomethylation), especially at repetitive sequences, is thought to be involved in the etiology of cancer (Esteller 2007; Berdasco and Esteller 2010). In contrast to irreversible genetic alterations (by mutations, deletions etc.), alterations in gene expression via epigenetic mechanisms are reversible. Consequently, aberrant methylation has been identified as an attractive target for cancer chemoprevention with dietary compounds.

18.1.2 Histone Modifications

Chromatin accessibility and gene expression is dynamically controlled by various post-translational modifications of N-terminal histone tails, including acetylation and methylation (Barnes et al. 2019; Kouzarides 2007; Soshnev et al. 2016). Histone acetylation of histone tails is catalyzed by histone acetyltransferases (HATs) that transfer acetyl groups from acetyl-CoA mainly to lysine residues, resulting in opening of the chromatin structure and facilitating transcription factor binding to promoter or enhancer regions to regulate transcription (Voss and Thomas 2018). Histone acetylation is reversed by histone deacetylases (HDACs) that remove histone acetyl groups, leading to chromatin condensation and transcriptional repression (Minucci and Pelicci 2006). Importantly, the catalytic activity of HATs and HDACs is not limited to histones, and numerous non-histone proteins, including cytoskeletal proteins, molecular chaperones, hormone receptors, nuclear import factors, and transcription factors such as p53 and NF-κB, have been identified as targets (Glozak et al. 2005; Kim et al. 2016). Besides the currently known HDACs 1-11, structurally unrelated sirtuins (SIRTs), which use NAD^+ as a cofactor, possess deacetylating activity (Seto and Yoshida 2014).

In contrast to histone acetylation, histone methylation can have activating or repressive effects on gene expression, dependent on which lysine residue is modified by methylation and how many methyl groups are transferred (Kouzarides 2007). Histone methylation by transfer of methyl groups from SAM to lysine residues is catalyzed by more than 30 histone methyltransferases (HMT) (Upadhyay and Cheng 2011; Allis et al. 2007) and removed by histone lysine demethylases. Again, these enzymes possess non-histone targets including p53, RB1 and STAT3 with important roles in carcinogenesis (Hamamoto et al. 2015). So far, the impact of chemical or natural product inhibitors of histone-modifying enzymes on non-histone proteins is likely largely underestimated in cancer prevention (Kim et al. 2016; Shortt et al. 2017).

18.1.3 Regulation of Gene Expression by Noncoding (Micro) RNAs

MicroRNAs (miRNAs or miRs) are short single stranded RNA oligonucleotides with a length of 20–23 nucleotides. They influence mRNA levels and translation by interacting with a target sequence often in the 3′ untranslated region of a gene, either by perfect base-pairing, leading to mRNA degradation, or by partial base-pairing that blocks translation. Each miRNA is estimated to control several hundred genes involved in key biological processes, including development, differentiation, apoptosis and proliferation (Calin and Croce 2006). The miRBase database currently lists about 1900 human, 1200 mouse, and 500 rat miRs (Kozomara et al. 2019). Biogenesis of miRNAs from RNA precursor structures is highly regulated and involves multiple steps [reviewed in Winter et al. (2009)]. Expression of many miRs is deregulated during cancer development. miRNAs have either tumor suppressive function, such as the miR-200 family (Park et al. 2008), or oncogenic functions (onco-miRs), such as miR-21 upregulated in many types of cancer (Wu et al. 2015). Major mechanisms contributing to their deregulation include genetic and epigenetic alterations such as DNA methylation, as well as defects in the miRNA processing machinery (Brait and Sidransky 2011).

18.2 Combination Effects Targeting the Epigenome

During the past 15 years, the influence of natural products and dietary chemopreventive agents on epigenetic mechanisms has gained major interest in the research community. Only recently, studies are emerging that are based on the combination of chemopreventive agents targeting the epigenome. Already about 40 years ago, Michael Sporn reported about the concept of 'combination chemoprevention of cancer' by combining two or more chemopreventive agents with complementary mechanisms of action to enhance efficacy while reducing toxicity (Sporn 1980). This concept has been taken up in a recent report on cancer chemoprevention by the Division of Cancer Prevention of the National Cancer Institute (Mohammed et al. 2019).

Agents investigated in combination studies with the aim to target two or more epigenetic mechanisms include green tea catechins and soy isoflavones, quercetin, resveratrol and pterostilbene, withaferin A (WA), the short chain fatty acid butyrate, sulforaphane (SFN), selenium, curcumin, synthetic triterpenoids, and docosahexaenoic acid (DHA) (Fig. 18.1).

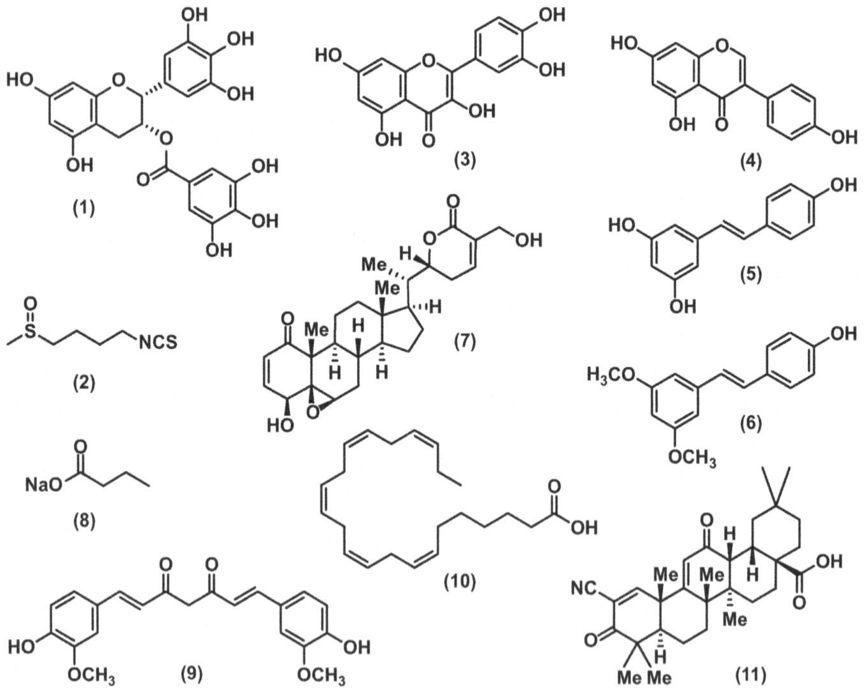

Fig. 18.1 Structures of chemopreventive agents tested in combination studies targeting epigenetic mechanisms. (1) Epigallocatechin gallate (EGCG), (2) sulforaphane (SFN), (3) quercetin, (4) genistein, (5) resveratrol, (6) piceatannol, (7) withaferin A (WA), (8) butyrate, (9) curcumin, (10) docosahexaenoic acid (DHA), (11) 2-cyano-3,12-dioxo-oleana-1,9(11)-dien-28-oic acid (CDDO)

These compounds have been tested in various combinations to explore potential additive or synergistic effects on epigenetic mechanisms, with a focus on breast and colon cancer, as outlined below. Before describing their combination effects, the compounds and their sources are briefly introduced, including a summary of their chemopreventive and epigenetic activities. For a general overview of effects of bioactive compounds on the epigenome, readers are referred to a number of recent review articles on nutri-epigenetics and cancer prevention (Link et al. 2010; vel Szic et al. 2010; Huang et al. 2011, 2019; Vanden Berghe 2012; Gerhauser 2013, 2014, 2018; Shukla et al. 2014; Aggarwal et al. 2015; Shankar et al. 2016; Carlos-Reyes et al. 2019; Gao and Tollefsbol 2015; Biersack 2016).

18.2.1 Breast Cancer Studies

With an estimated number of 2.09 million new cases and about 627,000 cancer deaths in 2018, breast cancer is worldwide the most common cancer in females (Bray et al. 2018). Based on characteristic gene expression patterns, breast cancer is clinically sub-grouped into at least five distinct subtypes (Sorlie et al. 2003). Luminal A/B breast cancers express the estrogen receptor (ER) and genes responsive to ER-signaling. HER2 tumors are characterized by amplification of the *ERBB2* gene, and patients respond to monoclonal antibody therapy with trastuzumab. Basal breast tumors express breast basal cell keratins 5/6 and 17 and overlap with the 'triple negative' breast cancer subtype (TNBC) that does not express ER, progesterone receptor (PR) and HER2, whereas gene expression patterns of the normal-like subtype resemble that of normal breast tissue (Sorlie et al. 2003; Perou et al. 2000). Anti-estrogenic therapies are used to treat luminal breast cancers, but they fail in ER-negative tumors. Epigenetic analyses have indicated that the ERα is epigenetically silenced by promoter methylation [reviewed in Hervouet et al. (2013)]. Combined in vitro treatment of the basal breast cancer cell line MDA-MB-231 with the DNMT inhibitor 5-aza-2′-deoxy-cytidine (decitabine, DAC) and the HDAC inhibitor trichostatin A (TSA) resulted in synergistic ~400-fold elevated ERα mRNA expression, indicating that chromatin de-condensation in combination with DNA demethylation was effective in ERα de-repression (Yang et al. 2001).

A number of studies have evaluated the combined effects of chemopreventive agents in in vitro and in vivo breast cancer models, especially combinations with green tea catechins or sulforaphane (SFN) (Table 18.1).

18.2.1.1 Combination of Green Tea Catechins with Broccoli Sprouts or Sulforaphane (SFN)

Green tea polyphenols (GTP) represent a mixture of compounds, including (−)-epigallocatechin 3-gallate (EGCG), epigallocatechin (EGC), epicatechin gallate (ECG) and epicatechin (EC). GTP and especially EGCG have a broad spectrum of

Table 18.1 Combination effects in breast cancer models in vitro and in vivo

Model and optimal treatment	Effects	References
In vitro		
MDA-MB-231, MDA-MB-453, MCF10A Green tea polyphenols (GTP) 20 μg/ml SFN 5 μM	⇧ synergistic reactivation of ERα expression in ER-negative breast cancer cell lines ⇧ activating histone marks to ERα promoter ⇩ repressive histone marks ⇩ DNA methylation at ERα promoter ⇧ sensitivity to tamoxifen (TAM) treatment	Meeran et al. (2012)
MDA-MB-231, MDA-MB-157 EGCG 20 μM SFN 10 μM	⇧ synergistic reactivation of ERα expression ⇩ HDAC1, DNMT1 expression	Li et al. (2017)
HMEC, SH and SHR breast cancer cells EGCG 20 μM SFN 10 μM	⇧ apoptosis, cell cycle arrest in S-phase ⇩ HDAC1, DNMT1 expression ⇧ H3 hyperacetylation ⇧ DNA hyper- and hypomethylation ⇧ DCBLD2 mRNA levels ⇩ Septin 9 mRNA	Li et al. (2016)
MDA-MB-231, MCF7, MCF-10A SFN 5 μM Withaferin A 1 μM	⇩ synergistic reduction of cell growth in MCF7 cells ⇧ induction of apoptosis ⇩ DNMT3A/B protein (MCF7) or mRNA expression (MDA-MB-231) ⇩ HDAC1 mRNA (MCF7) or protein expression (MDA-MB-231) ⇧ upregulation of pro-apoptotic BAX and downregulation of anti-apoptotic BCL2 in both cell lines	Royston et al. (2017)
MDA-MB-231, MCF7 SFN 5 μM Withaferin A 1 μM	⇧ induction of cell cycle arrest ⇩ reduction of Cyclin D1, CDK4, HDAC2 and 3 expression, RB phosphorylation, HDAC2 and 3 ⇧ induction of E2F and p21 expression ⇩ HMT activity ⇧ HAT activity	Royston et al. (2018)
MDA-MB-231, MCF7 SFN 5 μM Genistein 10, 15 μM	⇩ synergistic decrease in cell viability ⇧ synergistic induction of apoptosis ⇧ synergistic induction of G1 (MCF7) or G_2/M (MDA-MB-231) cell cycle arrest ⇩ synergistic reduction of HDAC and HMT activity ⇩ HDAC2 and HDAC3 mRNA and protein expression	Paul et al. (2018)

(continued)

Table 18.1 (continued)

Model and optimal treatment	Effects	References
MDA-MB-231, MDA-MB-157 Genistein 25 μM TSA 100 ng/ml	⇧ synergistic reactivation of ERα expression in ER-negative breast cancer cell lines ⇧ chemosensitivity to tamoxifen treatment Modulation of histone modifications at ERα promoter ⇩ HDAC activity	Li et al. (2013)
HCC1806, MDA-MB-157, MCF10A Resveratrol 15 μM Pterostilbene 5 μM	⇩ colony formation (MDA-MB-157) ⇧ apoptosis ⇧ G_2/M arrest (HCC1806), S-phase arrest (MDA-MB-157) ⇩ SIRT1 protein expression and activity ⇩ DNMT mRNA levels and DNMT activity ⇩ γH2AX foci as a measure of DNA damage and repair (DDR) response ⇩ hTERT mRNA levels and telomerase activity	Kala et al. (2015)
HCC1806, MDA-MB-157, MCF7 Resveratrol 15 μM Pterostilbene 5 μM	⇧ synergistic reactivation of ERα expression ⇧ acH3, acH4, H3K9ac at ERα promoter ⇩ DNMT activity and global DNA methylation (MDA-MB-157) ⇧ sensitivity to 4-hydroxytamoxifen (4-OHT) treatment Modulation of PGR mRNA expression in response to estradiol (E2) or 4-OHT treatment	Kala and Tollefsbol (2016)
Tumorospheres from MMTV-neu-Tg tumors Human breast cancer cell lines MCF10A4, CAL51, murine mammary tumor cell line 4 T1 3D cultures of MMTV-neu-Tg CSCs Butyrate 1 mM 5-Azacytidine 1 μg/ml	⇩ cancer stem cell (CSC) abundance in tumorospheres ⇩ colony formation Differential expression of genes involved in cell cycle regulation, cell division, kinetochore formation, chromosome segregation and mitosis	Pathania et al. (2016)
Raw264.7 murine macrophages, primary macrophages from PyMT mice CDDO-Ea 1, 3, 10 nM or CDDO-Me 1, 3, 10 nM SAHA 100, 300, 1000 nM	⇩ enhanced reduction of INF-γ- or LPS-induced inflammatory response (measured as nitrite) by combination relative to single compounds	Tran et al. (2013)

(continued)

Table 18.1 (continued)

Model and optimal treatment	Effects	References
In vivo		
Nu/nu mice, orthotopic injection of MDA-MB-231 cells into mammary fat pads Green tea polyphenols (0.3% in drinking water) Broccoli sprouts BSp (13% BSp seeds in AIN-93G diet)	⇧ inhibition of tumor growth by combination treatment ⇧ chemosensitivity to tamoxifen treatment ⇧ synergistic reactivation of ERα expression ⇩ HDAC1, DNMT1 expression ⇧ H3 hyperacetylation Modulation of histone marks at ERα promoter ⇧ binding of p300 at ERα promoter ⇩ binding of repressor at ERα promoter	Li et al. (2017)
Nu/nu mice, orthotopic injection of SHR cells into mammary fat pads Green tea polyphenols (0.5% in drinking water) Broccoli sprouts BSp (26% BSp seeds in AIN-93G diet)	Up to 94% inhibition of tumor growth by combination treatment	Li et al. (2016)
C3(1) SV40 TAg mouse model BSp (13% BSp seeds in AIN-93G diet) Genistein (250 mg/kg diet)	⇧ tumor latency ⇩ tumor and volume	Paul et al. (2018)
Nu/nu mice, orthotopic injection of MDA-MB-231 cells into mammary fat pads Genistein (250 mg/kg diet) alone and in combination with TAM (25 mg/pellet)	⇩ tumor growth by genistein alone and especially in combination with TAM, no effect of TAM alone ⇩ tumor weight ⇧ ERα mRNA and protein expression, especially in combination with TAM ⇩ DNMT1, HDAC1 mRNA and protein expression in combination with TAM ⇩ HDAC1 mRNA levels, genistein and TAM alone and in combination	Li et al. (2013)
C3(1) SV40 TAg mouse model Genistein (250 mg/kg diet) alone and in combination with TAM (25 mg/pellet)	⇧ tumor latency ⇧ sensitivity to TAM ⇧ ERα protein expression, alone and especially in combination with TAM ⇩ HDAC1 protein expression, alone and in combination with TAM ⇩ HDAC1 mRNA levels and activity, genistein and TAM alone and in combination ⇩ DNMT1 mRNA levels, genistein and TAM in combination, ⇩ DNMT1 activity, genistein alone and in combination with TAM	Li et al. (2013)

(continued)

Table 18.1 (continued)

Model and optimal treatment	Effects	References
Orthotopic 4 T1 cell injection in Balb/c mice Butyrate (10 mg/21 day release tablets) 5-Azacytidine (0.5 mg/21 day release tablets)	⇧ overall survival	Pathania et al. (2016)
Murine MMTV- polyomavirus middle T (PyMT) model of ER-negative mammary tumors CDDO-Ea 400 mg/kg diet or CDDO-Me 50 mg/kg diet + Suberoylanilide hydroxamic acid (SAHA) 250 mg/kg diet	⇧ efficacy in delaying tumor onset by either triterpenoid in combination with SAHA treatment ⇩ infiltration of tumor associated macrophages (TAM) by CDDO-Me + SAHA ⇩ secreted levels of pro-angiogenic MMP9 ⇩ INF-γ (10 ng/ml) or LPS (3 ng/ml)-induced nitric oxide levels in RAW 264.7 or isolated PyMT macrophages by combination of SAHA (30,100, 300 nM) with CDDO-Me (1,3,10 nM) or CDDO-Ea (3, 10, 30 nM)	Tran et al. (2013)

⇧ induction, enhancement, increase; ⇩ repression, inhibition, reduction; ⇔ no change

chemopreventive activities in vitro. They act as pro- and antioxidants, influence a series of signal-transduction pathways (MAPK, EGFR, NF-κB, IGF), and inhibit cell growth, angiogenesis, and the activity of enzymes relevant for drug metabolism and inflammation (Khan and Mukhtar 2008; Yang et al. 2009; Yang and Wang 2016). Recent research suggests that cancer stem cells are targeted by GTP and EGCG (Fujiki et al. 2018). GTP and EGCG were able to prevent cancer development in animal models of all major organ sites. Although human intervention studies with GTP have provided some promising results (Yang and Wang 2016; Fujiki et al. 2018; Yang et al. 2016), human epidemiological studies were less conclusive. This was attributed mainly to the low quantities of tea consumed (Yang et al. 2009, 2016). GTP have been tested in intervention studies and clinical trials for the prevention and treatment of breast, prostate, colorectal, bladder, lung, skin, esophageal, liver and thyroid cancer (National Library of Medicine 2019).

With respect to epigenetic mechanisms, ECGC and other GTP have been shown to inhibit the activity of DNMTs in vitro and to reduce their expression in cell culture (Carlos-Reyes et al. 2019). As a consequence, EGCG induced reexpression of genes regulating cell cycle progression (p16, p21), cell signaling (*RARβ*), WNT signaling (*WIF-1*), DNA repair (*MGMT, hMLH1*) and apoptosis (*DAPK*). In rodent models and in human epidemiological studies, the influence of EGCG on DNA methylation is inconsistent [review in Gerhauser (2014)]. With respect to posttranslational histone modifications, EGCG was shown to enhance the expression of HATs and to reduce the expression of HDACs, both resulting in increased levels of acetylation at histone as well as non-histone proteins (e.g., p53). Additionally, EGCG inhibited HAT activity and thereby reduced acetylation of important transcription factors including NF-κB p65 and androgen receptor (AR) [review in Gerhauser (2014) and Gao and Tollefsbol (2015)]. In addition to DNA methylation and histone modifications, EGCG also affected the expression of numerous miRNAs in various cancer cell lines, resulting in cell growth inhibition or induction of apoptosis (Gerhauser 2014; Biersack 2016).

Sulforaphane (SFN) is an isothiocyanate (ITC) found as a precursor glucosinolate in broccoli and other cruciferous vegetables (Verkerk et al. 2009). ITCs are thiol-reactive compounds and act by a broad range of cancer preventive activities, including induction of antioxidant and Phase 2 metabolizing enzymes via the NRF2/KEAP1 pathway (Qin and Hou 2016), induction of cell cycle arrest, apoptosis, and autophagy, as well as anti-inflammatory, anti-proliferative and anti-angiogenic activity (Thomson et al. 2010; Houghton et al. 2013). In addition, ITCs possess antimicrobial properties (Dufour et al. 2015). SFN and other ICTs are currently investigated in clinical trials for breast, prostate, lung and gastrointestinal cancers (National Library of Medicine 2019; Palliyaguru et al. 2018; Tortorella et al. 2015).

About 15 years ago, a cysteine metabolite of SFN was first described to inhibit HDAC activity in vitro (Myzak et al. 2004). This epigenetic effect was also demonstrated in vivo in various tissues and intestinal polyps in the $Apc^{Min/+}$ mouse model. In a small human trial, consumption of fresh broccoli sprouts resulted in rapid and transient inhibition of HDAC activity and histone hyper-acetylation in peripheral blood mononuclear cells (Dashwood and Ho 2007). In various hormone-dependent cancer cell lines SFN downregulated the expression of DNMTs and induced DNA methylation changes, e.g., of the cell cycle regulators cyclin D2 and p21, pro-apoptotic *BAX*, as well as of TSGs *PTEN, RARβ2, CDH1, DAPK1* and *GSTP1*, leading to cell cycle arrest and apoptosis induction [review in Tortorella et al. (2015) and Su et al. (2018)]. In addition, SFN and other ITCs affected the expression of noncoding RNAs, thereby inhibiting cell proliferation, cell migration, invasiveness and epithelial-to-mesenchymal transition (EMT) [reviewed in Martin et al. (2018)].

In 2012, Meeran et al. reported that incubation of ER-negative MDA-MB-231 cells with a green tea polyphenol (GTP) extract (20 μg/ml) in combination with 5 μM SFN for 72 h resulted in ERα reactivation at the mRNA and protein level (Meeran et al. 2012). The co-treatment led to a significant ~40% reduction of DNMT and HDAC activities in nuclear extracts. This was associated with a 40–65% reduction of DNMT1, 3a and 3b protein expression compared to control cells. Also, protein expression of HDAC1, 4, and 6 as well as of H3 lysine 9 methyltransferase SUV39H1 (also known as KMT1A) was strongly reduced. Consequently, global acetylation of histones H3 and H4 as well as the activating mark H3K9ac time-dependently increased at the ERα promoter, whereas the repressive mark H3K9me3 declined. Bisulfite sequencing indicated that GTP + SFN treatment lowered DNA methylation at the ERα core promoter. Chromatin immunoprecipitation (ChIP)-PCR experiments confirmed that the combined treatment significantly reduced binding of a repressor complex composed of the epigenetic writers DNMT1, HDAC1 and SUV39H1 as well as of the methyl-binding proteins MBD1 and MeCP2 to the ERα promoter. Epigenetic de-repression of ERα re-sensitized MDA-MB-231 cells to treatment with the selective estrogen receptor modulator (SERM) tamoxifen (TAM). This was indicated by significant ER-dependent induction of apoptosis by co-treatment with GTP, SFN and TAM (Meeran et al. 2012).

Similar results were obtained when MDA-MB-231 cells were treated with EGCG (20 μM) in combination with 10 μM SFN (Li et al. 2017). To confirm that the observations were relevant in vivo, Li et al. treated athymic nude mice with GTP (0.3% in drinking water) and broccoli sprouts BSp as a source of SFN (13% BSp in diet) alone and in combination for 2 weeks, and then injected MDA-MB-231 cells orthotopically into mammary fad pads. Both single as well as the combined treatment especially in combination with TAM significantly reduced xenograft growth. Consistent with the in vitro results, the combination treatment with GTP + BSp resulted in re-expression of ERα protein, reduction of HDAC1 and DNMT1 protein expression, elevated levels of H3ac, H4ac, H3K9ac and the histone acetyltransferase p300 at the ERα promoter, whereas SUV39H1 and H3k9me3 levels were reduced (Li et al. 2017). These results suggest that re-sensitizing TNBC cells to anti-hormonal therapy by combined opening of the chromatin and demethylation of the ER promoter is a feasible approach to reduce TNBC growth.

In a previous study, Li et al. had investigated the combination of EGCG and SFN in an in vitro model of early stages of breast cancer cellular transformation (Li et al. 2016). Normal human mammary epithelial cells (HMECs) were transfected with *SV40* and *hTERT* to generate ER-negative early transformed precancerous SH cells, or additionally with *H-Ras* to produce completely transformed breast cancer cells (SHR cells). Combined treatment with 20 μM EGCG and 10 μM SFN reduced cell growth in transformed cells, but not in normal HMECs, and induced apoptosis and cell-cycle arrest in S-phase. In SHR cells, EGCG and SFN alone and in combination reduced HDAC1 and DNMT1 mRNA expression and activity. SFN treatment alone and in combination with EGCG led to H3 hyper-acetylation. Genome-wide methylation changes at 485,000 CpG dinucleotides were assessed using Illumina 450k BeadChip arrays in SHR cells. Both compounds alone and in combination differentially affected DNA methylation at 266 CpG sites with methylation differences larger than 20%. The combination of EGCG and SFN induced more prominent changes (both hyper- and hypomethylation) than the single agents. Affected genes were enriched for chromosomal rearrangement, RNA binding, differentiation and development. In vivo, the combination of GTP (0.5% in drinking water) as a source of EGCG and BSp (26% BSp in the diet) as a source of SFN significantly and additively reduced SHR xenograft growth when the cells were injected into mammary fat pads of nude mice (Li et al. 2016).

Overall, these studies showed that dietary interventions targeting complementary epigenetic mechanisms can re-sensitize ER-negative tumors to anti-hormonal therapy. The results demonstrated that combined application of GTP + BSp in combination with anti-hormonal treatment might be a feasible treatment option for breast cancer patients with ER-negative tumors, which should be further evaluated in clinical trials.

18.2.1.2 Combination of SFN with Withaferin A (WA)

Withania somnifera, also known as Indian ginseng, is used in traditional Ayurvedic medicine to treat diseases with a broad spectrum of indications from diabetes to cancer (Vyas and Singh 2014; Gauttam and Kalia 2013; Palliyaguru et al. 2016). Beside other bioactive compounds (flavonoids, tannins), *Withania somnifera* is rich in steroidal lactones known as withanolides. Withaferin A (WA) bears a reactive α,β-unsaturated carbonyl group, which has been associated with its bioactivities by interaction with cysteine thiol-residues of intracellular signaling molecules (Lee and Choi 2016). WA affects a broad spectrum of chemopreventive mechanisms. Its pro-oxidative activity is linked to induction of apoptosis. WA also targets various signaling pathways, including KEAP1/NRF2 (Heyninck et al. 2016), NF-κB, STAT3, NOTCH, mitogen-activated protein kinase (MAPK), p53, and estrogen receptor signaling. Further, WA was shown to influence stress response by inducing heat shock response and to inhibit angiogenesis. Various studies have reported that WA inhibits carcinogenesis in chemically-induced rodents models for head and neck, mammary gland and skin cancer. It was also shown to suppress growth of prostate, breast, thyroid, cervical, lung and colon cancer cells in cancer xenograft models [reviewed in Vyas and Singh (2014), Palliyaguru et al. (2016), and Lee and Choi (2016)].

With respect to epigenetic mechanisms, WA reduced the expression of DNMTs in both ER-dependent and -independent breast cancer cell lines (Mirza et al. 2013). Conversely, WA treatment led to DNA hypermethylation and downregulation of selected genes related to cancer invasiveness in TNBC cells (Szarc Vel Szic et al. 2017). It was further shown to decreases histone H3 acetylation and transcription factor recruitment to the interleukin IL-6 gene promoter and thus abolished IL-6 gene expression in TNBC cells (Ndlovu et al. 2009).

SFN (5 μM) was tested in vitro in combination with WA (1 μM) in ER-positive (MCF7) and negative (MDA-MB-231) breast cancer cell lines (Royston et al. 2017, 2018). In both cell lines, the combination of SFN + WA reduced cell viability and induced apoptosis. The combination also lowered DNMT activity as well as DNMT1, 3a and 3b and HDAC1 mRNA and protein expression, often more effective than either compound alone. With respect to apoptosis induction, SFN + WA induced protein expression of pro-apoptotic BAX and reduced anti-apoptotic BCL-2 (Royston et al. 2017). The authors could further show that SFN + WA induced G1 cell cycle arrest by modifying the expression of cell cycle regulating genes, including p21. Further, protein expression of HDAC2 and 3 were lowered, histone methyl transferase (HMT) activity was reduced, and HAT activity was induced, especially in MDA-MB-231 cells (Royston et al. 2018).

These results indicate that by combining SFN and WA, cell growth inhibition by induction of cell cycle arrest and apoptosis was achievable at lower concentration than with either compound alone. Since both compounds possess a broad spectrum of bioactivities, the mechanism of inhibition induced by the combination should be further investigated in vitro and in animal models for breast cancer.

18.2.1.3 Combination of SFN with Soy Isoflavones

Soybean (*Glycine max* L.) and soy products contain high levels of isoflavones such as genistein and daidzein with phyto-estrogenic properties (Xiao et al. 2018). A traditional soy-rich, low-fat Asian diet is generally associated with a reduced risk for breast and prostate cancer (Xiao et al. 2018; Messina 2016; Mukund et al. 2017; Russo et al. 2016; Magee and Rowland 2012). Beside estrogen receptor-mediated signaling, genistein and other soy isoflavones act by additional chemopreventive mechanisms, including inactivation of carcinogens and reactive oxygen species as well as inhibition of cell-signaling, inflammation, angiogenesis, cell cycle progression, and induction of apoptosis (Magee and Rowland 2012; Steiner et al. 2008; Molinie and Georgel 2009). In various rodent models for cancer prevention, isoflavones have been shown to prevent major cancer types (Banerjee et al. 2008). Genistein is tested in various clinical trials for treatment and prevention of prostate, bladder, kidney, breast, colorectal, lung, pancreas and endometrial cancer (National Library of Medicine 2019; Taylor et al. 2009).

Isoflavone interaction with ER leads to recruitment of nuclear co-activators or co-repressors, which have histone modifying function and modulate the chromatin structure. Various in vitro and in vivo studies have demonstrated potential of genistein and soy isoflavones to target the activity or expression of enzymes functioning as epigenetic writers, readers and erasers and to influence miRNA expression. These activities affect genes associated with the major hallmarks of cancer, and lead to activation TSGs such as *RARβ2, BTG3, PTEN* and *ATM*, genes involved in DNA repair (*MGMT, BRCA1, BRCA2, GSTP1*), cell signaling (especially Wnt-signaling, e.g., *APC, SOX7, WIF1, DKK1, SFRP1, SFRP2*), epigenetic (*EZH2, SRC3, p300*) and cell cycle regulators (p16, p21), estrogen receptors (ER-α, ER-β) and genes associated with EMT (e.g., *ZEB1/2, VIM*). This is of relevance for all major cancer types [comprehensive review in Gerhauser (2014, 2018) and Pudenz et al. (2014)], although a causative link between the influence on epigenetic mechanisms and cancer prevention is still missing.

Similar to the study of SFN and WA (Royston et al. 2018), the combination of SFN (5 μM) with genistein (10 or 15 μM, respectively) was tested in ER-positive (MCF7) and negative (MDA-MB-231) breast cancer cell lines. SFN + genistein inhibited cell proliferation and induced apoptosis and cell cycle arrest of both cell lines (Paul et al. 2018). The authors reported reduced HDAC and HMT activity in MCF-7 and MDA-MB-231 cells treated with the combination, but not with either compound alone. Normal MCF10A cells were not affected. Also, mRNA and protein expression of HDACs 2 and 3 were most reduced by the combined compounds. In the C(3)1 SV40 TAg transgenic mouse model, combination of genistein (250 mg/kg diet) with BSp (13% in diet) (representing human daily consumption of about 2 g isoflavones and 2 cups of broccoli) most effectively increased tumor latency and reduced average tumor volume by about 50% (Paul et al. 2018).

These results support the enhanced benefit of combining a soy-based diet with cruciferous vegetables such as broccoli sprouts for the prevention of breast cancer development.

18.2.1.4 Combination of Genistein with the HDAC Inhibitor Trichostatin A (TSA)

Li et al. investigated the combination effects of genistein in combination with the HDAC inhibitor trichostatin A (TSA) (Li et al. 2013). TSA is an antifungal antibiotic with cytostatic and differentiating activity and is classified as a pan-HDAC inhibitor (Vigushin et al. 2001; Kim and Bae 2011). In vitro, treatment of MDA-M-231 cells with 25 μM genistein in combination with 100 ng/ml TSA resulted in synergistic ERα re-expression, reduced HDAC activity, reduced HDAC1 and DNMT1 expression and binding to the ERα promoter, as well as in elevated levels of activating histone marks (H3ac, H4ac, H3K9ac) at the ERα promoter.

In vivo, dietary genistein (250 mg/kg diet) fed for 2 weeks prior to orthotropic injection of MDA-MB-231 cells reduced xenograft growth. Importantly, genistein re-sensitized the tumor cells to treatment with TAM (25 mg pellet implanted 2 weeks after xenograft injection). Genistein intervention combined with TAM inhibited xenograft growth by >95%. In the C(3)1 SV40 TAg transgenic mouse model for basal breast cancer, genistein increased tumor latency and response to TAM treatment. Mechanistically, genistein alone and in combination with TAM inhibited tumor cell proliferation measured by PCNA staining and led to re-expression of ERα protein. In both the xenograft and the transgenic mouse model, genistein in combination with TAM significantly reduced DNMT1 and HDAC1 mRNA and protein expression and activity (Li et al. 2013).

This study is another demonstration that the ER can be re-activated in basal or TNBC models by combined treatment with HDAC inhibitors and compounds modulating DNA methylation, resulting in enhanced response to anti-hormonal treatment.

18.2.1.5 Combination of Two Stilbenes Resveratrol and Pterostilbene

Resveratrol and pterostilbene are plant-derived stilbene derivatives found in the skin of red grapes, blueberries and in other fruits (Rimando and Suh 2008). Resveratrol was first described as a cancer chemopreventive agent in 1997 and has a broad spectrum of health-beneficial effects, including anti-oxidant, cardio-protective and anti-tumor activities (Pezzuto 2008). Mechanistically, these activities have been linked to the interaction with hormone receptors, influence on drug metabolism, and anti-inflammatory, anti-proliferative, anti-angiogenic and anti-metastatic properties, as well as pro-apoptotic activity (Rimando and Suh 2008; Pezzuto 2008; Kundu and Surh 2008; Pavan et al. 2016). Resveratrol and pterostilbene have been shown to reduce inflammation and to prevent carcinogenesis in animal models for colon cancer, as well as some other cancer types (Rimando and Suh 2008). Resveratrol is rapidly metabolized and plasma levels after oral consumption are low (Baur and Sinclair 2006). Bioavailability can be modulated by various factors including formulation, matrix effects, time of consumption and combination with modulators of resveratrol metabolism (Ramirez-Garza et al. 2018). Resveratrol is currently tested in several human intervention trials, with a focus on colon cancer prevention, which does not require systemic uptake (National Library of Medicine 2019; Pezzuto 2008, 2019; Pavan et al. 2016).

In earlier reports, resveratrol had been described as an activator of SIRT1 activity (Bonkowski and Sinclair 2016). Some of these effects seem to be due to technical artifacts and should be considered with care (Pezzuto 2019). Nevertheless, SIRT1 activation by resveratrol in vivo was associated with longevity, beneficial effects on metabolic disorders, cardio- and neuroprotection (Fernandes et al. 2017).

Resveratrol has been shown to affect DNA methylation in vitro and in vivo and to reactivate the TSGs *PTEN, BRCA1* and *RASSF1A*, whereas methylation of cell cycle regulators *AURKA* and *CCNB1* was increased at high concentrations. Resveratrol also increased acetylation and activated p53 in prostate cancer cells. Expression of several oncogenic miRNAs was reduced by resveratrol, whereas expression of genes related to apoptosis, cell cycle regulation, cell proliferation and differentiation were predicted to be modulated by upregulation of miRNAs after resveratrol treatment. Pterostilbene similarly was shown to modulate miRNA expression, and it reduced migratory and invasive potential of TNBC cells [review in Lee et al. (2018)].

Kala et al. investigated the influence of a combination of resveratrol (15 μM) and pterostilbene (5 μM) on TNBC cells in vitro (Kala et al. 2015). The combinatorial treatment synergistically reduced cell viability and induced apoptosis in both HCC1806 and MDA-MB-157 TNBC cell lines, but not in MCF10A normal mammary cells. The combined treatment induced G_2/M- and S-phase cell cycle arrest in HCC1806 and MDA-MB-157 cells, respectively, and was more effective than either treatment alone. The combination reduced mRNA and protein expression of the SIRT1 histone deacetylase in both cell lines, leading to reduced SIRT1 activity. This resulted in reduced γ-H2AX as a marker of DNA damage response in combination-treated cells. The combination treatment lowered mRNA expression of DNMTs 1, 3A and 3B as well as DNMT activity. It also lowered mRNA expression of epigenetically regulated hTERT and reduced telomerase activity catalyzed by hTERT (Kala et al. 2015).

In a follow up study, resveratrol and pterostilbene in combination were found to reactivate ERα expression by increasing activating histone marks at the ERα promoter and by reducing DNMT activity and global DNA methylation levels. Combination treatment also re-sensitized the cells to either estrogen (E2, ER-agonist) or 4-hydroxy-tamoxifen (4-OHT, ER-antagonist) treatment, with increased/reduced cell viability after E2/4-OHT treatment and increased/reduced expression of the ER target gene PGR, respectively (Kala and Tollefsbol 2016).

This is another interesting example of combined dietary agents that re-activate ER expression and response to anti-hormonal therapy as a treatment approach for TNBC. Since polyphenols are less bioavailable than more lipophilic compounds such as SFN and WA and concentrations tested in this study were relatively high, it still needs to be demonstrated that effective doses can indeed be reached in mammary tumors in vivo.

18.2.1.6 Combination of Short Chain Fatty Acid Butyrate with the Demethylating Agent 5-Azacytidine

In the MMTV-neu-Tg mouse model, Her2 (neu) is under the control of the mouse mammary tumor virus (MMTV), and tumors arise from luminal progenitor and basal myoepithelial stem cells (Pathania et al. 2016). Pathania et al. tested a combination of the demethylating agent 5-azacytidine (5-Aza, 1 μg/ml) with the HDAC inhibitor butyrate (1 mM) (further information see Sect. 18.2.2.1). The combination reduced the number of primary and secondary tumorospheres derived from MMTV-neu-Tg tumors more than the compounds alone. The combination also strongly reduced the number and sizes of tumorospheres generated with the human breast cancer cell lines MCF10A4 (basal subtype), CAL51 (triple negative subtype) and the murine cell line 4T1 (triple negative subtype). When 4T1 cells were xenografted into mammary fat pads of Balb/c mice, implantation with tablets releasing 5-Aza (0.5 mg/21 days) and butyrate (10 mg/21 days) significantly prolonged the mean survival time, more than salinomycin (5 mg/kg, intraperitoneal injection), a known cancer stem cell inhibitor (Gupta et al. 2009). Self-renewing cancer stem cells were isolated from MMTV-neu-Tg tumors and cultured in 3D cultures. 5Aza + butyrate led to alterations in mRNA expression of genes enriched in cell cycle and cell division pathways. Downregulated genes were typically upregulated in human breast cancer samples, whereas transcript levels of upregulated genes were generally downregulated in human breast cancer. Among others, three genes with high expression in basal breast cancer (*RAD51AP1, NUSAP1, SPC25*) were downregulated by the combination treatment. *RAD51AP1* is associated with double strand break repair, whereas *SPC25* plays a role during cell division.

Overall, these results demonstrated that 5-Aza in combination with butyrate effectively reduced mammary tumorigenesis and tumorosphere-forming potential of tumor-propagating cells and might be a treatment alternative for basal breast cancer with high levels of cancer stem cells (Pathania et al. 2016).

18.2.1.7 Combination of Oleanane Triterpenoids with the HDAC Inhibitor SAHA

Synthetic oleanane triterpenoids are synthetic analogs of the natural triterpenoid oleanolic acid, which is widely distributed in the plant kingdom with highest concentrations found in olives (*Olea europea* L.) (Ziberna et al. 2017). Oleanane triterpenoids have anti-inflammatory and cyto-protective properties by targeting NRF2/KEAP1, NF-κB, TGF-β, and STAT signaling. These activities have been attributed to their high reactivity with protein thiol groups. Oleanane triterpenoids have been shown to induce cell differentiation and apoptosis and to inhibit cell proliferation. In vivo, they prevented or inhibited tumor growth in various animal models, especially the development of lung cancer (Liby et al. 2007; Liby and Sporn 2012). CDDO-Me (methyl-2-cyano-3,12-dioxooleana-1,9(11)-dien-28-oate, also known as bardoxolone methyl or RTA 402) has been tested or is currently undergoing testing in clinical trials for lymphoma (Hong et al. 2012) and pulmonary arterial hypertension (National Library of Medicine 2019). Clinical trials for chronic kidney disease were terminated because of a higher rate of cardiovascular events with bardoxolone methyl treatment compared to placebo treatment (de Zeeuw et al. 2013).

Anti-proliferative and apoptosis-inducing effects of CDDO-Me have been associated with the inhibition of human telomerase reverse transcriptase (hTERT) expression and activity, partly by downregulation of DNMTs and hypomethylation and reduced histone acetylation at the hTERT promoter (Deeb et al. 2014). In a rat model for aflatoxin B1 (AFB1)-induced liver carcinogenesis, CDDO-Im (1-[2-cyano-3-,12-dioxo-oleana-1,9(11)-dien-28-oyl]imidazole) abrogated AFB1-induced miRNA expression (Livingstone et al. 2017).

Tran et al. tested the combination of the HDAC inhibitor vorinostat (also known as SAHA, suberoylanilide hydroxamic acid) with either of the synthetic oleanane triterpenoids CDDO-Me or CDDO-Ea in the MMTV polyoma middle T (PyMT) mouse model of ER-negative mammary tumors (Tran et al. 2013). The combination was more effective than either compound alone in inhibiting pro-inflammatory nitrite production in Raw264.7 mouse macrophages or macrophages derived from the PyMT model, which were stimulated with interferon γ (IFN-γ) or lipopolysaccharides. The CDDO derivatives are potent inhibitors of NF-κB signaling. However, this anti-inflammatory mechanism was not enhanced by co-treatment with SAHA. The combination of SAHA (250 mg/kg diet) with either CDDO-Me (50 mg/kg diet) or CDDO-Ea (400 mg/kg diet) significantly prolonged tumor latency in the PyMT mouse model. This was accompanied by significantly reduced infiltration with tumor-associated marcrophages (TAM). Mechanistically, the combination significantly lowered the secretion of pro-angiogenic MMP9 expression from primary PyMT macrophages and was more effective than the individual compounds. Tissue and plasma levels of SAHA were measured in the range of 50 nM. Therefore, the observed anti-tumorigenic effects might be independent of its known HDAC inhibitory potential (Tran et al. 2013). Reactivation of the ER was not investigated in this study.

In summary, multiple studies have suggested that epigenetic mechanisms are involved in the reduced expression of the ER in TNBC. Several combinations of chemopreventive agents (GTP/EGCG + SFN, resveratrol + pterostilbene, genistein + TSA) led to reactivation of ER in ER-negative tumors and consequent reactivation of anti-estrogen sensitivity. This approach might be a feasible strategy in the clinical management of TNBC, which could be followed up in clinical trials. Also, the combination of chemopreventive agents with clinically approved epigenetic drugs resulted in improved efficacy at low doses in mouse models for breast cancer. Nonetheless, the studies did not prove a causal relationship of the measured effects. Although the combinations were demonstrated to affect epigenetic markers, additional mechanisms might underlie the observed enhancement of tumor latency or reduction in tumor growth and need to be further investigated.

18.2.2 Colorectal Cancer Studies

With 1.1 million estimated new cases and about 550,000 estimated cancer deaths in 2018, colorectal cancer is the third most common cancer type in both the male and female population worldwide (Bray et al. 2018). The great majority of colorectal tumors are adenocarcinomas. Five to 10% of all cases are based on hereditary conditions, including familial adenomatous polyposis (FAP) caused by a mutation in the TSG *APC* (Adenomatous polyposis coli) and non-polyposis colorectal cancer (HNPCC) linked to mutations in DNA repair genes, but the same genetic defects are also involved in the etiology of sporadic cases (World Cancer Research Fund International/American Institute for Cancer Research 2017). Also, chromatin regulators such as *ARID1A* (AT-rich interactive domain 1A), a component of the SWI/SNF chromatin remodeling complex, are frequently mutated in colorectal cancer (Vymetalkova et al. 2019). Driver genes inactivated by DNA hypermethylation include genes involved in Wnt signaling (*APC, SFRP1, SFRP2*), DNA repair (*MLH1, MGMT*), cell-cell adhesion (*CDH1, CDH13, TSP1*), cell signaling (*RASSF1A, RUNX3, ESR1, ID4, IRF8*) and others. Onco-*miR-21* is frequently upregulated in colorectal cancer, whereas the *miR200* family that negatively regulates EMT is frequently silenced by DNA methylation (Lao and Grady 2011).

A large meta-analysis of dietary patterns associated with cancer risk in epidemiological case-control and cohort studies found strong associations between food choice and both decreased and increased colon cancer risk (Grosso et al. 2017). There is increasing evidence that diet affects colonic health and cancer risk through its effects on colonic microbial metabolism, for example through the generation of short chain fatty acids (SCFAs) with HDAC inhibitory activity, but also via alterations in miR expression (O'Keefe 2016; Bultman 2017; Farhana et al. 2018). Most studies investigating combination effects for colorectal cancer prevention accordingly combined butyrate (in vitro) or dietary fiber (in vivo) with another chemopreventive agent (Table 18.2).

18.2.2.1 Combination of Butyrate with Green Tea Catechins

Dietary fiber is fermented by the gut microbiota to short chain fatty acids (SCFAs) including acetate, propionate and butyrate (O'Keefe 2016). In the healthy colon, butyrate is a major energy source for colonocytes (Bultman 2017; den Besten et al. 2013). As a colon cancer preventive agent, butyrate acts by reducing pro-inflammatory and pro-oxidative conditions and was shown to induce cell-cycle arrest, cell differentiation, and apoptosis [review in O'Keefe (2016), Guilloteau et al. (2010), and McNabney and Henagan (2017)]. Many of these activities have been linked to the potential of butyrate to inhibit HDACs, which was discovered almost 40 years ago [summary in Davie (2003)]. Recent studies indicate that butyrate effects on histone-modifying enzymes are concentration-dependent. At low concentrations such as in colonocytes at the base of the colonic crypt, butyrate increased the

Table 18.2 Combination effects in colon cancer models in vitro and in vivo

Model and treatment	Effects	References
In vitro		
HT29, Caco2 EC (100 μM) or EGCG, 20 μM Sodium butyrate 2 mM	Antagonistic activity of GTP on butyrate-induced differentiation ⇩ relocalization of butyrate transporter, independent of HDACi	Sanchez-Tena et al. (2013)
RKO, HT29, HCT116 EGCG 10 μM Butyrate 5 mM	⇧ apoptosis, cell cycle arrest, ⇩ colony formation ⇩ protein expression of HDAC1, DNMT1, survivin, NF-κB p65 ⇧ p21 mRNA and protein expression ⇩ DNA methylation ⇧ H3 hyperacetylation, DNA-damage (γH2AX)	Saldanha et al. (2014)
HCT116 Docosahexaenoic acid (DHA) 50 μM Butyrate 5 mM 5′aza-deoxycytidine 2 μM	⇧ apoptosis ⇩ DNA methylation of apoptosis-related genes: *BCL2l11, CIDEB, DAPK1, LTBR, TNFRSF25*	Cho et al. (2014)
Caco-2, HCT116 SFN or Iberin 6–8 μM Se-methylselenocysteine (SeSMC) or Na-selenite 0.2–5 μM Up to 12 days	⇔ no effect on p16 and *ESR1* promoter CpG islands or LINE1 methylation ⇩ transient reduction of DNMT mRNA levels in Caco2 cells ⇧ transient increase of DNMT mRNA levels in HCT116	Barrera et al. (2013)
In vivo		
Azoxymethane (AOM)-induced colon cancer in Sprague-Dawley rats Fish oil 11.5% + pectin 6% in the diet (FOP) vs. corn oil 15% + cellulose 6% (COC) diet	⇩ tumor incidence by FOP diet ⇧ apoptosis of DNA-damaged colon cells ⇧ anti-apoptotic Bcl2 promoter methylation ⇩ Bcl2 mRNA levels	Cho et al. (2012)
AOM-induced colon cancer in Sprague-Dawley rats Fish oil 11.5% + pectin 6% in the diet (FOP) vs. corn oil 15% + cellulose 6% (COC) diet	⇩ tumor incidence ⇩ inhibition of AOM-induced downregulation of let-7d, miR-15b, miR-107, miR-324-5p and miR-191 expression by fish oil	Davidson et al. (2009)
AOM-induced colon carcinogenesis in Sprague-Dawley rats (colon mucosa, 10 weeks) Fish oil 11.5% + pectin 6% in the diet (FOP) vs. corn oil 15% + cellulose 6% (COC) diet	⇧ miR-19b, miR-26b, miR-27b, and miR-203 expression by FOP diet ⇩ mRNA expression of miRNA targets Ptk2B, Igfr2, Pde4b2, Atp2b1, Tcf4 by FOP diet ⇩ protein expression of Ptk2b, Pde4b2 and Tcf4 by FOP diet	Shah et al. (2011)
AOM-induced colon cancer in Lgr5-EGFP-IRES-creER^{T2} mice Fish oil 11.5% + pectin 6% in the	⇩ number of aberrant crypt foci by FOP diet ⇧ upregulation of putative tumor	Shah et al. (2016a)

(continued)

Table 18.2 (continued)

Model and treatment	Effects	References
diet (FOP) vs. corn oil 15% + cellulose 6% (COC) diet	suppressor miRNAs in colonic mucosa ⇩ downregulation of mRNA expression of predicted target genes upon carcinogen exposure Differential miRNA expression in $Lgr5^{high}$ colonic stem cells vs. $Lgr5^{negative}$ differentiated cells: miR-19b, miR-26b, miR-203	
AOM-induced colon cancer in Sprague-Dawley rats Fish oil 11.5% + pectin 6% in the diet (FOP) vs. corn oil 15% + cellulose 6% (COC) diet	⇩ number of high multiplicity aberrant crypt foci by FOP diet Context-specific alterations in gene expression and chromatin structure ⇧ histone acetylation in AOM-treated FOP diet groups ⇧ combination of fish oil with pectin facilitates DHA-mediated stimulation of nuclear receptors upstream of lipid metabolism genes.	Triff et al. (2018)
AOM-induced colon cancer in Sprague Dawley rats Green tea extract (0.5% in diet) + selenium (1 ppm in diet)	⇩ additive inhibition of large aberrant crypt foci (ACF) and tumor incidence and multiplicity ⇩ DNMT1 expression by green tea extract ⇧ H3 acetylation by selenium ⇩ β-catenin nuclear translocation, cyclin D1 mRNA, proliferation (measured as Ki-67 expression) by selenium	Hu et al. (2013)

⇧ induction, enhancement, increase; ⇩ repression, inhibition, reduction; ⇔ no change

production of acetyl-CoA and stimulated HAT activity, with overall pro-proliferative effects. In colon cancer cells, accumulation of butyrate led to HDAC inhibition, increased acetylation of histones and non-histone proteins such as tubulin and p53, and resulted in inhibition of cell proliferation and cell cycle arrest [summary in Gerhauser (2018) and McNabney and Henagan (2017)]. Additionally, butyrate-mediated inhibition of miRNA expression has been associated with cell cycle arrest and inhibition of metastases [overview in Chen et al. (2019)]. Recently, it has been postulated that SCFA activities might be related to signal transduction through metabolite-sensing G-protein coupled receptors (GPCR) (Tan et al. 2017).

Sanchez-Tena et al. treated HT29 colon cancer cells with butyrate (2 mM) in combination with green tea catechins EC (100 μM) or EGCG (20 μM) (Sanchez-Tena et al. 2013). Interestingly, co-treatment with the polyphenols impaired butyrate-induced differentiation of HT29 cells, measured by alkaline phosphatase activity. This antagonistic effect was independent of HDAC activity. Instead, the green tea compounds inhibited butyrate entry into cells by reducing membrane localization of the butyrate transporter protein MCT1 (monocarboxylate transporter 1, also known as SLC16A1) (Sanchez-Tena et al. 2013).

Saldanha et al. investigated anti-proliferative potential of the combination of butyrate (5 mM) with EGCG (10 μM) in three colon cancer cell lines (Saldanha et al. 2014). In this study, the combination was more effective than either compound alone in inhibiting cell proliferation. Butyrate + EGCG induced apoptosis and cell cycle arrest and reduced colony formation. Mechanistically, the combination inhibited HDAC activity and induced protein levels of acetylated histone H3, p21, p53 and NF-κB p65. Levels of DNMT1 mRNA and DNMT3A and 3B protein were reduced, and consequently, global DNA methylation was lowered. The combination increased DNA damage, measured as γ-H2AX levels by western blotting and lowered the levels of survivin, which is a negative regulator of apoptosis and often overexpressed in colorectal cancer (Saldanha et al. 2014).

These studies with opposite effects indicate that the applied concentrations and ratio of butyrate and EGCG might influence the outcome of the studies.

18.2.2.2 Combination of Dietary Fiber with Fish Oil

Docosahexaenoic acid (DHA) is a long-chain omega-3 polyunsaturated fatty acid (ω3-FA) from cold-water fish and component of fish-oil. ω3-FAs are essential for human health (Berquin et al. 2008). They are incorporated into cellular membranes and have anti-oxidant and anti-inflammatory activities by activating the NRF2/KEAP1 pathway and reducing the production of pro-inflammatory prostaglandins (Yum et al. 2016; Saini and Keum 2018). In human studies, dietary intake of ω3-FA reduced the risk for chronic degenerative diseases including coronary heart disease, breast cancer and depression (Marventano et al. 2015).

Omega 3-FAs have been shown to target the epigenome at the levels of DNA methylation, histone methylation and miRNA expression [recent review in Lau et al. (2019)]. After intervention of pregnant mothers with DHA in several intervention studies, alterations in DNA methylation were detected in cord blood or blood spots derived from the babies. In vitro cell culture incubation with DHA resulted in downregulation of several HDACs, with potential impact on chromatin structure. DHA also lowered repressive H3K27me3 levels by reducing the protein expression of the histone methyltransferase EZH2 in breast cancer cell lines (Dimri et al. 2010). In addition, DHA treatment led to alterations in miRNA expression, including downregulation of oncogenic *miR-21* in breast and colon cancer, cholangiocarcinoma and neuroblastoma cell lines (Lau et al. 2019).

The group of Robert Chapkin investigated combined effects of pectin (giving rise to butyrate) and fish oil as a source of ω3-FA (fish oil/pectin, FOP diet) in several in vivo colon cancer prevention experiments (Triff et al. 2015). Control animals were fed a diet containing corn oil and cellulose (COC diet), and colorectal carcinogenesis was induced by injection of AOM. Early stages of tumorigenesis were analyzed in colonic mucosa 10 or 16 weeks after carcinogen injection, and tumors were collected after 34 weeks.

In a study by Cho et al. (2012), FOP diet significantly reduced colon cancer incidence and increased the apoptotic index (mean number of apoptotic cells vs. total number of cells per colon crypt) in rats. FOP diet also significantly reduced mRNA expression of the anti-apoptotic regulator *Bcl-2*, concomitant with increased promoter methylation (Cho et al. 2012).

To gain further mechanistic insight, Cho et al. incubated HCT116 cells with butyrate (5 mM) and DHA (50 μM) and measured promoter (de-)methylation of 24 selected apoptosis-related genes (Cho et al. 2014). Global DNA methylation was not altered by either compound or the combination. At a single gene level, butyrate treatment led to demethylation of *BCL2L11*, whereas DHA reduced methylation of the promoter regions of *CITEB, DAPK1* and *TNFRSF25*. All of these pro-apoptotic genes were methylated >60% in untreated control cells. In combination, butyrate and DHA demethylated *BCL2L11, CITEB, DAPK1, LTBR* and *TNFRSF25*. Butyrate alone and in combination with DHA transiently induced mRNA levels of *TNFRS25* and *DAPK1* after 48 h, but significantly reduced transcript levels after 96 h of incubation. Butyrate as an HDAC inhibitor also increased acetylation of histone H3, but there was no additive effect of the combination (Cho et al. 2014).

Davidson et al. studied the impact of FOP diet on the expression of non-coding microRNAs at early stages of tumorigenesis and in tumors (Davidson et al. 2009). Fish oil-containing diets significantly lowered the number of differentially expressed miRNAs in colonic mucosa 10 weeks after AOM injection, and in combination with pectin (FOP diet) significantly reduced tumor incidence. A tumorigenesis-associated reduction of *let-7d, miR-15b, miR-107, miR-324-5p* and *miR-191* expression was prevented by fish oil intervention (Davidson et al. 2009).

In a follow-up study, miRNA expression levels were correlated with mRNA expression of predicted target genes in colonic mucosa 10 weeks after AOM injection. FOP diet prevented the downregulation of *miR-19b, miR-26b, miR-27b*, and *miR-203*, with consequent reduced mRNA expression of the protein tyrosine kinase *Ptk2B*, insulin-like growth factor 2 receptor (*Igfr2*), phosphodiesterase *Pde4b2*, the plasma membrane pump *Atp2b1*, and transcription factor *Tcf4* involved in Wnt signaling. Expression of *Ptk2b, Pde4b2* and *Tcf4* was also reduced at the protein level by the FOP diet (Shah et al. 2011). The antagonistic link between *miR-19b, miR-26b* and *miR-203* and their predicted targets *Pde4b2* and *Tcf4* was confirmed in gain and loss of function studies (Shah et al. 2016a).

As further confirmation of these findings, Shah et al. analyzed the influence of fish oil/pectin combination on miRNA/mRNA expression in the stem cell niche of the mouse colonic crypt. As shown previously, FOP diet inhibited AOM-induced ACF by about 37% compared to the COC diet (Shah et al. 2016a). Sorted stem cells with high expression of the stem cell marker *Lgr5* showed elevated expression of *miR-125a-5p, miR-190b* and *miR-191* compared to $Lgr5^{low}$ cells. Different from the rat study (Shah et al. 2011), FOP reduced expression of *miR-19b, miR-26b* and *miR-203* in Lgr^{high} colonic stem cells of AOM injected animals (Shah et al. 2016b). Expression of the confirmed targets Ptk2b and Tcf4 did not change, and Pde4b was significantly upregulated by FOP diet. These data suggest that the response to AOM and diets might be different in the bulk cell population of the colon vs. stem cells

(Shah et al. 2016a). Also, the data indicated that it is still challenging to causally link miRNA expression changes with expression of target genes.

In a recent study, the spectrum of epigenetic mechanisms was extended to profiling of posttranslational histone modifications (Triff et al. 2018). In confirmation of earlier studies, fish oil-containing diets significantly lowered the number of high multiplicity (HM) aberrant crypts in colonic mucosa 10 weeks after AOM injection. The combination of fish oil with pectin was more efficient than either treatment separately. Gene expression in colonic mucosa was studied by RNA-seq. In AOM-treated animals, FOP diet significantly altered the expression of 83 genes predominantly associated with lipid metabolism (increased fatty acid catabolism, decreased accumulation of lipids, reduction of fatty acid synthesis), whereas fish oil and pectin diets separately altered only 1 or 0 genes, respectively. In the absence of carcinogen treatment, fish oil alone modulated more genes that in combination with pectin (63 vs. 14 genes), whereas pectin alone did not alter expression of any gene. These results indicated that the diets had a context specific effect. The authors also measured activating histone modifications including H3K9ac and H3K4me3 using ChIP-seq in colonic mucosa. In general, they observed poor correlation between the measured changes in histone marks and gene expression. After AOM treatment, none of the diets induced any change in H3K9ac. In the absence of the carcinogen, pectin alone induced more acetylation changes than in combination with fish oil or fish oil alone (24 vs. 15 vs. 4). Conversely, effects on H4K4me3 were stronger in AOM-treated animals than in the absence of the carcinogen and mainly induced by pectin diet (combination: 21 peaks, fish oil: 0 peaks, pectin: 15 peaks, false discovery rate 10%). Key affected pathways were related to metabolic disease, lipid metabolism and cell death and survival. An analysis of upstream regulators identified ligand activated nuclear receptors including PPARs, LXR, FXR, PXR, GCR and HNF4A as main targets. The authors postulated that the combination of fish oil with pectin facilitates stimulation of DHA-ligand activated nuclear receptors associated with lipid metabolism (Triff et al. 2018).

Overall, these studies demonstrated enhanced colon cancer chemopreventive efficacy by the combined intervention with fish oil and pectin and suggest plausible mechanisms of action via modulation of mRNA and miRNA expression and alterations of the chromatin structure, which seemed, however, not directly linked to changes in gene expression.

18.2.2.3 Combination of Isothiocyanates (ITCs) with Selenium

Selenium (Se) is an essential trace element and is incorporated as selenocysteine into selenoproteins, which are involved in redox control and protection from oxidative stress (Barrera et al. 2012; Rayman 2005). Epidemiological studies have associated Se deficiency with increased cancer risk. Supplementation with anorganic sodium selenite in experimental animal studies reduced tumor incidence, but this form of Se might not be representative for dietary organo-Se-compounds. Suggested mechanisms targeted by Se include carcinogen activation, DNA repair, cell proliferation, apoptosis, angiogenesis, and immune functions (Combs Jr. and Gray 1998; Jung and Seo 2010). Also, Se compounds were shown to affect DNA methylation by inhibition of DNMTs, resulting in upregulation of, e.g., *GSTP1*, *APC* and *CSR1*, in a prostate cancer cell line. Se also reduced HDAC activity and activated gene expression through increase in H3K9 acetylation and miRNA expression, partly through the activity of metabolites (Huang et al. 2011; Barrera et al. 2012). Lack of efficacy or even negative health effects of Se-methionine supplementation in the large Phase III "Selenium and Vitamin E Cancer Prevention Trial" (SELECT) for prostate cancer prevention reduced the hopes for Se as a human cancer chemopreventive agent, although it might still be valuable in geographic areas of Se-deficiency (Lippman et al. 2009; Lu et al. 2016; Vinceti et al. 2014).

Barrera et al. were interested in the combined effects of ITCs and selenium, based on their complementary mechanisms (Barrera et al. 2012). They treated colorectal cancer cell lines in vitro for up to 12 days with SFN or iberin (6–8 μM) in combination with an inorganic (selenite) or an organic (selenium methylselenocysteine, SeMSC) selenium source (0.2–5 μM) (Barrera et al. 2013). In both cell lines, neither single compounds nor the combination affected promoter methylation of *p16, ESR1, APC* and *MGMT*. Also, methylation of the repetitive element *LINE1* was not affected by the interventions. In Caco2 cells, iberin (8 μM) transiently induced mRNA levels of DNMT1, 3A and 3B after 4 days of treatment, whereas SFN treatment (8 μM) rather reduced the expression after 4 and 8 days of incubation. SeSMC had no significant effects and weakened the inhibition by SFN when used in combination. In HCT116 cells, both ITCs transiently induced DNMT1 and 3B mRNA levels after 4 days of culture. DNMT3B mRNA levels were also induced by combinations of both ITCs with either selenium source. Since translation to protein and global methylation changes were not analyzed, it is difficult to draw final conclusions from these observations (Barrera et al. 2013). Overall, the combination of ITCs and Se seemed to result in antagonistic rather than additive effects.

18.2.2.4 Combination of Selenium with Green Tea Catechins

Hu et al. tested selenium (1 ppm as selenium-enriched milk protein in the diet) and green tea extract (0.5% in the diet) individually and in combination to prevent azoxymethane (AOM)-induced colorectal cancer in rats (Hu et al. 2013). Both single interventions reduced the numbers of large aberrant crypt foci (ACF), and there was an additive increase in inhibition in the combination group. Tumor size, incidence and multiplicity was significantly reduced by around 40–50% in the Se diet group. In combination with green tea polyphenols, the Se effect was additively enhanced to 75–80% inhibition of all endpoints. In all groups receiving Se diet, histone H3 acetylation in colonic crypt sections was elevated. Conversely, DNMT1 protein expression was reduced by diets containing green tea extract. Se intervention reduced β-catenin nuclear translocation, Cyclin D1 expression and Ki-67 staining, indicating reduced proliferation (Hu et al. 2013). Overall, the study provided promising results that should be reproduced in additional models and with additional sources of Se.

Table 18.3 Combination effects in other cancer models

Model and treatment	Effects	References
Ovarian cancer		
SKOV3-ip1 (paclitaxel-sensitive), SKOV3TR-ip2 (paclitaxel-resistant) EGCG 20 μM SFN 10 μM	⇧ apoptosis, cell cycle arrest in S and G_2/M-phase ⇧ DNA-damage (pH2AX) ⇩ hTERT protein expression and activity ⇩ Bcl-2 protein levels ⇩ DNMT1 expression	Chen et al. (2013a)
A2780 (cisplatin-sensitive), A2780/CP20 (cisplatin-resistant) EGCG 2.5–40 μM SFN 2.5–20 μM	⇩ cell viability in both cell lines ⇧ cisplatin-induced apoptosis and G_2/M arrest ⇧ p21 expression	Chen et al. (2013b)
Lymphoma		
CA46 EGCG 6–48 μg/ml Trichostatin A (TSA) 3–48 ng/ml	⇩ cell proliferation ⇧ cell cycle arrest in G_0/G_1 and G_2/M ⇩ p16 promoter methylation ⇧ p16 mRNA + protein expression	Wu et al. (2013)
Prostate cancer		
PC3, DU145 Quercetin 5 μM Curcumin 5 μM	⇩ DNMT activity in both cell lines ⇩ DNA methylation at the promoter of the androgen receptor (AR) gene ⇧ reexpression of AR mRNA and protein ⇧ anti-androgen responsiveness ⇧ induction of apoptosis	Sharma et al. (2016)

⇧ induction, enhancement, increase; ⇩ repression, inhibition, reduction; ⇔ no change

18.2.3 Studies with Ovarian Cancer, Prostate Cancer and Lymphoma

Until now, only a few in vitro studies investigated combination effects via epigenetic mechanisms in tumor entities beside breast and colon cancer. Table 18.3 summarized combination studies targeting ovarian and prostate cancer and lymphomas.

18.2.3.1 Combination of EGCG with SFN in Chemotherapy-Resistant Ovarian Cancer Models

Ovarian cancer is the eighth most common cancer in females, with about 295,000 estimated new cases and 185,000 estimated cancer deaths worldwide in 2018 (Bray et al. 2018). Ovarian cancer mortality is relatively high due to a lack of screening options, late diagnosis, and the development of resistance against conventional chemotherapy.

In two studies by Chen et al., the effects of EGCG in combination with SFN were tested in chemotherapy-sensitive vs. resistant ovarian cancer cell lines (Chen et al. 2013a, b). In the first study, the combination of EGCG (20 μM) and SFN (10 μM)

efficiently reduced cell proliferation and induced cell cycle arrest in S and G_2/M phase and apoptosis in paclitaxel-resistant ovarian cancer cells. In addition, expression and activity of hTERT, the catalytic subunit of human telomerase that is often upregulated in cancer cells, as well as expression of the anti-apoptotic *Bcl-2* were reduced (Chen et al. 2013a). Combination of both compounds also effectively reduced DNMT1 expression in the ovarian cancer cell lines. As shown previously, hTERT expression is epigenetically regulated by DNA methylation at specific CpG sites in the promoter region. Loss of methylation at these sites allows interaction with the E2F repressive complex, resulting in hTERT down-regulation [summary in Gerhauser (2013)]. In the study by Chen et al., hTERT promoter methylation was not determined (Chen et al. 2013a).

In the second study, Chen et al. used a pair of cisplatin-sensitive and resistant cell lines to investigate cell growth inhibitory effects of the combination of EGCG (10 μM) and SFN (5 μM) (Chen et al. 2013b). Both compounds in combination reduced cell proliferation and induced apoptosis in both cell lines, and strongly increased sensitivity to cisplatin in the resistant cell line. EGCG + SFN, especially in combination with cisplatin (1.5 μM), also potently induced cell-cycle arrest in G_2/M phase, more than either compound alone. This was linked to up-regulation of cyclin-dependent kinase inhibitor p21 only in the cisplatin-sensitive cell line.

Since these interesting findings were limited to in vitro investigations, further work should demonstrate enhanced efficacy of chemotherapy in combination with EGCG + SFN in animal models for tumor resistance and clinical studies (Chen et al. 2013b).

18.2.3.2 Combination of EGCG with TSA in Lymphoma Cells

Burkitt lymphoma is a rare but highly aggressive subtype of B-cell non-Hodgkin lymphoma (NHL). With an estimated 510,000 new cancer cases and about 250,000 cancer death in 2018, NHL is the eighth most common cancer type in males and the tenth most common cancer type in females worldwide (Bray et al. 2018).

Wu et al. investigated the impact of EGCG (6 μg/ml) and the HDAC inhibitor TSA (15 ng/ml) on proliferation and cell cycle progression of CA46 lymphoma cells via epigenetic regulation of the cell cycle inhibitor $p16^{INK4A}$ (Wu et al. 2013). EGCG in combination with TSA inhibited cell proliferation more potently than either compound alone, and reduced the fraction of cells in S-phase of the cell cycle. The authors demonstrated by methylation-specific PCR that the cell-cycle inhibitor *p16* promoter was demethylated by EGCG in a dose-dependent manner. Co-treatment with TSA enhanced the demethylating effect of EGCG. Reduced methylation at the *p16* promoter was associated with enhanced *p16* mRNA and protein expression, with stronger effects by the co-treatment than with EGCG alone.

This study demonstrated increased cell growth inhibition by combining a demethylating agent (EGCG) with a potent chromatin modulator (TSA). The study focused on investigating the combination treatment effect on cell cycle inhibitor *p16*. It can be assumed that the combination will affect additional targets beside *p16*, which might contribute to the anti-proliferate activity.

18.2.3.3 Combination of Polyphenols Quercetin and Curcumin in Prostate Cancer

After lung cancer, prostate cancer is the second most common cancer types in males, with an estimated 1.27 million new cases and about 360,000 cancer death worldwide in 2018 (Bray et al. 2018). Prostate cancer cell proliferation is driven by androgen binding to the androgen receptor (AR). In a subset of prostate cancer cell lines and prostate tumors, *AR* is silenced by promoter methylation (Massie et al. 2017).

Quercetin-glycosides are flavonoids ubiquitously occurring in fruits, vegetables and beverages (Russo et al. 2012). Quercetin is regarded as a broad-spectrum cancer preventive agent: it has radical-scavenging potential and modulates signaling transduction pathways and transcription factors involved in detoxification, inflammation, cell cycle regulation, apoptosis, angiogenesis, autophagy, immune defense and senescence [reviewed in Kashyap et al. (2019) and Murakami et al. (2008)]. In rodent models, quercetin intervention prevented the development of colon, mammary gland, skin and lung cancers (Murakami et al. 2008). In humans, uptake of quercetin reduced markers of oxidative stress and inflammation (Russo et al. 2012).

With respect to epigenetic mechanisms, activation of HATs and sirtuins by quercetin was linked to anti-inflammatory activity by suppressing COX-2 expression, inhibition of NF-κB acetylation and activation of ERK/JNK signaling. Quercetin led to re-expression of cell cycle inhibitor *p16* through inhibition of promoter hypermethylation and inhibited the histone demethylase LSD1. Quercetin also modulated the expression of several miRNAs in various cancer cell lines [summary in Aggarwal et al. (2015) and Shankar et al. (2016)].

Curcumin (diferuloyl methane) is a yellow pigment found in turmeric (*Curcuma longa*). Curcumin has been used for centuries as a traditional medicine in India and other countries (Gupta et al. 2013). As an anti-inflammatory and cancer preventive agent, curcumin targets NF-κB and other signaling pathways (Pavan et al. 2016; Xu et al. 2018). It induced apoptosis and blocked invasion, metastasis, and angiogenesis in in vitro models, and prevented or inhibited tumor growth in rodent models essentially for all major tumor entities (Gupta et al. 2013; Huminiecki et al. 2017). Curcumin is well tolerated even at high concentrations up to 15 g/day (Gupta et al. 2013; Xu et al. 2018).

With respect to epigenetics, curcumin was shown to inhibit p300/CBP HAT activity and to reduce HDAC and DNMT expression. In addition to histone acetylation, curcumin also inhibited acetylation of non-histone targets such as p53 (Balasubramanyam et al. 2004). Effects on DNA methylation after long-term culture for 240 days with curcumin were interpreted as an indirect effect subsequent to changes in, e.g., NF-κB signaling (Huminiecki et al. 2017). Curcumin and derivatives have also been identified as potent modulators of miRNAs and long noncoding RNAs. Main targets in various tumor entities include *miR-21*/PTEN/Akt signaling, *miR19a/b*/Akt/MDM2/PTEN/p53 signaling, *miR15/16*/Bcl2 or WT1 signaling, and miRNA-mediated effects on EZH2, Wnt signaling, cell viability and apoptosis [extensive reviews in references Huminiecki et al. (2017) and Liu et al. (2019)].

Sharma et al. combined quercetin and curcumin to re-sensitize *AR*-negative prostate cancer cells to anti-androgen treatment by re-expression of AR (Sharma et al. 2016). PC3 and DU145 cells were treated with curcumin (12 μM), quercetin (14 μM) or a 1:1 mix of both compounds (10 μM) at the EC_{25} (effective concentration inhibiting 25% of cell growth). Both compounds alone, but more effectively in combination, reduced DNMT activity in both cell lines, especially after treatment for 72 h. Curcumin alone was more potent than the combination in reducing global methylation levels. The authors demonstrated that a region spanning 27 CpG sites in the AR promoter was methylated in both cell lines, leading to silencing of AR expression at the mRNA and protein level. The combination was significantly more effective in demethylating and re-expressing the AR than either compound alone. Using a luciferase reporter assay, the authors also demonstrated that the combination effectively re-sensitized the cell lines to androgen-stimulation. In both cell lines, the combination was more potent in inducing apoptosis than either compound alone, estimated by FITC-Annexin-V staining and flow cytometry. These findings should be confirmed in animal studies. Since the AR is not commonly deactivated by promoter methylation in human prostate tumors, the results might be limited to the in vitro model and lack relevance for the treatment or prevention of human prostate cancer.

18.3 Summary and Conclusions

The aim of this chapter was to give an overview of mostly diet-derived cancer chemopreventive agents that target epigenetic mechanisms and have been tested in combination to enhance their efficacy. Compounds covered in this chapter include some of the best investigated chemopreventive agents, including green tea catechins, soy isoflavones, quercetin, resveratrol and pterostilbene, the short chain fatty acid butyrate, sulforaphane, selenium, curcumin, synthetic triterpenoids such as CDDO, docosahexaenoic acid and withaferin A.

Many of the combinations have so far only been tested in vitro in cell culture models, with some limitations.

1. Most of the studies based the selection of concentrations used for combination interventions on dose-response analyses using anti-proliferative activity as an endpoint. Concentrations required to target epigenetic mechanisms might differ.
2. One of the main aims of combination studies is to reduce the doses necessary to achieve activity/efficacy. Only few of the studies considered whether the applied concentrations would be achievable in vivo.
3. An aim of combination studies is to combine compounds with complementary activity to enhance the biological effect, preferentially more than additively. To draw conclusions on synergism, additive effects or antagonism, ideally the study design should allow quantitative determination of the mode of interaction. This information is largely missing in the presented studies. A suitable approach is nonlinear modeling, which was reported to be advantageous in comparison to the

frequently used Combination Index according to Chou and Talalay [details in Chou (2010), Boik et al. (2008), and Ashton (2015)].

4. As seen with the combination of GTP and butyrate in colorectal cancer studies, depending on the concentrations tested, the outcome of the combination treatment might differ (Sanchez-Tena et al. 2013; Saldanha et al. 2014). Therefore the likely interactions of the tested compounds should be known to avoid antagonistic effects (DiMarco-Crook and Xiao 2015).
5. Most of the studies focused on preselected target genes. Monitoring of global gene expression changes by RNA-sequencing and gene set or pathway enrichment of differentially expressed genes might help in providing a more complete understanding of the mechanisms of interaction. Additional information might come from genome-wide-omics approaches to monitor changes in chromatin accessibility.

Despite of these limitations, the combination studies have provided interesting results which were often confirmed in animal models. Most of the described projects focused on breast and colorectal cancers. A common theme in breast cancer studies was the reactivation of epigenetically silenced ERα, re-sensitizing ER-negative TNBC to anti-hormonal treatment. Currently, no targeted therapy exists to treat TNBC, and only about 50% of TNBC cases respond to chemotherapy. Therefore, intervention with epigenetically active dietary agents to re-establish sensitivity to anti-hormonal therapy might be a strategy to manage TNBC worth being followed-up in clinical trials. Similarly, for ovarian cancer, increasing the susceptibility of resistant tumors to chemotherapy by co-treatment with epigenetically active compounds such as EGCG + SFN might be a promising strategy which should be further investigated in vivo.

For colorectal cancer prevention, treatment with dietary fiber, which is metabolized to SCFAs affecting chromatin compaction, in combination with additional chemopreventive agents such as DHA, has provided promising results in rodent models (Cho et al. 2012; Davidson et al. 2009; Shah et al. 2011, 2016a; Triff et al. 2018). Advanced –omics technologies including genome-wide DNA methylation analyses, miRNA expression analyses, RNA-sequencing and chromatin immunoprecipitation coupled with sequencing (ChIP-seq) have been employed to allow integrative analyses of multiple epigenetic mechanisms. Overall, these studies have indicated that linking miRNA expression or alterations in DNA methylation and chromatin accessibility with expression of associated target genes is still challenging in dietary intervention studies with weak and infrequent treatment-induced effects, compared to cancer-induced epigenetic alterations. Integration and interpretation of results is aggravated by variation in treatment response observed in individual animals and a lack in statistical power when genome-wide analyses are performed with small numbers of animals per group and results are corrected for multiple testing. Translation of results from animal studies with dietary fiber to the human situation might additionally be complicated by the heterogeneity of the human gut microbiota and varying levels of butyrate-producing bacteria, which adds another level of complexity to human intervention studies with the aim of colon cancer prevention.

In conclusion, combination of epigenetic agents that target the epigenome to enhance efficacy is a promising strategy in cancer chemoprevention. We are beginning to understand how chemopreventive agents affect DNA methylation, histone modifications or miRNA expression in vivo, and how alterations of these epigenetic mechanisms by combination treatments will affect gene expression and can be translated to chemopreventive efficacy. Genome-wide analyses and more systems biology-based approached might be required to fully comprehend the compounds' interactions affecting the epigenome.

References

Aggarwal R et al (2015) Natural compounds: role in reversal of epigenetic changes. Biochemistry (Mosc) 80(8):972–989

Allis CD et al (2007) New nomenclature for chromatin-modifying enzymes. Cell 131(4):633–636

Ashton JC (2015) Drug combination studies and their synergy quantification using the Chou-Talalay method—letter. Cancer Res 75(11):2400

Balasubramanyam K et al (2004) Curcumin, a novel p300/CREB-binding protein-specific inhibitor of acetyltransferase, represses the acetylation of histone/nonhistone proteins and histone acetyltransferase-dependent chromatin transcription. J Biol Chem 279(49):51163–51171

Banerjee S et al (2008) Multi-targeted therapy of cancer by genistein. Cancer Lett 269(2):226–242

Barnes CE, English DM, Cowley SM (2019) Acetylation & Co: an expanding repertoire of histone acylations regulates chromatin and transcription. Essays Biochem 63(1):97–107

Barrera LN et al (2012) Epigenetic and antioxidant effects of dietary isothiocyanates and selenium: potential implications for cancer chemoprevention. Proc Nutr Soc 71(2):237–245

Barrera LN et al (2013) Colorectal cancer cells Caco-2 and HCT116 resist epigenetic effects of isothiocyanates and selenium in vitro. Eur J Nutr 52(4):1327–1341

Baur JA, Sinclair DA (2006) Therapeutic potential of resveratrol: the in vivo evidence. Nat Rev Drug Discov 5(6):493–506

Berdasco M, Esteller M (2010) Aberrant epigenetic landscape in cancer: how cellular identity goes awry. Dev Cell 19(5):698–711

Berquin IM, Edwards IJ, Chen YQ (2008) Multi-targeted therapy of cancer by omega-3 fatty acids. Cancer Lett 269(2):363–377

Biersack B (2016) Current state of phenolic and terpenoidal dietary factors and natural products as non-coding RNA/microRNA modulators for improved cancer therapy and prevention. Noncoding RNA Res 1(1):12–34

Boik JC, Newman RA, Boik RJ (2008) Quantifying synergism/antagonism using nonlinear mixed-effects modeling: a simulation study. Stat Med 27(7):1040–1061

Bonkowski MS, Sinclair DA (2016) Slowing ageing by design: the rise of NAD(+) and sirtuin-activating compounds. Nat Rev Mol Cell Biol 17(11):679–690

Brait M, Sidransky D (2011) Cancer epigenetics: above and beyond. Toxicol Mech Methods 21 (4):275–288

Bray F et al (2018) Global cancer statistics 2018: GLOBOCAN estimates of incidence and mortality worldwide for 36 cancers in 185 countries. CA Cancer J Clin 68(6):394–424

Bultman SJ (2017) Interplay between diet, gut microbiota, epigenetic events, and colorectal cancer. Mol Nutr Food Res 61(1)

Calin GA, Croce CM (2006) MicroRNA signatures in human cancers. Nat Rev Cancer 6 (11):857–866

Carlos-Reyes A et al (2019) Dietary Compounds as Epigenetic Modulating Agents in Cancer. Front Genet 10:79

Chen H et al (2013a) Epigallocatechin gallate and sulforaphane combination treatment induce apoptosis in paclitaxel-resistant ovarian cancer cells through hTERT and Bcl-2 down-regulation. Exp Cell Res 319(5):697–706
Chen H et al (2013b) Enhancement of cisplatin-mediated apoptosis in ovarian cancer cells through potentiating G2/M arrest and p21 upregulation by combinatorial epigallocatechin gallate and sulforaphane. J Oncol 2013:872957
Chen J, Zhao KN, Vitetta L (2019) Effects of intestinal microbial(−)elaborated butyrate on oncogenic signaling pathways. Nutrients 11(5):E1026
Cho Y et al (2012) A chemoprotective fish oil/pectin diet enhances apoptosis via Bcl-2 promoter methylation in rat azoxymethane-induced carcinomas. Exp Biol Med (Maywood) 237 (12):1387–1393
Cho Y et al (2014) Colon cancer cell apoptosis is induced by combined exposure to the n-3 fatty acid docosahexaenoic acid and butyrate through promoter methylation. Exp Biol Med (Maywood) 239(3):302–310
Chou TC (2010) Drug combination studies and their synergy quantification using the Chou-Talalay method. Cancer Res 70(2):440–446
Combs GF Jr, Gray WP (1998) Chemopreventive agents: selenium. Pharmacol Ther 79(3):179–192
Dashwood RH, Ho E (2007) Dietary histone deacetylase inhibitors: from cells to mice to man. Semin Cancer Biol 17(5):363–369
Davidson LA et al (2009) n-3 Polyunsaturated fatty acids modulate carcinogen-directed non-coding microRNA signatures in rat colon. Carcinogenesis 30(12):2077–2084
Davie JR (2003) Inhibition of histone deacetylase activity by butyrate. J Nutr 133(7 Suppl):2485S–2493S
de Zeeuw D et al (2013) Bardoxolone methyl in type 2 diabetes and stage 4 chronic kidney disease. N Engl J Med 369(26):2492–2503
Deeb D et al (2014) Induction of apoptosis in pancreatic cancer cells by CDDO-Me involves repression of telomerase through epigenetic pathways. J Carcinog Mutagen 5:177
den Besten G et al (2013) The role of short-chain fatty acids in the interplay between diet, gut microbiota, and host energy metabolism. J Lipid Res 54(9):2325–2340
DiMarco-Crook C, Xiao H (2015) Diet-based strategies for cancer chemoprevention: the role of combination regimens using dietary bioactive components. Annu Rev Food Sci Technol 6:505–526
Dimri M et al (2010) Dietary omega-3 polyunsaturated fatty acids suppress expression of EZH2 in breast cancer cells. Carcinogenesis 31(3):489–495
Dufour V, Stahl M, Baysse C (2015) The antibacterial properties of isothiocyanates. Microbiology 161(Pt 2):229–243
Esteller M (2007) Cancer epigenomics: DNA methylomes and histone-modification maps. Nat Rev Genet 8(4):286–298
Farhana L et al (2018) Role of microbiome in carcinogenesis process and epigenetic regulation of colorectal cancer. Methods Mol Biol 1856:35–55
Feinberg AP, Koldobskiy MA, Gondor A (2016) Epigenetic modulators, modifiers and mediators in cancer aetiology and progression. Nat Rev Genet 17(5):284–299
Felsenfeld G (2014) A brief history of epigenetics. Cold Spring Harb Perspect Biol 6(1):a018200
Fernandes GFS et al (2017) Epigenetic regulatory mechanisms induced by resveratrol. Nutrients 9 (11):E1201
Fujiki H et al (2018) Cancer prevention with green tea and its principal constituent, EGCG: from early investigations to current focus on human cancer stem cells. Mol Cells 41(2):73–82
Gao YF, Tollefsbol TO (2015) Impact of epigenetic dietary components on cancer through histone modifications. Curr Med Chem 22(17):2051–2064
Gauttam VK, Kalia AN (2013) Development of polyherbal antidiabetic formulation encapsulated in the phospholipids vesicle system. J Adv Pharm Technol Res 4(2):108–117
Gerhauser C (2013) Cancer chemoprevention and nutriepigenetics: state of the art and future challenges. Top Curr Chem 329:73–132

Gerhauser C (2014) Epigenetics, (poly) phenolics and cancer prevention. In: Romani A, Quideau S (eds) Recent advances in polyphenol research, vol 4. Wiley, New York, pp 143–207
Gerhauser C (2018) Impact of dietary gut microbial metabolites on the epigenome. Philos Trans R Soc Lond Ser B Biol Sci 373(1748):20170359
Glozak MA et al (2005) Acetylation and deacetylation of non-histone proteins. Gene 363:15–23
Grosso G et al (2017) Possible role of diet in cancer: systematic review and multiple meta-analyses of dietary patterns, lifestyle factors, and cancer risk. Nutr Rev 75(6):405–419
Guil S, Esteller M (2009) DNA methylomes, histone codes and miRNAs: tying it all together. Int J Biochem Cell Biol 41(1):87–95
Guilloteau P et al (2010) From the gut to the peripheral tissues: the multiple effects of butyrate. Nutr Res Rev 23(2):366–384
Gupta PB et al (2009) Identification of selective inhibitors of cancer stem cells by high-throughput screening. Cell 138(4):645–659
Gupta SC et al (2013) Multitargeting by turmeric, the golden spice: from kitchen to clinic. Mol Nutr Food Res 57(9):1510–1528
Hamamoto R, Saloura V, Nakamura Y (2015) Critical roles of non-histone protein lysine methylation in human tumorigenesis. Nat Rev Cancer 15(2):110–124
Hervouet E et al (2013) Epigenetic regulation of estrogen signaling in breast cancer. Epigenetics 8 (3):237–245
Heyninck K et al (2016) Withaferin A induces heme oxygenase (HO-1) expression in endothelial cells via activation of the Keap1/Nrf2 pathway. Biochem Pharmacol 109:48–61
Hong DS et al (2012) A phase I first-in-human trial of bardoxolone methyl in patients with advanced solid tumors and lymphomas. Clin Cancer Res 18(12):3396–3406
Houghton CA, Fassett RG, Coombes JS (2013) Sulforaphane: translational research from laboratory bench to clinic. Nutr Rev 71(11):709–726
Hu Y et al (2013) Combination of selenium and green tea improves the efficacy of chemoprevention in a rat colorectal cancer model by modulating genetic and epigenetic biomarkers. PLoS One 8 (5):e64362
Huang J, Plass C, Gerhauser C (2011) Cancer chemoprevention by targeting the epigenome. Curr Drug Targets 12(13):1925–1956
Huang D et al (2019) An overview of epigenetic agents and natural nutrition products targeting DNA methyltransferase, histone deacetylases and microRNAs. Food Chem Toxicol 123:574–594
Huminiecki L, Horbanczuk J, Atanasov AG (2017) The functional genomic studies of curcumin. Semin Cancer Biol 46:107–118
Jones PA (2012) Functions of DNA methylation: islands, start sites, gene bodies and beyond. Nat Rev Genet 13(7):484–492
Jung HJ, Seo YR (2010) Current issues of selenium in cancer chemoprevention. Biofactors 36 (2):153–158
Kala R, Tollefsbol TO (2016) A novel combinatorial epigenetic therapy using resveratrol and pterostilbene for restoring estrogen receptor-alpha (ERalpha) expression in ERalpha-negative breast Cancer cells. PLoS One 11(5):e0155057
Kala R et al (2015) Epigenetic-based combinatorial resveratrol and pterostilbene alters DNA damage response by affecting SIRT1 and DNMT enzyme expression, including SIRT1-dependent gamma-H2AX and telomerase regulation in triple-negative breast cancer. BMC Cancer 15:672
Kashyap D et al (2019) Fisetin and quercetin: promising flavonoids with chemopreventive potential. Biomol Ther 9(5):174
Khan N, Mukhtar H (2008) Multitargeted therapy of cancer by green tea polyphenols. Cancer Lett 269(2):269–280
Kim HJ, Bae SC (2011) Histone deacetylase inhibitors: molecular mechanisms of action and clinical trials as anti-cancer drugs. Am J Transl Res 3(2):166–179

Kim E et al (2016) Histone and non-histone targets of dietary deacetylase inhibitors. Curr Top Med Chem 16(7):714–731

Kouzarides T (2007) Chromatin modifications and their function. Cell 128(4):693–705

Kozomara A, Birgaoanu M, Griffiths-Jones S (2019) miRBase: from microRNA sequences to function. Nucleic Acids Res 47(D1):D155–D162

Kundu JK, Surh YJ (2008) Cancer chemopreventive and therapeutic potential of resveratrol: mechanistic perspectives. Cancer Lett 269(2):243–261

Lao VV, Grady WM (2011) Epigenetics and colorectal cancer. Nat Rev Gastroenterol Hepatol 8 (12):686–700

Lau ATY, Yu F-Y, Xu Y-M (2019) Epigenetic effects of essential fatty acids. Curr Pharmacol Rep 5(1):68–78

Lee IC, Choi BY (2016) Withaferin-A--A natural anticancer agent with pleitropic mechanisms of action. Int J Mol Sci 17(3):290

Lee PS et al (2018) Chemoprevention by resveratrol and pterostilbene: targeting on epigenetic regulation. Biofactors 44(1):26–35

Li Y et al (2013) Epigenetic reactivation of estrogen receptor-alpha (ERalpha) by genistein enhances hormonal therapy sensitivity in ERalpha-negative breast cancer. Mol Cancer 12:9

Li Y et al (2016) Combinatorial epigenetic mechanisms and efficacy of early breast cancer inhibition by nutritive botanicals. Epigenomics 8(8):1019–1037

Li Y, Meeran SM, Tollefsbol TO (2017) Combinatorial bioactive botanicals re-sensitize tamoxifen treatment in ER-negative breast cancer via epigenetic reactivation of ERalpha expression. Sci Rep 7(1):9345

Liby KT, Sporn MB (2012) Synthetic oleanane triterpenoids: multifunctional drugs with a broad range of applications for prevention and treatment of chronic disease. Pharmacol Rev 64 (4):972–1003

Liby KT, Yore MM, Sporn MB (2007) Triterpenoids and rexinoids as multifunctional agents for the prevention and treatment of cancer. Nat Rev Cancer 7(5):357–369

Link A, Balaguer F, Goel A (2010) Cancer chemoprevention by dietary polyphenols: promising role for epigenetics. Biochem Pharmacol 80(12):1771–1792

Lippman SM et al (2009) Effect of selenium and vitamin E on risk of prostate cancer and other cancers: the Selenium and Vitamin E Cancer Prevention Trial (SELECT). JAMA 301(1):39–51

Liu Y et al (2019) The targeting of noncoding RNAs by curcumin: Facts and hopes for cancer therapy (Review). Oncol Rep 42(1):20–34

Livingstone MC et al (2017) Profound changes in miRNA expression during cancer initiation by aflatoxin B1 and their abrogation by the chemopreventive triterpenoid CDDO-Im. Mol Carcinog 56(11):2382–2390

Lu J et al (2016) Cancer chemoprevention research with selenium in the post-SELECT era: promises and challenges. Nutr Cancer 68(1):1–17

Magee PJ, Rowland I (2012) Soy products in the management of breast cancer. Curr Opin Clin Nutr Metab Care 15(6):586–591

Martin SL, Royston KJ, Tollefsbol TO (2018) The role of non-coding RNAs and isothiocyanates in cancer. Mol Nutr Food Res 62(18):e1700913

Marventano S et al (2015) A review of recent evidence in human studies of n-3 and n-6 PUFA intake on cardiovascular disease, cancer, and depressive disorders: does the ratio really matter? Int J Food Sci Nutr 66(6):611–622

Massie CE, Mills IG, Lynch AG (2017) The importance of DNA methylation in prostate cancer development. J Steroid Biochem Mol Biol 166:1–15

McNabney SM, Henagan TM (2017) Short chain fatty acids in the colon and peripheral tissues: a focus on butyrate, colon cancer, obesity and insulin resistance. Nutrients 9(12):E1348

Meeran SM et al (2012) Bioactive dietary supplements reactivate ER expression in ER-negative breast cancer cells by active chromatin modifications. PLoS One 7(5):e37748

Messina M (2016) Soy and health update: evaluation of the clinical and epidemiologic literature. Nutrients 8(12):754

Minucci S, Pelicci PG (2006) Histone deacetylase inhibitors and the promise of epigenetic (and more) treatments for cancer. Nat Rev Cancer 6(1):38–51
Mirza S et al (2013) Expression of DNA methyltransferases in breast cancer patients and to analyze the effect of natural compounds on DNA methyltransferases and associated proteins. J Breast Cancer 16(1):23–31
Mohammed A, Fox JT, Miller MS (2019) Cancer chemoprevention: preclinical in vivo alternate dosing strategies to reduce drug toxicities. Toxicol Sci 170:251–259
Molinie B, Georgel P (2009) Genetic and epigenetic regulations of prostate cancer by genistein. Drug News Perspect 22(5):247–254
Mukund V et al (2017) Genistein: its role in metabolic diseases and cancer. Crit Rev Oncol Hematol 119:13–22
Murakami A, Ashida H, Terao J (2008) Multitargeted cancer prevention by quercetin. Cancer Lett 269(2):315–325
Myzak MC et al (2004) A novel mechanism of chemoprotection by sulforaphane: inhibition of histone deacetylase. Cancer Res 64(16):5767–5774
National Library of Medicine (NLM) (2019), Clinicaltrial.gov
Ndlovu MN et al (2009) Hyperactivated NF-{kappa}B and AP-1 transcription factors promote highly accessible chromatin and constitutive transcription across the interleukin-6 gene promoter in metastatic breast cancer cells. Mol Cell Biol 29(20):5488–5504
O'Keefe SJ (2016) Diet, microorganisms and their metabolites, and colon cancer. Nat Rev Gastroenterol Hepatol 13(12):691–706
Palliyaguru DL, Singh SV, Kensler TW (2016) *Withania somnifera*: from prevention to treatment of cancer. Mol Nutr Food Res 60(6):1342–1353
Palliyaguru DL et al (2018) Isothiocyanates: translating the power of plants to people. Mol Nutr Food Res **62**(18):e1700965
Park SM et al (2008) The miR-200 family determines the epithelial phenotype of cancer cells by targeting the E-cadherin repressors ZEB1 and ZEB2. Genes Dev 22(7):894–907
Pathania R et al (2016) Combined inhibition of DNMT and HDAC blocks the tumorigenicity of cancer stem-like cells and attenuates mammary tumor growth. Cancer Res 76(11):3224–3235
Paul B, Li Y, Tollefsbol TO (2018) The effects of combinatorial genistein and sulforaphane in breast tumor inhibition: role in epigenetic regulation. Int J Mol Sci 19(6):E1754
Pavan AR et al (2016) Unraveling the anticancer effect of curcumin and resveratrol. Nutrients 8 (11):628
Perou CM et al (2000) Molecular portraits of human breast tumours. Nature 406(6797):747–752
Pezzuto JM (2008) Resveratrol as an inhibitor of carcinogenensis. Pharm Biol 46(7–8):443–573
Pezzuto JM (2019) Resveratrol: twenty years of growth, development and controversy. Biomol Ther (Seoul) 27(1):1–14
Pudenz M, Roth K, Gerhauser C (2014) Impact of soy isoflavones on the epigenome in cancer prevention. Nutrients 6(10):4218–4272
Qin S, Hou DX (2016) Multiple regulations of Keap1/Nrf2 system by dietary phytochemicals. Mol Nutr Food Res 60(8):1731–1755
Ramirez-Garza SL et al (2018) Health effects of resveratrol: results from human intervention trials. Nutrients 10(12):1892
Rayman MP (2005) Selenium in cancer prevention: a review of the evidence and mechanism of action. Proc Nutr Soc 64(4):527–542
Rimando AM, Suh N (2008) Biological/chemopreventive activity of stilbenes and their effect on colon cancer. Planta Med 74(13):1635–1643
Royston KJ et al (2017) A novel combination of withaferin A and sulforaphane inhibits epigenetic machinery, cellular viability and induces apoptosis of breast cancer cells. Int J Mol Sci 18 (5):1092
Royston KJ et al (2018) Withaferin A and sulforaphane regulate breast cancer cell cycle progression through epigenetic mechanisms. Exp Cell Res 368(1):67–74

Russo M et al (2012) The flavonoid quercetin in disease prevention and therapy: facts and fancies. Biochem Pharmacol 83(1):6–15
Russo M et al (2016) Understanding genistein in cancer: the "good" and the "bad" effects: a review. Food Chem 196:589–600
Saini RK, Keum YS (2018) Omega-3 and omega-6 polyunsaturated fatty acids: dietary sources, metabolism, and significance - a review. Life Sci 203:255–267
Saldanha SN, Kala R, Tollefsbol TO (2014) Molecular mechanisms for inhibition of colon cancer cells by combined epigenetic-modulating epigallocatechin gallate and sodium butyrate. Exp Cell Res 324(1):40–53
Sanchez-Tena S et al (2013) Green tea phenolics inhibit butyrate-induced differentiation of colon cancer cells by interacting with monocarboxylate transporter 1. Biochim Biophys Acta 1832 (12):2264–2270
Seto E, Yoshida M (2014) Erasers of histone acetylation: the histone deacetylase enzymes. Cold Spring Harb Perspect Biol 6(4):a018713
Shah MS et al (2011) Integrated microRNA and mRNA expression profiling in a rat colon carcinogenesis model: effect of a chemo-protective diet. Physiol Genomics 43(10):640–654
Shah MS et al (2016a) Comparative effects of diet and carcinogen on microRNA expression in the stem cell niche of the mouse colonic crypt. Biochim Biophys Acta 1862(1):121–134
Shah MS et al (2016b) Data describing the effects of dietary bioactive agents on colonic stem cell microRNA and mRNA expression. Data Brief 6:398–404
Shankar E et al (2016) Dietary phytochemicals as epigenetic modifiers in cancer: promise and challenges. Semin Cancer Biol 40-41:82–99
Sharma V et al (2016) Sensitization of androgen refractory prostate cancer cells to anti-androgens through re-expression of epigenetically repressed androgen receptor - Synergistic action of quercetin and curcumin. Mol Cell Endocrinol 431:12–23
Shortt J et al (2017) A chemical probe toolbox for dissecting the cancer epigenome. Nat Rev Cancer 17(3):160–183
Shukla S, Meeran SM, Katiyar SK (2014) Epigenetic regulation by selected dietary phytochemicals in cancer chemoprevention. Cancer Lett 355(1):9–17
Sorlie T et al (2003) Repeated observation of breast tumor subtypes in independent gene expression data sets. Proc Natl Acad Sci U S A 100(14):8418–8423
Soshnev AA, Josefowicz SZ, Allis CD (2016) Greater than the sum of parts: complexity of the dynamic epigenome. Mol Cell 62(5):681–694
Sporn MB (1980) Combination chemoprevention of cancer. Nature 287(5778):107–108
Steiner C et al (2008) Isoflavones and the prevention of breast and prostate cancer: new perspectives opened by nutrigenomics. Br J Nutr 99(E Suppl 1):ES78–E108
Stirzaker C et al (2014) Mining cancer methylomes: prospects and challenges. Trends Genet 30 (2):75–84
Su X et al (2018) Anticancer activity of sulforaphane: The epigenetic mechanisms and the Nrf2 signaling pathway. Oxid Med Cell Longev 2018:5438179
Szarc Vel Szic K et al (2017) Epigenetic silencing of triple negative breast cancer hallmarks by Withaferin A. Oncotarget 8(25):40434–40453
Tan JK et al (2017) Metabolite-sensing G protein-coupled receptors-facilitators of diet-related immune regulation. Annu Rev Immunol 35:371–402
Taylor CK et al (2009) The effect of genistein aglycone on cancer and cancer risk: a review of in vitro, preclinical, and clinical studies. Nutr Rev 67(7):398–415
Thomson CA, Dickinson S, Bowden GT (2010) Cruciferous vegetables, isothiocyanates, indoles, and cancer prevention. In: Milner JA, Romagnolo DF (eds) Bioactive compounds and cancer. Humana, Totowa, NJ, pp 535–566
Tortorella SM et al (2015) Dietary sulforaphane in cancer chemoprevention: the role of epigenetic regulation and HDAC inhibition. Antioxid Redox Signal 22(16):1382–1424
Tran K et al (2013) The combination of the histone deacetylase inhibitor vorinostat and synthetic triterpenoids reduces tumorigenesis in mouse models of cancer. Carcinogenesis 34(1):199–210

Triff K, Kim E, Chapkin RS (2015) Chemoprotective epigenetic mechanisms in a colorectal cancer model: modulation by n-3 PUFA in combination with fermentable fiber. Curr Pharmacol Rep 1 (1):11–20

Triff K et al (2018) Dietary fat and fiber interact to uniquely modify global histone post-translational epigenetic programming in a rat colon cancer progression model. Int J Cancer 143 (6):1402–1415

Upadhyay AK, Cheng X (2011) Dynamics of histone lysine methylation: structures of methyl writers and erasers. Prog Drug Res 67:107–124

Vanden Berghe W (2012) Epigenetic impact of dietary polyphenols in cancer chemoprevention: lifelong remodeling of our epigenomes. Pharmacol Res 65(6):565–576

vel Szic KS et al (2010) Nature or nurture: let food be your epigenetic medicine in chronic inflammatory disorders. Biochem Pharmacol 80(12):1816–1832

Verkerk R et al (2009) Glucosinolates in Brassica vegetables: the influence of the food supply chain on intake, bioavailability and human health. Mol Nutr Food Res 53(Suppl 2):S219

Vigushin DM et al (2001) Trichostatin A is a histone deacetylase inhibitor with potent antitumor activity against breast cancer in vivo. Clin Cancer Res 7(4):971–976

Vinceti M et al (2014) Selenium for preventing cancer. Cochrane Database Syst Rev 2014(3): CD005195

Voss AK, Thomas T (2018) Histone lysine and genomic targets of histone acetyltransferases in mammals. BioEssays 40(10):e1800078

Vyas AR, Singh SV (2014) Molecular targets and mechanisms of cancer prevention and treatment by withaferin A, a naturally occurring steroidal lactone. AAPS J 16(1):1–10

Vymetalkova V et al (2019) DNA methylation and chromatin modifiers in colorectal cancer. Mol Aspects Med 69:73–92. https://doi.org/10.1016/j.mam.2019.04.002

Winter J et al (2009) Many roads to maturity: microRNA biogenesis pathways and their regulation. Nat Cell Biol 11(3):228–234

World Cancer Research Fund International/American Institute for Cancer Research (2017). Continuous update project report: diet, nutrition, physical activity and colorectal cancer. Available at: wcrf.org/colorectal-cancer-2017

Wu DS et al (2013) Epigallocatechin-3-gallate and trichostatin A synergistically inhibit human lymphoma cell proliferation through epigenetic modification of p16INK4a. Oncol Rep 30 (6):2969–2975

Wu K, Li L, Li S (2015) Circulating microRNA-21 as a biomarker for the detection of various carcinomas: an updated meta-analysis based on 36 studies. Tumour Biol 36(3):1973–1981

Xiao Y et al (2018) Comprehensive evaluation of the role of soy and isoflavone supplementation in humans and animals over the past two decades. Phytother Res 32(3):384–394

Xu XY et al (2018) Bioactivity, health benefits, and related molecular mechanisms of curcumin: current progress, challenges, and perspectives. Nutrients 10(10):1553

Yang CS, Wang H (2016) Cancer preventive activities of tea catechins. Molecules 21(12):1679

Yang X et al (2001) Synergistic activation of functional estrogen receptor (ER)-alpha by DNA methyltransferase and histone deacetylase inhibition in human ER-alpha-negative breast cancer cells. Cancer Res 61(19):7025–7029

Yang CS et al (2009) Cancer prevention by tea: animal studies, molecular mechanisms and human relevance. Nat Rev Cancer 9(6):429–439

Yang CS et al (2016) Lessons learned from cancer prevention studies with nutrients and non-nutritive dietary constituents. Mol Nutr Food Res 60(6):1239–1250

Yum HW, Na HK, Surh YJ (2016) Anti-inflammatory effects of docosahexaenoic acid: implications for its cancer chemopreventive potential. Semin Cancer Biol 40-41:141–159

Ziberna L et al (2017) Oleanolic acid alters multiple cell signaling pathways: implication in cancer prevention and therapy. Int J Mol Sci 18(3):E643

Chapter 19
Perspective: A Positive Cocktail Effect of the Bioactive Components in the Diet

John M. Pezzuto and Ole Vang

Abstract Throughout this book the power of combination chemoprevention is highlighted. Even individual agents that function by virtue of pleiotropic mechanisms of action portray a combination effect. In this final chapter, we offer a brief perspective on the concept of combining numerous (e.g., 10–25) dietary agents for the creation of a cocktail capable of mediating a broad-based cancer chemopreventive response. The challenges of logically and systematically founding a cocktail comprised of 10–25 dietary chemopreventive components functioning in an additive or synergistic manner are addressed. Obviously, this is no mean task. Some technological advances are necessary, such as creating in vitro systems engineered to encompass several hallmarks of cancer, and animal models that generically correlate with the genesis of human cancer. Nonetheless, as illustrated by the cogent, on point contributions presented in this book, over the past several decades, we have already acquired the knowledge and skill necessary for accomplishing this vast undertaking. Given the current day morbidity and mortality associated with malignant metastatic cancer, and future projections of even greater devastation, all of humanity would benefit by a holistic approach utilizing the tools provided to us by Nature.

19.1 Introduction

Around 50 years ago, the conceptual underpinning of cancer chemoprevention was tied to epidemiological evidence suggesting an inverse correlation between diet and cancer. In particular, a lower incidence of colorectal cancer in Japan that shifted upward subsequent to adopting a 'western diet', and a lower incidence of cancer

J. M. Pezzuto (✉)
Arnold & Marie Schwartz College of Pharmacy and Health Sciences, Long Island University, Brooklyn, New York, USA
e-mail: john.pezzuto@liu.edu

O. Vang
Department of Science and Environment, Roskilde University, Roskilde, Denmark
e-mail: ov@ruc.dk

J. M. Pezzuto, O. Vang (eds.), *Natural Products for Cancer Chemoprevention*,
https://doi.org/10.1007/978-3-030-39855-2_19

among Seventh-Day Adventists, many of whom are vegetarian or vegan. The most recent update on the diet–cancer relation from AICR/WCRF showed there is strong evidence that dietary fruit decreased the risk of cancers of lung as well as of mouth, pharynx and larynx, and dietary vegetables decreased the risk of cancers of mouth, pharynx and larynx (Summary of global evidence on cancer prevention 2017). The same update verified strong evidence of cancer prevention by whole grains and fibers for colorectal cancer. Based on these promising observations, the AICR/WCRF recommends "Eat a wide variety of wholegrains, vegetables, fruit and pulses such as beans" (Summary of global evidence on cancer prevention 2017), which also may be beneficial for human health in general.

Recommendations of this type represent a good common sense approach for disease prevention. However, on an individual level, it is difficult to expect a predictable outcome based on recommending that the human population should increase the intake of fruits, vegetables, wholegrains and pulses. First of all, the content of bioactive components diverges from one variety of a given vegetable to the next, and the content varies based on different growing and handling conditions. One broccoli is different from another broccoli, one tomato is different from another tomato, etc. Therefore, the level of exposure for specific bioactive compounds is difficult to regulate, which makes estimates of relevant compounds, and subsequent response, uncertain.

Next, experimental researchers have focused mainly on single compounds to analyze the health promoting effect of a given bioactive component. Based on such single compounds, clinical studies as well as in vitro and in vivo data have shown health promoting effects, but often at very high concentrations that cannot be achieved by dietary means. In general, bioactive compounds are only present in small amounts in a plant-based diet.

Thus, the hypothesis of a single dietary bioactive component lowering the risk of developing a chronic disease is questionable. It is relatively clear that regular consumption of fruits, vegetables, and whole grains is associated with reduced risk of developing chronic diseases, but individual bioactive components do not show consistent beneficial effects. Further, dietary supplements alone do not explain the observed health benefits of diets rich in fruits, vegetables, and whole grains (Liu 2013).

This leads to the idea of a combined effect resulting from a myriad of bioactive components in the diet. The concept is not new but often times overlooked. The present book includes many examples of bioactive components present in many different plant-based sources. It helps to guide us in a way to view cancer chemoprevention mediated by dietary constituents from a more holistic point-of-view (Fig. 19.1).

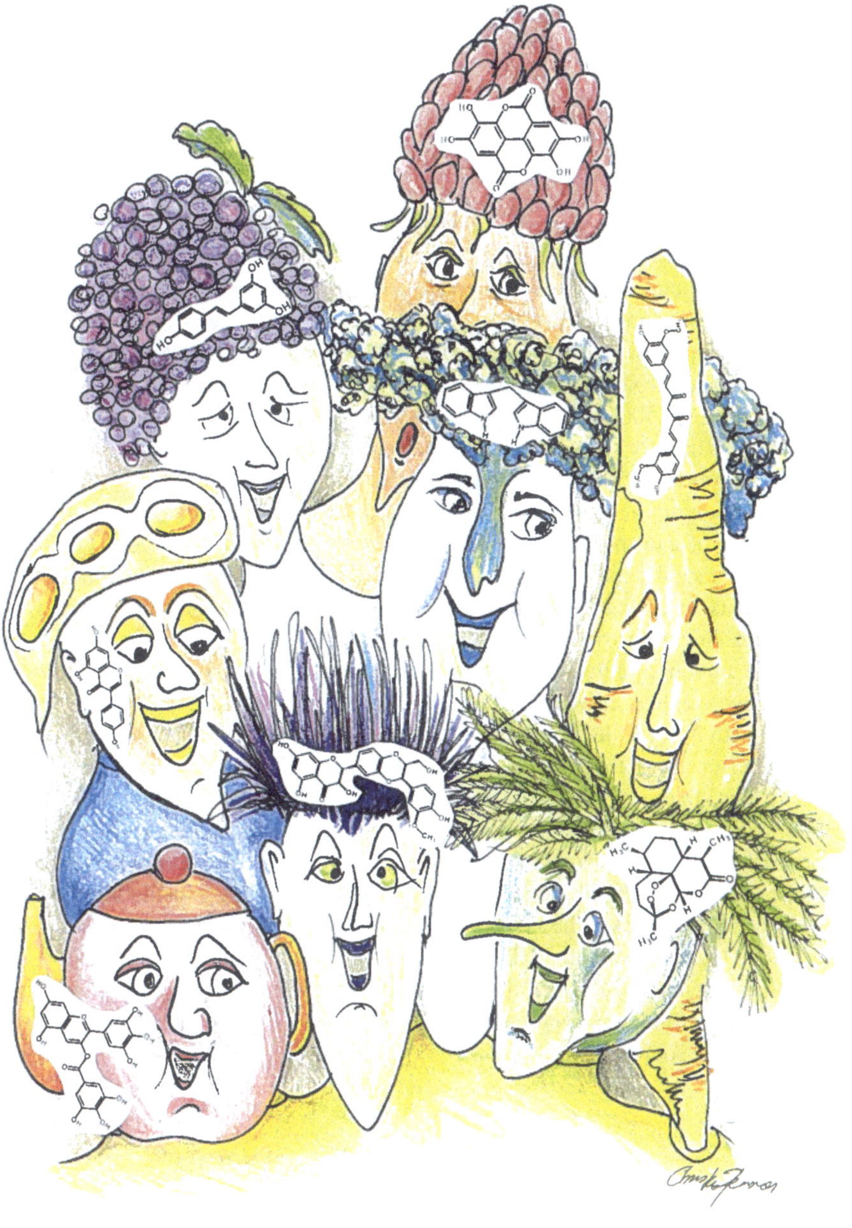

Fig. 19.1 A montage of humanity depicting the concept of "You are what you eat" [Anthelme Brillat-Savarin, *The Physiology of Taste*, 1826; and subsequently many others]. The human diet, now known to contain a variety of biologically active phytochemicals, is associated with disease prevention and good health. Here we portray individuals consuming diets containing resveratrol (grapes), ellagic acid (raspberry), genistein (soy), 3,3′-diindoylmethane (broccoli), curcumin (turmeric), EGCG (tea), silbinin (milk thistle), or artemisinin (sweet wormwood). As described in this *Perspective*, a cocktail is feasible that could yield much greater efficacy than the heltar-skelter doses delivered by dietary friuts and vegetables. Artwork courtesy of Christa Persson, Roskilde University

19.2 Bioactive Compounds Are Present in All Plant-Based Diets

19.2.1 Bioactive Components Are Present in Small Amounts in the Diet

Since bioactive compounds are found in low levels in plant-based diets, unrealistically high intake would be necessary to achieve the levels found to be active with in vivo experiments. For example, pterostilbene is found in grape berries and blueberries (Levenson and Kumar, Chap. 3). Levels may greatly vary, but upper limits are around 520 ng/g in blueberries and 530 ng/g in grapes (Levenson and Kumar, Chap. 3). Experiments where mice were exposed to 10 mg Pter/kg bw (corresponding to 500 g of blueberries/day/mouse) in combination with SAHA showed a significantly reduced prostate cancer burden (Butt et al. 2017). Obviously, daily consumption of 500 g by a 25 g mammal is not practicable.

Consider curcumin as another example. The level of curcumin has been estimated at up to 2.5% of a turmeric powder or 0.6% of curry powder (Tayyem et al. 2006). However, in recent experiments conducted with rats treated with benzo(*a*)pyrene, improvements in lung biochemical and biophysical indices were observed when treated with curcumin (60 mg/kg bw) or resveratrol (5.7 μg/mL water) (Liu et al. 2019). The amount of curcumin corresponds to around 2 g curry powder/day/rat; the responses were enhanced when both agents were administered in combination.

Along with this, results from Lau and Yue (Chap. 7) indicate that turmeric extract shows superior anti-tumor effects in tumor-bearing mice compared with curcumin alone. In fact, there are numerous examples in the scientific literature wherein an extract containing bioactive compounds is more potent compared with the single compounds. Some plants contain several derivatives of the same compound that may have the same or nearly the same response. Therefore, in only considering the level of resveratrol (Chap. 2) as the stilbenoid in grape juice and wine, one is overlooking compounds like pterostilbene (Chaps. 3 and 12), isorhapontigenin, piceatannol and vineferins (Fernandez-Marin et al. 2012), and underestimating the combined effect of stilbenoids in grapes. Therefore, high doses, beyond those feasibly obtainable from the natural source, are often necessary to obtain the physiological effects by the single bioactive compound.

19.2.2 Bioactive Dietary Compounds Often Showed Lower Activities with No Toxic Effects

The activities of bioactive phytochemicals found in the human diet are generally weak in comparison with designer or prescription drugs. The fabricated drugs are intended to interact with one specific molecular target but, most often, unintended targets are affected as well, causing side effects. For example, resveratrol inhibits

COX-1 and COX-2 in the 2–20 μM range (Handler et al. 2007; Jang et al. 1997; Kutil et al. 2015; Seaver and Smith 2004; Waffo-Teguo et al. 2001; Willenberg et al. 2015), whereas an NSAID such as indomethacin is more potent. However, resveratrol is not known to generate gastric ulcers or induce cardiotoxicity as is the case with some 'specific' COX-2 inhibitors. As another example, ribociclib (Chap. 15), a selective CDK4 and CDK6 inhibitor, reduces the proliferation of MCF7 cells with an IC_{50} around 4 μM (Jansen et al. 2017), whereas 3,3′-diindolylmethane affects MCF-7 cells growth with an IC_{50} in the range of 30–60 μM (Jin 2011). Ribociclib has also been related to cardiotoxicity whereas no toxic effects have been described for 3,3′-diindolylmethane.

19.2.3 Broader Activities Are Mediated by Bioactive Components

Another important aspect is that bioactive components from plant-based diets generally have many cellular and molecular targets. Resveratrol is a prime example (Chap. 2). As another example, tea catechins (Chap. 8) show many different activities. They act as anti- and pro-oxidants and enhance phase II metabolic enzymes. Beside these 'rough' effects, specific protein targets have been identified for EGCG, including vimentin, IGF1R, FYN, glucose-regulated protein 78 kDa, ZAP70 and Ras-GTPase-activating protein SH3 domain-binding protein 1 (Shim et al. 2010) (Yang, Chap. 8). Further, a long list of enzyme activities are inhibited by EGCG, including mitogen-activated protein (MAP) kinases, protein kinase B (AKT), chymotryptic activity of 20S proteasomes, MMP2, MMP9, DNMT1, dihydrofolate reductase, glucose-6-phosphate dehydrogenase, glyceraldehyde-3-phosphate dehydrogenase, carbonyl reductase and receptor tyrosine kinases (Yang and Wang 2016) (Yang, Chap. 8).

In addition, the same targets may have a number of 'ligands'. Sundar and Firestone (Chap. 15) clearly show that among other naturally occurring bioactive compounds, 3,3′-diindolylmethane, artemisinin, resveratrol, curcumin and EGCG modulate CDK function and expression. Likewise, modulation of the NF-κB pathway is a common target of various dietary chemicals, such as pterostilbene (Chap. 3), isothiocyanates (Chap. 9), resveratrol (Chaps. 2 and 12), silibinin (Chap. 6), and several anthocyanins (Chap. 11). In a similar sense, Neophytou et al. (Chap. 16) described different compounds that induce apoptosis (tocopherols, curcumin, EGCG, quercetin, resveratrol, genistein), and Monteillier and Cuendet (Chap. 17) described several compounds with anti-inflammatory effects (resveratrol, curcumin, parthenolide, artesunate, isothiocyanates, green tea catechins). Also, various recent reviews have pointed out such multi-ligand effects of dietary components, e.g., for inhibition of PI3K in relation to cancer development (Suvarna et al. 2017) or inhibition of the epithelial-to-mesenchymal transition (Avila-Carrasco et al. 2019).

19.3 Combinatory Effects

19.3.1 Definition of Synergy

Synergy or synergistic effect mediated by dietary components are common terms used in the area of health promotion. The term 'synergy' is defined in the Cambridge Dictionary as "the combined power of a group of things when they are working together that is greater than the total power achieved by each working separately". In other words, the combinatory effects, when synergy is achieved, is greater than the sum of the single effects.

19.3.2 Synergy and Other Interactions in Phytomedicines

It is often observed that a mixture (e.g., an extract) shows a stronger response than adding the single active components together. As such, individual pomegranate phytochemicals were only modestly effective compared with the pomegranate extract in inhibiting cell proliferation (Chap. 13) (Nair et al. 2011). This exemplifies that an active component can be overlooked in an extract or an interaction between several compounds is necessary for a strong effect.

However, some claims of synergy based on a stronger effect of the mixture compared with the effect of the single compounds can be problematic. A water-soluble derivative of propolis (mostly polyphenols) was found to have a stronger effect than the components, but it was not clearly demonstrated that the combined effect was synergistic (Orsolic et al. 2005). A similar claim of synergism based on tests of different pomegranate extracts (Lansky et al. 2005) is problematic, as no comparative tests were performed. In other examples, it was claimed that supplementation of curcumin and resveratrol maintain adequate zinc levels and reduced cyclooxygenase activity synergistically in benzo(*a*)pyrene treated mice (Malhotra et al. 2011), and it was claimed that resveratrol, glucan and vitamin C acted synergistically in increasing the phagocytosis effect of isolated granulocytes (Vetvicka and Vetvickova 2012), without showing any tests for synergy. In cases such as these, the claim of synergistic effects may be correct, but would need to be proven using a reliable combination model.

In sum, there are numerous claims of synergy in the literature; some are documented but many are not proven. The onus should be placed on the research community to prove claims of synergy or to demonstrate the true nature of combinatory effects. It is therefore not surprising that the term synergy is used without scrutiny in the general population.

Nonetheless, the stronger effect of a mixture (full extract) relative to single compound brings us to the idea of having a "positive cocktail effect". The cocktail effect was originally introduced in ecotoxicology as the combined toxic effect of multiple toxicants present at levels wherein toxicity was not mediated with the individual toxicants (Holzman 2000; Kortenkamp 2007).

19.3.3 How to Determine Synergy

Various models for synergy determination have been devised. They originally focused on the effect of drug interactions, and not on compounds with multiple targets and weak interactions. In short, as described by Berenbaum (1989) and Williamson (2001), different models have been suggested.

19.3.3.1 Summation of Effects Model

The model predicts synergy when the total effect of a combination of compound *a* and compound *b* is greater than expected from the sum of their effects

$$E\ (da, db) = E\ (da) + E(db),$$

where E is the observed effect at the doses (da and db) of agents *a* and *b*. The summation of effects model depends on the mechanism of action of each component, and assumes linear responses for each effect. This model or derivatives of the model have been used in many reports. So, the combination of sulforaphane and myricetin was found to act synergistically on cell viability (Yao et al. 2018). Also, the antioxidant activity of a combination of catechin and quercetin-3-β-glucoside was found to be synergistic based on the summation effect method (Hidalgo et al. 2010). The combined effect of ellagic acid and quercetin on the induction of $p21^{waf1/cip1}$ was claimed synergistic based on summation of effects (Mertens-Talcott et al. 2005). The described examples of synergistic effects noted above are likely synergistic but should be proven by using a more realistic (non-linear) model. Further, the summation of effects model is generally not applicable with complex mixtures.

19.3.3.2 Effect of One Compound in Addition to a Fixed Dose of Another Component

This has similar disadvantages to the ‘summation of effects model’.

19.3.3.3 Comparison of the Effect of a Combination With That of Each of Its Components

By this method, synergy is deemed present if the effect of a combination is greater than that of each of the individual agents:

$$E(da, db) > E(da) \text{ and } E(da, db) > E\ (db).$$

The advantage of this model is that it is independent of knowledge of the mechanism of action, but fails if an effect less than the sum of the effects of compounds *a* and *b* is claimed to be synergistic.

19.3.3.4 Isobole Method

The isobole model was originated by Loewe in 1926–1927 (Williamson 2001) and is now the method of choice as it is independent of the mechanism of action and applies under most conditions. Further, the model makes no assumptions in regard to the performance of the agent and is therefore applicable to multiple component mixtures. An isobole is a "same-effect" curve, where the effect of a combination of the constituents (da, db) is shown on a graph where the axes are thc dose-axes of the individual agents (da and db). With no interaction, the curve (the line joining the points representing the combination to those on the dose axes representing the individual doses with the same effect as the combination) will be a straight line. If synergy is occurring, i.e., the effect of the combination is greater than expected from their individual dose-response curves, the dose of the combination will show the same effect at lower doses than the sum of the individual components; the curve will be 'concave'. For antagonism, the dose of the combination is greater than expected to obtain the same effects, and produces a 'convex' isobole. It is necessary to keep in mind that it is possible, with the same mixture of compounds, to observe synergy at one dose combination and antagonism at another. This would produce a complicated isobole with a wave-like or even elliptical appearance.

This model was further developed by Chou (2006), based on the median-effect equation for a single compound, which has been extended to the multiple-drug effect equation for *n* drugs. For two compounds:

$$CI = \frac{D1}{d1} + \frac{D2}{d2}$$

where D1 and D2 are the doses of the single compounds alone, to produce a chosen effect level (usually IC_{50}), and d1 and d2 are the doses of the individual constituents in the combination giving the same effect.

The combination index (CI)-isobologram equation allows quantitative determination of drug interactions, where CI <1, =1, or >1, indicates synergism, additive effect, or antagonism, respectively. The model is developed for interactions of two drugs, but the number of compounds included in the model may be greater than two. Then

$$^{n}(CI)x = \sum_{j=1}^{n} \frac{(D)j}{(d)j} \text{ for } n \text{ compounds.}$$

The challenge is that upon addition of each new compound, the number of possible combinations that should be tested will increase to an unlimited number.

CI values may be determined using different software programs [CalcuSyn (http://www.biosoft.com); CompuSyn (http://www.combosyn.com)]. A sampling of reports where combinations of dietary bioactive components have been tested for interactions and analyzed using the CalcuSyn or ComboSyn software packages is given below. Only a limited number of compounds have been found and included in the table: resveratrol, pterostilbene, curcumin, quercetin and fisetin and the combinations only contained two compounds at one time (Table 19.1). The calculated CI values showed synergistic to additive effect, but in some cases (resveratrol + quercetin) a significant antagonism was observed.

Beside these examples using CalcuSyn or ComboSyn software packages, others have calculated the CI values 'by hand': Combinations of 3,3′-diindolylmethane and sulphoraphane (1:1) showed antagonism at effects below 0.5 (below 50% inhibition) whereas additivity was observed under different experimental conditions. The report showed CI values for other combinations of 3,3′-diindolylmethane and sulphoraphane, but the general picture was the same (Pappa et al. 2007). In addition, the combination of 4-methoxy-indole-3-ylcarbinol and indole-3-ylcarbinol (both found in cruciferous vegetables) showed additive combination with some synergistic action in two different colon cell lines (Kronbak et al. 2010).

19.3.4 Is Synergy Better than Additivity?

As the plant-based diet may contain numerous bioactive substances, any of which may play a part in the process of the cancer prevention, by similar or different mechanisms, a synergistic effect is not necessary. For example, a mixture of 10 bioactive substances may each contribute to 1/10 of the final response without having more than an additive effect.

Based on observations of the cocktail effect in ecotoxicology, the funnel hypothesis was derived by Warne and Hawker (1995). The Toxicity Enhancement Index (TEI) can increase with an increasing number of components, with the overall response going toward additive effects. If a similar response is found when studying the positive cocktail effect of bioactive components in the diet (unpublished data), the overall additive response should be the result of the combinatory effect of many components.

19.4 Hallmarks of Cancer

Establishment of the six hallmarks of cancer (Hanahan and Weinberg 2000) and extension with an additional four hallmarks (Hanahan and Weinberg 2011) points out some central processes in cancer development. If the diet contains bioactive

Table 19.1 Studies showing drug combination on cell proliferation/cytotoxicity with resveratrol (and derivatives) as one of the compounds and using CompuSyn or CalcuSyn software to calculate the CI values

Cell lines and type of assay	Compounds (numbers in combination)	Concentrations, time	Calculated CI (Fa low → high)	References
HTC-116, MTT assay	Resveratrol + Curcumin (2)	2.5–40 μM 2.5–40 μM, 48 h	0.43–0.90	Majumdar et al. (2009)
MCF-7 MTT assay	Resveratrol + Curcumin (2)	1–94 μM, 1–94 μM, 72 h	1:1: 0.9–1.1; 1:3: 0.8–0.3; 3:1: 0.9–0.2	Pushpalatha et al. (2017)
HCC1806, MDA-MB-157, MTT assay	Pterostilbene + Resveratrol (2)	0–15 μM 0–20 μM, 24 and 72 h	0.41–1.85 0.46–1.11	Kala et al. (2015)
Human VSMC, BrdU assay	Resveratrol + Quercetin (2)	0.5–5 μM 0.25–5 μM, 24 h	0.15–1.0	Khandelwal et al. (2012)
Rat VSMC, BrdU assay	Resveratrol + Quercetin (2)	0.5–50 μM 0.5–50 μM, 48 h	0.21–9.9	Kleinedler et al. (2011)
Rat macrophages, BrdU assay	Resveratrol + Quercetin (2)	5.5–50 μM 0.5–10 μM, 48 h	0.27–3.1	Kleinedler, et al. (2011)

compounds capable of modulating each of these hallmarks at various steps, it seems logical that a combinatory cancer preventive effect of dietary bioactive compounds may be obtained. Such an effect is likely since human dietary intake is life-long.

A supplementary issue of *Seminars in Cancer Biology* 2015 (Bishayee and Block 2015) addresses this idea nicely. As described in the summary by Block et al. (2015), it is possible to envision many bioactive compounds from plants (mostly edible) that interact with one or several of the hallmarks. Given below is a brief summary of this treatise dealing with the possible bioactive compounds interacting with the hallmarks along with some additions from the literature.

1. **Genomic instability** is reduced by vitamin D, B vitamins, carotenoids, resveratrol, and isothiocyanates.
2. **Sustained proliferative signaling** is downregulated by compounds like EGCG, curcumin, genistein and resveratrol.
3. **Evading growth suppressors** is counteracted by EGCG, luteolin, curcumin, genistein, resveratrol, withaferin A, and deguelin (Amin et al. 2015).
4. **Resistance to cell death** (apoptosis): There is a long list of bioactive dietary compounds capable of inducing apoptosis and many have been described in this book. Pro-apoptosis is nicely addressed by Neophytou et al. (Chap. 16). Additionally, single compounds are shown to induce apoptosis: Pterostilbene (Chap. 3), silibinin (Chap. 6), curcumin (Chap. 7), tea polyphenols including EGCG (Chap. 8), isothiocyanates (Chap. 9), anthocyanins (Chap. 10) grape constituents (Chap. 12).
5. **Enabling replicative immortality**: Some compounds capable of mediated such an effect are described in this book, including indole-3-carbinol, EGCG (Chap. 8), resveratrol (Chap. 2), pterostilbene (Chap. 3), curcumin, sulforaphane (Chap. 9), silibinin (Chap. 6) and quercetin. Ganesan and Xu (2017) summarized a longer list of telomerase inhibitors isolated from plant sources, such as diosgenin, gingerol, resveratrol, crocin, luteolin-7-*O*-glucoside, genistein, saponins, tanshinones, baicalin, wogonoside, gossypol, silymarin and berberine among others. To our knowledge, these compounds have not been tested in combination in relation to their potency on telomerase inhibition.
6. **Deregulation of cellular energetics** may be targeted by resveratrol, which activates Sirt1, modulates mitochondrial activity and/or the mTOR cascade. All three targets may have an impact on the metabolism. In addition, fisetin (Adhami et al. 2012), curcumin (Lin 2007), a combination of indole-3-ylcarbinol and genistein (Nakamura et al. 2009), and plumbagin (Zhou et al. 2015) inhibit the mTOR cascade.
7. **Tumor-promoting inflammation** may be regulated by curcumin, resveratrol, EGCG, genistein, lycopene, and anthocyanins, and additional compounds active in modulation of inflammation as described by Monteillier and Cuendet (Chap. 17).
8. **Induction of angiogenesis** is modulated by pterostilbene (Chap. 3), silibinin (Chap. 6) and some grape constituents (stilbenes, flavonols, catheins and anthocyanins) (Chap. 12).

9. **Tissue invasion and metastasis**. Here, extracts of *Agaricus blazei*, *Albatrellus confluens*, *Cordyceps militaris*, *Ganoderma lucidum*, *Poria cocos* and *Silybum marianum* (containing silibilin) are active in inhibiting the hallmark. In addition, tissue interactions in the tumor microenvironment is inhibited by compounds like berberine, resveratrol, desoxyrhapontigenin, onionin A, EGCG, genistein, naringenin, piperine and zerumbone.
10. **Avoiding immune destruction:** Besides astaxanthin, extracts of *Ganoderma lucidum*, *Trametes versicolor*, *Astragalus membranaceus*, and *Lentinus edodes* have been identified as active.

A few compounds have shown interactions with most of the hallmarks of cancer: curcumin, EGCG, genistein and resveratrol (Block et al. 2015), but more compounds will be included in this multi-potent list in the future.

19.5 How to Prove the Concept?

A multitude of primary reports and reviews have described compelling biological activities that are mediated by a large number of dietary compounds in the prevention of cancer. As illustrated by the chapters presented in this book, we know of a number of dietary compounds that may impact the combined effect of plant-based diets. Considering the magnitude of the cancer problem, and the opportunity for making a far-reaching advancement, it seems rational to consider a logical and systematic approach for taking the next steps of testing the combinatory effect of these bioactive components.

One of the most profound challenges in suggesting that a chemopreventive effect in humans is actually facilitated by the combination of numerous of bioactive compounds in the diet is simply how to prove the hypothesis. The situation goes from difficult to virtually impossible when taking into account the need for acknowledging the effect is mediated by life-long exposure.

In any case, it is apparent that use of in vitro tests would be obligatory in any approach designed to prove combinatory concepts. The combination index as described by Chou is useful for multiple compounds although other non-linear mathematical models to forecast the combinatory effect should be established and included as well. Nonetheless, consider the example of evaluating four compounds of interest, each known to be independently active. As described by Chou, for determining synergism or antagonism, the knowledge of 'mechanisms' for each drug alone is not required. Thus, working with more than two active compounds, isobolograph analysis by combining the agents is completely feasible.

Working with four bioactive compounds **A**, **B**, **C**, and **D**, the initial analyses would involve six unique combinations (**A** + **B**, **A** + **C**, **A** + **D**, **B** + **C**, **B** + **D**, and **C** + **D**). The analyses would establish if the sets of agents function in an additive or synergistic manner but, of utmost importance, ascertain they do not function in an antagonistic manner. Once a set of agents is found to behave in an appropriate manner, sets of the compounds can be evaluated with a third agent. This results in up to 12 additional tests [(**A** + **B**) + **C**, (**A** + **B**) + **D** (**A** + **C**) + **B**, (**A** + **C**) + **D**, (**A** + **D**) + **B**, (**A** + **D**) + **C**, (**B** + **C**) + **A**, (**B** + **C**) + **D**, (**B** + **D**) + **A**, (**B** + **D**) + **C**, (**C** + **D**) + **A**, and (**C** + **D**) + **B**], when is not assumed the combinations are equivalent [e.g., (**A** + **B**) + **C** ≠ (**A** + **C**) + **B**]. In other words, this hierarchy of testing will show how the third compound affects the CI of the two compound combination. Again, the experiments can be performed to investigate additive or synergistic responses, and to establish the lack of an antagonistic response. Finally, the fourth agent can be added to the combination and tested. For this test, there are four unique combinations [(**A** + **B** + **C**) + **D**, (**A** + **B** + **D**) + **C**, (**A** + **C** + **D**) + **B**, and (**B** + **C** + **D**) + **A**]. Given the availability of high-throughput technology, these up to 22 experiments can readily be completed. Such an experimental paradigm has been discussed in great detail by Chou (2006). It should be noted that the number of tests is based on the evaluation of a single concentration of each compound, and a change from antagonism to synergism may be observed from one concentration to the next. Therefore, dose-dependent analysis must be performed for the single compounds and the six 2-compound combinations illustrated above.

In a similar fashion, additional dietary bioactive compounds can be tested, again, starting with the dose-response effects of the single compounds. Of course, the in vitro test used for such an analyses should have sufficient screening power to generate a high number of data points. Moreover, the mixtures should be tested in a system that reflects all (or most of) the hallmarks of cancer. It is difficult to envision such an in vitro system, but sufficient technology and knowledge are available to enable creating such a system through means such as genetic engineering taking cancer hallmarks into account.

Once a promising cocktail of dietary chemopreventive agents is identified, one could speculate about testing efficacy in humans. But, of course, this is not realistic since such a protocol might involve exposing a large number of healthy humans to the mixtures for years until a substantial number of cases have developed. In addition to the large number of participants, it would take many years to obtain reliable data. Obviously, the next logical step is exposure of experimental animals to the mixture. As a general axiom, chemopreventive agents effective in human beings are also effective in animal models. The converse is also correct, given, for example, β-carotene failed in human trials to prevent lung cancer, and likewise failed in experiments conducted with laboratory animals. Nonetheless, in animal chemopreventive experiments, it is only sensible to test a few mixtures. Thus, the 'optimal' mixture must first be established with in vitro models. However, similar to the scrutiny to which in vitro models will be subjected, given that human preventive trials are unrealistic, the animal models will be subject to question. Perhaps testing of the relevant mixtures in a pig model (Neff 2019) should be considered.

In any case "The journey of a thousand miles begins with one step" [Lao Tzu], and the first step of obtaining proof or disproof of the idea of chemopreventive effect of mixtures of dietary components will not be without challenge. Some examples of issues that need to be solved properly follow.

- The number of bioactive compounds to be selected among is very high, but at the current time we only have enough data to include a few. The remaining compounds have to be included based on some tangible indication of their activity.
- The number of combinations becomes very high with 10–25 different compounds. The initial tests will need to be designed to distinguish the value of adding more-and-more compounds to the cocktail. Even with 10 compounds, the number of combinations is high. It would not be prudent to have too few compounds included, but the value of adding more compounds needs to be clear as well.
- The in vitro models need to have enough screening power to manage the high number of samples to be tested, but the models must reflect several of the hallmarks of cancer.
- The cost for evaluating not one but 10–25 compounds together with in vitro and in vivo models will be high.

However, we know cancer cells are insidious. Over the decades, we have learned the ability of cancer cells to evade our therapeutic strategies has proven uncanny. In searching for the favorable cocktail of chemopreventive agents, we may consider taking a lesson from a flock of geese flying in autumn from the north to the south to escape the bitter cold winter. By flying together in a V-formation, it has been estimated that the flock may fly 70% faster than a single goose flying alone. This is due to additional lift and reduction in air resistance. Similarly, cancer chemoprevention is a heavy burden to be carried out in a sustained manner by as single agent that is otherwise viewed as innocuous, so teamwork is viewed with utmost importance. The lead goose in a V-formation requires greater effort but, when necessary, the goose will drop out of formation and take a position requiring less effort. Another goose will take over and keep the flock moving seamlessly on track. In chemoprevention, if one agent were serving to block cellular transformation, for example, and the process being ameliorated by that particular agent became fatigued, the action of another agent could step in, take the lead, and continue allowing the cocktail to succeed. As with the geese, each component of the cocktail may have an opportunity to take the lead, and successfully sustain the overall protective response.

To conclude, we acknowledge the effort proposed here to proof or disproof the chemopreventive effect of mixtures is enormous. However, based on our current knowledge, the task could be successfully managed by a multi-laboratory, multinational effort. The beneficiary would be all of humanity.

References

Adhami VM, Syed DN, Khan N, Mukhtar H (2012) Dietary flavonoid fisetin: a novel dual inhibitor of PI3K/Akt and mTOR for prostate cancer management. Biochem Pharmacol 84:1277–1281

Amin AR, Karpowicz PA, Carey TE, Arbiser J, Nahta R, Chen ZG, Dong JT, Kucuk O, Khan GN, Huang GS et al (2015) Evasion of anti-growth signaling: a key step in tumorigenesis and potential target for treatment and prophylaxis by natural compounds. Semin Cancer Biol 35: S55–S77

Avila-Carrasco L, Majano P, Sanchez-Tomero JA, Selgas R, Lopez-Cabrera M, Aguilera A, Gonzalez MG (2019) Natural plants compounds as modulators of epithelial-to-mesenchymal transition. Front Pharmacol 10:715

Berenbaum MC (1989) What is synergy? Pharmacol Rev 41:93–141

Bishayee A, Block K (2015) A broad-spectrum integrative design for cancer prevention and therapy. Semin Cancer Biol 35:S1–S304

Block KI, Gyllenhaal C, Lowe L, Amedei A, Ruhul Amin ARM, Amin A, Aquilano K, Arbiser J, Arreola A, Arzumanyan A et al (2015) Designing a broad-spectrum integrative approach for cancer prevention and treatment. Semin Cancer Biol 35:S276–S304

Butt NA, Kumar A, Dhar S, Rimando AM, Akhtar I, Hancock JC, Lage JM, Pound CR, Lewin JR, Gomez CR et al (2017) Targeting MTA1/HIF-1alpha signaling by pterostilbene in combination with histone deacetylase inhibitor attenuates prostate cancer progression. Cancer Med 6:2673–2685

Chou TC (2006) Theoretical basis, experimental design, and computerized simulation of synergism and antagonism in drug combination studies. Pharmacol Rev 58:621–681

Fernandez-Marin MI, Guerrero RF, Garcia-Parrilla MC, Puertas B, Richard T, Rodriguez-Werner MA, Winterhalter P, Monti JP, Cantos-Villar E (2012) Isorhapontigenin: a novel bioactive stilbene from wine grapes. Food Chem 135:1353–1359

Ganesan K, Xu B (2017) Telomerase inhibitors from natural products and their anticancer potential. Int J Mol Sci 19:13

Hanahan D, Weinberg RA (2000) The hallmarks of cancer. Cell 100:57–70

Hanahan D, Weinberg RA (2011) Hallmarks of cancer: the next generation. Cell 144:646–674

Handler N, Jaeger W, Puschacher H, Leisser K, Erker T (2007) Synthesis of novel curcumin analogues and their evaluation as selective cyclooxygenase-1 (COX-1) inhibitors. Chem Pharm Bull 55:64–71

Hidalgo M, Sanchez-Moreno C, De Pascual-Teresa S (2010) Flavonoid-flavonoid interaction and its effect on their antioxidant activity. Food Chem 121:691–696

Holzman DC (2000) Chemical mixtures. Chemical cocktails: are mixed pesticides more potent? Environ Health Perspect 108:A114

Jang M, Cai L, Udeani GO, Slowing KV, Thomas CF, Beecher CW, Fong HH, Farnsworth NR, Kinghorn AD, Mehta RG et al (1997) Cancer chemopreventive activity of resveratrol, a natural product derived from grapes. Science 275:218–220

Jansen VM, Bhola NE, Bauer JA, Formisano L, Lee KM, Hutchinson KE, Witkiewicz AK, Moore PD, Estrada MV, Sanchez V et al (2017) Kinome-wide RNA interference screen reveals a role for PDK1 in acquired resistance to CDK4/6 inhibition in ER-positive breast cancer. Cancer Res 77:2488–2499

Jin Y (2011) 3,3′-Diindolylmethane inhibits breast cancer cell growth via miR-21-mediated Cdc25A degradation. Mol Cell Biochem 358:345–354

Kala R, Shah HN, Martin SL, Tollefsbol TO (2015) Epigenetic-based combinatorial resveratrol and pterostilbene alters DNA damage response by affecting SIRT1 and DNMT enzyme expression, including SIRT1-dependent gamma-H2AX and telomerase regulation in triple-negative breast cancer. BMC Cancer 15:672

Khandelwal AR, Hebert VY, Kleinedler JJ, Rogers LK, Ullevig SL, Asmis R, Shi R, Dugas TR (2012) Resveratrol and quercetin interact to inhibit neointimal hyperplasia in mice with a carotid injury. J Nutr 142:1487–1494

Kleinedler JJ, Foley JD, Alexander JS, Roerig SC, Hebert VY, Dugas TR (2011) Synergistic effect of resveratrol and quercetin released from drug-eluting polymer coatings for endovascular devices. J Biomed Mater Res B Appl Biomater 99:266–275

Kortenkamp A (2007) Ten years of mixing cocktails: a review of combination effects of endocrine-disrupting chemicals. Environ Health Perspect 115:98–105

Kronbak R, Duus F, Vang O (2010) Effect of 4-methoxyindole-3-carbinol on the proliferation of colon cancer cells in vitro, when treated alone or in combination with indole-3-carbinol. J Agric Food Chem 58:8453–8459

Kutil Z, Kvasnicova M, Temml V, Schuster D, Marsik P, Cusimamani EF, Lou JD, Vanek T, Landa P (2015) Effect of dietary stilbenes on 5-lipoxygenase and cyclooxygenases activities in vitro. Int J Food Prop 18:1471–1477

Lansky EP, Jiang W, Mo H, Bravo L, Froom P, Yu W, Harris NM, Neeman I, Campbell MJ (2005) Possible synergistic prostate cancer suppression by anatomically discrete pomegranate fractions. Investig New Drugs 23:11–20

Lin JK (2007) Molecular targets of curcumin. Adv Exp Med Biol 595:227–243

Liu RH (2013) Health-promoting components of fruits and vegetables in the diet. Adv Nutr 4:384s–392s

Liu D, He B, Lin L, Malhotra A, Yuan N (2019) Potential of curcumin and resveratrol as biochemical and biophysical modulators during lung cancer in rats. Drug Chem Toxicol 42:328–334

Majumdar AP, Banerjee S, Nautiyal J, Patel BB, Patel V, Du J, Yu Y, Elliott AA, Levi E, Sarkar FH (2009) Curcumin synergizes with resveratrol to inhibit colon cancer. Nutr Cancer 61:544–553

Malhotra A, Nair P, Dhawan DK (2011) Curcumin and resveratrol synergistically stimulate p21 and regulate cox-2 by maintaining adequate zinc levels during lung carcinogenesis. Eur J Cancer Prev 20:411–416

Mertens-Talcott SU, Bomser JA, Romero C, Talcott ST, Percival SS (2005) Ellagic acid potentiates the effect of quercetin on $p21^{waf1/cip1}$, p53, and MAP-kinases without affecting intracellular generation of reactive oxygen species in vitro. J Nutr 135:609–614

Nair V, Dai Z, Khan M, Ciolino HP (2011) Pomegranate extract induces cell cycle arrest and alters cellular phenotype of human pancreatic cancer cells. Anticancer Res 31:2699–2704

Nakamura Y, Yogosawa S, Izutani Y, Watanabe H, Otsuji E, Sakai T (2009) A combination of indol-3-carbinol and genistein synergistically induces apoptosis in human colon cancer HT-29 cells by inhibiting Akt phosphorylation and progression of autophagy. Mol Cancer 8:100

Neff EP (2019) Cancer modeling thinks big with the pig. Lab Anim 48:75–78

Orsolic N, Kosalec I, Basic I (2005) Synergystic antitumor effect of polyphenolic components of water soluble derivative of propolis against Ehrlich ascites tumour. Biol Pharm Bull 28:694–700

Pappa G, Strathmann J, Lowinger M, Bartsch H, Gerhauser C (2007) Quantitative combination effects between sulforaphane and 3,3′-diindolylmethane on proliferation of human colon cancer cells in vitro. Carcinogenesis 28:1471–1477

Pushpalatha R, Selvamuthukumar S, Kilimozhi D (2017) Comparative in silico docking analysis of curcumin and resveratrol on breast cancer proteins and their synergistic effect on MCF-7 cell line. J Young Pharm 9:480–485

Seaver B, Smith JR (2004) Inhibition of COX isoforms by nutraceuticals. J Herb Pharmacother 4:11–18

Shim JH, Su ZY, Chae JI, Kim DJ, Zhu F, Ma WY, Bode AM, Yang CS, Dong Z (2010) Epigallocatechin gallate suppresses lung cancer cell growth through Ras-GTPase-activating protein SH3 domain-binding protein 1. Cancer Prev Res 3:670–679

Summary of global evidence on cancer prevention (2017) World Cancer Research Fund/American Association of Cancer Research

Suvarna V, Murahari M, Khan T, Chaubey P, Sangave P (2017) Phytochemicals and PI3K inhibitors in cancer-an insight. Front Pharmacol 8:916

Tayyem RF, Heath DD, Al-Delaimy WK, Rock CL (2006) Curcumin content of turmeric and curry powders. Nutr Cancer 55:126–131

Vetvicka V, Vetvickova J (2012) Combination of glucan, resveratrol and vitamin C demonstrates strong anti-tumor potential. Anticancer Res 32:81–87

Waffo-Teguo P, Hawthorne ME, Cuendet M, Merillon JM, Kinghorn AD, Pezzuto JM, Mehta RG (2001) Potential cancer-chemopreventive activities, of wine stilbenoids and flavans extracted from grape (*Vitis vinifera*) cell cultures. Nutr Cancer 40:173–179

Warne MS, Hawker DW (1995) The number of components in a mixture determines whether synergistic and antagonistic or additive toxicity predominate: the funnel hypothesis. Ecotoxicol Environ Saf 31:23–28

Willenberg I, Meschede AK, Gueler F, Jang MS, Shushakova N, Schebb NH (2015) Food polyphenols fail to cause a biologically relevant reduction of COX-2 activity. PLoS One 10: e0139147

Williamson EM (2001) Synergy and other interactions in phytomedicines. Phytomedicine 8:401–409

Yang CS, Wang H (2016) Cancer preventive activities of tea catechins. Molecules 21:1679

Yao AJ, Shen YZ, Zhang ZW, Zou ZQ, Wang AS, Chen SY, Zhang HQ, Chen F, Zhao JS, Chen ZM et al (2018) Sulforaphane and myricetin act synergistically to induce apoptosis in 3T3-L1 adipocytes. Mol Med Report 17:2945–2951

Zhou ZW, Li XX, He ZX, Pan ST, Yang Y, Zhang X, Chow K, Yang T, Qiu JX, Zhou Q et al (2015) Induction of apoptosis and autophagy via sirtuin1- and PI3K/Akt/mTOR-mediated pathways by plumbagin in human prostate cancer cells. Drug Des Devel Ther 9:1511–1554

The manufacturer's authorised representative in the EU is Springer Nature Customer Service Centre GmbH, Europaplatz 3, 69115 Heidelberg, Germany. If you have any concerns regarding our products, please contact ProductSafety@springernature.com

Printed and bound by CPI Group (UK) Ltd, Croydon, CR0 4YY
05/10/2026
02228123-0017